Cancer in children

Cancer in children
Clinical management

SIXTH EDITION

Michael C. G. Stevens
Professor of Paediatric Oncology,
University of Bristol
and Consultant Paediatric Oncologist,
Bristol Royal Hospital for Children
Bristol, UK

Hubert N. Caron
Professor of Paediatric Oncology,
Emma Children's Hospital AMC
University of Amsterdam, Amsterdam, The Netherlands

Andrea Biondi
Professor of Pediatrics, University of Milano-Bicocca
Director, Department of Pediatrics, Hospital S.Gerardo/
Fondazione MBBM, Monza, Italy

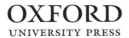
OXFORD
UNIVERSITY PRESS

OXFORD

UNIVERSITY PRESS

Great Clarendon Street, Oxford OX2 6DP

Oxford University Press is a department of the University of Oxford.
It furthers the University's objective of excellence in research, scholarship,
and education by publishing worldwide in

Oxford New York

Auckland Cape Town Dar es Salaam Hong Kong Karachi
Kuala Lumpur Madrid Melbourne Mexico City Nairobi
New Delhi Shanghai Taipei Toronto

With offices in

Argentina Austria Brazil Chile Czech Republic France Greece
Guatemala Hungary Italy Japan Poland Portugal Singapore
South Korea Switzerland Thailand Turkey Ukraine Vietnam

Oxford is a registered trade mark of Oxford University Press
in the UK and in certain other countries

Published in the United States
by Oxford University Press Inc., New York

© Oxford University Press, 2012

The moral rights of the authors have been asserted
Database right Oxford University Press (maker)

First edition published 1975
Second edition published 1986
Third edition published 1992
Fourth edition published 1998
Fifth edition published 2005
Sixth edition published 2012

British Library Cataloguing in Publication Data
Data available

Library of Congress Cataloging in Publication Data
Data available

Typeset in Minion by Cenveo, Bangalore, India
Printed and bound by
CPI Group (UK) Ltd, Croydon, CR0 4YY

ISBN 978–0–19–959941–7

10 9 8 7 6 5 4 3 2 1

Foreword

The treatment of children and young people with cancer has shown enormous progress since the first edition of this book was published in 1975. In economically privileged countries, overall survival rates now approach 80% at 5 years from diagnosis and most of these young people will become long term survivors. Such progress has been achieved by the willingness of the paediatric oncology community to collaborate and to commit to clinical trials which have achieved step wise improvements in outcome for many diagnoses.

It is now possible to cure some children with less intensive therapy than previously used, with less risk of important late effects of treatment. At the same time, cure is now a real possibility for some diseases which were once associated with a very poor outcome. In many less privileged countries, however, and for the majority of children with cancer in the world, there is still much to be done to achieve such standards. The international authorship of this 6th Edition of Cancer in Children illustrates how paediatric oncology works as a global community with a common aim—that no child should die of cancer.

State of the art descriptions of the approach needed for the optimal management of children with cancer are a key feature of this textbook, with revised guidance about current treatments in light of the advances made over the past decade. The challenges ahead will include how to ensure that current knowledge is made available everywhere and how best to incorporate new techniques and technologies into established therapies.

As President of the International Society of Paediatric Oncology, I welcome the new edition of this well known textbook and I am sure that it will serve its readers well.

Gabriele Calaminus
Münster, Germany, 2011

Preface from the Editors

This is the 6th edition of this book, first published in 1975. Since that time great progress has been made in the treatment of children with cancer. Much of this progress has derived from the friendship and collaboration of paediatric oncologists across the world who have built an enviable reputation for international collaboration in clinical trials and in basic and clinical research.

The 21st century brings the challenge of how best to harness the enormous progress made in the molecular and genetic understanding of the diseases we see and how to achieve cure at least cost in terms of the damage that can result from the cancer and its treatment. Cancer in children represents only a small fraction of the global burden of cancer but it contributes an increasingly important component of those who live beyond their cancer in adult life.

We hope that this book will offer readers a clear understanding of what is now possible and what is still needed to take things forward into the future.

We would like to thank the contributors to this edition, our colleagues and collaborators, and all others who have helped with the preparation of this book.

We dedicate this edition to the memory of Tom Voute, previous editor and a tireless advocate for the care of children with cancer throughout the world.

Mike Stevens
Huib Caron
Andrea Biondi
2011

Contents

Contributors

Maurizio Aricó
Director, Department Pediatric Hematology
Oncology, Azienda Ospedaliero-
Universitaria Meyer,
Florence, Italy

Christophe Bergeron
Paediatric Oncologist and Head of Institut
d'Hématologie et d'Oncologie Pédiatrique,
Lyon, France

Mark Bernstein
Division of Pediatric Hematology-Oncology,
IWK Health Centre, Dalhousie University,
Halifax, Canada

Stefan Bielack
Klinikum Stuttgart,
Zentrum für Kinder- und
Jugendmedizin – Olgahospital Pädiatrie 5
(Onkologie, Hämatologie, Immunologie;
Allgemeine Pädiatrie, Gastroenterologie,
Rheumatologie)
Stuttgart, Germany

Andrea Biondi
Professor of Pediatrics,
University of Milano-Bicocca, Director,
Department of Pediatrics,
Hospital S.Gerardo/Fondazione MBBM,
Monza, Italy

Gianni Bisogno
Hematology Oncology Division,
Department of Pediatrics,
University Hospital of Padova,
Padova, Italy

Tom Boterberg
Department of Radiation Oncology,
Ghent University Hospital,
Ghent, Belgium

Franck Bourdeaut
Department of Paeditric Oncology &
INSERM U830,
Institut Curie, Paris, France

Gabriele Calaminus
Consultant Pediatric Hematologist/Oncologist,
University Childrens Hospital Münster,
Department of Pediatric Hematology and
Oncology,
Münster, Germany

Hubert N. Caron
Professor of Paediatric Oncology,
Department of Paediatric Oncology,
Emma Children's Hospital AMC,
University of Amsterdam,
Amsterdam, The Netherlands

Guillermo Chantada
Principal Physician,
Hemato-oncology service,
Hospital JP Garrahan,
Buenos Aires, Argentina

Julia Chisholm
Paediatric Oncologist,
Royal Marsden Hospital,
Sutton, UK

Finella Craig
Lead Palliative Care Consultant,
Department of Palliative Care,
Great Ormond Street Hospital for Children,
London, UK

Beatriz de Camargo
Pediatric Hematology-Oncology Program,
Instituto Nacional do Cancer,
Rio de Janeiro, Brazil

Francois Doz
Department of Paediatric Oncology,
Institut Curie,
and Professor of Paediatrics,
University Paris Descartes, Sorbonne Paris
Cité, France

R. Maarten Egeler
Professor of Paediatrics,
University of Toronto,
Director, Stem Cell Transplantation,
The Hospital for Sick Children,
Toronto, Canada

Angelika Eggert
Professor of Pediatrics,
University Children's Hospital Essen,
Germany

Andrea Ferrari
Pediatric Oncology Unit,
Fondazione IRCCS Istituto Nazionale
Tumori,
Milan, Italy

Alberto Garaventa
Oncology Unit,
Department of Pediatric Haematology-
Oncology,
Giannina Gaslini Children's Hospital,
Genova, Italy

Mark Gaze
Department of Oncology,
University College London Hospitals NHS
Foundation Trust and Great Ormond Street
Hospital for Children NHS Trust,
London, UK

Norbert Graf
Director of the Department for Pediatric
Hematology and Oncology,
Saarland University, Medical Faculty,
Homburg, Germany

Martha Grootenhuis
Psychosocial Department,
Emma Children's Hospital AMC,
University of Amsterdam,
Amsterdam, The Netherlands

Thomas Gross
Gordon Teter Chair for Pediatric Cancer
Research, and Professor,
Department of Pediatrics,
OSU School of Medicine,
Nationwide Children's Hospital,
Columbus, USA

Rupert Handgretinger
Chairman, Department of Hematology/
Oncology and General Pediatrics,
Children's University Hospital,
Tuebingen, Germany

Henrik Hasle
Professor, Department of Pediatrics,
Aarhus University Hospital Skejby,
Aarhus, Denmark

Riccardo Haupt
Consultant Pediatrician,
Epidemiology and Biostatistics Section,
Scientific Directorate,
G. Gaslini Children's Hospital,
Genova, Italy

Lars Hjorth
Consultant Paediatric Oncology &
Haematology,
Department of Paediatrics, Skåne
University Hospital,
Clinical Sciences Lund University,
Lund, Sweden

Scott Howard
Department of Oncology and International
Outreach Program,
St Jude Children's Research Hospital,
Memphis, USA

Thierry A.G.M. Huisman
Professor of Radiology and Radiological
Science,
Director, Division of Pediatric Radiology,
Russell H. Morgan Department of Radiology
and Radiological Science,
Johns Hopkins Hospital,
Baltimore, USA

Shai Izraeli
Associate Professor of Pediatrics,
Tel Aviv University,
Pediatric Hemato-Oncology,
Sheba Medical Center, Israel

Momcilo Jankovic
Pediatric Oncologist,
Department of Paediatrics,
University of Milano-Bicocca,
Hospital San Gerardo/Fondazione MBBM,
Monza, Italy

Robert Johnston
Consultant in Paediatric Oncology,
Royal Belfast Hospital for Sick Children,
Belfast, UK

Herbert Jürgens
Universitätsklinikum Münster,
Klinik und Poliklinik für Kinderheilkunde -
Päd. Hämatologie/Onkologie,
Münster, Germany

Gertjan Kaspers
Pediatric Oncology/Hematology,
VU University Medical Center,
Amsterdam, The Netherlands

Michelle Koh
Palliative Care Consultant,
Department of Palliative Care,
Great Ormond Street Hospital for Children,
London, UK

Dieter Korholz
Professor of Pediatrics,
Director Clinic for Children and Adolescents,
Martin Luther University Halle/Wittenberg,
Halle, Germany

Heinrich Kovar
Professor of Molecular Biology,
Children's Cancer Research Institute,
St Anna Children's Hospital,
Wien, Austria

Leontien Kremer
Department of Paediatric Oncology,
Emma Children's Hospital AMC,
University of Amsterdam,
The Netherlands,
and Coordinator Editor of the
Cochrane Childhood Cancer Group

Kieran McHugh
Consultant Paediatric Radiologist,
Great Ormond Street Hospital for Children,
London, UK

Esther Meijer-van den Bergh
Clinical Psychologist,
Department of Medical Psychology,
University Medical Centre St Radboud,
Nijmegen, The Netherlands

Elizabeth Molyneux
Professor of Paediatrics,
College of Medicine, Blantyre 3, Malawi

James Nicholson
Consultant Paediatric Oncologist,
Cambridge University Hospitals,
NHS Trust, UK

Charlotte Niemeyer
University Children's Hospital,
University of Freiburg, Germany

Daniel Orbach
Pediatric Department,
Institut Curie, Paris, France

Michael Paulussen
Medical Director,
Vestische Kinder- und Jugendklinik Datteln,
Germany,
and Chair of Paediatrics,
Faculty of Health,
Witten/Herdecke University

Giorgio Perilongo
Pediatric Oncology Department,
Centre Hospitalier Universitaire,
Angers, France

Robert S. Phillips
Centre for Reviews and Dissemination,
University of York,
and Paediatric Oncologist,
Leeds Children's Hospital,
Leeds General Infirmary,
Leeds, UK

Rob Pieters
Department of Pediatric Oncology/
Hematology,
Erasmus MC-Sophia Children's Hospital,
Rotterdam,
The Netherlands

Kathy Pritchard-Jones
Professor of Paediatric Oncology,
University College London Institute of Child
Health and Consultant Paediatric Oncologist,
Great Ormond Street Hospital for Children,
London, UK

Yves Reguerre
Oncologic Pediatric Department,
Centre Hospitalo-Universitaire,
Angers, France

Dirk Reinhardt
Pediatric Oncology/Hematology,
Medical School Hannover, Germany

Carlos Rodríguez-Galindo
Department of Pediatric Oncology,
Dana-Farber/Children's Hospital
Cancer Center,
Associate Professor of Pediatrics,
Harvard Medical School, Boston, USA

Angelo Rosolen
Hemato-Oncology Unit,
Department of Pediatrics,
University of Padova, Padova, Italy

Frank Saran
Consultant Clincial Oncologist,
Department of Paediatric Oncology,
The Royal Marsden NHS Foundation Trust,
Sutton, UK

Martin Schrappe
Director, and Professor of Pediatrics,
Department of General Pediatrics,
University Hospital Schleswig-Holstein,
Kiel, Germany

Anjali Shah
Childhood Cancer Research Group,
University of Oxford and
London School of Hygiene and Tropical
Medicine, UK

Rod Skinner
Consultant/Clinical Senior Lecturer in
Paediatric & Adolescent Oncology/BMT,
Department of Paediatric & Adolescent
Haematology Oncology,
and Children's BMT Unit,
Great North Children's Hospital,
Royal Victoria Infirmary,
Newcastle upon Tyne, UK

Stuart Smith
Children's Brain Tumour Research Centre,
School of Clinical Sciences, University of
Nottingham, UK

Michael C.G. Stevens
Professor of Paediatric Oncology,
University of Bristol
and Consultant Paediatric Oncologist,
Bristol Royal Hospital for Children,
Bristol, UK

Charles Stiller
Childhood Cancer Research Group,
University of Oxford, UK

Maria Grazia Valsecchi
Professor of Medical Statistics,
Center of Biostatistics for Clinical
Epidemiology,
Department of Clinical Medicine and
Prevention,
University of Milano-Bicocca, Italy

Marianne van de Wetering
Department of Paediatric Oncology,
Emma Children's Hospital AMC,
University of Amsterdam,
Amsterdam, The Netherlands

Arnauld Verschuur
Département de Cancérologie Pédiatrique,
Hôpital d'Enfants de La Timone,
Marseille, France
and Department of Paediatric Oncology,
Emma Children's Hospital AMC,
University of Amsterdam,
Amsterdam, The Netherlands

Jantien Vrijmoet-Wiersma
Health Psychologist, Den Haag,
The Netherlands

David Walker
Children's Brain Tumour Research Centre,
School of Clinical Sciences,
University of Nottingham, UK

Hamish Wallace
Professor of Paediatric Oncology,
Royal Hospital for Sick Children,
Edinburgh, UK

Sheila Weitzman
Associate Director (Clinical),
Division of Hematology/Oncology,
The Hospital for Sick Children,
Toronto; and Professor of Pediatrics,
University of Toronto, Canada

Joanne Wolfe
Director, Pediatric Palliative Care,
Children's Hospital Boston; Division Chief,
Pediatric Palliative Care Service,
Department of Psychosocial Oncology
and Palliative Care,
Dana-Farber Cancer Institute, Boston, USA

Jozsef Zsiros
Department of Paediatric Oncology,
Emma Children's Hospital AMC,
University of Amsterdam,
Amsterdam, The Netherlands

Michel Zwaan
Associate Professor of Pediatric Oncology,
Department of Pediatric Oncology,
Sophia Children's Hospital/Erasmus MC,
Rotterdam, The Netherlands

Abbreviations

17-AAG	17-amino-allyl geldanamycin	BMD	bone mineral density
17-DMAG	17-(dimethylaminoethylamino)-17-demethoxygeldanamycin	BSA	body surface area
		BW	body weight
6-MP	6-mercaptopurine	BWS	Beckwith–Wiedemann syndrome
6-TG	6-thioguanine	C	cyclophosphamide
A	actinomycin D	C-ALCL	primary cutaneous anaplastic large cell lymphoma
A-RMS	alveolar rhabdomyosarcoma		
ABVD	doxorubicin, bleomycin, vinblastine, dacarbazine	CAM	complementary and alternative medicine
aCPP	atypical choroid plexus papillomas	CBV	cyclophosphamide, BCNU, and etoposide
ADV	adenovirus		
AER	absolute excess risk	CCG	Children's Cancer Group
AF	aggressive fibromatosis	CCNU	procarbazine, 6-thioguanine, dibromodulcitol, and lomustine
AFP	alpha fetoprotein		
AJCC	American Joint Committee on Cancer	CCS	childhood cancer survivors
ALCL	anaplastic large cell lymphoma	CCSS	Childhood Cancer Survivor Study
ALK	anaplastic lymphoma kinase	Cen	centromeric
ALL	acute lymphoblastic leukaemia	CEVAIE	carboplatin, epirubicin, vincristine, actinomycin D, ifosfamide, and etoposide
alloHSCT	allogenic HSCT		
AML	acute myeloid leukaemia		
AMPK	activation of AMP-activated protein kinase	CGH	comparative genomic hybridization
		CHC	choriocarcinoma
APL	acute promyelocytic leukaemia	CHOP	cyclophosphamide, doxorubicin, vincristine, and prednisolone
APO	adriamycin (doxorubicin), prednisone, and vincristine		
		CHS	Chédiak-Higashi syndrome
ASR	Age-standardized rate	CI	confidence interval
ATRA	all-*trans* retinoic acid	CML	chronic myelogenous leukaemia
ATRT	atypical teratoid rhabdoid tumours	CMML	chronic myelomonocytic leukaemia
BCD	bleomycin, cyclophosphamide, and actinomycin D	CMN	congenital mesoblastic nephromas
		CMV	cytomegalovirus
		CNS	central nervous system
BCH	benign cephalic histiocytosis	COG	Children's Oncology Group
BCRP	breast cancer resistance protein	COJEC	cisplatin, vincristine, carboplatin, etoposide, and cyclophosphamide
BEACOPP	bleomycin, etoposide, doxorubicin, cyclophosphamide, vincristine, prednisolone and procarbazine		
		COMP	cyclophosphamide, vincristine, methotrexate, and prednisone
BEAM	BCNU, etoposide, cytarabine, and melphalan	COPAD	cyclophosphamide, vincristine, prednisone, and doxorubicin
BEP	cisplatin, etoposide and bleomycin	COPDAC	vincristine, cyclophosphamide, dacarbazine, and prednisone
BFM	Berlin-Frankfurt-Munster		
BL	Burkitt lymphoma	COPP	vincristine, cyclophosphamide, procarbazine, and prednisone
BM	bone marrow		

CPC	choroid plexus carcinomas
CPP	choroid plexus papillomas
CPT	choroid plexus tumours
CRT	conformal radiotherapy
CsA	cyclosporin A
CSC	cancer stem cells
CSF	cerebrospinal fluid
CT	computed tomography
CTL	cytotoxic lymphocytes
CTV	clinical target volume
CWS	German Soft Tissue Sarcoma Cooperative Group
CXR	chest X-ray
D	doxorubicin
DC	dyskeratosis congenita
DDS	Denys–Drash syndrome
DEXA	dual X-ray absorptiometry
dFdC	2',2'-difluorodeoxycytidine
DFS	disease-free survival
DI	diabetes insipidus
DIA/DIG	Desmoplastic infantile astrocytoma/ganglioglioma
DIPG	diffuse intrinsic pontine glioma
DLBCL	diffuse large B-cell lymphoma
DLI	donor lymphocyte infusions
DLT	dose limiting toxicity
DM	double minute
DNET	Dysembryoplastic neuroepithelial tumour
DS	Down syndrome
DSRCT	Desmoplastic small round cell tumour
DVH	dose volume histograms
E	etoposide
e IPV	enhanced inactivated polio vaccine
E-RMS	embryonal rhabdomyosarcoma
EBM	evidence-based medicine
EBRT	external beam radiotherapy
EBV	Epstein–Barr virus
EC	embryonal carcinoma
EFS	event-free survival
EGF	epidermal growth factor
EGFR	epidermal growth factor receptor
EICNHL	European Intergroup for Childhood Non-Hodgkin Lymphoma
EMA	epithelial membrane antigen

ENSG5	European Neuroblastoma Group Fifth Study
EpSSG	European paediatric Soft tissue sarcoma Study Group
ES	Ewing sarcoma
ESFT	Ewing sarcoma family of tumours
ESR	erythrocyte sedimentation rate
EU CTD	EU Clinical Trials Directive
EVD	external ventricular drain
FA	fibrillary astrocytomas
FAB	French–American–British
FAP	familial adenomatous polyposis
FDA	Federal Drug Agency
FDG	18-fluorodeoxyglucose
FHL	familial haemophagocytic lymphohistiocytosis
FISH	fluorescent *in situ* hybridization
FL	follicular lymphoma
FN	febrile neutropenia
FNCLCC	French system for grading tumours
G-CSF	granulocyte colony-stimulating growth factor
GA	general anaesthetic
GBM	glioblastoma multiforme
GCT	germ cell tumour
GD2	disialoganglioside
GFAOP	Groupe Franco-Africaine d'Oncologie Pediatrique
GFAP	glial fibrillary acidic protein
GIST	gastrointestinal stromal tumour
GM-CSF	granulocyte macrophage colony-stimulating growth factor
GNB	ganglioneuroblastoma
GSII	Griscelli syndrome type II
GTV	gross tumour volume
GvH	graft-versus-host
GvL	graft-versus-leukaemia
GvT	graft-versus-tumour
HbF	fetal haemoglobin
HBV	hepatitis B virus
HC	haemorrhagic cystitis
HCG	β-human chorionic gonadotropin
HCV	hepatitis C virus
HDAC	histone deacetylase
HDCT	high-dose chemotherapy
HGG	high grade gliomas
HHV8	human herpesvirus 8

HIC	high-income countries	ITCC	Innovative Therapies for Children with Cancer
HIV	human immunodeficiency virus		
HL	Hodgkin lymphoma	ITD	internal tandem duplication
HLA	human leukocyte antigen	ITT	insulin tolerance test
HLH	hemophagocytic lymphohistiocytosis	IVADo	ifosfamide, vincristine, actinomycin D, and doxorubicin
HPA	hypothalamic pituitary axis		
HPV	human papilloma virus	JEB	carboplatin, etoposide and bleomycin
HR	hypophosphataemic rickets	JMML	juvenile myelomonocytic leukaemia
HRS	Hodgkin/Reed Sternberg	JPA	juvenile pilocytic astrocytomas
HSCR	haematopoietic stem cell rescue	JXG	juvenile xanthogranuloma
HSCT	haematopoietic stem cell transplantation	KIR	killer-cell immunoglobulin-like receptor
HSR	homogeneously staining region	L-MTP-PE	liposomal muramyl tripeptide phenol ethanolamine (mifurmatide)
HSV	herpes simplex virus		
HVA	homovanillic acid	LAE	late adverse events
HvG	host-versus-graft	LAIP	leukaemia-associated immunophenotype
I	ifosfamide		
i.v.	intravenous	LCH	Langerhans cell histiocytosis
ICCC-3	International Classification of Childhood Cancer, Third Edition	LD-PCR	long-distance polymerase chain reaction
ICD-O	International Classification of Diseases for Oncology	LDH	lactate dehydrogenase
		LFS	leukaemia-free survival
ICE	ifosfamide, carboplatin, and etoposide	LGA	low-grade astrocytoma
ICG	Italian Cooperative Group	LL	lymphoblastic lymphoma
ICP	intracranial pressure	LMIC	low- and middle-income countries
IDRFs	image-defined risk factors	LOH	loss of heterozygosity
IEP	ifosfamide, etoposide, and prednisolone	LOI	loss of imprinting
		LRP	lung resistance-related protein
IESS	Intergroup Ewing Sarcoma	LSC	leukaemic stem cell
IFS	infantile fibrosarcoma	LTFU	long-term follow up
IGF	insulin-like growth factor	LyP	lymphoid papulosis
IGFBP	IGF binding proteins	MAHO	German protocols for testicular GCT
IGRT	image guided radiotherapy	MAKEI	German protocols for non-testicular GCT
IMRT	intensity modulated radiotherapy		
INPC	International Neuroblastoma Pathology Classification	MALT	mucosa-associated tissue lymphoma
		MAPK	mitogen-activated protein kinase
INRG	International Neuroblastoma Risk Group	MAS	macrophage activation syndrome
		MBEN	medulloblastoma with extensive nodularity
INRGSS	International Neuroblastoma Risk Group Staging System		
		MDP	methylene-diphosphonate
INSS	International Neuroblastoma Staging System	MDR	multidrug resistance
		MDS	myelodysplastic syndrome
IPSS	International Prognostic Scoring System	MF	mycosis fungoides
		MFD	matched family donor
IR	intervention radiology	MGCT	malignant germ cell tumours
IRS	insulin receptor substrates	mHag	minor histocompatibility antigen
IRS	Intergroup Rhabdomyosarcoma Study	MHC	major histocompatibility complex

MIBG	metaiodobenzylguanidine
miRNAs	microRNAs
ML-DS	myeloid leukaemia of Down syndrome
MLC	multi-leaf collimators
mMLC	mini multi-leaf collimators
MMR	measles, mumps, rubella
MMT	Malignant Mesenchymal Tumour Committee
MoAbs	monoclonal antibodies
MPNST	malignant peripheral nerve sheath tumours
MPO	myeloperoxidase
MRD	minimal residual disease
MRI	magnetic resonance imaging
MRP	multidrug resistance protein
MRT	malignant rhabdoid tumour
MS	metabolic syndrome
MSD	matched sibling donor
MSKCC	Memorial Sloan-Kettering Cancer Center
MSTS	Musculoskeletal Tumor Society
MTD	maximum tolerated dose
mTOR	mammalian target of rapamycin
MTP-PE	muramyl tripeptide
MTX	methotrexate
MUD	matched unrelated donor
MZL	marginal zone lymphoma
NBO	neurofibromatous bright object
NCI	National Cancer Institute
NCR	natural cytotoxicity receptor
NDI	nephrogenic diabetes insipidus
NF1	neurofibromatosis
NGGCT	non-germinomatous germ cell tumours
NGS	next generation sequencing
NHEJ	non-homologous end joining
NHL	non-Hodgkin lymphoma
NK	natural killer
NLPHL	nodular lymphocyte predominant Hodgkin lymphoma
NMA	*MYCN* amplification
NMDA	N-methyl-D-aspartate
NMSC	non-melanomatous skin cancer
NMZL	nodal marginal zone lymphoma
NOPHO	Nordic Society of Paediatric Haematology and Oncology
NOS	not otherwise specified

NPM	nucleophosmin
NPM1	nucleophosmin-1
NRSTS	non-rhabdomyomatous soft tissue sarcomas
NS	Noonan syndrome
NSE	neuron-specific enolase
NTV	neuroendoscopic third ventriculostomy
OEPA	vincristine, etoposide, prednisone, and adriamycin
OMS	opsoclonus-myoclonus syndrome
OS	overall survival
OS	osteosarcoma
PA	pilocytic astrocytomas
$paCO_2$	arterial carbon dioxide tension
PAS	periodic-acid-Schiff
PBSC	peripheral blood stem cells
PCNSL	primary central nervous system non-Hodgkin lymphomas
PCR	polymerase chain reaction
PCU	paediatric cancer unit
PCV	CCNU/procarbazine, and vincristine
PDGF	platelet-derived growth factor
PDGFR	platelet derived growth factor receptor
PEI	ifosfamide, cisplatin, and etoposide
PET	positron emission tomography
PFS	progression-free survival
PFT	pulmonary function test
PGC	primordial germ cell
PHPV	persistent hyperplastic primary vitreous
PI3K	phosphatidylinositol-3-kinase
PIS	patient information sheets
PLAP	placental alkaline phosphatase
PMBL	primary mediastinal large B-cell lymphoma
PNET	primitive neuro-ectodermal tumours
pNT	peripheral neuroblastic tumour
POG	Paediatric Oncology Group
PPB	peuropulmonary blastoma
pPNET	peripheral primitive neuroectodermal tumour
PPTP	preclinical paediatric testing program
PRETEXT	pre-treatment extent
PTCL	peripheral T-cell lymphomas
PTSD	post traumatic stress disorder

PTV	planning target volume		SMN	secondary malignant neoplasm
PVB	cisplatin, vinblastine, and bleomycin		SMR	standardized mortality ratio
PXA	pleomorphic xanthoastrocytoma		SPTL	subcutaneous panniculitic T-cell lymphoma
QoL	quality of life		STS	soft tissue sarcoma
R–E	Reese–Ellsworth		STSC	Soft Tissue Sarcoma Committee
RA	refractory anaemia		SVC	superior vena cava
RAEB	refractory anaemia with excessive blasts		TAM	transient abnormal myelopoiesis
RAEB-t	refractory anaemia with excessive blasts in transformation		tAML	treatment-related AML
			TBI	total body irradiation
RANK	receptor activator for nuclear factor \ kappa-B		TCR	T-cell receptor
			TdT	terminal deoxynucleotidyl transferase
RARS	refractory anaemia with ringed sideroblasts		Tel	telomeric
RC	refractory cytopenia		TKI	tyrosine kinase inhibitors
RCC	refractory cytopenia of childhood		TLCT	transitional liver cell tumour
RCC	renal cell carcinoma		TLS	tumour lysis syndrome
RCT	randomized controlled clinical trials		TMD	transient congenital myeloid proliferative disease
RDD	Rosai-Dorfman disease		TMP/SMZ	trimethoprim–sulfamethoxazole
REAL	Revised European-American Lymphoma Classification of HL		TNFR	tumour necrosis factor receptor
RFS	relapse-free survival		TNM	tumour-node-metastasis
RIC	reduced-intensity conditioning		TPMT	thiopurine methyltransferase
RMS	rhabdomyosarcoma		TRM	transplant-related mortality
RNAi	RNA interference		TSH	thyroid-stimulating hormone
ROS	reactive oxygen species		UCB	umbilical cord blood
RR	relative risk		UCH	uncommon histiocytosis
RT	radiotherapy		UICC	International Union Against Cancer
RTA	renal tubular acidosis		UNCRC	UN Convention of the Rights of the Child
RTK	rhabdoid tumours of the kidney		US	ultrasound
RTK	receptor tyrosine kinase		V	vincristine
SCF	stem cell factor		VAC	vincristine, actinomycin, and cyclophosphamide
SCN	severe congenital neutropeni		VDC-IE	vincristine, doxorubicin, cyclophosphamide, ifosfamide, and etoposide
SDD	selective decontamination of the digestive tract			
SDS	Shwachman-Diamond syndrome		VEGF	vascular endothelial growth factor
SEER	surveillance, epidemiology, and end results		VIP	vasoactive intestinal peptide
SEGA	subependymal giant cell astrocytoma		VIP	vinblastine, ifosfamide, and cisplatin
SEN	sub-ependymal nodules		VMA	vanillylmandelic acid
SHML	sinus histiocytosis with massive lymphadenopathy		VOD	venous occlusive disease
SIg	suface immunoglobin		VTC	topotecan, cyclophosphamide, and vincristine
SIOP	International Society of Paediatric Oncology		VZV	varicella zoster virus
SIOPEL	International Childhood Liver Tumor Strategy Group		WAGR	Wilms tumour, aniridia, genital deformity, retardation
siRNas	small interfering RNAs			

WBC	white blood cell count	XLP	X-linked lymphoproliferative syndrome
WCC	World Child Cancer		
WHO	World Health Organization	YST	yolk sac tumour
WT	Wilms tumour		

Chapter 1

The epidemiology of cancer in children and adolescents

Charles Stiller and Anjali Shah

Introduction

Childhood and adolescent cancers account for less than 2 per cent of all cancer in industrialized countries, but the young age at which they occur means that they account for a much larger proportion of total population life-years potentially lost to cancer. In this chapter we consider the classification of childhood and adolescent cancer, incidence and survival rates, late effects, and aetiology.

Classification

The current standard classification for those under the age of 15 years is the *International Classification of Childhood Cancer, Third Edition (ICCC-3)*, with groups defined by the codes for morphology and topography in the third edition of the *International Classification of Diseases for Oncology* (ICD-O). Most of these groups are limited to malignant neoplasms, but benign and unspecified intracranial and intraspinal tumours are also included, since they are recorded by many cancer registries.

In the most recent version of the standard classification for cancers of adolescents and young adults (15–24 years), diagnostic groups are defined by morphology and topography codes in the second edition of ICD-O. The grouping of diagnoses is more logical than ICCC-3 for cancers affecting adolescents and young adults especially at age 20–24 years, but some comparability with data on childhood cancer is thereby sacrificed.

Incidence

Incidence in the UK

Table 1.1 gives numbers of cases and incidence rates for the main groups and principal subgroups of ICCC-3 among children aged 0–14 years in the UK during 1996–2005. The pattern of incidence is typical of that found among mainly White populations of industrialized countries. The total age-standardized rate (ASR) was 142 per million children, giving a cumulative risk of 1 in 484 of developing cancer during the first 15 years of life.

Overall, incidence is 20 per cent higher in boys than in girls. The male excess is greatest for lymphomas. Extracranial germ cell tumours, melanoma, and carcinomas of several sites are markedly more frequent in girls than in boys. Within childhood, total incidence of cancer is highest in the first 5 years of life. There are also marked early age peaks for acute lymphoblastic leukaemia (ALL) and for all the distinctive embryonal tumours. In contrast, Hodgkin lymphoma and bone sarcomas are virtually never seen before the age of 2 years, and their incidence increases

Table 1.1 Childhood cancer in the UK, 1996–2005. Numbers of registrations, age-specific and age-standardized (World Standard Population) incidence rates, and sex ratio of age-standardized rates (not calculated for groups with fewer than 20 registrations)

Diagnostic group	Total registrations	Annual rates per million by age group			Age-standardized rate per million	Sex ratio (M/F)
		0–4 years	5–9 years	10–14 years		
All cancers	15165	192.0	108.5	112.7	142.1	1.2
Leukaemias, myeloproliferative and myelodysplastic diseases	4851	72.3	35.4	25.3	46.8	1.2
Lymphoid leukaemias	3780	57.4	29.1	17.3	36.6	1.2
Acute myeloid leukaemias	724	9.7	4.6	5.5	6.8	1.0
Chronic myeloproliferative diseases	104	0.8	0.6	1.5	0.9	1.2
Myelodysplastic syndrome and other myeloproliferative diseases	194	3.7	1.0	0.7	1.9	1.1
Unspecified and other specified leukaemias	49	0.8	0.2	0.3	0.5	0.7
Lymphomas and reticuloendothelial neoplasms	1520	6.6	12.5	21.4	12.8	2.0
Hodgkin lymphomas	687	1.2	4.2	12.7	5.5	1.6
Non-Hodgkin lymphomas including Burkitt lymphoma	814	5.1	8.2	8.5	7.1	2.4
Miscellaneous lymphoreticular neoplasms	6	0.2	–	–	0.1	–
Unspecified lymphomas	13	0.1	0.1	0.2	0.1	–
Central nervous system and miscellaneous intracranial and intraspinal neoplasms	3752	37.9	34.8	29.0	34.3	1.1
Ependymomas and choroid plexus tumour	371	6.0	2.5	1.7	3.6	1.4
Astrocytomas	1614	15.2	15.4	13.1	14.6	1.0
Intracranial and intraspinal embryonal tumours	709	8.4	7.0	4.0	6.6	1.5
Other gliomas	386	3.3	4.2	2.9	3.5	1.1
Other specified intracranial and intraspinal neoplasms	506	3.1	4.5	5.9	4.4	1.2
Unspecified intracranial and intraspinal neoplasms	166	1.9	1.3	1.4	1.5	1.0

Neuroblastoma and other peripheral nervous cell tumours	934	22.4	3.1	0.7	9.9	1.1
Neuroblastoma and ganglioneuroblastoma	922	22.3	3.1	0.5	9.8	1.1
Other peripheral nervous cell tumours	12	0.1	0.1	0.2	0.1	–
Retinoblastoma	395	10.5	0.5	0.1	4.3	0.9
Renal tumours	855	18.3	4.3	1.2	8.8	0.9
Wilms tumour and other nonepithelial renal tumours	835	18.3	4.2	0.9	8.7	0.9
Renal carcinomas	17	0.1	0.0	0.3	0.1	–
Unspecified malignant renal tumours	3	–	0.1	–	0.0	–
Hepatic tumours	163	3.7	0.3	0.5	1.7	1.4
Hepatoblastoma	132	3.5	0.2	0.1	1.4	1.6
Hepatic carcinomas	28	0.2	0.1	0.4	0.2	0.8
Unspecified malignant hepatic tumours	3	0.1	–	–	0.0	–
Malignant bone tumours	602	0.8	4.6	10.5	4.8	1.0
Osteosarcomas	318	0.1	2.4	5.9	2.5	0.9
Chondrosarcomas	14	–	0.0	0.3	0.1	–
Ewing tumour and related bone sarcomas	244	0.6	1.9	4.0	2.0	1.1
Other specified malignant bone tumours	17	0.1	0.1	0.3	0.1	–
Unspecified malignant bone tumours	9	0.1	0.1	0.1	0.1	–
Soft tissue and other extraosseous sarcomas	999	10.8	7.9	8.4	9.2	1.3
Rhabdomyosarcomas	513	7.0	4.7	2.4	4.9	1.5
Fibrosarcomas, peripheral nerve sheath tumours and other fibrous neoplasms	72	0.7	0.3	1.0	0.6	0.9
Kaposi sarcoma	3	–	0.0	0.1	0.0	–
Other specified soft tissue sarcomas	344	2.3	2.5	4.4	3.0	1.1
Unspecified soft tissue sarcomas	67	0.7	0.5	0.6	0.6	1.1

(continued)

Table 1.1 (continued)

Diagnostic group	Total registrations	Annual rates per million by age group				Age-standardized rate per million	Sex ratio (M/F)
		0–4 years	5–9 years	10–14 years			
Germ cell tumours, trophoblastic tumours and neoplasms of gonads	504	6.1	2.0	5.5	4.6	0.8
Intracranial and intraspinal germ cell tumours	164	0.9	1.1	2.4	1.4	1.5
Malignant extracranial and extragonadal germ cell tumours	135	3.4	0.1	0.3	1.4	0.4
Malignant gonadal germ cell tumours	197	1.8	0.7	2.7	1.7	0.7
Gonadal carcinomas	4	–	0.1	0.1	0.0	–
Other and unspecified malignant gonadal tumours	4	0.0	0.0	0.1	0.0	–
Other malignant epithelial neoplasms and malignant melanomas	502	1.7	2.6	9.0	4.1	0.7
Adrenocortical carcinomas	28	0.6	0.2	0.1	0.3	0.4
Thyroid carcinomas	106	0.2	0.6	2.0	0.9	0.5
Nasopharyngeal carcinomas	23	–	0.1	0.5	0.2	2.2
Malignant melanomas	122	0.6	0.6	2.1	1.0	0.7
Skin carcinomas	98	0.2	0.6	1.8	0.8	1.1
Other and unspecified carcinomas	125	0.1	0.7	2.5	1.0	0.7
Other and unspecified malignant neoplasms	88	0.9	0.4	1.1	0.8	1.0
Other specified malignant tumours	18	0.3	0.1	0.2	0.2	–
Other unspecified malignant tumours	70	0.6	0.3	0.9	0.6	1.0

Source: National Registry of Childhood Tumours.

steeply throughout childhood and adolescence. Gonadal germ cell tumours are most frequent among boys in early childhood, whereas among girls they are rare until the postpubertal increase, which begins at an earlier age than among boys.

Table 1.2 gives numbers of cases and incidence rates for the main groups and subgroups of the Birch classification among adolescents aged 15–19 years in England during 1996–2005. The total annual incidence was 169 per million. About 25% of all adolescent cancers are lymphomas, predominantly Hodgkin lymphoma. Leukaemias, central nervous system tumours, and carcinomas each account for about 14 per cent of all cancers, germ cell tumours for 12%, and bone tumours for 10%.

Table 1.2 Adolescent cancer in England, 1996–2005. Numbers of registrations, age-specific incidence rates, and sex ratio (not calculated for groups with fewer than 20 registrations)

Diagnostic group	Total registrations	Annual rates per million 15–19 years	Sex ratio (M/F)
All cancers	5682	169.4	1.3
Leukaemias	757	22.6	1.5
Acute lymphoblastic leukaemia	417	12.4	2.0
Acute myeloid leukaemia	237	7.1	1.0
Chronic myeloid leukaemia	68	2.0	1.1
Other and unspecified leukaemia	35	1.0	1.7
Lymphomas	1,383	41.2	1.3
Non-Hodgkin's lymphoma	462	13.8	2.0
Hodgkin's lymphoma	921	27.5	1.0
Central nervous system and other intracranial and intraspinal neoplasms	762	22.7	1.2
Astrocytoma	297	8.9	1.4
Other glioma	96	2.9	1.3
Ependymoma	39	1.2	1.4
Medulloblastoma	55	1.6	1.3
Other tumours	237	7.1	1.0
Tumours of unknown morphology	38	1.1	1.0
Bone tumours	582	17.4	1.6
Osteosarcoma	287	8.6	1.8
Chondrosarcoma	30	0.9	2.8
Ewing sarcoma	236	7.0	1.4
Other bone tumours	29	0.9	1.1
Soft tissue sarcomas	331	9.9	1.4
Fibrosarcoma	43	1.3	1.3
Rhabdomyosarcoma	90	2.7	2.9
Other soft tissue sarcomas	138	4.1	1.0
Unspecified soft tissue sarcomas	60	1.8	1.3

(continued)

Table 1.2 (continued)

Diagnostic group	Total registrations	Annual rates per million 15–19 years	Sex ratio (M/F)
Germ cell tumours	663	19.8	5.1
Gonadal	586	17.5	5.3
Non-gonadal	77	2.3	4.1
Melanoma	394	11.7	0.6
Carcinomas	730	21.8	0.5
Thyroid	204	6.1	0.2
Other head and neck carcinomas	110	3.3	1.1
Lung	25	0.7	1.5
Breast	13	0.4	–
Genito-urinary tract	174	5.2	0.1
Gastro-intestinal tract	162	4.8	1.0
Other carcinomas	42	1.3	1.1
Miscellaneous, specified	63	1.9	1.0
Unspecified	17	0.5	–

Source: Data collected by the nine regional cancer registries in England and collated by the UK Association of Cancer Registries (Robert Alston, personal communication).

International variations

Total incidence of cancer in children and adolescents tends to be higher in industrialized countries and in parts of tropical Africa, and lower in developing countries in other regions of the world. The relative frequencies of different types of cancer also vary considerably between world regions and between ethnic groups in the same country.

Leukaemia

In the industrialized countries of all continents, leukaemias form the largest diagnostic group of childhood cancer, with an ASR of 40–50 per million, and often account for one-third of all malignancies. Incidence is lower in less industrialized countries of Asia and Africa, and among black children in the United States. ALL is the most commonly occurring leukaemia, and variation in the magnitude of the early childhood peak accounts for much of the international variation in total incidence.

Incidence of leukaemia among adolescents ranges from under 10 per million in some African countries to over 35 per million in United States Hispanics, and variations are again mostly attributable to ALL. There is little international variation in the incidence of acute myeloid leukaemia, the second most frequent subtype in children and adolescents.

Lymphomas

Incidence of lymphomas in childhood is highest in parts of tropical Africa, with an ASR of 30–60 per million. They account for 30–40% of all childhood cancers in Africa, compared with 15–25% in Latin America, Asia, and the Middle East, and about 10% in industrialized countries. The most common type in the countries with highest incidence is Burkitt lymphoma but other types of non-Hodgkin lymphoma (NHL) are also seen. Hodgkin lymphoma is rare among children in tropical Africa and East Asia. In developing countries the incidence of Hodgkin lymphoma sometimes peaks at 5–9 years, whereas in developed countries it increases more steeply at the onset of adolescence.

In adolescence, incidence of lymphomas is highest among Jews in Israel and lowest in East Asia and parts of sub-Saharan Africa. In industrialized countries, including Israel, Hodgkin lymphoma is more common than NHL. Elsewhere in the world NHL predominates, with Hodgkin lymphoma occurring rarely in some parts of Asia and Africa. Hodgkin lymphoma is around twice as frequent among boys under 15 years of age as it is among girls, but at age 15–19 incidence among females is usually at least as high as among males. NHL is nearly everywhere more frequent among males than females throughout childhood and adolescence.

Brain and spinal tumours

In industrialized countries brain and spinal tumours are the second most frequent childhood cancer, accounting for 20–25% of all cases. They also occur in substantial numbers in adolescence. Incidence in the United States in both children and adolescents is highest in whites and lowest in blacks. Recorded incidence is lower in developing countries, where under-diagnosis is likely to be a factor.

Neuroblastoma

Neuroblastoma occurs most frequently in infancy. Its incidence is higher in industrialized countries than in developing countries, probably in large part because of a higher rate of diagnosis of asymptomatic tumours. Recorded incidence is lowest in sub-Saharan Africa, where the risk may also be lower. Higher incidence among infants has been found in several industrialized countries compared with the UK, possibly because of increased detection of otherwise silent tumours at routine health checks. Mass screening for neuroblastoma proved to be ineffective, resulting in especially high incidence in infants, but without lowering the incidence of advanced stage neuroblastoma at older ages.

Retinoblastoma

Bilateral retinoblastoma, which is always heritable, has relatively constant incidence worldwide, whereas incidence of the unilateral, predominantly non-heritable form is more variable, with rates as high as 20 per million children in some developing countries.

Wilms tumour

Incidence of Wilms tumour tends to depend on ethnicity rather than geographic area. Incidence is highest in black populations with an ASR of 9–12 per million and lowest in those of Asian origin with an ASR of under 5 per million.

Liver tumours

Hepatoblastoma has constant incidence worldwide. The incidence of hepatocellular carcinoma in young people is highest in regions where there is a high proportion of chronic carriers of hepatitis B in the population, namely East Asia, Melanesia, and sub-Saharan Africa.

Bone tumours

Incidence of malignant bone tumours increases with age, reaching a peak in late adolescence. The two most common bone tumours of children and adolescents are osteosarcoma and Ewing sarcoma. Osteosarcoma has fairly constant incidence worldwide, whereas Ewing sarcoma is extremely rare in East Asian and black populations.

Soft tissue sarcomas

In parts of East and Central Africa with high levels of human herpesvirus 8 (HHV8) infection, Kaposi sarcoma is the most frequent cancer in young people, with incidence sometimes above 40 per million in children and adolescents. Elsewhere, incidence of soft tissue sarcomas in childhood rarely exceeds 10 per million and rhabdomyosarcoma is the most frequent type. Children of Asian origin have a lower incidence of soft tissue sarcoma.

Germ cell tumours

Childhood germ cell tumours are most frequent in East Asia. In adolescence, testicular cancer has an incidence of 25–30 per million in Europe, North America, and Oceania, and less than 10 per million in most other populations. Ovarian germ cell tumours have an incidence of 5–10 per million at age 15–19 years and are one of the very few types of cancer whose peak incidence occurs in this age group. Intracranial and intraspinal germ cell tumours have an incidence of 1–3 per million among adolescents worldwide.

Trends in incidence

The best-documented trend concerns ALL, the most common childhood cancer in all developed countries. The early childhood peak started to emerge in mortality data in England and Wales in the 1930s, and was well established among white children in the USA by the early 1940s. Incidence continued to rise, particularly in early childhood, in some western countries until at least the end of the 20th century. Small increases have also been observed in western populations for a wide range of other childhood cancers, but it is not clear how much they are attributable to changes in diagnostic practice rather than in underlying risk. Incidence of thyroid carcinoma rose steeply in areas heavily contaminated by radiation from the Chernobyl nuclear reactor explosion, but has returned to normal levels among children conceived since the accident.

Survival rates

The past decades have seen dramatic increases in survival rates for most types of childhood cancer. In Europe, 5-year survival from all childhood cancers combined had reached 80% by 2000. Figure 1.1 shows 5-year survival rates for the most frequent types of childhood cancer in Europe in 2000–2002. Broadly similar results have been observed in other industrialized countries. The proportion of children 'cured' of leukaemia in Britain, that is who survive until they no longer experience excess mortality compared with the general population, had reached 68% by 1995 and was predicted to increase since then.

In Europe and the US overall survival among adolescents with cancer has improved to about 73–78%. Adolescents have substantially lower survival rates than children for ALL, NHL, bone tumours, and soft tissue sarcomas, which may be due to differences in biology, treatment, psychosocial characteristics, and participation in clinical trials.

Follow-up

Continuing improvement in survival from childhood cancer has led to a great increase in long-term survivors, including substantial numbers of adults. For childhood cancer overall, excess mortality continues beyond 25 years from diagnosis, principally due to second primary cancers and circulatory diseases. The risk of developing a second primary cancer is about six times that in the general population, but it varies according to type of first cancer and treatment given. The risk is highest in those who received radiotherapy and among survivors of heritable retinoblastoma.

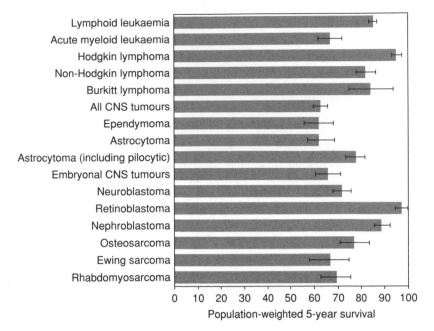

Fig. 1.1 Population-based 5-year survival (%) with 95% confidence intervals for 15 common cancers diagnosed among children (0–14 years) in Europe in 2000–2002 using period analysis. Data source: EUROCARE-4 (Gatta et al., 2009).

Survivors of childhood and adolescent cancer are at increased risk of a range of chronic diseases, which are discussed in other chapters.

Aetiology of cancer in children and adolescents

The causes of the great majority of cases of childhood cancer remain unknown, despite intensive investigation since the mid 20th century.

Environmental factors

Ionizing radiation

Exposure to ionizing radiation is one of the few factors generally accepted to increase the risk that a child will develop cancer. Recent studies do not themselves show an association with antenatal diagnostic X-ray exposure but they are consistent with earlier, more powerful studies that do. In the past, antenatal radiography probably caused at most about 5 per cent of childhood cancers, even when it was more widely used and doses were higher than they are now. The much larger doses of radiation given during radiotherapy are also carcinogenic but can only account for a tiny proportion of all childhood cancers. Naturally occurring background radiation is largely unavoidable and 15–20% of childhood leukaemia in Britain may be attributable to this source of exposure.

Non-ionizing radiation

Ultraviolet radiation from sunlight can cause melanoma and other skin cancers. Concern has been expressed for more than 20 years over possible carcinogenic effects of electromagnetic fields arising from electric power transmission and use. There is no evidence of raised risk of childhood leukaemia with exposure to power frequency fields at the levels experienced by more than 95 per cent of children in western countries. A doubling of risk has been consistently found at the very highest exposure levels but the explanation is unknown, and only a tiny fraction of childhood leukaemia cases could be attributable to electromagnetic fields. There is no apparent association of childhood leukaemia with radio frequency fields.

Infections

Worldwide, the most frequent virus-associated cancers among children and adolescents are Burkitt lymphoma, Hodgkin lymphoma and nasopharyngeal carcinoma (Epstein–Barr virus), liver carcinoma (hepatitis B), Kaposi sarcoma (HHV8 and human immunodeficiency virus, HIV) and cervical carcinoma (human papilloma virus, HPV). For Hodgkin lymphoma, 60% of cases in children of 0–14 years in developed countries and 80% of cases in children aged 0–14 in developing countries can be attributed to Epstein–Barr virus, but only 30% of cases in people aged 15–44.

It is likely that infection is sometimes involved in the aetiology of childhood leukaemia, especially ALL. Two main hypotheses are supported by substantial epidemiological evidence. About 1% of children are born with a pre-malignant clone with the potential to develop into precursor B-cell ALL. Under the 'delayed infection' hypothesis, if they are protected from exposure to infection in infancy then heightened immune response to infection later in childhood acts as a promoter of leukaemia. Evidence supporting this hypothesis includes consistent associations of breastfeeding and attendance at day-care in early childhood with a reduced risk of leukaemia, particularly common ALL.

Under the 'population mixing' hypothesis, childhood leukaemia is an unusual response to one or more specific but as yet unidentified infectious agents, with higher risk occurring when susceptible and infected people are brought together. This is supported by numerous studies in which childhood leukaemia rates have increased when people from different areas come together.

Chemical exposures

In 1998, a review of 48 published studies found some biologically plausible associations of parental occupation with childhood cancer but insufficient evidence that any were causal.

Other factors associated with pregnancy and birth

There is considerable evidence that high birth weight is associated with a raised risk of leukaemia and several other cancers in childhood, possibly as a result of increased antenatal growth rate. The largest study of parental age confirmed previous findings of slightly increased risk of leukaemia with older maternal age, and indicated a similar effect for most other common types of childhood cancer. Children who are twins have a risk of cancer that is about 80 per cent that in singletons.

A meta-analysis of studies published to 2005 found no evidence of increased risk of cancer amongst children born following assisted reproductive technology. The largest study to date found a statistically significant excess of cancer in children born after *in vitro* fertilization, but the numbers of cases of specific types of cancer were low and the association could well have been due to confounding with other factors.

Genetic epidemiology

The most obvious example of a genetically determined cancer is retinoblastoma. About 40 per cent of cases have the heritable form of this disease. The pattern of inheritance is autosomal dominant, but in fact the gene *RB1* is the first example of a tumour suppressor gene; about 90 per cent of individuals who inherit the mutated form of this gene from a parent subsequently suffer a mutation of the wild-type (normal) allele, leading to loss of heterozygosity and the development of retinoblastoma. These individuals are also at increased risk of a variety of other cancers.

Wilms tumour is associated with an especially wide range of syndromes and congenital anomalies, but the pattern of inheritance in Wilms tumour is a great deal more complicated and the proportion of clearly hereditary cases is much smaller.

A variety of childhood cancers and some adult cancers, notably premenopausal breast cancer, are observed in Li-Fraumeni syndrome. The risk of childhood cancer is roughly 20 times that in the general population. Germ-line mutations of the *TP53* tumour suppressor gene are responsible for the high risk and distinctive pattern of cancer in many Li-Fraumeni families, but other genes have been implicated in some families apparently without *TP53* mutations.

Some familial aggregations arise through the association of childhood and adult tumours with known genetic disease such as neurofibromatosis, tuberous sclerosis, Fanconi anaemia, ataxia telangiectasia, xeroderma pigmentosum, and Bloom syndrome, although the actual number of cases of childhood cancer in which these conditions occur is rather small. There are also well-documented associations with chromosomal abnormalities; the strongest association is with Down syndrome, which occurs in a small percentage of cases of childhood leukaemia.

Relatives of affected children

If one child in a family has malignant disease, then, in the absence of any further information about the existence of genetic disease in that family, and excluding twins and retinoblastoma, that child's siblings have approximately double the risk of the general population for developing childhood cancer, i.e. a risk of approximately 1 in 250 compared with the average risk of about 1 in 500. As more has become known about the genetic element in childhood cancer, the risk estimates have increased for families where familial syndromes have been identified, while those for the remaining families have decreased. Indeed, the excess of cancer among siblings of children and adolescents with cancer could well be entirely accounted for by familial syndromes. It should be emphasized that the risk is less than 1 in 250 for siblings who are a few years old when the affected child is diagnosed. The estimated risk is also lower if there are other children in the family who are not affected.

The risk that the co-twin of a twin with cancer will also be affected is of particular concern, especially if the twins are monozygous. In general, both twins and childhood cancer are too rare for risk estimates to be made. Nearly all published cases of childhood cancer in twins are like-sexed pairs and are known or assumed to be monozygous. The fact that the co-twins of the great majority of cases do not develop cancer implies that the risk to co-twins is, in general, not very high. The exception is childhood leukaemia, where up to 25 per cent of co-twins of monozygotic cases also develop the disease. However, these cases are usually due to *in utero* transfer of leukaemic or pre-leukaemic cells rather than being genetically determined.

There is no evidence of a raised risk of cancer or genetic disease among the offspring of survivors who do not themselves have a hereditary cancer syndrome. There is no evidence that the parents of children with cancer have an increased risk of cancer in the absence of known hereditary syndromes.

Genetic susceptibility

A rapidly growing body of research has investigated the possibility that polymorphic variants of certain genes affect the risk of various cancers, including some affecting children. A recent meta-analysis of gene association studies found significantly raised or reduced risk of childhood ALL with specific variants in eight different genes, but these results should be interpreted cautiously since the false-positive report probabilities were all quite high. Several studies have been reported on other childhood cancers but they have often involved small numbers of cases and as yet few have been replicated.

Further reading

Barr RD, Holowaty EJ, Birch JM (2006) Classification schemes for tumours diagnosed in adolescents and young adults. *Cancer* **106**, 1425–30.

Caughey RW, Michels KB (2009) Birth weight and childhood leukemia: a meta-analysis and review of the current evidence. *Int J Cancer* **124**, 2658–70.

Colt JS, Blair A (1998) Parental occupational exposures and risk of childhood cancer. *Environ Health Perspect* **106**, 909–25.

de Klerk N, Milne E (2008) Overview of recent studies on childhood leukaemia, intra-uterine growth and diet. *Radiat Prot Dosimetry* **132**, 255–58.

Desandes E (2007) Survival from adolescent cancer. *Cancer Treat Rev* **33**, 609–15.

Draper GJ, Sanders BM, Brownbill PA, Hawkins MM (1992) Patterns of risk of hereditary retinoblastoma and applications to genetic counselling. *Br J Cancer* **66**, 211–9.

Gatta G, Zigon G, Capocaccia R, Coebergh JW, Desandes E, Kaatsch P, Pastore G, Peris-Bonet R, Stiller CA, the Eurocare Working Group (2009) Survival of European children and young adults with cancer diagnosed 1995–2002. *Eur J Cancer* **45**, 992–1005.

Infante-Rivard C (2008) Chemical risk factors and childhood leukaemia: a review of recent studies. *Radiat Prot Dosimetry* **132**, 220–7.

Jenkinson HC, Hawkins MM, Stiller CA, Winter DL, Marsden HB, Stevens MCG (2004) Long-term population-based risks of second malignant neoplasms after childhood cancer in Britain. *Br J Cancer* **91**, 1905–10.

Kaatsch P, Steliarova-Foucher E, Crocetti E, Magnani C, Spix C, Zambon P (2006) Time trends of cancer incidence in European children (1978–1997): Report from the Automated Childhood Cancer Information System project. *Eur J Cancer* **42**, 1961–71.

Linabery AM, Ross JA (2008a) Childhood and adolescent cancer survival in the US by race and ethnicity for the diagnostic period 1975–1999. *Cancer* **113**, 2575–96.

Linabery AM, Ross JA (2008b) Trends in childhood cancer incidence in the US (1992–2004). *Cancer* **112**, 416–32.

Lindor NM, McMaster ML, Lindor CJ, Greene MH (2008) Concise handbook of familial cancer susceptibility syndromes. Second edition. *J Natl Cancer Inst Monogr* **38**, 1–93.

Little J (1999) *Epidemiology of Childhood Cancer*. Lyon: IARC.

Magnani C, Pastore G, Coebergh JWW, Viscomi S, Spix C, Steliarova-Foucher E (2006) Trends in survival after childhood cancer in Europe, 1978–1997: Report from the Automated Childhood Cancer Information System project (ACCIS). *Eur J Cancer* **42**, 1981–2005.

McNally RJQ, Eden TOB (2004) An infectious aetiology for childhood acute leukaemia: a review of the evidence. *Br J Haematol* **127**, 243–63.

Olsen JH, Boice JD, Seersholm N, Bautz A, Fraumeni JF (1995) Cancer in the parents of children with cancer. *N Engl J Med* **333**, 1594–9.

Parkin DM, Kramárová E, Draper GJ, Masuyer E, Michaelis J, Neglia J, Qureshi S, Stiller CA, Kramárová E, Draper GJ (1998) *International Incidence of Childhood Cancer, Volume 2*. IARC Scientific Publications, No 144. Lyon: IARC.

Reulen RC, Winter DL, Frobisher C, Lancashire ER, Stiller CA, Jenney ME, Skinner R, Stevens MC, Hawkins MM, for the British Childhood Cancer Survivor Study Steering Group (2010) Long-term cause-specific mortality among survivors of childhood cancer. *JAMA* **304**, 172–9.

Sankila R, Olsen JH, Anderson H, Garwicz S, Glattre E, Hertz H, Langmark F, Lanning M, Moller T, Tulinius H, for the Association of the Nordic Cancer Registries and the Nordic Society of Paediatric Haematology and Oncology (1998) Risk of cancer among offspring of childhood-cancer survivors. *N Engl J Med* **338**, 1339–44.

Shah A, Stiller CA, Kenward MG, Vincent T, Eden TOB, Coleman MP (2008) Childhood leukaemia: long-term excess mortality and the proportion 'cured'. *Br J Cancer* **99**, 219–23.

Steliarova-Foucher E, Stiller C, Lacour B, Kaatsch P (2005) International Classification of Childhood Cancer, third edition. *Cancer* **103**, 1457–67.

Stiller CA (2005) Constitutional chromosomal abnormalities and childhood cancer. *Ital J Pediatr* **31**, 347–53.

Stiller CA (2007) International patterns of cancer incidence in adolescents. *Cancer Treat Rev* **33**, 631–45.

Vijayakrishnan J, Houlston RS (2010) Candidate gene association studies and risk of childhood acute lymphoblastic leukemia: a systematic review and meta-analysis. *Haematologica* **95**, 1405–14.

Winther JF, Sankila R, Boice JD, Tulinius H, Bautz A, Barlow L, Glattre E, Langmark F, Møller TR, Mulvihill JJ, Olafsdottir GH, Ritvanen A, Olsen JH (2001) Cancer in siblings of children with cancer in the Nordic countries: a population-based cohort study. *Lancet* **358**, 711–7.

Chapter 2

The biology of cancer in children

Heinrich Kovar and Shai Izraeli

General mechanisms and theories of cancer evolution

The disruption of tissue homeostasis

Starting from a single fertilized egg, the human body ends up comprised of an estimated 10^{14} cells and distinguishable cell types as a result of a complex and marvellous development. This process is subject to a genetically predefined, continuous remodelling program, in which increases in cell number are balanced by the elimination of cells through programmed cell death. Even in an adult, 10^8 cells are lost and renewed per minute. Consequently, a total of about 10^{17} cells are produced during a typical human lifetime.

This astronomic number may imply an infinite ability of somatic cells to divide. However, the ability of a cell to replicate is limited by an inner clock; telomeres at the end of each chromosome shorten with every cell division until a critical minimum length is achieved. For fibroblasts in culture, replicative senescence, a state of permanent growth arrest in which cells can remain metabolically active almost indefinitely, occurs after about 50 to 100 population doublings. Moreover, cells adopt special functions characteristic of their host tissue, and this differentiation also limits their capacity to divide. Thus, the potential to produce progeny cells that retain the capability of differentiation and self perpetuation is restricted to a relatively small number of cells, called tissue stem cells. These cells, although aging with the body, maintain their replicative potential by halting the inner clock at a critical minimum telomere length that is maintained by the activity of the enzyme telomerase, a specialized reverse transcriptase that adds nucleotide repeats to telomeres.

Importantly, the decision to divide or not depends on information exchanged between various cells in a tissue via signalling networks, orchestrating tissue development and remodelling. It is a subtle equilibrium between mechanisms that increase cell numbers such as the limited proliferation of differentiated cells and the activity of stem cells, and of mechanisms restricting cell numbers, such as differentiation, replicative senescence, and apoptosis that guarantee tissue homeostasis. Cancer happens if this equilibrium is permanently disrupted.

Erroneous repair and replication as the source of cancer-causing mutations

Every cell division requires the faithful replication of all of the DNA in the genome which, in humans, is comprised of ~3×10^9 nucleotide base pairs. During this process, the replication apparatus is confronted with a large amount of spontaneously occurring and environmentally induced DNA damage, the majority of which is repaired by built-in correction mechanisms. The fidelity of DNA repair is not absolute and may result in erroneous corrections, which are perpetuated upon cell division. In addition, the replication process in itself is prone to error due to the presence of unrepaired DNA damage. Such DNA damage occurs in every cell stochastically, and results in an estimated 2.4×10^{10} mutations occurring in a human body per day. Environmental and lifestyle factors increase this number and lead to a gradual accumulation of mutations with aging. This results in an increasing chance that some mutations affect genes involved in the maintenance of tissue homeostasis and cause hyperplasia.

Fortunately this terrifying number of potentially harmful genetic aberrations is counteracted by a complex system of intracellular and immune surveillance mechanisms which maintain genetic integrity, the correct protein make-up of the cell, and the function of a cell. The problem is that these safeguard mechanisms are themselves encoded by the genome and are thus at risk of being affected by mutations. In the worst case scenario, an aberration affects a gene involved in DNA repair thus dramatically increasing the number of mutations. This is not only the case in inheritable, cancer-predisposing, repair deficiency syndromes including xeroderma pigmentosa, ataxia teleangiectasia, Bloom syndrome, and Fanconi anaemia, it also occurs spontaneously at different stages of tumour development. It increases the likelihood of mutations striking genes involved in the subtle balance between proliferation and cell death. If such a cell stops responding to external growth inhibitory signals and manages to escape detection and/or elimination by the immune system, it will ultimately result in an unscheduled net increase in cell mass and thus tumour formation.

Escape from microenvironmental surveillance

Still, this is not yet cancer. Even if cells escaped growth control, they may still be responsive to differentiation-inducing signals that will ultimately result in a block to further tumour growth and tumour regression.

The best example for this is neuroblastoma, a remarkably heterogenous paediatric cancer. Neuroblastomas expressing the neutrophin receptor TrkA are prone to spontaneous regression or neuronal differentiation, depending on the absence or presence of its ligand, nerve growth factor (NGF), in the microenvironment. In contrast, the closely related TrkB receptor signals cell survival when interacting with its ligand brain derived neurotrophic factor (BDNF), which is produced by the tumour cells themselves in an autocrine or paracrine loop, resulting in aggressive neuroblastoma. This example demonstrates that malignant tumour cells are not just innocent victims of stochastic mutations, but actively engage into mechanisms promoting cellular autonomy and survival.

Metabolic switch

Normal differentiated cells use most of their oxygen supply for energy production by mitochondrial oxidative phosphorylation to generate ATP and do not take up nutrients from their environment unless stimulated to do so by growth factors. However, massively proliferating cells require an adaptation of their metabolic pathways to fuel the rapid increase in biomass. The biosynthesis of amino acids, long fatty acid chains and other macromolecules requires rich carbon sources. A proliferating cell uses glucose (and glutamine) mostly for the biosynthesis of acetyl-coenzyme A as the building block of carbon chains. This is achieved by glycolysis, independent of the availability of oxygen (the 'Warburg effect'), which occurs not only in cancer, but also in embryonic development and the immune response. This metabolic switch from oxidative phosphorylation to anerobic glycolysis, is triggered by many growth factor signalling pathways including the phosphoinositide 3-kinase (PI3K) and several receptor tyrosine kinase (RTK) pathways. In cancer, many oncogenic mutations result in the cell-autonomous activation of these pathways. rendering them non-responsive to microenvironmental growth control but making them dependent on high glucose flux, a therapeutically exploitable Achilles´ heel.

Angiogenic switch

Initially, the growth of a tumour is fueled by nearby blood vessels. When the cell mass of a tumour increases, these are no longer sufficient and the inner areas suffer from malnutrition and hypoxia. Such metabolic stress will result in the production of potentially mutagenic reactive oxygen species (ROS), and in consequence to cell death and tumour shrinkage, unless tumour cells switch to anaerobic glycolysis and take action to secure fueling of tumour growth.

In 1971, Dr Judah Folkman published a landmark article in the *New England Journal of Medicine*, with the hypothesis that solid tumours cause new blood vessel growth (angiogenesis) in the tumour microenvironment. This ability of a tumour to induce the formation of vasculature, termed the 'angiogenic switch', is stimulated by proangiogenic factors secreted from the tumour cells. Tumour cells can mimic microvascular endothelial cells and form vessel-like structures. Sustained angiogenesis is among the six essential 'hallmarks' or processes that are required for the transformation of a normal cell to a cancer cell (see below).

Because angiogenesis is a key process in tumour growth, and a limited process in healthy adults, a number of angiogenesis inhibitors have entered clinical trials as anticancer agents, although sustained responses remain scarce. This may be due in part to the largely irregular microvascular network structure in a tumour that leaves areas of hypoxia with increased selective pressure for autonomy-conferring mutations.

Models of carcinogenesis

Our knowledge about the mechanisms of malignancy is greatly biased by observations from epithelial cancers, the typical cancers in adults that develop through a series of steps from premalignant benign lesions to metastatic cancer. A general model of cancer proposed by Hanahan and Weinberg states that six functional pathways need to be activated during carcinogenesis:

1. Sustaining proliferative signalling
2. Evading growth suppressors
3. Resisting cell death
4. Enabling replicative immortality
5. Inducing angiogenesis
6. Activating invasion and metastasis.

For epithelial cancers, a conceptual model of carcinogenesis is now well documented experimentally and encompasses at least three distinct steps: initiation, promotion, and progression. Initiation is the consequence of a mutation and results in little or no observable changes in the cellular or tissue morphology but does confer a permanent increase in susceptibility to cancer formation. Tumour promotion requires non-mutagenic tissue disruption by wounding or inflammation and results in formation of a non-malignant tumour which may regress without further stimulus. Subsequent tumour progression and malignant transformation requires multiple additional mutations and further interactions with the tumour microenvironment.

Cancer stem cells

There is also increasing evidence that cancer cells in individual patients are phenotypically heterogeneous and only a subset has the competence to propagate the disease through self renewal. This subset is commonly called cancer stem cells (CSC) or tumour initiating cells to account for their unique property of giving rise to tumours when injected at low cell counts into immune-compromised mice. Similar to tissue stem cells, CSC have been defined as asymmetrically dividing cells which give rise to cells with limited life span and proliferation capacity, and to self-propagating CSC with an indefinite life span and the capability to repopulate a tumour. Based on xeno-transplantation assays in mice, their frequency has been estimated to be between 0.0001 and 0.1 per cent. This concept has been recently challenged by the finding that the tumour-initiating ability of melanoma or childhood ALL cells is dependent on the choice of the mouse strain and its residual immune system, and may be as high as 25 per cent.

Cancer stem cells share many properties with tissue stem cells. Since the tumour stem cell concept has pronounced consequences for cancer therapy, large efforts have been undertaken recently to isolate and characterize CSC from many tumours. The problem with many childhood cancers is that, in contrast to carcinomas, they are intrinsically undifferentiated and even the bulky tumour mass retains stem-cell properties. Thus, to which childhood tumours the cancer stem cell concept may apply remains an unanswered question. However, phenotypic and genotypic tumour hetero-geneity remains an important issue in paediatric oncology.

Modelling cancer for research

Research on primary cancer cells has been limited by the scarcity of these cells and by the inability to propagate most of primary cancers *in vitro*. Cancer cell lines are immortalized cells derived from primary cancers. Although relatively few cell lines exist from each type of cancer and although they have been propagated for years *in vitro*, they have been instrumental in deciphering cancer biology and development of new therapeutics. A program for the most abundant paediatric cancers, supported by the US National Cancer Institute (NCI), has been installed at St Jude Children´s Research Hospital. The Preclinical Pediatric Testing Program (PPTP; *http://pptp. nchresearch.org/index.html/*) systematically tests 10–12 agents or combinations of agents annually in *in vitro* and *in vivo* preclinical models of common childhood cancers. The cell line panel has been characterized extensively on the genomic level and the data is publically available (http://pptp. nchresearch.org/data.html).

Cell lines are also easily amenable to genetic manipulations and high-throughput screens. Thus genes blocking differentiation or enhancing survival and growth can be identified by a screen of cancer cell lines with a library of small interference RNAs (siRNAs).

Mouse models of cancer are divided into two general groups: mouse cancers and growth of human cancers in mice. Powerful genetic tools developed during the last two decades have enabled the generation of sophisticated transgenic mouse models of cancer. Conditional induci-ble expression of an oncogene within a mouse tissue allows, for example, testing its importance during different stages of tissue development. Using this approach, it was demonstrated that fusion oncogenes generated by specific chromosomal translocations in childhood leukae-mias (i.e *MLL–ENL, ERG*) act in a tissue-specific way by transforming only permissive cells. Importantly, it was learned from these studies that leukaemia-initiating cells can be generated from lineage-committed cells, and that the oncogene can cause lineage reassignment if the chromosome translocation occurred in a lineage-noncommitted progenitor cell.

Primary human cancers can now be explanted in immunodeficient mice in the proper micro-environment (orthotopically), for example human breast cancer cells are transplanted into the mouse breast buds, or childhood bone sarcoma cells are transplanted into the mouse tibia. New molecular tools allow manipulation of gene expression in primary human cells before or after their transplantation into mice.

Another approach is transformation of primary human cells by forced expression of oncogenes or silencing of tumour suppressor genes and orthotopically transplanting these cells into immu-nodeficient mice.

Cancer as a genetic disease of the somatic cell

Gatekeepers, driver and passenger mutations

The process of tumorigenesis is initiated when a replication-competent cell (stem cell or partially differentiated descendent of a stem cell) acquires a mutation in a 'gatekeeping' pathway that endows it with a selective growth advantage. Many of the known gatekeepers were identified through the study of unusual families with predispositions to specific types of cancers. The uncertainty about the true number and type of mutations in a cancer genome is the consequence of the low resolution of methods for genome-wide mutation detection available at the time. The recent rapid developments in high throughput DNA sequence determination technology— known as next-generation (NextGen, NGS) or massive parallel sequencing—has already resulted in the description of what is called the 'genomic landscape' of several tumours, including breast, colon, brain, lung, and liver cancer. The genomic landscape of a typical cancer genome comprises 'hills' and 'mountains', representing low and high frequency mutations, respectively: A typical adult cancer harbours about 80 non-silent mutations. Although almost 10 per cent of all genes may be affected, there are only a handful of commonly mutated genes represented by the mountains. These are considered 'driver' mutations involved in initiation and progression of the disease. The large majority of mutations, however, is found in 'hills' and most likely has nothing to do with the pathogenesis of the disease. These are therefore called 'passenger' mutations and increase with age. The only paediatric tumour sequenced so far is medulloblastoma. Consistent with the early onset of disease, the number of mutations was found to be five to ten times less than in an adult cancer (B. Vogelstein, personal communication).

Types of genetic and molecular abnormalities identified in cancer

Most driver genes in cancerogenesis can be classified as either oncogenes, tumour-suppressor genes or genomic stability genes.

Oncogene activations by mutations can result from chromosomal translocations, from gene amplifications or from subtle intragenic mutations affecting crucial residues that regulate the activity of the gene product.

In contrast, tumour-suppressor genes are inactivated by mutations. Such alterations arise from missense mutations at residues that are essential for its activity, from mutations that result in a truncated protein, from deletions or insertions of various sizes, or from epigenetic silencing.

Genomic stability genes include the mismatch, nucleotide-excision and base-excision repair genes responsible for correcting subtle mistakes made during normal DNA replication or induced by exposure to mutagens, genes responsible for recombination repair, mitotic recombination and chromosomal segregation, and genes responsible for recognition of DNA damage. Genomic stability genes keep genetic alterations to a minimum, and thus when they are inactivated, mutations in other genes occur at a higher rate. Therefore, they are also termed 'caretakers'.

These three categories apply not only to protein coding genes but also to non-coding RNA genes, in particular genes for microRNAs (miRNAs) which serve as negative post-transcriptional regulators of gene expression. About 50 per cent of miRNAs are aligned to genomic fragile sites or regions associated with cancers, and there is evidence that DNA copy number abnormalities are involved in miRNA deregulation.

This division to categories is a bit artificial and a certain gene may be classified to more than one category. A good example is the famous *TP53*, also named 'guardian of the genome' to account for its 'caretaker' function on metabolic and genotoxic stress. The wild-type gene behaves as a typical tumour suppressor. When activated during stress response or senescence, it triggers growth arrest and/or apoptosis. Heterozygous point mutations in *TP53* predispose to a wide spectrum of early onset cancer in patients with Li-Fraumeni syndrome, and complete loss of TP53 wild-type function allows for unrestricted proliferation. TP53 is activated by protein modification and stabilization in response to DNA double strand breaks and, as a 'caretaker', prohibits replication of severely damaged DNA. If TP53 is inactivated, this important checkpoint function is lost, resulting in genomic instability and consequently the rapid acquisition of additional mutations. However, not all *TP53* mutations result in loss of protein function. Many frequent *TP53* mutants show an oncogenic gain of function by activating some of its target genes more efficiently than the wild-type protein and conferring further aggressive oncogenic properties such as exacerbated malignant transformation and metastatic phenotype. *TP53* is the most frequently mutated gene in adult cancers (>50 per cent). However, in childhood cancer, *TP53* mutations are generally rare, with only few exceptions.

Cytogenetically, cancer genomes of adult cancers are usually very complex with a plethora of both numerical and structural chromosome aberrations. This may at least in part be explained by the high rate of *TP53* inactivation. Yet, the majority (~90 per cent) of mutations identified by NGS of adult cancer genomes are single-base pair substitutions. In contrast, most childhood cancer genomes are comparably simple and karyotype studies are characterized by few recurrent and tumour-specific chromosome aberrations, in line with the rarity of *TP53* alterations. Exceptions to this are osteosarcoma and glioblastoma multiforme which are characterized by a general genetic instability that is otherwise typical of carcinomas with disruption of stability genes. It is therefore not surprising, that in these diseases *TP53* alterations are a lot more frequent than in other childhood cancers.

Chromosomal translocations

Distinct recurrent reciprocal chromosome translocations typically characterize leukaemia, lymphoma and childhood sarcoma types, but also occur in solid tumours of the adult. Illegitimate V(D)J recombination, class switch recombination, homologous recombination, non-homologous end-joining (NHEJ) and genome fragile sites (explained below) all have potential roles in the production of non-random chromosomal translocations. In addition, mutations in DNA repair pathways have been implicated in the production of chromosomal translocations in humans, mice, and yeast. The detection of DNA sequence patterns that are typical for NHEJ repair at the respective gene fusion sites render it likely that this is the predominant route for the generation of the majority of leukaemia- and sarcoma-associated chimeric fusion genes. This is supported by the observation of increased risk for secondary leukaemias with an *MLL* gene rearrangement in cancer patients who had previously been treated with topoisomerase II inhibitors. Such treatment results in the persistence of non-random DNA double strand breaks that will be repaired by NHEJ.

Chromosome translocations result in either abnormal expression of a structurally normal gene from the cis-regulatory transcriptional elements of the translocation partner, or in the fusion of the coding regions of two unrelated genes to produce a chimeric protein with novel properties (Table 2.1). The first molecularly characterized example of the former is the t(8;14) chromosomal translocation in Burkitt lymphoma, in which the *c-MYC* oncogene is inserted into the immunoglobulin heavy chain (IgH) enhancer region on the long arm of chromosome 14. These types of translocations are especially common in lymphomas and in lymphoid leukaemia (in particular T-cell leukaemias) and result from DNA breakage and joining at the immunoglobulin and T-cell receptor genes in developing lymphocytes necessary to generate the immunological diversity. There are additional examples for this type of translocations that do not involve immune gene receptors. In up to 25 per cent of T-cell acute lymphoblastic leukaemia (T-ALL), a microdeletion on the short arm of chromosome 1 juxtoposes the *TAL1* gene (also known as *SCL*) to the promoter of the *STIL* gene (also known as *SIL*) leading to the aberrant leukemogenic expression of *SCL*. More recently, a similar microdeletion was described on chromosome X which places the cytokine receptor gene *CRLF2* under the regulation of an upstream promoter of *P2RY8*.

Usually, the involved genes and the structure of chromosomal translocations associated with specific cancer types display a high degree of specificity. For instance, Ewing sarcoma is tightly characterized by gene fusion of the *EWSR1* gene with an ETS transcription factor gene, while *EWSR1* fusions to other types of transcription factors tightly associate with other sarcoma or leukaemia entities. On the other hand, there are highly promiscuous genes that are found fused to a multitude of different genes encoding proteins of different function and structure. Among them, the *MLL* gene is the most promiscuous and is found with more than 100 different fusion partners in childhood acute leukaemias. Although about 10 per cent of acute leukaemias as a whole, *MLL* gene rearrangements are particularly prevalent in infant leukaemia (80 per cent of cases) and are associated with dismal outcome.

The DNA binding protein MLL (with DNA methyl transferase activity, see below) binds to non-methylated CpG motifs in gene promoter regions. Despite this high diversity in fusion partners, there appears to be a common theme in *MLL* gene fusions: the amino-terminal portion of MLL serves as a targeting unit to direct MLL oncoprotein complexes to their target loci through DNA binding whereas the fusion partner portion serves as an effector unit that causes aberrant regulation of the target gene. This chimeric structure of a transcription factor is shared by the gene products of most chromosomal translocations that lead to the fusion of coding gene regions.

Among the best investigated examples in this respect are the *EWS–FLI1* gene fusion resulting from the t(11;22)(q24;q12) translocation in Ewing sarcoma, *PAX3/7–FOXO1*, the molecular equivalents of the alternative t(2;13)(q35;q14) and t(1;13)(p36;q14) translocations in alveolar rhabdomyosarcoma, and *ETV6–RUNX1* corresponding to the t(12;21)(p13;q22) translocation in B-cell precursor ALL. In all these instances, the DNA binding portion of a DNA-binding protein (most frequently a transcription factor) is unhinged from its normal effector context and fused to an unrelated functional domain which, in the new context of the chimeric protein, engages in unscheduled aberrant regulation of a large number of genes.

Another type of chromosomal translocation leads to the constitutive activation of a kinase. Kinases are the receptors and effectors of signal integration. Upon ligand binding (or phosphorylation by another kinase), a conformational switch in protein structure enables the hydrolysis of ATP bound in a pocket domain of the kinase resulting in transfer of a phosphate group to a variety of downstream molecules. Depending on the amino acid specificity of the enzyme, there are kinases targeting either serine and threonine, or tyrosine residues.

Several chromosome translocations activate the kinase domain of receptor tyrosine kinases (RTK). RTKs multimerize in response to ligand binding, leading to kinase activation by auto-phosphorylation. Chromosomal translocations commonly generate chimeric proteins consisting of the cytoplasmic domain of RTKs and the dimerization or multimerization motif of the fusion partner, resulting in the constitutive dimerization of RTKs. The most prominent and historic example is the Philadelphia chromosome, t(9;22)(q34;q11), in chronic myelogenous leukaemia (CML) and in about 5 per cent of childhood ALL, which leads to the activation of the Abelson protein (ABL1) by fusion to the 'breakpoint cluster region 1' (BCR1). See Table 2.1 for additional examples. Constitutively activated RTKs are very attractive targets for therapeutic small molecule inhibitors that compete with ATP for binding to the ATP-binding pocket. Several such broad-spectrum RTK inhibitors have already been successfully introduced into clinical trials. The prototype example is Imatinib mesylate (Gleevec) which has been developed to treat CML patients with rearrangements with great success.

Table 2.1 Examples for chromosomal translocations in childhood cancers

Chromosomal translocation	Gene product	Disease
Translocation into a regulatory element		
	Increased expression of MYC	Burkitt lymphoma
		T-ALL
Chr 1p32 microdeletion	STIL–SCL rearrangment	T-ALL
Chimeric DNA binding proteins		
t(11;22)(q24;q12)	*EWSR1–FLI1*	Ewing sarcoma
t(2;13)(q35;q14)	*PAX3–FOXO1*	Alveolar rhabdomyosarcoma
t(12;21)(p13;q22)	*ETV6–RUNX1*	B cell precursor (B) ALL
Chimeric activated kinases		
t(9;22)(q34;q11)	*BCR1ABL1*	Chronic myeloid leukaemia and B-ALL
t(2;5)(p23;q35)	*NPM–ALK*	Non Hodgkin lymphoma
t(9;12)(p24;p13)	*ETV6–JAK2*	Leukaemias

Gene rearrangements not only provide insight into the etiology of the disease, but also act as ideal diagnostic markers. Due to the *de novo* combination of otherwise unrelated DNA that is restricted to the tumour cells, and the high specificity of individual chromosome translocations for certain cancer types, subtypes, or even prognostic groups, they can be easily exploited for highly specific and sensitive monitoring of tumour cells in tissue sections, blood, bone marrow, and even patient serum using molecular techniques (polymerase chain reaction and fluorescence *in situ* hybridization). Most recently, NGS technology has been adapted to the detection of gene rearrangements, leading to the identification of a plethora of novel chromosome translocations even in adult solid tumours.

Chromosomal aneuploidy

The genome of a somatic human cell comprises two copies of each parentally inherited chromosome. A diploid human karyotype therefore contains 46 chromosomes. Deviations from this number, which are termed aneuploidy, are frequently found in cancer. It has been debated if chromosomal aneuploidy is the cause of cancer or simply reflects one of the consequences of inherent genomic instability of the tumour cell. A repeated theme in this chapter is the importance of rare paediatric syndromes as models to understand cancer biology. Some of such syndromes are described in Table 2.2. Mosaic variegated aneuploidy is a rare inherited syndrome caused by mutations in *BUBR1*, a mitotic checkpoint gene. Defects in regulation of chromosomal segregation in mitosis cause chromosomal aneuploidy in the somatic cells of these patients. Fifty per cent of them develop cancer during childhood. This observation strongly suggests that chromosomal aneuploidy directly contributes to the development of cancer.

The importance of aneuploidy in tumorigenesis is also supported by the specific associations between aneuploidy of certain chromosomes and specific types of cancers. For childhood cancer, three extraordinary types of aneuploidy are of particular interest: constitutional trisomy 21, hyperdiploid ALL, and pseudotriploid neuroblastoma.

Children with constitutional trisomy 21 (Down syndrome) have a markedly increased risk for a self-limiting transient congenital myeloid proliferative disease (TMD) as well as to acute

Table 2.2 Selected examples of rare childhood cancer syndromes

Syndrome	Childhood cancers	Mutated gene(s) and comments
Fanconi anaemia	Myeloid leukaemias	**Several Fanconi genes**. A genomic instability syndrome. Increased risk for head and neck and gynecological cancers in adults
Ataxia telangectasia	Lymphoid malignancies	***ATM***. A genomic instability syndrome. The association with lymphoid malignancies demonstrate the importance of *ATM* in prevention of oncogenic accidents in V(D)J recombination during lymphoid development
Mosaic variegated aneuploidy	Gliomas, sarcomas, leukaemias	***BUBR1***. Defects in regulation of chromosomal segregation in mitosis cause chromosomal aneuploidy. Chromosomal aneuploidy is very common in cancer and this syndrome demonstrates that it can cause cancer
Familial retinoblastoma	Retinoblastoma and osteosarcoma	***Rb***. First tumour suppressor described. Somatic mutations in Rb-related protein observed in most cancers
Li- Fraumeni syndrome	Leukaemias, brain tumours, sarcomas, adrenal carcinoma	***TP53***. Somatic mutations common in adult but rare in childhood cancers
Adenomatous polyposis syndrome	Medulloblastoma, colon polyps and cancer	***APC***. Somatic mutations universal in colon cancer
Neurofibromatosis type I	Optic glioma, juvenile myelomonocytic leukaemia (JMML) and other leukaemias	***NF1***. A negative regulator of the RAS pathway, which is commonly mutated in cancers
Gorlin syndrome	Medulloblastoma, basal cell carcinomas	***PTCH1***. A negative regulator of the Hedgehog pathway which is commonly activated in brain, lung and gastrointestinal cancers
Noonan syndrome	JMML and other leukaemias. neuroblastoma	***PTPN11*, *KRAS***. Somatic mutations activating RAS pathway in multiple cancers
Down syndrome	Leukaemias	**Constitutional trisomy 21**. Decreased risk of epithelial cancers in adults with Down Syndrome. Somatic trisomy 21 is common in leukaemias
Beckwith–Wiedemann syndrome	Wilms tumour, hepatoblastoma, neuroblastoma, adrenocortical carcinoma, Rhabdomyosarcoma	**Loss of imprinting 11p15.5**. An epigenetic syndrome. Cancer may be caused by the overexpression of IGF-2. Somatic loss of imprinting and activation of IGF pathway are commonly observed in sarcomas and other cancers

myeloid and lymphoid leukaemias. The specific leukemogenic role of trisomy 21 is underscored by the decreased risk for adult cancers in Down syndrome. Recent research uncovered several somatic mutations that cooperate with trisomy 21 in the pathogenesis of these leukaemias, but the role of the trisomy is still unclear. Possibly the increased risk of childhood leukaemia may relate to an effect of trisomy 21 on fetal hematopoietic development.

The extraordinary biology and behaviour of neuroblastoma ranges from life-threatening progression to maturation into ganglioneuroblastoma and spontaneous regression.[16] The latter is one of the most unusual aspects of infants with stage IV-S, a disseminated disease form that may involve liver, skin, and/or bone marrow, but not cortical bones or distal lymph nodes. Genetically, these tumours are characterized by a pseudotriploid karyotype that usually consists of pure non-random numerical changes. Specifically, they also lack the typical markers for progressive and late stages, such as MYCN amplification and 1p deletions. Moreover, such favourable neuroblastomas rarely, if ever, evolve into unfavourable ones. When, how, and why pseudotriploidy arises remains as enigmatic as its role in the unusual disease process.

Amplifications

In contrast to whole chromosome gains, amplifications multiply up to several hundred fold small chromosomal regions, resulting in a significant increase in dosage of affected genes. Gene amplifications appear in two cytogenetically identifiable structures: extrachromosomal double minutes (DMs) and the chromosomal homogeneously staining region (HSR). DMs are composed of autonomously replicating circular DNA of genomic origin. They are unequally distributed to the daughter cells of a dividing tumour cell, and may be eliminated from the cell upon entrapment into micronuclei and active expulsion. HSR contain multiple copies of the amplified genomic region in a tandem arrangement integrated into the genome. The mechanism of gene amplification is still incompletely understood but, similar to chromosomal translocations, is initiated by a DNA double-strand break. The prevalent hypothesis for gene amplification is that extrachromosomal elements excised from the chromosome arm might generate DMs, and HSRs are generated from DMs by DNA double-strand breakage–fusion cycles.

The size of the amplified genomic region may vary and can include single or multiple genes. Among the best studied examples for the role of gene amplification in oncogenesis are the *MYC* genes. MYC proteins (MYCC, MYCN, and MYCL) regulate processes involved in many, if not all, aspects of cell fate including cell growth and metabolism, proliferation, senescence, apoptosis, DNA damage response, and stem-cellness. As such, *MYC* genes represent hubs in gene regulatory networks and deregulation of their expression severely impairs tissue homeostasis. Among childhood tumours, *MYCN* amplification at chromosome band 2p24 has been known since the 1980s to occur in about 20 per cent of neuroblastomas and to be associated with a particularly poor outcome, therefore still serving as the only accepted molecular prognostic marker stratifying for high-dose chemotherapy in this disease. Similarly, *MYCN* but also *MYCC* (chromosome 8q24) amplifications are bad prognostic markers in medulloblastoma occurring at frequencies of 8 per cent and 6 per cent, respectively. In this disease, recent observations suggest that also low level *MYC* copy number changes may already be of prognostic impact. Amplifications of *MYCN* have also been reported in retinoblastoma and in both alveolar and embryonal rhabdomyosarcoma.

Epigenetic mechanisms

While genes and their natural polymorphisms and pathologic mutations carry all the information for the normal or aberrant function of a cell, it is the dynamic plasticity of the chromatin organization which exerts a profound control over gene expression. Within the nucleus of a cell, DNA is tightly packed with proteins and wrapped around regularly spaced repeated structures known as nucleosomes. Nucleosome cores are composed of eight histone proteins (octamers). Nucleosomes reduce the binding of a variety of DNA regulatory proteins including transcription, DNA repair, and recombination machinery. Derepression of these processes requires chromatin remodelling by effective shifting of nucleosomes along the length of the DNA molecule to expose segments of DNA that can interact with gene expression or DNA repair machinery. Regulatory mechanisms of gene expression that are independent of DNA sequence are called 'epigenetic' modifications and govern the flexible conversion of the DNA-encoded information into cell- and tissue-specific gene activity patterns. By the cooperation of multiple processes, including noncoding RNAs, covalent modifications of chromatin (acetylation, deacetylation, and/or methylation of histone proteins), physical alterations in nucleosomal positioning, and DNA methylation, they orchestrate key biological processes, including differentiation, imprinting, and silencing of large chromosomal domains.

Epigenetic abnormalities in cancer comprise a multitude of aberrations in virtually every component of chromatin involved in packaging the human genome. Since epigenetic silencing processes are mitotically heritable, they can play the same roles and undergo the same selective processes as genetic alterations in the development of a cancer. Alterations in gene expression induced by epigenetic events, which give rise to a cellular growth advantage, are therefore selected for in the host organ, resulting in the progressive uncontrolled growth of the tumour. DNA methylation is one form of epigenetic gene silencing, occurring at cytosine residues predominantly in CpG islands of gene regulatory regions. Cytosine methylation attracts methylated DNA binding proteins and histone deacetylases to methylated CpG islands during chromatin compaction and gene silencing.

Monoallelic methylation of a gene as an inheritable mark of parental origin is called imprinting. In humans, about 70 genes are known to be imprinted, the chromosomal 11p15 region containing the gene for insulin-like growth factor *IGF2* and *H19* being among the best-studied examples. Normally, *IGF2* is only expressed from the chromosome transmitted by the father, while *H19* is expressed solely from the maternal allele. The uncoordinated expression of these and other genes can cause various developmental disturbances and diseases, including overgrowth and tumour-predisposition syndromes, the prototype of which is the well-known Beckwith–Wiedemann syndrome. In Wilms tumour, a paediatric kidney cancer, the maternal *IGF2* allele becomes activated due to loss of imprinting, thus increasing gene dosage of this proliferation-promoting growth factor.

While cancer genomes appear generally undermethylated compared to their normal counterparts, presumably as a reflection of their metabolic activity and immature phenotype, regional hypermethylation has been considered a mechanism for the inactivation of tumour suppressor and apoptosis pathways in many types of cancer. In aggressive neuroblastoma, DNA methylation was identified responsible for the silencing of caspase 8 involved in the initiation of extrinsic cell death. The cell cycle inhibitor gene *CDKN2A* is a frequent target of aberrant methylation which occurs in many solid tumours and haematologic malignancies including childhood *ALL*.

Epigenetic mechanisms are also affected by mutations of genes involved in chromatin modification. In mixed lineage leukaemia of children, the histone methyltransferase MLL is rearranged by chromosome translocation with a variety of different fusion partners that destroy normal histone methyltransferase function of MLL and replace it by heterologous functions contributed by the fusion partner. The resulting chimeras are transcriptional regulators that take control of targets normally controlled by MLL.

The mammalian SWI/SNF complex is a chromatin remodelling complex that uses the energy of ATP hydrolysis to facilitate access of transcription factors to regulatory DNA sequences. The gene *INI1* (*hSNF5/SMARCB1*) encodes a subunit of the human chromatin remodelling SWI/SNF complex. Bi-allelic *INI1* mutations are the rate-limiting mutations characterizing rhabdoid tumours, a very aggressive form of paediatric cancer.

Childhood cancer as a developmental disease

Initiation of cancer during fetal development

A simple comparison between the common types of cancers in children and adults is quite revealing. Childhood cancers are closely linked to development of certain tissues while most adult cancers evolve through the interaction of epithelial cells with environmental carcinogens, with the internal endocrine cycles, and with the process of aging.

In children, the primary initiating event resulting in a growth of a precancerous lesion may occur during embryonic development. This is evident for some embryonic tumours such as Wilms tumour, medulloblastoma, and neuroblastoma, but has also been shown for a 'non-embryonic' tumour such as childhood ALL. Prompted by the unusual high concordance of ALL in identical twins, Mel Greaves proposed that a preleukaemic clone is initiated *in utero* in one twin and transferred to the other twin before birth via the common placental vascular connections. He later confirmed this suggestion by demonstrating the same initiating genetic lesion (for example the *ETV6–RUNX1* fusion translocation) in pre-B cells in both twins. This observation was extended to a general model of the development of childhood ALL in which an initiating somatic genetic event occurs during embryonic development and leads to a growth of a preleukaemic clone. Additional somatic genetic progression events occurring after birth in such pre-leukaemic clones are required for the evolution to a full-blown leukaemia. Without such additional events, the pre-leukaemic clone eventually disappears. The model is now generally accepted due to several studies demonstrating the presence of specific clonal somatic abnormalities in blood samples collected at the time of birth for routine neonatal screening ('Guthrie Cards') in the majority of children with ALL.

It is tempting to speculate that most childhood cancers develop in a similar fashion through precancerous fetal tumours. Screening of urine catecholamines in babies tripled the incidence of infant neuroblastomas without changing the incidence of clinically significant neuroblastomas. This observation suggests the relatively common presence of neonatal pre-cancerous lesions similar to the pre-leukaemic clones.

Mechanisms linking childhood development and cancer

What is the mechanism responsible for the unique spectrum of childhood cancers? Does embryonic development of certain tissues increase the mutational risk, or are certain developing tissues more sensitive to neoplastic transformation caused by specific mutations? Both scenarios are probably correct.

The clearest example of mutational pressure caused by a developmental process relates to lymphoid development. For generation of immunological diversity, the genes coding the immune receptors are modified through a process of DNA breakage and gene fusion known as V(D)J recombination. This process involves lymphoid-specific enzymes, RAG1 and RAG2, and the general machinery of error-prone non-homologous end joining (NHEJ) DNA repair. It is thought that many of the genomic aberrations observed in ALL are caused by 'accidents' in this process as we have described above. Inherited abnormalities in the regulation of V(D)J recombination such as ataxia telangiectasia are associated with both immunodeficiency and increased risk of lymphoid malignancies. Indeed, given the extent of lymphoid development during the fetal and early childhood period, it is quite surprising that only one of every 2000 children develops leukaemia.

While the lymphoid system is the only tissue whose development is directly associated with genomic instability, an association between development and sensitivity to specific oncogenic mutations is possibly relevant to most childhood cancers. This is evident from the patterns of cancers in rare inherited or congenital syndromes (Table 2.2).

Somatic mutations in the tumour suppressor gene *TP53* are very common in most adult and relatively rare in childhood tumours. Children with a germline mutation in *TP53* (Li-Fraumeni syndrome) are at increased risk for multiple typical childhood cancers such as rhabdomyosarcoma, gliomas and leukaemias, childhood cancers that are not associated usually with somatic mutations in *TP53*. Those who survive to adulthood are at increased risk for typical adult malignancies such as breast cancers. Thus, this syndrome demonstrates the age-dependent sensitivity of different tissues to an oncogenic mutation.

An example directly linking the role of a gene in embryonic development to cancer is the increased risk of medulloblastomas in children with a germline mutation in the *PTCH1* gene encoding the Patched protein. Patched is a receptor that inhibits the Hedgehog signalling pathway, a critical developmental pathway that also regulates cerebellar development. Loss of one allele of *PTCH1* leads to overgrowth of the precursors of cerebellar neurons. This overgrowth results in medulloblastomas in some of the children. Not unexpectedly, activating somatic mutations in the Hedgehog pathway are also identified in sporadic medulloblastomas which is the most common malignant childhood brain tumour.

Studies of these rare syndromes in humans coupled with biological research in experimental animals demonstrate that the pathogenesis of childhood cancers is influenced by specific interactions between cancer-causing mutations and tissue growth and development.

Convergence of the somatic alterations into functional oncogenic pathways: specific examples

Cancer etiology is currently viewed as the result of successive clonal expansions driven by cells that acquire a selective advantage through mutations, and that a large number of mutations, each associated with a small fitness advantage, drive tumour progression. But while the number of potential driver genes is large (>100 000), changes appear to occur in a much more limited number of 'driver' pathways (<20). The elucidation of cancer-associated pathways is highly relevant for the development of targeted therapy.

Cell cycle checkpoint control

At the heart of these pathways are two intermingled cell-cycle regulatory circuits which are controlled by the retinoblastoma susceptibility protein pRb1 and the TP53 tumour suppressor protein (Fig. 2.1).

The retinoblastoma susceptibility protein pRb1 controls cell cycle progression at the restriction point, the transition from growth factor dependency to autonomous entry into the replication (synthesis, S) phase of mitosis. TP53 controls the DNA damage checkpoint, an emergency break to halt progression through the cell cycle after cells passed through the restriction point in order to inhibit potentially mutagenic replication of damaged DNA and to eliminate genetically aberrant daughter cells. TP53 also provides a safeguard mechanism counteracting proliferative signals from aberrant oncogene activation. Upon such oncogenic stress, TP53 triggers apoptosis to eliminate potentially neoplastic cells. Thus, oncogene-driven carcinogenesis requires mechanisms to eliminate or circumvent the TP53 checkpoint. Human Adenovirus E1A and E1B, E6 and E7 proteins from human papillomavirus, and large and small T antigens from SV40 inactivate pRb1 and TP53, respectively, allowing for self-sufficiency in DNA replication and the rapid accumulation of mutations. Due to their central position in mechanisms regulating tissue homeostasis, pRb1 and TP53 integrate a large number of environmental and cellular signals via protein modifications, mostly phosphorylations, and microRNAs that regulate their expression, activity, and stability. As such, *RB1* and *TP53* represent highly connected network hubs. It is therefore not surprising that a still increasing number of diverse driver gene alterations in sporadic cancers interfere with TP53 and/or pRb1 function.

In addition, they always seem to go together in oncogenesis. Even in retinoblastoma, which is caused by biallelic disruption of *Rb1*, amplification of TP53 regulatory *MDM4* and *MDM2* genes has been described in 65 per cent and 10 per cent of cases, respectively, resulting in destabilization

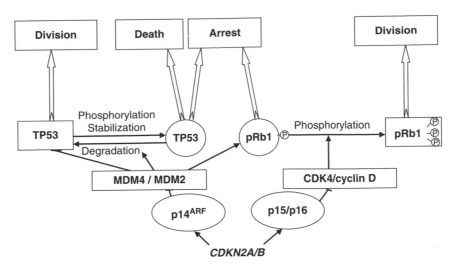

Fig. 2.1 The central players in growth and cell cycle checkpoint control, pRb and TP53, and their regulation by *CDKN2A/B* and *MDM2/4* genes. The tumour suppressive function of TP53 is activated by cellular stress, leading to phosphorylation and stabilization of the protein. Oncogenic regulators of p53, such as MDM2 and MDM4 degrade and/or inhibit TP53, promoting cell growth. The CDKN2A-encoded p14^ARF blocks the MDM2/MDM4 complex, supporting the tumour-suppressive function of TP53. On the other hand, pRb1 in its partially phosphorylated form prevents cell cycle entry. When hyperphosphorylated in response to growth factor signals, pRb1 allows for transition of the cell cycle into S phase. CDKN2A/B gene products p16 and p15 negatively regulate pRb1, phosphorylating kinases, and thus suppress cell growth.

of TP53. In osteosarcoma, in which recurrent genetic aberrations have not been detected so far, the only consistent pattern is that of *TP53* and *Rb1* alterations.

Although direct mutation of the *TP53* gene is the prevalent mechanism of TP53 inactivation in adult cancers, it is comparably rare in childhood cancers with only few exceptions, a phenomenon that is not well understood. However TP53 activity is reduced by alternative mechanisms in childhood cancer. The chromosome translocation products of Ewing sarcoma, EWS-FLI1, and of acute leukaemias, AML-ETO and MLL gene fusion proteins were shown to impact TP53 activity by distinct mechanisms. The resulting decrease in TP53 activity allows survival and proliferation of cells under oncogenic stress.

Mutations in TP53 are associated with resistance to chemotherapy. The sensitivity of many childhood cancers to chemotherapy may be explained by the absence of such mutations. Conversely, mutations in TP53 may explain the resistance of a lethal subset of childhood malignancies.

An alternative mechanism of TP53 disruption which concomitantly jeopardizes cell cycle control by pRb1 is frequently seen in several paediatric malignancies including Ewing sarcoma, childhood ALL, childhood cutaneous melanoma, and rhabdomyosarcoma: homozygous deletion or heterozygous deletion with inactivation of the normal allele by either gene mutation or promoter methylation of the *CDKN2A* gene on chromosome 9p21.

CDKN2A is a unique gene in that it encodes two proteins from two overlapping but distinct reading frames: p16 (INK4A), a cyclin-dependent kinase inhibitor that prevents Rb1 from phosphorylation thus keeping cells in a quiescent state, and p14 (alternative reading frame product ARF), which interacts with MDM2 thus preventing degradation of TP53 and consequently supporting cell cycle arrest. Inactivation of *CDKN2A* therefore unleashes cell proliferation. It is not surprising that heterozygous germline mutations of this gene as seen in hereditary melanoma heavily predispose to cancer development. But also common natural polymorphisms in the *CDKN2A* gene were demonstrated to increase the risk of developing childhood ALL and glioma.

Frequently, 9p21 deletions encompass not only *CDKN2A* but also the neighbouring *CDKN2B* gene encoding a related cyclin-dependent kinase inhibitor p15 (INK4B) that has also been shown to have tumour suppressive activity, acting as a back-up to p16. Thus, 9p21 deletions eradicate three tumour suppressor proteins in one strike.

Differentiation

Most childhood cancers, particularly embryonal tumours and leukaemias, arise from very young and immature progenitor cells. These are frequently still uncommitted and retain the ability to differentiate along several distinct pathways. In embryonal tumours and leukaemias, the immature phenotype is at least partially retained suggesting that the transforming hits block terminal differentiation of the tumour progenitor.

A paradigmatic example for this phenomenon is Ewing sarcoma, which was originally described as endothelioma of bone, based on histology and subsequently for many years on immunohisto-chemistry, Ewing sarcoma was considered of neuroectodermal origin because of the variable expression of neural marker proteins. In fact, Ewing sarcoma-like bone tumours with the highest number of neural markers were for a long time considered a distinct entity named peripheral primitive neuroectodermal tumour (pPNET) or neuroepthelioma. However, genetic studies revealed that Ewing sarcoma and pPNET are actually two extremes of one disease, today known as the Ewing sarcoma family of tumours (ESFT), positioned along a gradient of increasing neural differentiation, but sharing the same molecular cause, an *EWS–ETS* gene rearrangement. Functional genomics studies discovered that ESFT are most highly related to mesenchymal stem cells and that the partial neuronal and endothelial phenotype of Ewing sarcoma and pPNET are the consequence of aberrant neural and endothelial gene expression patterns imposed by the chimeric ETS transcription factor. ESFT remain largely undifferentiated tumours which do not respond to any stimuli that induce differentiation of mesenchymal stem cells. However, when EWS–FLI1 expression is experimentally suppressed, ESFT cells gain adipogenic, neuronal, and osteogenic differentiation potential due to the upregulation of otherwise EWS–FLI1 suppressed developmental genes.

Often differentiation is arrested or diverted in cancer by abnormal expression of transcription factors. For example, the two chromosomal translocations characterizing alveolar rhabdomyosarcoma involve *PAX3* or *PAX7* which encode two transcription factors important in normal muscle differentiation. The same phenomenon is frequently observed in acute leukaemias too. For example, many of childhood B cell precursor leukaemias display deletions or mutations in transcription factor genes such as *PAX5* or *IKZF1* that regulate B cell differentiation. About two thirds of T-ALL harbour somatic activating mutations in NOTCH1, a receptor that upon proteolytic cleavage becomes a transcription factor, enhances proliferation of T-cell precursors and blocks their maturation. A major regulator of hematopoiesis, RUNX1 affects both myeloid and lymphoid development. It is commonly involved in mutations and translocations in leukaemias. Each RUNX1 abnormality is associated with a specific subtype of leukaemia.

Another mechanism that interferes with normal differentiation is misexpression of a transcription factor in the wrong lineage. For example TAL1 (SCL) is important for the erythro-megakaryocytic lineage. Misexpression of TAL1 (for example by the *STIL-TAL1* microdeletion described in this chapter) in early T lymphocytes blocks their maturation leading to T-ALL.

Escape from senescence and cell death

Tumour cells expand their lifespan and reduce their apoptotic rates by various mechanisms to increase in mass. Oncogenic, metabolic, chemo- and radiotherapeutic stress select for tumour cells with acquired mutations in cell death and senescence pathways. This may be true only for the small number of tumour initiating cells, but also for progeny cells.

Mitochondria are the metabolic center of the cell and the warehouse for molecules instrumental in the execution of cell death. They sense metabolic stress and the dangerous production of potentially mutagenic reactive oxygen species (ROS). TP53 as a transcription factor and sensor of DNA damage in the nucleus is involved in the communication between mitochondria and the nucleus and signals to mitochondria by transcription independent interaction with members of the Bcl2 family. This family encodes proteins that insert into the mitochondrial membrane to either form an open (pro-apoptotic) or closed (anti-apoptotic) pore for the breakdown of mitochondrial membrane potential that ceases energy (ATP) production, and the release of pro-apoptotic factors from the intermembrane space of mitochondria to execute apoptosis.

TP53 regulates the expression of several proapoptotic Bcl2 related proteins (e.g. BAX, Puma). It also regulates the expression of tumour necrosis factor receptor (TNFR) related cell death receptors on the cell surface [e.g. CD95 (FAS/APO-1), DR5 (TRAIL receptor)]. These receptors integrate extrinsic death-inducing signals by activating so-called initiator caspases (such as caspase 8) which, by proteolytic cleavage, not only directly activate cell death execution caspases in the cytoplasm but also trigger mitochondrial apoptosis by activating the proapoptotic Bcl2 protein BID.

Thus, there are many entry sites for cancer-associated mutations to affect programmed cell death, and only few examples are listed here. The initiator caspase 8 gene is frequently silenced in neuroblastoma. The antiapoptotic IAP Survivin is overexpressed in many cancers including precursor B-cell ALL and childhood AML as the result of aberrant transcription factor activity or loss of negative regulatory microRNA activity. The expression of the anti-apoptotic protein MCL1 may explain resistance of some ALLs to prednisone. Mutations in CD95 were identified in childhood T-ALL and Hodgkin lymphoma. In general, every aberration that affects the subtle balance between pro- and anti-apoptotic molecules or proteins involved in the sensing of cellular stress will have an effect on a cell´s ability to properly respond to intrinsic and extrinsic cell death signals.

To unbalance tissue homeostasis and surveillance of genomic integrity, a tumour cell not only has to escape cell death but also to bypass replicative senescence triggered by telomere shortening. When telomere length approaches a critical size, activation of telomerase can rescue genomic stability and the self-renewal capacity of a cell. Telomerase is a ribonucleoprotein enzyme with two components: a constitutively expressed small RNA component (TERC) which serves a template for the reverse transcriptase activity that adds *de novo* telomere repeats to the chromosome ends, and the catalytic protein component (TERT) whose expression is tightly regulated in the cell. Unscheduled expression of TERT by mostly unknown mechanisms is a hallmark of many cancers, including childhood leukaemia and embryonal tumours.

Aberrant signalling

According to the Hanahan–Weinberg model, the first two conditions a cancer cell has to fulfill are self-sufficiency in growth signals and insensitivity to antigrowth signals.[2] Growth factors and anti-growth factors signal to the cell via receptors on the cell surface. Many different growth factor pathways converge on few intracellular signalling pathways, among them the phosphatidylinositol-3-kinase (PI3K), the mitogen-activated protein kinase (MAPK), and the JAK/STAT pathways, which play central roles in the regulation of cell growth, proliferation, survival, differentiation, and invasion. Here we describe several examples for deregulation of these pathways in childhood cancer.

In solid tumours, specifically in sarcomas, the IGF signalling pathway upstream of PI3K and MAPK activities has been recognized as a frequent target of oncogenic alterations and therefore as a promising drug target. The IGF system consists of three ligands (IGF-1, IGF2 and insulin), four cell membrane receptors [IGF-1R, insulin receptor isoform A (IR-A), hybrid receptors and IGF receptor type 2 (IGF-2R)] and six modulatory IGF binding proteins (IGFBPs). Upon activation and autophosphorylation of the receptor, adaptor proteins (insulin receptor substrates, IRS1–4) are recruited to the cytoplasmic domain and activate the PI3K pathway. In humans, IGF-2 is the predominant circulating IGF, with plasma levels three to seven-fold higher than IGF-1. Both, IGF-1 and IGF-2 bind to the IGF-1R receptor.

In normal tissues, the *IGF-2* gene on chromosome 11p15.5 is imprinted. In tumours, however, loss of imprinting is frequent, resulting in enhanced IGF-2 levels due to bi-allelic expression. Some sarcoma subtypes (e.g. embryonal rhabdomyosarcoma) show loss of the maternal 11p15.5 locus, causing loss of heterozygosity (LOH). LOH is associated with duplication of the paternal allele of *IGF2* (paternal isodisomy), resulting in the expression of two paternal genes. The IGF receptor, IGF-1R, is overexpressed in cancer due to either amplification or transcriptional deregulation, either loss of repressors such as TP53 (by mutation or *MDM2* amplification) or increased expression of transcriptional activators such as EWS–WT1 fusion protein in desmoplastic small round cell tumour, and PAX3–FOXO1 and PAX7–FOXO1 transcription factors in alveolar rhabdomyosarcoma.

Taken together, the IGF signalling pathway emerges as an attractive therapeutic target in many cancers and several phase 2 clinical trials with IGF-1R targeting antibodies and small molecule inhibitors have been initiated with promising results particularly in Ewing sarcoma.

Receptor tyrosine kinases (RTK) belong to another group of receptors that is frequently targeted by oncogenic activating mutations. Self-sufficiency is achieved when RTKs multimerize in the absence of a growth regulating ligand and consequently initiates sustained downstream signalling. Constitutive activation of RTKs may be achieved by gene rearrangements that result in ligand-independent oligomerization, but more frequently it is the consequence of subtle point mutations of either the activation loop of the kinase domain or in the juxtamembrane or extracellular domains, which normally prevent the activation loop from adopting an active configuration. Constitutive activation of the stem cell factor receptor c-Kit, the platelet derived growth factor receptors PDGFR, and the fms-like receptor FLT3 are very frequently found in hematopoietic malignancies and occasionally in solid tumours such as gastrointestinal stromal tumours (GISTs).

RTK point mutations may also predispose to malignancy. Recently, several groups have reported in parallel the presence of *ALK* kinase domain mutations in cases of familial neuroblastoma. In sporadic cases, *ALK* mutations have been observed in low and high risk neuroblastoma at an overall frequency of ~8 per cent. However, deregulated ALK expression is probably more generally involved in neuroblastoma pathogenesis, since it is also found amplified and/or overexpressed at a much higher rate than its mutation frequency in poor prognosis neuroblastoma. This may in part be related to the close proximity of the *ALK* gene to *MYCN* and its probable co-amplification with this oncogene, which has been known for a long time to be associated with dismal outcome in this disease.

Cytokine receptors that do not have kinase activity often recruit intracellular kinases for intracellular transmission of the signal. While somatic mutations in these receptors are only rarely found in cancers, they are commonly found within the signalling proteins. A recent example is the activating mutations identified in the JAK family of kinases. Upon interaction between various cytokine receptors and their ligands, JAK kinases (JAK1–3 and additional related kinases) bind to the cytoplasmic domain of the receptors and phosphorylate one or more STAT proteins. Phosphorylated STAT proteins translocate to the nucleus where they bind to DNA and regulate specific gene expression. Constitutive phosphorylation of STAT3 and STAT5 is often observed in solid and hematopoietic tumours respectively. Mutations in JAK1, JAK2 or JAK3 causing ligand-independent constitutive activation have been recently described in several hematopoietic malignancies including myeloproliferative neoplasms and acute lymphoid and myeloid leukaemias. Inhibitors of JAK-STAT signalling are already in clinical trials.

Analysis of a rare childhood cancer, juvenile myelomonocytic leukaemia (JMML), provides an extraordinary example of how seemingly unrelated different mutations activate the same cytokine signalling pathway (Fig. 2.2). JMML is a type of leukaemia involving mature malignant monocytes in very young children and is currently curable only by hematopoietic stem cell transplantation. Uniquely, these monocytes proliferate *in vitro* in the presence of extremely small concentrations of the cytokine GM-CSF. Despite extensive research, no mutations have been identified in the receptor to GM-CSF. Over the last few years a series of mutations downstream to this receptor have been identified in genetic syndromes associated with JMML and in sporadic JMML. Three of the genes, *KRAS*, *NF1* and *PTPN11*, encode proteins that regulate the transmission of signals through the RAS pathway. The RAS proteins mediate a critical signalling pathway downstream to many receptors. RAS proteins resonate between an active GTP and an inactive GDP bound state. Activating oncogenic mutations in RAS that keep it in the GTP state are very common in cancer, in particular the typical carcinomas of adults but also in childhood leukaemias. Germline inactivating mutations in NF1, a protein that inactivates RAS, are found in neurofibromatosis. PTPN11 is a phosphatase important in transmitting signals from the GM-CSF receptor to RAS. Germline activating mutations in *PTPN11* or in *KRAS* cause Noonan syndrome. Importantly somatic mutations in JMML in *RAS*, *NF1* or *PTPN11* are mutually exclusive, implying that mutation in one of these genes is enough to constitutively activate signalling and to endow these malignant monocytes with extreme sensitivity to GM-CSF. Recently, germline and somatic mutations were identified in the *CBL* gene, encoding an E3 ubiquitin ligase that normally degrades the GM-CSF (and other) receptor. Loss of function of CBL enhances the level of the receptor, further augmenting the sensitivity to GM-CSF.

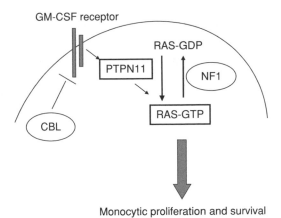

Monocytic proliferation and survival

Fig. 2.2 A highly simplified and schematic demonstration of mutations activating the granulocyte–macrophage colony-stimulating factor (GM-CSF) receptor–RAS pathway in juvenile myelomonocytic leukaemia. Oncogenes are boxed and tumour suppressors are circled.

The convergence of cancer-associated mutations into relatively few pathways is an evolving general paradigm of cancer. The nodes and hubs of these pathways are important targets for future cancer therapeutics.

Translation of biology into the clinic: promises and challenges

We are in the midst of a revolution in cancer medicine. We used to know very little about cancer biology. The enormous progress in curing children with cancer has until recently been the result of carefully conducted, empirically based clinical trials with very little biological information. Nowadays the stream of biological information is increasing exponentially. The challenge for the clinician is how to harness this stream for the benefit of children with cancer, rather than sinking under the overwhelming information.

Impact on diagnosis, risk classification, and personalized therapy

The realization that at least some tumours can be defined by their common genetic abnormality have aided tremendously pathological diagnosis, as described in detail above for the Ewing sarcoma family of tumours. Similarly, the various pathological subtypes of Burkitt lymphoma were unified by the diagnostic requirement for the presence of MYC translocations. Exploiting a tumour-defining molecular abnormality is important in distinguishing between different types of tumours with similar morphological appearance. For example, Ewing sarcoma, Burkitt lymphoma, rhabdomyosarcoma and neuroblastoma are often morphologically very similar and classified as 'small-round-blue-cell-tumours'. The presence of *EWS–ETS* translocations, *IgH–MYC* translocations, *PAX3/7* translocations or *NMYC* amplification, respectively, is an important diagnostic aid.

Another important diagnostic application is the recognition of specific tumour genetic subtypes for risk classification and adjustment of therapy. Among numerous examples we mention the identification of the *BCR1–ABL1* and the *ETV6—RUNX1* rearrangements as poor and good prognostic markers, respectively, in B-ALL, the poor prognostic significance of *MYCN* amplification in neuroblastoma, or the presence of *PAX3* or *PAX7* translocation in alveolar rhabdomyosarcoma. The current challenge, however, is to optimally select the diagnostic molecular markers for prognostic applications. This is essential also because of the limited amount of biological material available from diagnosis and the important issue of costs.

When reviewing suggestions for introduction of new prognostic or risk classification markers it is important to consider several important parameters:

1. **Were the tumour specimens analysed derived from a representative population of patients?** Often analysis has been restricted on tumours arbitrarily kept in the laboratories. This 'available sample bias' is an important factor that is often mistakenly ignored. Usually 'leftovers' from tumours or leukaemias represent cancers with higher cell load, and thus more advanced tumours. Research based on prospectively curated tumour banks has a better chance to be translated into the diagnostic arena.

2. **Treatment is the most important prognostic factor**. The prognostic significance of any clinical or biological tumour marker critically depends on the type of treatment received. An excellent example is the poor prognosis previously associated with the *E2A–PBX1* chromosomal translocation in B-ALL in older, less intensive treatment protocols. Thus the prognostic evaluation of a novel biomarker must be performed prospectively in a clinical trial. The universality of its prognostic significance can be determined by comparison of its impact on patients' outcome to several types of treatments. For example *MYCN* amplification in neuroblastoma retains its prognostic significance regardless of the treatment protocols.

3. **Prognostic significance in a multivariate analysis with other risk classifying factors**. The decision on a clinical application of risk-classifying criteria is a practical one and is also based on the relative predicting power of a novel marker. For such a marker to enter the diagnostic arena, it needs to demonstrate an advantage by a multivariate analysis of its effect (preferably in analysis of data derived from a prospective clinical trial) in comparison with standard criteria.

4. **Direct impact on therapy**. For example, the determination of *BCR1–ABL1* fusion gene in acute lymphoblastic leukaemia is imperative because specific inhibitors are available and need to be combined in therapy. Conversely, with the entrance of many targeted drugs into the clinic, it may become necessary to exclude the presence of an abnormality that might block drug activity. For example, as treatment with novel EGFR inhibitors has been shown to be active only in colon cancers lacking *RAS* mutations, it is now recommended to determine the status of RAS before commencement of such treatment.

5. **Practical issues**. Development of a reliable diagnostic test is usually done by the commercial sector. These issues are important for example in development (or the lack of) diagnostic applications of microarrays for paediatric cancers.

The molecular diagnostic tools are varied and evolve rapidly. Classical cytogenetics have been largely replaced by molecular approaches such as fluorescent *in situ* hybridization (FISH) for diagnosis of specific structural or numerical chromosomal rearrangements. Novel methodologies for extraction of RNA from paraffin-embedded tissues have increased the range of potential applications of the polymerase chain reaction (PCR), especially for microRNA detection. Gene arrays have been widely used for research and have proven their applicability for diagnosing specific tumour subtypes and for prognostication. However their entrance so far to the paediatric oncology diagnostic arena (compared for example with breast and colon cancers) has been delayed also because of commercial considerations.

Impact on novel therapies

The identification of cancer-specific abnormalities has raised hopes for the development of specifically targeted therapies. Such therapies are commonly expected to be highly effective and highly selective against cancer without any side effects, truly a 'magic bullet', while classical cytotoxic chemotherapy is frequently considered just 'non specific poison'.[24] This view has been fueled by the successful development of an inhibitor of the BCR1-ABL1 kinase (Imatinib) and its magical effects on CML. Several such biologically targeted therapies have been already introduced to the clinic and may be relevant for childhood cancer.

'Targeted therapy' is not without side effects. The pathways modulated in cancer are important for growth, development, and differentiation of normal tissues. Thus, like cytotoxic chemotherapy, side effects on normal tissues are expected from novel targeted drugs. For example there are concerns that the BCR1-ABL1 inhibitor Imatinib cannot be administered chronically in children because of its growth inhibitory effects. The clinical trials with inhibitors of the Notch pathway had to be stopped and modified because of intractable diarrhea. This diarrhea was caused by differentiation to Goblet cells induced by inhibition of the Notch pathway in the large intestine. Thus, like any other drug, the success of an anti cancer 'targeted' therapy will depend on its therapeutic ratio.

The tremendous heterogeneity of cancer and the selective evolutionary forces in a cancer under treatment almost inevitably result in the emergence of mutant clones that prohibit access of specifically targeted small molecule inhibitors to their targets, leading to relapse. This has been clearly shown with Imatinib therapy of CML. Imatinib is not effective against the leukaemia stem cells and cells with point mutations in the kinase domain of the BCR-ABL kinase emerge. For CML, the solution is currently chronic therapy with second or third generation RTK inhibitors but for *BCR1-ABL1* acute leukaemia a combination therapy with traditional cytotoxic drugs is both essential and effective.

The dramatic cures of the majority of childhood cancers, however, have been achieved with empirically developed chemotherapies. Many of the new effective drugs (e.g. topoisomerase I inhibitors and new nucleoside analogs) are in fact rationally developed cytotoxic chemotherapies. Hence it is worthwhile to study the biological basis for the dramatic sensitivity of some childhood cancers to chemotherapy. Little is known, for example, why anti-mitotic therapy with anti-microtubule agents (e.g. vinca alkaloids or taxanes) is so effective and relatively non-toxic. The general notion that cancer cells respond to chemotherapy because of their faster proliferation rate is incorrect as many skin, intestinal and hematopoietic normal cells proliferate faster than most cancer cells. It is likely that the same precancerous lesions in the DNA maintenance and repair machinery and in cell cycle checkpoints that enable the rapid evolution of cancer cells act also as their Achilles' heel in enhancing the cytotoxicity of chemotherapy. The lack of *TP53* mutations and the relative genomic simplicity possibly explain why paediatric cancers are so much more sensitive to cyto-toxic chemotherapy compared with cancers in adults.

Biological targets have been traditionally classified either as 'drugable' and 'non-drugable'. The first category includes oncogenic kinases and also surface molecules that may be targeted by antibodies. For example, an anti-CD20 antibody rituximab has transformed the treatment of non-Hodgkin lymphoma mostly in adults but occasionally in children. We have already men-tioned the ongoing trials with anti-IGFR1 antibodies for treatment of paediatric sarcomas. Antibodies can also be coupled to either cytotoxic molecules or to other molecules that could attract the immune system to the tumour cells.

Transcription factors have been considered typical 'non drugable' targets. This vision is chang-ing however. First, drugs that modify the metabolism of oncogenic transcription factors or modify their effect on chromatin and gene expression have either entered clinical trials or already been approved for clinical use. Examples include the inhibitors of histone deacetylase and DNA methyltransferase which have already been introduced to the clinic.

The second approach to target non-enzymatic molecules is by designing small molecules or pep-tides inhibiting interactions between these molecules and other proteins critical to its function. This approach has been already shown experimentally for blocking the activity of EWS-FLI1 in Ewing sarcoma, and for blocking BCL6 activity in lymphoma. The same approach was used for creation of pro-apoptotic drugs that mimic the BH3 domain shared by anti and pro-apoptotic molecules. It is highly likely that these approaches will eventually result in clinically translatable therapies.

The third approach, in earlier stages of clinical development, is based on evolving small inter-fering RNA (siRNA) therapy. Theoretically, every RNA and protein may be specifically inhibited by small (up to 22 base pair) double stranded oligonucleotides. One can imagine. for example, the specific targeting of a cancer-associated chimeric transcription factor by a siRNA directed against the fusion region, a treatment that should be free from side effects. Although numerous chal-lenges such as specificity and delivery into cancer cells exist, significant progress in preclinical trials suggests that clinical trials with siRNA targeting oncogenic molecules will commence during the lifetime of the current edition of this textbook.

Further reading

Albihn A, Johnsen JI, Henriksson MA (2010) MYC in oncogenesis and as a target for cancer therapies. *Adv Cancer Res* **107**, 163–224.

Aplan PD (2006) Causes of oncogenic chromosomal translocation. *Trends Genet* **22**, 46–55.

Bercovich D, Ganmore I, Scott LM, et al. (2008) Mutations of JAK2 in acute lymphoblastic leukaemias associated with Down's syndrome. *Lancet* **372**, 1484–92.

Bourquin JP, Izraeli S (2010) Where can biology of childhood ALL be attacked by new compounds? *Cancer Treat Rev* **36**, 298–306.

Brodeur GM (2003) Neuroblastoma: biological insights into a clinical enigma. *Nat Rev Cancer* **3**, 203–16.

Deininger M, Buchdunger E, Druker BJ (2005) The development of imatinib as a therapeutic agent for chronic myeloid leukemia. *Blood* **105**, 2640–53.

Fearon ER, Vogelstein B (1990) A genetic model for colorectal tumorigenesis. *Cell* **61**, 759–67.

Folkman J. (1971) Tumour angiogenesis: therapeutic implications. *N Engl J Med* **285**, 1182–6.

Greaves M (2010) Cancer stem cells: back to Darwin? *Semin Cancer Biol* **20**, 65–70.

Greaves MF, Wiemels J (2003) Origins of chromosome translocations in childhood leukaemia. *Nat Rev Cancer* **3**, 639–49.

Hahn WC, Weinberg RA (2002) Rules for making human tumour cells. *N Engl J Med* **347**, 1593–603.

Hanahan D, Weinberg RA (2011) Hallmarks of cancer: the next generation. *Cell* **144**, 646–74.

Hanks S, Coleman K, Reid S, et al. (2004) Constitutional aneuploidy and cancer predisposition caused by biallelic mutations in BUB1B. *Nat Genet* **36**, 1159–61.

Harris TJ, McCormick F (2010) The molecular pathology of cancer. *Nat Rev Clin Oncol.* **7**, 251–65.

Heyer J, Kwong LN, Lowe SW, Chin L (2010). Non-germline genetically engineered mouse models for translational cancer research. *Nat Rev Cancer* **10**, 470–80.

Izraeli S (2008) Trisomy 21 tilts the balance. *Blood* **112**, 4361–2.

Jain RK (2008) Lessons from multidisciplinary translational trials on anti-angiogenic therapy of cancer. *Nat Rev Cancer* **4**, 309–16.

Jones PA, Baylin SB (2007) The epigenomics of cancer. *Cell* **128**, 683–92.

Knudson AG, Jr (1971)_Mutation and cancer: statistical study of retinoblastoma. *Proc Natl Acad Sci USA* **68**, 820–3.

Kovar H (2010) Downstream EWS/FLI1 - upstream Ewing´s sarcoma. *Genome Med* **2**, 8.

Lessnick SL, Dei Tos AP, Sorensen PH, et al. (2009) Small round cell sarcomas. *Semin Oncol* **36**, 338–46.

Mullighan CG, Goorha S, Radtke I, et al. (2007) Genome-wide analysis of genetic alterations in acute lymphoblastic leukaemia. *Nature* **446**, 758–64.

Strebhardt K, Ullrich A (2008) Paul Ehrlich's magic bullet concept: 100 years of progress. *Nat Rev Cancer* **8**, 473–80.

Vogelstein B, Kinzler KW (2004) Cancer genes and the pathways they control. *Nat Med* **10**, 789–99.

Wood LD, Parsons DW, Jones S, et al. (2007) The genomic landscapes of human breast and colorectal cancers. *Science* **318**, 1108–13.

Chapter 3

Imaging in paediatric oncology

Kieran McHugh and Thierry A.G.M. Huisman

Introduction

Some general principles regarding the radiology approach apply to all masses, despite the diverse range of pathologies seen in different body parts. Suspected abdominal and pelvic masses must be examined by ultrasound (US) first, and this may be all that is necessary to evaluate benign masses. Superficial lesions or palpable lumps should also be assessed by US initially. Lesion vascularity can be easily evaluated by Doppler interrogation, increased vascularity being an important finding with proliferating haemangiomas in infancy, lesions that could otherwise mimic more sinister pathology. Further cross-sectional imaging largely to determine lesion extent will be guided by the US findings, tumour location and local availability of magnetic resonance imaging (MRI). The reliable interpretation of imaging requires a radiologist with sufficient experience and expertise in paediatric oncology, particularly with the more advanced technologies such as X-ray computed tomography (CT), MRI and positron emission tomography (PET).

Imaging modalities

Plain Radiography

Plain films play a very limited role in the diagnostic work up of new paediatric mass lesions. The major exception to this is with bone tumours, both benign processes and malignant lesions. In this setting, the plain X-ray probably has a bigger role in suggesting the proper diagnosis than other techniques. Bone lysis with ill-defined margins is highly suggestive of an aggressive process such as osteomyelitis or tumour, which may be indistinguishable on imaging, but often have very different clinical presentations. Sclerotic well-defined margins in an osseous mass suggest a benign process. The dilemma of benign versus malignant for bone tumours is usually relatively straightforward at plain radiography, and the role of MRI in this setting is largely to define the extent of the lesion, and to evaluate for a soft tissue mass which is likely to be underestimated on plain radiographs.

Although the chest X-ray (CXR) is performed routinely and plays an important role in staging for metastatic disease at diagnosis, particular reliance is placed on chest CT to exclude pulmonary metastases in virtually all extra-cranial malignancies, with the exception of neuroblastoma. Posterior rib erosion and separation with an obvious chest mass are virtually pathognomic of a neurogenic tumour such as neuroblastoma. Another important role for the plain CXR, notably the lateral film, is assessing for airway compression from an anterior mediastinal mass. Follow-up during treatment and later surveillance for metastatic relapse is also performed with serial CXRs. The CXR is also useful in detecting secondary infection or other complications of treatment, such as rib osteochondromas secondary to irradiation, during follow-up.

Ultrasound

Ultrasound (US) entails no radiation burden and so can be done repeatedly without harm. Soft tissue masses can be easily evaluated to assess their cystic or solid nature, and presence of calcification. US is a dynamic real-time examination. With large abdominal masses, invasion into other organs can be difficult to interpret on CT or MRI, but may be easily evaluated with US. Movement of the liver separate from a renal mass is a reliable sign of non-invasion of the liver by the mass. With additional Doppler assessments, the degree of vascularity of a mass lesion can be identified. US is the best technique for detecting and excluding tumour thrombus extension into the inferior vena cava from a renal or adrenal tumour. US is the most sensitive technique in the detection of early fungal infiltration of the liver or spleen in the immunocompromIzed, best evaluated with linear-array high-resolution transducers. Most percutaneous imaging-guided biopsies are done simply with US guidance.

CT

The size and extent of large masses are easily assessed with CT but with that comes the added radiation burden of CT. The newer multi-detector CT scanners are extremely fast at examining any body region, avoiding the need for sedation or anaesthesia in many circumstances. CT is the optimal method for assessing the lung parenchyma. Calcification in a mass, often not apparent on MRI, is easily detected with CT. For chest and abdominal scanning in children, non-contrast enhanced CT studies are usually of little help due to children's lack of mediastinal or retroperitoneal fat. Thus, for paediatric chest and abdominal CT, single-phase post contrast-enhanced images are all that is generally required to evaluate a mass lesion. Bone detail is very well demonstrated on CT such that, for example with skull base tumours, an MRI to assess soft tissue extent and a CT to assess erosion of the skull base or facial bones may be necessary.

MRI

MRI is the ideal imaging modality because of its better characterization of tissues, multi-planar capabilities and lack of ionizing radiation. Tumour extent is best assessed with MRI, although for large masses CT can be as accurate. As MRI is sensitive to oedema (seen as hyperintense or bright signal on T2 sequences), it is generally impossible to differentiate tumour margins from oedema. In addition, at the end of treatment or after surgery MRI often cannot distinguish residual fibrosis or benign residual tissue from residual tumour. MRI studies generally take a minimum of 30 minutes, which means that most children less than 6 years of age need general anaesthesia or sedation for the MRI examination.

Nuclear medicine

Wilms tumours and hepatoblastoma seldom metastasize to bone and so do not merit routine bone scanning with technetium[99]-MDP (methylene-diphosphonate). Suspected neuroblastoma metastases are best assessed with iodine[123]-MIBG (metaiodobenzylguanidine) scans—if the primary tumour is not avid for MIBG then a bone scan is recommended to evaluate for skeletal metastases in this setting. For primary neuroblastoma non-avid for MIBG, it is likely that PET-CT or whole body MRI will prove to be more sensitive in the detection of distant metastatic spread than bone scanning. Most sarcomas and other solid tumours usually require routine bone scans for staging at diagnosis. PET-CT may well make bone scanning obsolete for many sarcomas and other tumours in time, but insufficient evidence exists at present to omit routine bone scans for paediatric sarcomas.

Interventional radiology

Paediatric interventional radiology (IR) has developed remarkably in the past 20 years. All children's oncology centres should have access to IR services. These services should include common procedures such as tumour biopsy, line placement, angiography, gastrostomy insertion and abscess drainage. More complicated procedures such as such as pre-operative tumour embolization to reduce haemorrhage at surgery, radiofrequency ablation, and chemo-embolization techniques should also ideally be available in the bigger centres.

Tumours outside the central nervous system

The differential diagnosis of masses in childhood is largely influenced by the age of a child and the organ of origin or location of the lesion. Calcification in a neuroblastoma or fat plus calcium in a teratoma are useful in suggesting a diagnosis but the imaging characteristics of the majority of tumours are in general relatively non-specific . Most tumours are, for example, hypovacular on contrast-enhanced CT with areas of low attenuation and heterogeneity. Homogeneous imaging appearances of a paediatric mass suggest a benign cause, such as haemangioma or fibromatosis in infancy. Tumours are typically of low signal on T1-weighted (T1W) MRI sequences and high signal on T2W MRI, again with variable contrast enhancement after gadolinium administration. Calcification typically has no inherent signal at MRI scanning such that calcification in mass lesions is missed or underestimated at MRI. Some densely fibrotic lesions may be of low signal (hypointense) on both T1W and T2W MR images. Some of the most important issues to consider when imaging tumours beyond the central nervous system (CNS) will be addressed in this section.

Renal tumours

Ultrasound should be utilized first to assess the origin of a potential renal tumour, tumour thrombus in the renal vein and/or IVC, the contralateral kidney, and liver. Dynamic real-time ultrasound is a very useful method for assessing tumour invasion of the liver or other organs, but tends to be under-utilized in this context. Abdominal CT should be performed only after intravenous contrast medium enhancement. Ipsilateral and contralateral small lesions or foci of nephroblastomatosis may be seen with Wilms tumour (nephroblastoma). A chest CT is required to detect or exclude pulmonary metastases. The diameter of pulmonary nodules should be measured on lung window settings, and these same settings should be used at follow up. MRI ideally is preferred over CT in evaluating the primary tumour due to its superior contrast resolution and lack of radiation. Tumour extent is equally assessed by CT or MRI, but foci of nephroblastomatosis are much better visualized with MRI (Fig. 3.1). All renal tumours in childhood have similar radiological appearances and age at presentation is the most important factor in the differential diagnosis. Clear cell sarcoma, because of its propensity to skeletal metastatic spread, merits radionuclide bone scanning. Renal cell carcinoma, which usually manifests in adolescence, demonstrates calcification in approximately 25 per cent of cases.

Neuroblastoma

Encasement of the aorta and upper abdominal arteries is the hallmark of the majority of abdominal neuroblastoma (Fig. 3.2), in contrast to renal tumours which tend to displace the aorta and IVC. Confinent to the suprarenal area is more often seen in infants. MS (formerly 4S) disease causes hepatomegaly and diffuse hepatic infiltration by tumour. The infiltration may be subtle

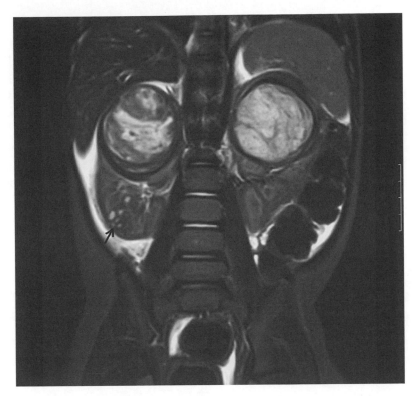

Fig. 3.1 Nephroblastoma (Wilms tumour). Wilms tumours in the upper poles of both kidneys are seen as hyperintense heterogenous round masses on coronal T2W MRI. A third possible tumour is seen in the right lower pole as a smaller cystic lesion (arrow).

however, and may only be appreciated with a higher resolution linear array US transducer. MRI and CT are probably equivalent when assessing the primary tumour, but MRI is superior at evaluating for intraspinal disease and allows easier depiction of marrow metastases. Some surgeons prefer contrast-enhanced CT prior to surgery as CT tends to give a more reliable surgical roadmap of the vasculature, and more clearly demonstrates the extent of tumour calcification. MIBG scanning is crucial for staging at diagnosis and for assessing response in patients with metastatic disease.

Rhabdomyosarcoma

Skull base tumours often need CT to assess the bony erosion and MR to evaluate the soft tissue extent. MRI is also superior in demonstrating tumour involvement of the neural foramina and intracranial spread. Orbital tumours rarely have lymphatic loco-regional spread. US evaluation of the cervical chain of nodes is probably underutilized for head and neck tumours. Cervical lymph nodes metastases are often difficult to identify on all modalities and a low threshold for biopsy is advisable. MRI is the modality of choice for assessing genito-urinary primaries, after initial assessment with US (Fig. 3.3). US of the liver should be performed in all patients to detect or exclude metastases. US of the retroperitoneal area should be performed in all patients with pelvic or lower limb primaries. Limb primary tumours (leg or arm) should also have US of the inguinal region or axilla to detect or exclude regional lymphadenopathy.

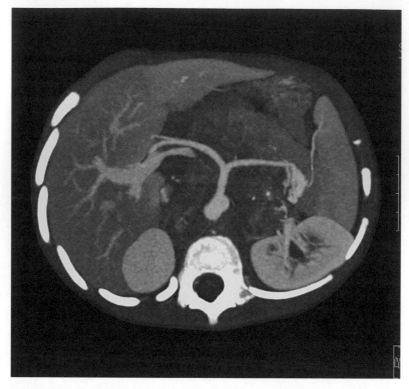

Fig. 3.2 Neuroblastoma. Maximum intensity projection (summated image), of a CT in the axial plane post intravenous contrast-enhancement. This shows anterior displacement and encasement of the aorta, coeliac, hepatic and splenic arteries by a large faintly calcified retroperitoneal mass.

Liver tumours

Between 60 and 70 per cent of all primary liver tumours in children are malignant, with hepato-blastoma and hepatocellular carcinoma constituting the vast majority of these malignancies. Haemangioendothelioma/haemangioma lesions and mesenchymal hamartoma account for nearly all the non-malignant tumours in children. The pre-treatment extent (PRETEXT) staging system used by the International Childhood Liver Tumor Strategy Group (SIOPEL) for hepatob-lastoma has gained widespread acceptance. PRETEXT is used to describe tumour extent before any therapy, thus allowing comparison between studies conducted by different collaborative groups. PRETEXT staging is based on Couinaud's system of liver segmentation. The liver seg-ments are grouped into four sections: segments 2 and 3 (left lateral section), segments 4a and 4b (left medial section), segments 5 and 8 (right anterior section), and segments 6 and 7 (right posterior section). Involvement of only one section by a hepatoblastoma mass is denoted as a PRETEXT I tumour, more involvement by a tumour to involve two, three or all four sections is classified as PRETEXT II, III or IV respectively. Increasing PRETEXT number gives, very roughly, an estimate of the difficulty of the planned surgical procedure. US is particularly useful is assessing portal or hepatic venous, or biliary ductal, invasion by tumour. MRI is superior to CT in evaluating liver segmental involvement by tumour (Fig. 3.4). Hepatocellular carcinoma occurs in children older than 5 years, often on a background of pre-existing cirrhosis.

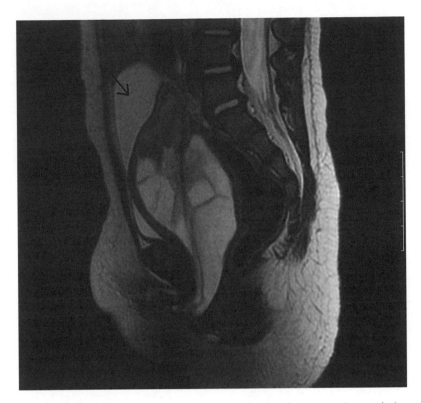

Fig. 3.3 Rhabdomyosarcoma. Sagittal T2W midline pelvis image shows a cystic mass lesion with septations in the vagina distorting the cervix and uterus. The fluid-filled bladder in seen anteriorly (arrow). Gas in the rectum returns dark signal.

Germ cell tumours

Midline germ cell rests are thought to arise in arrested migration from the hind gut yolk sac to the genital ridge. Germ cell tumours (GCT) are thus commonly found in the pineal gland, neck, mediastinum, retroperitoneum, and sacrococcygeal area. All GCT show mixed cystic and solid areas, often with foci of fatty attenuation and/or calcification. A mass lesion that contains both fatty tissues and calcification is virtually always a GCT. Fat, and calcification in particular, are easily evaluated with CT such that CT is more reliable than MRI in defining the extent of most GCT, with the possible exception of ovarian tumours. Rupture of a mediastinal teratoma may result in a pleural or pericardial effusion. Alternatively, pericardial invasion by tumour may cause a pericardial effusion. Radiology cannot differentiate a benign tumour from a malignant GCT. Of the malignant GCT, dysgerminoma and yolk sac tumours are the most common, with elevated alpha fetoprotein (AFP) and human chorionic gonadotropin (HCG) levels. The latter tumour markers are so reliable that post-operative routine radiological surveillance is generally not required.

Lymphomas

In the abdomen, a non-Hodgkin lymphoma (NHL) may present as a mass or intussusception, usually identifiable by US. NHL in the mediastinum may cause airway compression such that CT in the supine position may be dangerous. Clinical airway assessment and a lateral chest X-ray to

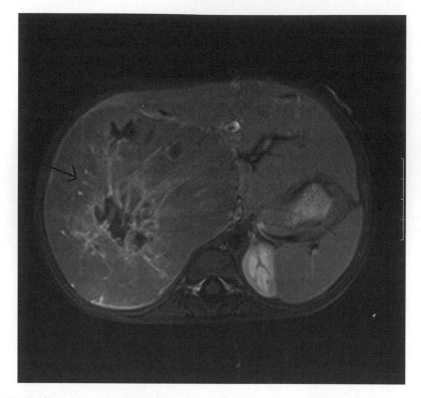

Fig. 3.4 Hepatoblastoma. Right lobe liver tumour (arrow) on a fat-suppressed T1 weighted MRI after gadolinium enhancement. Poor enhancement in the central tumour was due to necrosis. The middle and left hepatic veins were free of tumour which was classified as PRETEXT 2.

evaluate the trachea are warranted prior to a routine staging CT. NHL in Waldeyer's ring manifests as tonsillar enlargement and a nasopharyngeal mass. That mass tends to be associated with little if any adjacent osseous destruction, unlike rhabdomyosacoma in the nasopharynx which typically causes much skull base erosion.

At initial presentation, Hodgkin lymphoma merits high-resolution US to evaluate for splenic infiltration and a chest CT is necessary to evaluate the lung parenchyma. MRI of the neck and abdomen is as sensitive as CT for lymphadenopathy and would reduce the radiation burden in young patients. Increasing reliance is now being placed within clinical trials on PET-CT at diagnosis and follow-up, in assessing response to therapy.

Non-rhabdomyosarcomatous soft tissue tumours

Approximately half of paediatric soft tissue tumours are non-rhabdomyomatous soft tissue sarcomas (NRSTS). They are a heterogeneous group of tumours, all of mesenchymal origin, that share some biological characteristics but differ histologically. The most common NRSTS are synovial cell sarcoma (17–42 per cent), followed by fibrosarcoma (13–15 per cent), malignant fibrous histiocytoma (12–13 per cent) and malignant peripheral nerve sheath tumours (10 per cent). The frequency of most of these tumours is age dependent. Fibrosarcomas occur more commonly in children under 1 year of age, with synovial sarcomas and malignant peripheral nerve sheath tumours (MPNST) being more common in children over 10 years. These lesions generally have non-specific radiological findings of a soft tissue mass. Like most paediatric tumours, they are hypovascular at Doppler US evaluation, and more usually solid than cystic in appearance. The lesions are isointense (similar signal intensity) to muscle on T1W MRI, hyperintense on T2W and show variable enhancement after gadolinium administration. Locoregional adenopathy should be sought or excluded in all cases.

Bone tumours

Osteosarcomas mainly occur around the knee (in the metaphyses of the distal femur or proximal tibia) in adolescence. Radiation-induced sarcomas are rare in childhood. The Ewing's family of tumours, including primitive neuroectodermal tumours, tend to occur in children less than 10 years of age in either a flat bone (pelvis, scapula) or in the diaphysis of a long bone. Plain films are more reliable in assessing the aggressive nature of a lytic bone lesion. MRI is best at depicting tumour extent, the associated soft tissue mass, involvement of the neurovascular bundle and spread of tumour across the growth plate into the epiphysis. Some centres report dynamic contrast enhanced MRI is useful at predicting percentage tumour necrosis after initial chemotherapy but the technique is not widely available.

Tumours within the central nervous system in children

The frequently used phrase 'children are not small adults' is pertinent for pediatric radiology in general and pediatric neuroradiology in particular. Pediatric CNS tumours have multiple characteristic features that differ significantly from their adult counterparts (Chapter 20).

In pediatric neuroradiology, the age and the gender help to narrow the differential diagnosis. Each age group has typical tumours and certain tumours are more frequent in boys than in girls. Especially in the posterior fossa, this is helpful. The most frequent posterior fossa tumours are juvenile pilocytic astrocytomas (JPA) (35 per cent), primitive neuro-ectodermal tumours (PNET)/ medulloblastoma (25 per cent), brainstem gliomas (25 per cent) and ependymomas (12 per cent). These tumours represent 97 per cent of all posterior fossa tumours. If this 'frequency list' is combined with the gender of the patient, the tumour type can frequently be predicted. In the supratentorial brain the variety of tumours is greater. Astrocytomas are the most frequent tumours (30 per cent) followed by craniopharyngeomas (15 per cent) and hypothalamic/optic pathway gliomas (15 per cent).

The distribution of supra- versus infratentorial tumours also varies with age. In the first 2 years of life, supratentorial tumours are more frequent than infratentorial tumours; between 2 and 10 years infratentorial tumours outweigh supratentorial tumours while in children 10 years and older, supra- and infratentorial tumours are equally frequent.

Functional prognosis in children may be better because of the larger functional plasticity at younger age. On the other hand, treatment options may be more limited because the brain is more vulnerable for the potential deleterious effects of the various treatment options. For example, radiotherapy is frequently contra-indicated in the very young patients. In addition, radiotherapy may induce secondary neoplasm later in life.

Infratentorial tumours

As mentioned earlier the most frequent posterior fossa tumours in children are the cerebellar astrocytomas, PNET/medulloblastomas, brainstem gliomas, and ependymomas. Of course many less frequent tumours may be found including atypical teratoid rhabdoid tumours (ATRT), hemangioblastomas, cerebellar gangliocytomas, etc. It would go beyond the scope of this chapter to discuss all these less frequent tumours.

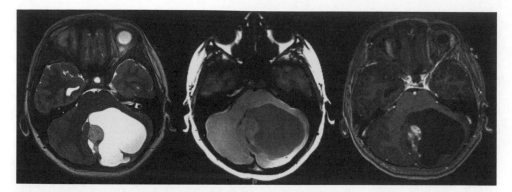

Fig. 3.5 Axial T2-, T1- and contrast enhanced T1-weighted imaging of child with a partially solid, predominantly cystic juvenile pilocytic astrocytoma within the left cerebellar hemisphere and vermis. The fourth ventricle is compressed and displaced to the right.

Cerebellar astrocytomas

Cerebellar astrocytomas can be subdivided in the frequent juvenile pilocytic astrocytoma (JPA) and the less common fibrillary astrocytoma. JPA is a unique form of astrocytoma which is rather benign and has a good prognosis if the tumour is recognized early and completely resected. Pilocytic astrocytomas may be seen in neurofibromatosis (NF1) patients. The so-called 'epicenter' of the tumour is frequently within the cerebellar vermis, followed in frequency by the cerebellar hemisphere. Most children present with symptoms related to an obstructive hydrocephalus. Pilocytic astrocytomas are usually well demarcated, have a solid, strongly contrast enhancing tumour component and a cystic component which does not or minimally enhance (Fig. 3.5). The cyst may be significantly larger than the solid tumour nodule. Calcifications are seen in approximately 20 per cent of cases, vasogenic edema is usually mild or minimal. The tumour typically compresses or displaces adjacent structures including the brainstem and fourth ventricle resulting in a supratentorial hydrocephalus. The imaging features resemble hemangioblastomas. Hemangioblastomas are however significantly rarer, occur usually as part of the von Hippel Lindau syndrome, tumour nodules are usually multiple, and dilated feeding and draining vessels may be seen. Next to the 'benign' pilocytic astrocytomas, each grade of astrocytomas (WHO I-IV) may be encountered in the posterior fossa. Frequently, lesions start as a lower grade lesion and on follow up de-differentiation into higher grade astrocytomas may occur. High grade or anaplastic astrocytomas may show diffuse infiltrative, ill-defined tumour components and are due to their close proximity to the fourth ventricle and subarachnoid space at risk for leptomeningeal cerebrospinal fluid (CSF) seeding. Consequently metastatic lesions should be searched for along the entire neuroaxis including the most distal tip of the dural sack. Unfortunately, grade III and IV astrocytomas have a poor prognosis.

Medulloblastomas

Medulloblastomas are also known as infratentorial PNET. The majority of lesions originate from the vermis (75–90 per cent), with 10–15 per cent primarily located within the cerebellar hemispheres (lateral medulloblastoma). In the vermian location, the tumour is located dorsally to the fourth ventricle; the anterior medullary velum and fourth ventricle are pushed anteriorly. Most clinical symptoms are related to an obstructive hydrocephalus as well as tumour infiltration of cerebellar structures. The tumour is most frequently encountered in the first decade of life (75 per cent) and boys are three times more frequently affected than girls. The lesion is typically hyperdense on CT due to its high cellularity. On MR examination, the tumour is solid, predominantly

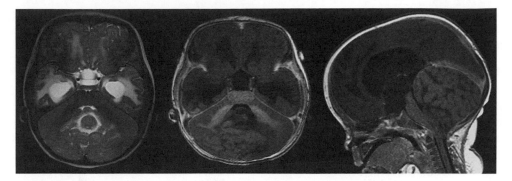

Fig. 3.6 Axial T2-, contrast enhanced axial and sagittal T1-weighted MRI of a child with a desmoplastic medulloblastoma. The epicentre of the tumour is dorsally to the anteriorly displaced and compressed fourth ventricle. Moderate supratentorial hydrocephalus is noted.

T1-hypointnese and T2-iso- or hyperintense (Fig. 3.6). Depending on the histological subtype, various degrees of contrast enhancement are noted. The most important imaging clue for diagnosis is the location of the tumour dorsally to the fourth ventricle, which helps to differentiate the lesion from fourth ventricle ependymomas. However, in advanced stages, the tumour may invade the fourth ventricle making differentiation less reliable. If the fourth ventricle is invaded, CSF seeding of the neuroaxis must be excluded. Spinal imaging should preferably be done preoperatively, because a mild postoperative leptomeningeal enhancement may mimic tumour seeding.

Brainstem gliomas

Brainstem gliomas can be classified upon their primary location into (a) diffuse infiltrative brainstem glioma (also known as pons glioma), (b) exophytic glioma of the medulla oblongata, and (c) tectal glioma. Clinical symptoms are determined by the primary location and degree of infiltration or compression of adjacent functional centers. Gliomas usually develop and grow slowly over a long time period before they become symptomatic. A sudden increase in size is usually an indication for increasing malignant degeneration. Patients may present with isolated or combined cranial nerve palsies as well as ataxia. Because these gliomas grow slowly, hydrocephalus is only encountered late in disease progression. Most gliomas are recognized between 3 and 10 years of age. Long-term prognosis of the diffuse infiltrative brainstem glioma is poor. These brainstem gliomas have a low sensitivity for chemotherapy and the young age of most patients as well as the central location of the tumour prevents high dose radiotherapy or surgical exploration/resection. The exophytic glioma of the medulla oblongata has a much more favorable prognosis; histological they usually belong to the group of pilocytic astrocytomas and they are more accessible to surgical resection. Tectal gliomas usually have an excellent prognosis, may remain stable for many decades and usually only require symptomatic treatment. The proximity to the Sylvian aqueduct usually results in an obstructive hydrocephalus which can be treated by a ventriculo-peritoneal shunt or a third ventriculostomy. Because of the stability of the lesions, several groups have discussed if a tectal glioma should be considered to be a variant hamartoma. On MRI, most gliomas are T1-hypointense, T2-hyperintense and show no or minimal contrast enhancement. Tectal gliomas are usually recognized as a 'thick/bulky' quadrigeminal plate. The exophytic glioma of the medulla oblongata is usually characterized by a large exophytic component attached to the medulla oblongata. The MR imaging features of the diffuse infiltrative brainstem glioma are considered to be sufficient to establish diagnosis. Typically, the lesion is centered in a diffuse enlarged pons, preserved fibre tracts may be seen as linear signal intensities within the lesion (especially well seen on T2-weighted imaging), the basilar artery is typically embraced and depending on the grade of malignancy multifocal areas of contrast enhancement may be observed. These gliomas may extend into the lower brainstem as well as into the mesencephalon and diencephalon.

Ependymoma

Ependymomas typically originate from the ependymal lining of the fourth ventricle (60–70 per cent). In contrast to the medulloblastoma, the 'epicenter' of the ependymomas is within the fourth ventricle. Ependymomas rarely infiltrate the vermis, brainstem or cerebellum. Ependymomas typically respect the boundaries of the ventricular system and extend along the various outlet channels of the fourth ventricle (foramen of Luschka and Magendie) along the brainstem into basal cisterns and spinal canal. CSF seeding may occur early due to the intraventricular location. Clinically, most children present with signs of an obstructive hydrocephalus or compression of the brainstem and cranial nerves. On imaging, ependymomas are solid, T1-iso- or hypointense, T2-iso- or hyperintense with a variable degree of contrast enhancement. Calcifications are seen in 50 per cent, cysts in 20 per cent and hemorrhage in 10 per cent of cases.

Supratentorial tumours

In contrast to the posterior fossa, the variation of tumours is higher in the supratentorial region.

Astrocytomas

Astrocytomas (WHO I-IV) are the most frequent supratentorial tumours in children (30 per cent). Clinical symptoms are determined by the primary location, degree of infiltration, and compression of functional centers. Focal functional deficits may be seen next to epileptic seizures and more general signs of increased intracranial pressure. Most pediatric astrocytomas are low grade, however in rare cases grade IV glioblastoma multiforme occurs. Pilocytic astrocytomas are much rarer in the supratentorial brain compared to the posterior fossa. Next to white matter locations, astrocytomas may also be located within the thalami and basal ganglia. On CT and MRI, depending on their WHO grade, the imaging appearance may differ. Low grade astrocytomas are T1-hypointense and T2-hyperintense with no or minimal contrast enhancement or mass effect. High-grade gliomas typically show an intense, inhomogeneous contrast enhancement with areas of necrosis within the center of the tumour (Fig. 3.7). Diffusion weighted imaging may be helpful to differentiate between a necrotic tumour and an abscess.

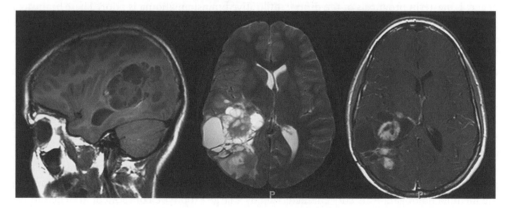

Fig. 3.7 Sagittal T1-, axial T2 and contrast enhanced T1-weighted MRI of a child with a glioblastoma multiforme. A large, inhomogeneous, partially multicystic, partially solid, contrast-enhancing tumour is seen within the right parieto-occipital region.

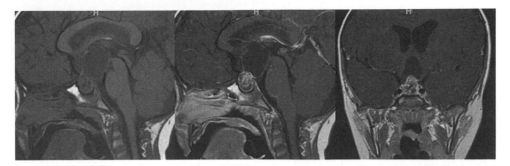

Fig. 3.8 Sagittal T1, contrast enhanced sagittal and coronal T1- weighted MRI of a child with a sellar/suprasellar craniopharyngeoma. The lesion shows an inhomogeneous contrast enhancement with a large cyst protruding into the third ventricle. The optic chiasm is pushed anteriorly.

Craniopharyngeomas

Craniopharyngeomas are seen in 15 per cent of children. They are most frequently seen between 10 and 14 years of age and are typically located in the sellar/suprasellar region along the axis between hypothalamus and pituitary gland. These tumours most likely originate from residual pluripotent cells after the development of the hypothalamus/pituitary gland. Clinical symptoms are related to compression of the optic chiasm/optic pathway, pituitary gland/hypothalamus or infiltration of the connection between hypothalamus and pituitary gland. Craniopharyngeomas are easily identified on CT/MRI. They are usually heterogeneous with sold and cystic components, as well as variable degree of calcifications and contrast enhancement (Fig. 3.8). The sella may be enlarged.

Optic pathway gliomas

Optic pathway gliomas represent a separate group of astrocytomas and are usually seen in NF1-patients. Histologically, they represent pilocytic astrocytomas. Non- or minimally enhancing optic nerve gliomas can be seen next to T2-hyperintense, strongly enhancing hypothalamic/chiasmatic tumours. These tumours may be stable for many years but typically present with slowly progressive blindness and pituitary/hypothalamic dysfunction.

Supratentorial ependymomas and PNET

Supratentorial ependymomas and PNET are rare tumours in childhood. Of all ependymomas, only 20–40 per cent are located within the supratentorial brain. Supratentorial ependymomas are most frequently located within the periventricular white matter; intraventricular ependymomas are much rarer. Local compression may result in trapped ventricles with asymmetrical hydrocephalus. Supratentorial PNETs are also rare, less than 5 per cent of all supratentorial tumours are PNETs. These tumours are usually large on initial presentation, heterogeneous and may be located within the white matter as well as in the ventricles. Differentiation from other rare tumours like ATRT or intraventricular meningeomas may be challenging.

Further reading

Abdel Razek AA, Gaballa G, Elhawarey G, Megahed AS, Hafez M, Nada N (2009) Characterization of pediatric head and neck masses with diffusion-weighted MR imaging. *Eur Radiol.* **19**, 201–8.

Brenner DJ, Elliston CD, Hall EJ, et al. (2001) Estimated risks of radiation-induced fatal cancer from pediatric CT. *Am J Roentgenol* **176**, 289–96.

Chowdhury T, Barnacle A, Haque S, Sebire N, Gibson S, Anderson J, Roebuck D (2009) Ultrasound-guided core needle biopsy for the diagnosis of rhabdomyosarcoma in childhood. *Pediatr Blood Cancer* **53**, 356–60.

Defachelles AS, Rey A, Oberlin O, Stevens MC (2009) Treatment of nonmetastatic cranial parameningeal rhabdomyosarcoma in children younger than 3 years old: International society of Paediatric Oncology Studies MMT 89 and 95. *J Clin Oncol* **27**, 1310–1315.

Lloyd C, McHugh K (2010) The role of radiology in head and neck tumours in children. *Cancer Imaging* **10**, 49–61.

Monclair T, Brodeur GM, Ambros PF et al. (2009) The International Neuroblastoma Risk Group (INRG) Staging System: an INRG Task Force Report. *J Clin Oncol* **27**, 298–303.

Roebuck DJ, Perilongo G (2006) Hepatoblastoma: an oncological review. *Pediatr Radiol* **36**, 183–6.

Silva CT, Amaral JG, Moineddin R, Doda W, Babyn PS (2010) CT characteristics of lung nodules present at diagnosis of extrapulmonary malignancy in children. *Am J Roentgenol* **194**, 772–8.

Smets AM, de Kraker J (2010) Malignant tumours of the kidney: imaging strategy. *Pediatr Radiol* **40**, 1010–18.

Chapter 4

Chemotherapy: current knowledge and new perspectives

Arnauld Verschuur and Michel Zwaan

Introduction

In contrast to many types of cancer arising in adults, the majority of those occurring in childhood are sensitive to cytotoxic chemotherapy. This is generally attributed to the high proliferation rate of childhood malignancies and the propensity of the malignant cells to undergo apoptosis- features that may be linked to the embryonal origin of many of these tumour types. Chemotherapy therefore, has a major role in treatment and contributes significantly to the generally good outcome for the majority of paediatric malignancies.

Chemotherapy is used either as the only treatment modality, or in combination with surgery and/or radiotherapy. However, some diseases remain or become refractory to chemotherapy and evidence for the long-term toxicity of some chemotherapeutic compounds has emerged. Thus, there is a necessity to understand the mechanisms both of therapeutic failure and long-term toxicity as the unravelling of these may lead to the development of novel treatment modalities. Taking into account biological and pathological differences between paediatric and adult cancer, it is clear that specific drug development programs are needed to identify new drugs for children in the future. Moreover, given the potential differences in drug metabolism at different ages, dosing may differ from adults even when the same drug is used. Young children may also need specific formulations. Fortunately, these challenges are now being addressed by the development of specific regulations facilitating pediatric drug development both in the United States and in Europe.

The first part of this chapter will summarize the current knowledge of conventional chemotherapeutic agents and their application. The second part will focus on the development of novel compounds in pediatric oncology.

Conventional chemotherapeutic agents

Overview

Chemotherapy is the key-element in the treatment of pediatric hematological malignancies, such as leukaemia and lymphoma. In acute lymphoblastic leukaemia (ALL) treatment consists of multiple agents given in combination for total treatment duration of 2–3 years. Central to this is multiagent induction treatment followed by a phase using intrathecal and intravenous chemotherapy to avoid leukaemia relapse in the central nervous system (CNS). Depending on the protocol and/or patient risk characteristics, further blocks of consolidation or reinduction therapy are introduced before the start of a prolonged phase of maintenance therapy that aims to eradicate minimal residual disease (MRD). In contrast, treatment duration is short in acute myeloid leukaemia (AML), (most protocols contain four or five blocks of chemotherapy) but very intensive.

In both diseases, many treatment optimization studies have been performed over the last decades, fine-tuning the application of conventional chemotherapy. These have included studies implementing new analogues of existing compounds with greater potency or with better pharmacological properties. Examples include asparaginase (erwinase, *E. coli* derived asparaginase, pegylated asparaginases and, recently, recombinant asparaginase) and corticosteroids (prednisone being replaced by dexamethasone). Nevertheless, a small subset of patients still fail to achieve a cure with current therapy and new agents with distinct modes of action are needed to improve outcomes for these individuals.

In pediatric solid tumours, chemotherapy is generally adapted to the diagnosis and stage of the malignancy. It is often used to obtain regression of the primary tumour in order to facilitate local tumor control by surgery and/or radiotherapy. Preoperative chemotherapy of this type, referred to as 'neoadjuvant' chemotherapy, also allows evaluation of the chemosensitivity of a particular tumour in a specific patient which may influence the choice of postoperative treatment. An example of this therapeutic approach is that used in the treatment of osteogenic sarcoma (see Chapter 22) and of Wilms tumour (see Chapter 23). Postoperative 'adjuvant' chemotherapy is used in these and other diagnoses to treat presumed or possible microscopic metastases or remaining viable tumor after incomplete local therapy. In other tumours, the primary approach is surgical removal of the localized primary tumour after which adjuvant chemotherapy is given (sometimes in conjunction to radiotherapy) in order to achieve optimal local control and to treat undetectable metastases. An example of this approach would be that used for medulloblastoma (see Chapter 20).

Chemotherapy regimes usually consist of combinations of two or more cytotoxic agents given as sequential courses often using different combinations in order to augment the probability of destroying the maximum number of malignant cells. In most treatment schedules, different classes of drugs with distinct mechanisms of action are used together in an attempt to achieve synergism and reduce the likelihood of chemoresistance. The choice of the chemotherapeutic agents depends on several factors such as tumour type, preclinical evidence of *in vitro* cytotoxicity and *in vivo* activity of a specific drug, and on the expected toxicity of the proposed combination. Sometimes preclinical data provide evidence of a synergistic effect between two or more compounds, although most of the standard chemotherapy regimens developed during the last three decades have been developed empirically and have not been evaluated in pediatric tumour models before their clinical use.

Classification of chemotherapeutic agents

There are several classes of anticancer drugs that are defined by their mode of action. In general, drugs of different classes are chosen for combination regimens. The classification used for drugs most frequently used in paediatric oncology is summarized in Table 4.1.

Routes of administration

Most chemotherapy agents are given intravenously (IV), for which children usually are provided with a central venous device such as a Port-a-cath® or Cellsite® catheter or a Hickman® or Broviac® tunneled central line. Some drugs are administered orally, either as tablets, capsules or liquid preparations. Hospital pharmacies sometimes develop dose-adapted capsules or liquid preparations for compounds that are not commercially available in the correct doses or formulation required by young children. In some mainly younger children, nasogastric or enterostomy tubes may need to be placed for drug administration as well as for nutritional support. Subcutaneous and intramuscular dosing is less acceptable in children. Intrathecal administration

Table 4.1 Classification of chemotherapeutic drugs

Class	Mode of action	Examples
Alkylating agents	Form covalent bonds between alkyl groups and nucleotides in DNA	Mechlorethamine, cyclophosphamide, ifosfamide, melphalan, busulfan, thiotepa,
	Alkylation alters DNA and its replication	Nitrosureas: carmustine (BCNU) and lomustine (CCNU)
	May induce mutations in DNA	Procarbazine and dacarbazine (DTIC)
		Temozolomide
Platinum compounds	Form covalent bonds between platinum atoms and DNA, resulting in intrastrand adducts or interstrand crosslinks, leading to DNA damage	Cisplatin, carboplatin, oxaliplatin
Anti-metabolites	Interfere with synthesis of DNA/RNA precursors	Purine analogs (mercaptopurine, thioguanine, fludarabine, clofarabine)
	Enzyme inhibition (e.g. dihydrofolate reductase or thymidylate synthetase)	Pyrimidine analogs (cytarabine, gemcitabine, 5-fluorouracil)
		Anti-folates (methotrexate, pemetrexed, trimetrexate)
Anti-microtubule compounds	Interfere with the formation of microtubules during cell division	Vinca alkaloids (vincristine, vinblastine, vinorelbine)
		Taxanes (paclitaxel, docetaxel)
		Ixabepilone
Topoisomerase I inhibitors	Inhibition of topoisomerase I	Irinotecan (CPT-11) and topotecan
		Diflomotecan, gimatecan
Epipodo-phyllotoxins	Topoisomerase II inhibitors	Etoposide (VP16), teniposide (VM26)
Antibiotics: Anthracyclines	Topoisomerase II inhibitors, but act also through DNA intercalation	Daunorubicin, doxorubicin, epirubicin, idarubicin
Anthracenediones	Oxidative DNA intercalation	Mitoxantrone
Others	DNA binding drug and inhibitor of RNA and protein synthesis	Bleomycin,
		Dactinomycin
MISCELLANEOUS:		
Corticosteroids	Induction of apoptosis	Prednisolone, dexamethasone
Asparaginase	Inhibits asparagine synthetase and depletes intracellular asparagine levels	L-Asparaginase, erwsiniase, PEG-asparginase
Differentiation-inducing agents	Inhibitor of ribonucleotide reductase	Hydroxyurea
	Induces differentiation of promyeloctes or neuroblasts	Cis-retinoic acid, all-trans-retinoic acid, fenretinide

of chemotherapy is used in leukaemia and most subtypes of non Hodgkin lymphoma (NHL), and is sometimes also applied in children with brain tumors either to treat leptomeningeal disease or in an attempt to avoid craniospinal irradiation in young children. Other specialized routes of administration which may be occasionally encountered include isolated limb perfusion for refractory sarcoma or intra-arterial administration of chemotherapy in hepatic tumours.

Toxicity of chemotherapy

The side effects induced by chemotherapy can be divided into acute and long-term toxicities. The latter become more relevant with increasing cure rates and because of the young age of most patients. Since most chemotherapeutic compounds have their mode of action on proliferating cells, some normally dividing tissues are especially at risk for the toxicity of chemotherapy. This includes the bone marrow, gastrointestinal mucosa and hair follicles, and most compounds lead to transient toxicity on these organs. Some drugs may also have a specific toxicity on one or more organ functions, often with implications in the mid to long term. For example, the anthracyclines are well known for their potential cardiac toxicity but this is rarely evident at the time of treatment. Cisplatin and, to a lesser extent, carboplatin may be ototoxic and/or nephrotoxic, whereas the newly developed oxaliplatin lacks this toxicity profile. Methotrexate may have acute renal, liver or CNS toxicity but this is generally not of long-term significance. The use of alkylating agents may result in secondary malignancy and fetility damage: this effect depends on the type and cumulative dose of the alkylating agent used. Epipodophyllotoxins may induce secondary myelodysplasia and/or AML.

The risk of severe late effects may be avoided by reducing cumulative dose exposures or by avoiding the use of compounds with unfavourable toxicity profiles if this can be achieved without compromising cure rates. This also reinforces the need to develop new drugs with novel mechanisms of action, directed against specific biological targets characteristic of a given cancer type (also referred to as targeted therapy). Targeted compounds may induce fewer side effects on healthy tissues although experience in children is still very limited and new (especially long-term) toxicities may emerge. The toxicity profile of the various compounds most commonly used in paediatric oncology is described in Table 4.2. The severity of chemotherapy-induced toxicity can be classified using the system of toxicity developed by the National Cancer Institute, the NCI Common Toxicity Criteria (NCI-CTC available at:http://ctep.cancer.gov/reporting/ctc.html).

Dose intensity

In general, given the dose–effect relationship of a chemotherapeutic compound and its narrow therapeutic window, chemotherapy is usually delivered at maximum tolerated dose (MTD) in order to obtain maximum anti-tumour effect. The concept of dose intensity is defined as the amount of drug administered per unit of time. Strategies which incorporate high-dose intensity have shown proven benefit in several paediatric tumours, for example in Burkitt lymphoma where more than 90 per cent of the patients can now be cured by intensive combination regimens of relatively short duration (see Chapter 17). Dose-intensive regimens demand the shortest intervals possible between sequential courses of treatment and may cause severe toxicity. Improved supportive care protocols (anti-emetic therapy, haematopoietic growth factors, antibiotic and antifungal prophylaxis, transfusion support, etc) have been developed (see Chapter 8), which has allowed further dose intensification without increasing treatment related mortality.

More recently there has been increased interest in metronomic chemotherapy. This is based on the chronic administration of chemotherapeutic agents at relatively low, minimally toxic doses, and without prolonged drug-free breaks. The precise mechanism of action is uncertain and is likely to be multifactorial. Recent findings suggest that, in addition to inhibiting tumour angiogenesis, metronomic chemotherapy might also restore anticancer immune response and induce tumour maturation.

High-dose chemotherapy

Several cytotoxic compounds have a (nearly) linear dose–effect relationship. These compounds are suitable for administration at high doses, especially when the toxicity of these drugs is

Table 4.2 Specific adverse effects of cytotoxic compounds commonly used in pediatric oncology categorized as short-term (days to weeks) and long-term (months to years) side effects. General adverse effects such as bone marrow suppression, gastrointestinal toxicity, and alopecia are not include as these are considered as common to all forms of chemotherapy

Drug	Short-term side effects	Long-Term Side Effects
Asparaginase	Clotting disorders, anaphylactic reactions, pancreatitis, hyperglycemia	Unknown
Bleomycin	Fever, malaise, skin rash	Pulmonary fibrosis
Busulfan	Veno-occlusive disease, seizures, hyperpigmentation	Hyperpigmentation, pulmonary fibrosis, fertility disorders
Carboplatin	Ototoxicity, allergic reactions	Ototoxicity
Cisplatinum	Renal toxicity, ototoxicity, radiosensitization	Renal toxicity, ototoxicity
Cyclophosphamide	Hemorrhagic cystitis	Fertility disorders, secondary leukemia
Cytarabine	Mucositis, rash, conjunctivitis, fever, encephalopathy, seizures, pancreatitis	Encephalopathy
Dactinomycin	Jaundice, veno-occlusive disease, radiosensitization	Unknown
Daunorubicin	Mucositis, cardiomyopathy, radiosensitization	Cardiomyopathy, secondary leukemia
Dexamethasone	Mood disorders, increased appetite, Cushingoid appearance, muscular atrophy, bone demineralization, skin disorders	Bone fractures, avascular femoral head necrosis, vertebral collapse, adrenal suppression
Doxorubicin	Mucositis, cardiomyopathy, radiosensitisation	Cardiomyopathy, secondary leukemia
Epirubicin	Mucositis, cardiomyopathy, radiosensitization	Cardiomyopathy, secondary leukemia
Etoposide (VP 16)	Allergic reactions, mucositis	Secondary leukemia
Fludarabine	Mucositis, fever, pneumonitis, neurotoxicity, hepatitis	Unknown
Idarubicin	Mucositis, cardiomyopathy, radiosensitisation	Cardiomyopathy, secondary leukemia
Ifosfamide	Hemorrhagic cystitis, tubulopathy, encephalopathy, seizures	Tubular and glomerular toxicity, fertility disorders
Irinotecan	Abdominal pain, diarrhea, sweating, hyperlacrimation, salivary excess	Unknown
Melphalan	Mucositis, interstitial pneumonitis	Pulmonary fibrosis, fertility disorders
6-Mercaptopurine	Hepatitis	Unknown
Methotrexate	Hepatitis, mucositis, encephalopathy, renal toxicity	Liver fibrosis, encephalopathy
Mitoxantrone	Mucositis, cardiomyopathy	Cardiomyopathy

(Continued)

Table 4.2 (Continued) Specific adverse effects of cytotoxic compounds commonly used in pediatric oncology categorized as short-term (days to weeks) and long-term (months to years) side effects. General adverse effects such as bone marrow suppression, gastrointestinal toxicity, and alopecia are not include as these are considered as common to all forms of chemotherapy

Drug	Short-term side effects	Long-Term Side Effects
Prednisolone	Mood disorders, increased appetite, Cushingoid appearance, muscular atrophy, bone demineralisation, skin disorders	Bone fractures, avascular femoral head necrosis, vertebral collapse, adrenal suppression
Procarbazine	Allergic reactions, hepatic dysfunction, headache, paresthesia, hallucinations	Fertility disorders
Temozolomide	Lymphocytopenia	Secondary malignancy
Teniposide (VM 26)	Allergic reactions, mucositis	Secondary leukemia
6-Thioguanine	Hepatitis	Unknown
Thiotepa	Headache, encephalopathy, dizziness, allergic reactions, skin rash, fever	Fertility disorders
Topotecan	Mucositis, radiosensitising	Unknown
Vinblastine	Paresthesia, neuralgia, sensory disorders, hypertension, Raynaud's phenomenon	Raynaud's phenomenon
Vincristine	Paresthesia, neuralgia, muscular weakness, sensory disorders, constipa tion, ileus, abdominal cramps, seizures, SIADH	Neurotoxicity

essentially haematological. The use of such high-dose (myeloablative) chemotherapy requires autologous or allogeneic haematopoietic stem cell support, which assures reconstitution of hae-matopoiesis, preventing severe and long-lasting neutropenia with its associated infectious complications. Maximum therapeutic effect is obtained and non-haematological toxicity becomes the dose-limiting factor. High-dose chemotherapy strategies are mostly applied in situations where very good partial or complete remission can be achieved in a chemotherapy-sensitive tumour but with a high risk of relapse. The favourable dose–effect relationship increases the probability of destroying residual malignant cells and/or overcoming cellular mechanisms of drug resistance. The most common examples of chemotherapeutic agents used for high-dose chemotherapy are the alkylating compounds such as cyclophosphamide, busulfan, melphalan, and thiotepa. In relapsed or high-risk leukaemia, myeloablative regimens may also include total body irradiation and immunosuppressive drugs such as fludarabine or monoclonal antibodies directed against T cells. In paediatric solid tumours, high-dose chemotherapy is most often used in neuroblastoma and Ewing sarcoma. Where allogeneic stem cell support is used, predominantly in acute leukaemia, a graft-versus-leukaemia effect may have additional anti-tumour effects beside the cytotoxic effects of chemotherapy and total body irradiation.

Drug resistance

There are several important mechanisms of drug resistance of which the multidrug resistance (MDR) phenotype expressed by some cancer cells is the best characterized. This is caused by the enhanced expression of drug-efflux pumps on the cancer cell membrane. Several proteins are implicated including P-glycoprotein, multidrug resistance proteins 1–8 (MRP), breast cancer resistance protein (BCRP) and the lung resistance-related protein (LRP). High expression of these membrane proteins in the tumour cells has been correlated with a poor outcome in some malignancies in paediatric oncology although the value of such observations remains controversial. Various preclinical models have been developed to circumvent the MDR-related mechanism of drug resistance but clinical trials using MDR blocking agents (for example, verapamil, ciclosporin A, PSC 833) have so far failed to demonstrate a clinical benefit. It is likely that other mechanisms are concurrently or sequentially involved in the development of drug resistance and that these are not circumvented by MDR blocking agents.

Dosing of drugs in paediatric oncology

Body surface area (BSA)

The principle of using BSA for dosing chemotherapeutic compounds in oncology results from pharmacological research between species and between adults and children. These data show that the most reliable method of comparing physiological variables, such as glomerular filtration rate, cardiac output and basal metabolic rate between species and across ages, is by correcting for BSA. Use of body weight instead of BSA results in an unreliable interspecies correction of all mechanisms contributing to the clearance and metabolism of drugs. Although the use of BSA is controversial in adult oncology, the variability of weight and height is so great in children that prescriptions are almost always based on BSA. Moreover, by prescribing cytotoxic drugs per m^2 it remains easier to determine a starting dose for phase I clinical trials in human beings based on the data reported in the toxicological studies in animal models.

BSA can be calculated by formulas or by using nomograms. The 'gold standard' formula was described by Dubois in 1916. Although very reliable, this formula is not easy to use and many other formulas have been validated since, taking into account either weight and height/length or weight only (Table 4.3).

Chemotherapy in infants

Tolerance to chemotherapy at a given dose is poorer in infants when compared to older children and adults. Maturation of the physiological mechanisms that contribute to the pharmacokinetics of drug handling occurs during the first year of life. For example, the water content of the human body decreases from 75 per cent at birth to 60 per cent at 1 year and 55 per cent in adult life. The content of plasma proteins also changes during the first year of life and hepatic drug-metabolizing enzymes (cytochrome P450 isoenzymes, UDP glucuronyltransferase, glutathione metabolizing enzymes) achieve their full physiological activity between 6 and 12 months of age. Glomerular filtration rate attains values comparable to that in adults at the age of 5 months. All these factors contribute to the poorer tolerance of infants to chemotherapy and doses should be reduced in their treatment.

Table 4.3 Formulas for calculating body surface area (BSA), body mass index (BMI) and ideal body weight

Dubois' formula	$BSA = W^{0.425} \times L^{0.725} \times 0.007184$
Mosteller's formula	$BSA = \sqrt{W} \times L/3600$
Formula without using length	$BSA = (4\,W + 7)/(W + 90)$
Body mass index	$BMI\ (kg/m^2) = W/L^2$
Lawrence's formula	Ideal body weight (kg) = $[L-100]-[(L-150)/K]$

Key: BSA = body surface area in m^2; W = body weight in kg; L = body length in cm; K = 4 for males and 2 for females.

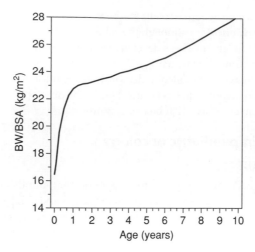

Fig. 4.1 Development of body weight (BW) to body surface area (BSA) ratio during childhood.

In general, chemotherapy in infants should be prescribed as mg/kg body weight instead of mg/m^2 since the relationship between body weight and BSA is different in infants as compared to older children (Fig. 4.1). A dose prescribed in mg/m^2 in an infant will lead to a higher dose than one prescribed in mg/kg (Table 4.4). In very young children (<3 months) even greater caution is required and additional dose reductions are frequently applied.

Chemotherapy in obese patients

Obesity is associated with modifications in body composition that may change the pharmacokinetics of cytotoxic compounds and may result either in inadequate dosing or in increased toxicity. Increased body fat mass will alter the distribution volume of a drug depending on its affinity for fatty tissues and plasma proteins. Fatty degeneration of liver tissue may also modify hepatic metabolizing capacity in obese patients.

The diagnosis of obesity is defined by an increased body mass index (BMI) (Table 4.3). Upper reference values for adults (>18 years) are 23 kg/m^2 in males, and 21 kg/m^2 in females. Overweight and obesity are defined by a BMI >25 and >30 kg/m^2, respectively. In children, BMI changes with increasing age. Upper reference values of BMI which define obesity therefore depend on age. For most cytotoxic compounds, no pharmacokinetic data are available in obese patients and thus it is recommended that chemotherapy is prescribed according to ideal body weight instead of actual body weight to avoid excessive toxicity. In adolescents and young adults, ideal body weight can be

Table 4.4 Comparison between dose prescribed in mg/m^2 *versus* dose in mg/kg in children

Child's characteristics			Dose calculated as		Dose reduction from calculation using mg/kg compared to BSA
Age	Weight	BSA	100 mg/m^2	3.33 mg/kg	
10 year	30 kg	1 m^2	100 mg	100 mg	0%
1 year	10 kg	0.46 m^2	46 mg	33 mg	28%
3 months	6 kg	0.29 m^2	29 mg	20 mg	31%

Key: BSA = body surface area in m^2.

calculated according to the formula by Lawrence (Table 4.3). In younger children the ideal body weight is best determined by the body weight corresponding to the centile of height.

Prescribing chemotherapy in difficult situations

Some patients may require chemotherapy in an acute situation where organ failure (most typically hepatic or renal failure), due either to the malignancy or as a result of previous treatment, limits the clearance of chemotherapy. In such situations chemotherapy doses should be reduced taking into account the type of drug and the mechanisms of clearance that are relevant for that drug. In addition, the potential additional toxicity on the affected organ should be taken into account. Detailed recommendations about dose adaptations are available from other sources.

Intrathecal chemotherapy

It is important to recognize that, compared to adults, the central nervous system (CNS) compartment in a child is proportionally larger than the rest of the body. For example, a child of 4–6 years has a CNS volume of 80–90 per cent compared to the adult brain, while adult BSA is only attained at 16–18 years. This physiological phenomenon requires the prescription of intrathecal therapy (such as methotrexate) in an absolute dose (mg) depending on the age of the patient rather than in mg/m^2.

Pharmacogenetics and drug interactions

Intracellular metabolism contributes to the clearance of drugs by transforming them to metabolites in order to facilitate renal or biliary excretion. Generally, drug metabolites have less or no therapeutic activity although some metabolites may still have a strong cytotoxic effect. Many enzymes are implicated in the biotransformation of drugs, of which the cytochrome P450 isoenzymes, the glucuronidation pathways, and detoxifying enzymes implicated in glutathione metabolism are most relevant. The activity of these enzymes influences the plasma concentration of drugs and thus their concentrations in the tumour tissue.

It is useful to know the metabolic pathways of drugs in order to identify potential drug interactions. Hepatic mechanisms, such as CYP450 enzyme induction or inhibition may dramatically alter the effect of a cytotoxic drug. Phenobarbitone, carbamazepine and phenytoin are all drugs that may induce the activity of the CYP3A4 and CYP2C9 isoenzymes and thus increase the biotransformation and clearance of many cytotoxic drugs. On the other hand, drugs such as fluconazole and itraconazole may inhibit the activity of several CYP isoenzymes, resulting in higher plasma concentrations and increasing toxicity of cytotoxic drugs metabolized by these pathways. Drug interactions should be taken into account when prescribing both chemotherapeutic and other drugs used for supportive care.

As the influence of these pharmacokinetic modifying enzymes has emerged, population-based studies of pharmacogenetics have been undertaken. Genetic polymorphisms of these or other enzymes may result in variable phenotypes resulting in different enzyme activities from patient to patient, and thus in differences in drug clearance. An example of pharmacogenetic variability is encountered in the metabolism of 6-mercaptopurine (6-MP). This drug is inactivated by the enzyme thiopurine methyltransferase (TPMT) and patients with TPMT mutations should therefore be treated with lowered dosages of 6-MP to avoid excessive haematological toxicity. Another example consists of polymorphisms in the gene *UGT1A1* that lead to large differences in the glucuronidation of irinotecan metabolites, and thus in differences in systemic exposure of the active metabolite SN38. Future insights into the genetic polymorphisms of enzymes or receptors implicated in the metabolism of cytotoxic and non-cytotoxic agents may lead to patient-adapted prescription of cytotoxic therapy.

Drug development in pediatric oncology

Overview

There are several factors that influence the development of novel compounds, analogues or formulations for children with cancer:

1. The need for proper safety and efficacy studies in the pediatric population with histologically different subtypes of cancer compared to adults

2. Evaluating outcome when adding a novel compound to an existing treatment regimen

3. Reduction of side effects and studying the effect on growth and development

4. Development of age-adapted pediatric formulations

5. Pharmacokinetic aspects, especially in children below the age of 2 years

6. Market authorization/regulatory factors.

Potential pharmacokinetic differences between children and adults need to be evaluated to ensure pediatric dosing schedules are safe and effective. The use of population pharmacokinetic models has enabled the feasibility of such studies with limited sampling, and is being applied in pediatric oncology. However, in most studies the differences in pharmacokinetic properties between adults and older children are limited and there is a relatively high correlation between the adult and pediatric maximum tolerated dose (MTD). This may be different in very young patients. However, until a few years ago, there was limited interest from the pharmaceutical industry to perform clinical trials in children. By 2003, of more than 100 drugs that had been approved by the Federal Drug Agency (FDA) for the treatment of cancer, information about paediatric use was available in less than 50 per cent of those commonly used in the treatment of pediatric malignancies (see Hirschfield *et al.* 2003 in Further reading). In 2007, following an earlier similar initiative in the USA, new legislation governing the development and authorization of all medicines for use in children, aged 0–17 years, was introduced in the European Union. Regulation EC no. 1901/2006 (the 'Pediatric Regulation') obliges pharmaceutical companies to explore pediatric indications when they want to have a new medicinal product authorized by the regulatory authorities. Early evidence suggests that the regulation is beginning to positively influence industry interest in paediatric drug development.

During the past two decades many new anti-cancer drugs have been developed for adults with (refractory) cancer. Although a minority of these compounds has so far been explored in paediatric oncology, the number of new compounds being evaluated in paediatric oncology is increasing. This is a direct result of the achievements of major academic collaborative groups such as the European consortium 'Innovative Therapies for Children with Cancer' (ITCC) and the phase I consortium of the Children's Oncology Group in North America.

Novel compounds can be broadly classified into the following groups:

1. New cytotoxics or improved analogues of older compounds

2. Targeted compounds (defined by their site of action):
   - Inhibitors of vascular endothelial growth factor (VEGF) signalling
   - Inhibitors of signal transduction pathways, including inhibitors of receptor tyrosine kinases (monoclonal antibodies, small molecules)
   - Compounds acting on cell cycle checkpoints
   - Compounds acting on tumour cell invasion

3. Miscellaneous

Recently developed cytotoxic drugs

Several new cytotoxic compounds and improved analogues have been developed during the past decades. Most new compounds have a slightly different cytotoxic mechanism of action and/or better pharmacological properties as compared to the conventional chemotherapy of the class to which they belong.

The alkylating agent temozolomide (Temodal®, Temodar®) now has an established therapeutic role in the treatment of high-grade glioma with concurrent radiotherapy, although its single-agent activity against high-grade glioma and brainstem glioma is limited (response rates of 5–20 per cent). It is possible that new metronomic dosing schedules may improve efficacy and/or may be more compatible with concurrent radiotherapy. Temozolomide also seems to be active against medulloblastoma, although it has not yet been integrated into first-line chemotherapeutic regimens and is mostly used as salvage regimen.

The taxanes (paclitaxel, docetaxel) inhibit tubulin depolymerization and have been investigated in several early clinical trials in paediatrics. The dose-limiting toxicities observed in phase I clinical trials are fatigue, neutropenia, rash, myalgia (docetaxel) and neutropenia, fatigue, peripheral neuropathy (paclitaxel). Although the anti-tumour activity of the taxanes has not been fully explored, the response rate in the phase II clinical trials is limited and their role has not been established in paediatric oncology. Other tubulin-inhibiting agents such as ixabepilone have also been explored in paediatric oncology with the recent accomplishment of a phase I and phase II clinical trial but its single drug activity seems limited in paediatric solid tumours.

The nucleoside analogue gemcitabine (2',2'-difluorodeoxycytidine, dFdC) has been studied both in leukaemia and solid tumours. In phase I, in ALL and AML, a maximum tolerated dose (MTD) was established at 3600 mg/m^2 when administered weekly for 3 weeks with 1 week rest between courses. Haematological toxicity was dose-limiting. Other toxicities included elevation of serum transaminases, nausea, vomiting, and rash/desquamation. However, a phase II study in ALL and AML concluded that gemcitabine was not effective at the dose and schedule studied. Gemcitabine has also been tested in solid tumours using several schedules. The MTD of gemcitabine given weekly for 3 weeks was 1200 mg/m^2/dose. In a 2-weekly every 4 weeks schedule, doses up to 2100 mg/m^2/dose were considered tolerable. The major toxicity was myelosuppression and the anti-tumour efficacy was limited.

The new platinum compound oxaliplatin has been explored in two phase I clinical trials with distinct schedules, and the recommended dose was determined at 130 mg/m2 every 3 weeks and 90 mg/m2/weekly. DLTs consisted of myelosuppression and sensory neuropathy similar to that observed in adults. Its efficacy as a single agent is limited in pediatric solid tumours. The same conclusion was reached in a recently completed ITCC phase II study of gemcitabine in combination with oxaliplatin in relapsed solid tumours.

Targeted compounds

Kinase inhibitors (monoclonal antibodies, small molecules)

Kinases are also known as phosphotransferases and are enzymes that activate substrates by phosphorylating them. The largest group consists of the protein kinases, including the serine/threonine kinases and the tyrosine kinases. Many tyrosine kinases are transmembrane receptors that transfer information from the extracellular environment to the nucleus. Activation by mutations may lead to constitutive autophosphorylation, and result in proliferation as seen in cancer. Some of these kinases have gained much interest as attractive targets for new anti-cancer treatment strategies. Kinase inhibitors may have several mechanisms of action:

- binding/neutralizing the ligand of the receptor
- inhibition of receptor dimerization
- binding of the receptor often through interfering with the ATP-binding pocket of the transmembrane or intracellular receptor domain
- interfering with intracellular activating phosphorylation steps.

Tyrosine kinase inhibitors (TKI) inhibiting ABL

Imatinib mesylate is a small molecule drug and the prime example of successful inhibition of the tyrosine kinase ABL, which is constitutively active as a result of a translocation between the *BCR* gene on chromosome 22 and the *ABL* gene on chromosome 9 (the Philadelphia chromosome) in chronic myelogenous leukaemia (CML) or Philadelphia-chromosome positive ALL. Only a few phase I and II studies have been performed in pediatrics and approval of imatinib for use in children was mainly granted on extrapolating adult data. In pediatric CML, as in adults, imatinib has changed the existing paradigms of treatment with cytarabine/interferon followed by stem-cell transplantation, and is now a first-line treatment for this disease, achieving high rates of morphological and cytogenetic remissions. In Philadelphia-chromosome positive ALL single agent activity is less marked, but a recent Children's Oncology Group (COG) study combining imatinib with chemotherapy showed a clear improvement in outcome for children treated with the combination compared to historical data.

Imatinib also inhibits the target c-Kit, the receptor for stem cell factor (SCF), and PDGFR-α and -β, a finding which led to its successful introduction in specific solid tumours, notably gastrointestinal stromal tumours (GIST). The mechanism of action of imatinib in solid tumours is probably through inhibition of angiogenesis by decreasing signalling via PDGFR in tumor cells, and, more importantly, in pericytes of tumour vascular stroma. The role of imatinib has been studied in several paediatric tumour types such as Ewing sarcoma and neuroblastoma. Ewing sarcoma cell lines were sensitive to imatinib-mediated apoptosis at clinically achievable concentrations and, in a xenograft model, imatinib treatment resulted in the regression or control of primary Ewing sarcomas. In neuroblastoma, imatinib appeared to have a cytotoxic effect *in vitro* and to increase the efficacy of chemotherapy in neuroblastoma models both *in vitro* and *in vivo*. Despite these data, clinical studies of paediatric patients with refractory or recurrent solid tumours have been disappointing showing very limited efficacy.

Despite the success story of imatinib in CML, it was quickly apparent that new drugs might also give rise to old problems, i.e. the development of resistance, in this case through mutations in *ABL*. These mutations prohibit effective binding of imatinib to the kinase pocket and hence cause resistance. Several second-generation kinase inhibitors are now available, which can still bind despite the presence of a mutation. The best studied second generation inhibitor is dasatinib. Two phase I/II studies in children have been performed, one including mainly solid tumours and one including haematological malignancies only. In general, the drug was well tolerated and appeared effective as salvage treatment in CML and Philadelphia-chromosome positive ALL, although responses were of short duration in the latter group. Tolerability was better than in adults.

Dasatinib targets a variety of other tyrosine kinases, such as c-Kit, SRC, PDGFRβ, and the ephrin receptors EphA and EphB. The SRC family of kinases has been associated with malignant behaviour of many different tumours. SRC is involved in processes such as adhesion, invasion and motility of tumour cells, which contribute to the metastatic potential of tumour cells. Dasatinib shows selective *in vitro* activity with high sensitivity in cell lines of AML (with a gain-of-function *c-Kit* mutation) and rhabdoid tumour although *in vivo,* it had limited activity against solid tumour xenografts. A phase I study in children with solid tumours has recently been completed.

TKIs targeting angiogenesis

Several strategies have been developed to interfere with the process of tumour angiogenesis. Such compounds may decrease signalling through VEGF/VEGFR by inhibiting either the ligand VEGF or one of the receptors of VEGF (flt-1, KDR, flt-4), or inhibit the signalling pathways through platelet-derived growth factor (PDGF) and its receptors (PDGFRα and β). Other compounds may principally target endothelial cells of tumour vessels and some compounds may have multiple effects by acting through various targets, including mechanisms not yet understood.

The humanized anti-VEGF antibody bevacizumab (Avastin®) was the first to demonstrate clinical proof of principle, and has been approved by the US Food and Drug Administration for use in adults at doses of 5–15 mg/kg. Bevacizumab is currently being used in an increasing number of indications in medical oncology. Several preclinical investigations were performed on paediatric tumour models and bevacizumab induced inhibition of tumour angiogenesis in preclinical models of a variety of paediatric tumours with tumour growth reduction in neuroblastoma. A paediatric phase I trial was conducted with bevacizumab by the North American Children's Oncology Group. Bevacizumab was administered intravenously every 2 weeks in 28-day courses with dose-escalation (5, 10, 15 mg/kg) to 21 children with refractory solid tumours. No dose-limiting toxicities were observed and adverse events included infusion reaction, rash, mucositis, proteinuria, and lymphocytopenia. There was neither haemorrhage nor thrombosis. There were no complete or partial responses, but one stable disease lasting more than 6 months was observed in a patient with chondrosarcoma. Further experience in a small series of 10 children with multiply recurrent low-grade gliomas who were treated with the combination of bevacizumab and irinotecan reported substantial responses. It is now being evaluated in combination with standard chemotherapy in patients with metastatic soft tissue sarcoma and high-grade glioma.

Sunitinib (SU11248, Sutent®) is an orally bio available, multi-target TKI with selectivity for VEGFR-1 and -2, PDGFR-α and -β, stem cell factor receptor (KIT) and Fms-like tyrosine kinase-3 (FLT3). Sunitinib has demonstrated clinical efficacy for various adult cancers and is registered in adults for use in metastatic renal cancer and GIST. Sunitinib was explored preclinically in a variety of paediatric tumour models with significant anti-tumour activity against 14 of 34 tested solid tumour xenografts, including 4 of 6 rhabdomyosarcoma, 4 of 5 Ewing sarcoma, and 2 of 3 rhabdoid tumour xenografts. The anti-tumour activity was predominantly tumour growth delay. The clinical experience with sunitinib thus far published is limited to a small series of seven patients with imatinib-resistant GIST. A phase I clinical trial has recently been accomplished within the COG consortium.

Sorafenib (BAY 43–9006, Nexavar®) was initially developed as a targeted compound against melanoma given its selectivity against *BRAF*, especially its mutant variant V300 E. However, the compound proved to be a multitarget TKI, with broad selectivity against the receptor tyrosine kinases VEGFR-1 and -2, PDGFR, c-KIT and RET which are involved in tumour growth, angiogenesis, invasion, and metastasis. Sorafenib is active against renal cell carcinoma and hepatocarcinoma and currently evaluated in clinical trials against other adult cancers. Sorafenib significantly reduced the growth of all paediatric cell lines in a dose-dependent manner. Subtypes of medulloblastoma appeared highly sensitive. Rhabdomyosarcoma, neuroblastoma, and Ewing sarcomas were significantly sensitive *in vitro* to sorafenib at concentrations that are cytostatic to the sensitive adult tumour types. Comparable results were observed with growth inhibition *in vivo* in a variety of paediatric solid tumour models. A phase I clinical trial with sorafenib is being under-taken in paediatric patients with solid tumours in the US.

TKIs targeting EGFRs

Several compounds targeting the epidermal growth factor receptors (EGFRs Her1–4) have been developed in clinical trials in medical oncology. Those compounds that target her1 only are erlotinib (Tarceva®) and gefitinib (Iressa®). The potential role of these compounds in paediatric oncology seems to be limited to high-grade glioma and maybe in extracranial tumours like neuroblastoma. Other compounds target specifically her-2 of which the monoclonal antibody trastuzumab (Herceptin®) is the best-known example with a clear benefit for patients with high-risk breast cancer. The role of trastuzumab in paediatric malignancies has still to be established. A phase II clinical trial with trastuzumab and chemotherapy is ongoing in adolescents and young adults with metastatic osteosarcoma.

Other compounds may have a dual inhibitory effect on Her1 and Her2 (lapatinib) with a potential role in paediatric high grade glioma and/or ependymoma (phase I evaluation is ongoing, see clinicaltrial.gov NCT00095940).

TKIs targeting IGF1R

Since 2008, various compounds targeting the insulin growth factor receptor IGF1R have been investigated in phase I/II trials in paediatrics, since there is growing preclinical evidence that IGF1R signalling seems to contribute to the malignant behaviour of various sarcomas (Ewing sarcoma, osteosarcoma and soft tissue sarcoma). At least five different monoclonal antibodies developed by various companies targeting IGF1R have recently been tested or are being tested in early clinical trials. The results of these trials are currently not publically available and it is still too early to confirm the IGF1R pathway as a valid therapeutic target.

Compounds acting on cell cycle checkpoints

A variety of specific enzymes contribute to the G2/M cell cycle checkpoint. These enzymes have led to therapeutic tools resulting to a mitotic arrest and/or apoptosis. The inhibitors of these enzymes with the most advanced clinical development in medical oncology are the compounds targeting the Polo-like kinases 1–4 and the Aurora kinases A, B or C (predominantly A and B). A phase I trial with AT9283 is underway and it is to be expected that a number of agents acting on the cell cycle will be developed for use in paediatric oncology in the near future.

Monoclonal antibodies in haematological malignancies

Several antibodies are being tested in various stages of development. Rituximab, a chimeric monoclonal antibody directed against CD20, has been used in salvage treatment for CD20-positive NHL, in combination with ICE (ifosfamide, carboplatin, etoposide) chemotherapy, leading to a 60 per cent response rate. In a phase II window study in 136 children with newly diagnosed Burkitt lymphoma or diffuse large B-cell NHL, rituximab was well tolerated, with a response rate of 41.4 per cent. However, to date there are no randomized studies proving that rituximab increases survival in pediatric NHL.

The same is true for gemtuzumab ozogamicin, an anti-CD33 antibody linked to the cytotoxic compound calicheamicin, which has been so far been mainly tested as a single-agent or in combi-nation with standard chemotherapy in pediatric AML. Safety data of combination chemotherapy (cytarabine, mitoxantrone or cytarabine/asparaginase) with gemtuzumab are also available. Despite clear efficacy in these early clinical studies, gemtuzumab was recently taken of the market outside Japan, and it is unclear whether it will be available at a later stage. Of interest is the development of a combination of an anti-CD22 antibody linked to calicheamicin (inotuzumab ozogamicin), which will be evaluated in pediatric ALL, after initial studies showing tolerance and efficacy in adult NHL. Epratuzumab is a naked antibody directed against CD22, which is being tested, but results are not yet available.

Miscellaneous

Differentiation induction, resulting in a maturation of tumor cells, has been utilized as a strategy both in acute promyelocytic leukaemia (APL) and in neuroblastoma. In APL, the value of all-*trans* retinoic acid is mainly in reducing early death by quickly diminishing the bleeding tendency that is characteristic of this disease. Moreover, data from the use of 13-*cis*-retinoic acid in neuroblastoma, given in minimal residual disease setting, now shows clear evidence of survival benefit.

Some compounds may act on mechanisms of tumour tissue integrity and tissue invasion, acting on target such as integrins. Integrins are heterodimer transmembrane receptors for the extracellular matrix that play a role in (endothelial) cell adhesion and cell migration. Cilengitide (EMD 121974) is an inhibitor of integrins and is in early clinical development in (brainstem) high-grade glioma.

Other compounds may decrease tumour cell capacity to repair DNA, for example, PARP1-inhibitors. These compounds may act synergistically with some DNA-damaging agents especially in tumour types that already have a modified capacity for DNA repair (e.g. *BRCA*-mutated tumours).

An example of a compound that may increase the cytotoxicity of conventional chemotherapy (or even of targeted agents) is the inhibitor of heat-shock protein 90 (Hsp-90), a chaperone protein which plays a role in maintaining several signal transduction proteins in a stable conformation. Compounds that target HSP90 are 17-amino-allyl geldanamycin (17-AAG) and 17-(dimethylaminoethylamino)-17-demethoxygeldanamycin (17-DMAG) both of which have so far been developed predominantly in medical oncology.

Inhibitors of intracellular signal transduction pathways such as PI3K inhibitors and mTOR inhibitors (sirolimus, everolimus, and temsirolimus) are being developed in paediatric oncology based on preclinical evidence of activity. The former may play a role in the treatment of relapsed high-grade glioma, the latter is being explored in combination with chemotherapy in various sarcomas. Clinical experience with these compounds is still limited, though rapidly increasing.

Finally, compounds inhibiting proteins involved in apoptosis-regulation (BCL-2, survivin) are also being explored in preclinical paediatric tumour models. There is so far no firm clinical experience with these compounds.

Conclusion

Chemotherapy has a prominent role in the treatment of paediatric malignancies. Several pharmacokinetic and pharmacodynamic mechanisms must be taken into account when administering chemotherapy. These mechanisms may contribute to the clearance, toxicity and/or efficacy of cytotoxic drugs. Examples are age, sex, body composition, genetic polymorphisms, and co-administered drugs.

A new era is emerging characterized by the development of many new agents as a result of advances in molecular biology. Directing drugs against the abnormalities identified only in tumour cells is known as targeted therapy. Such compounds ought to have a better anti-tumour effect and safety profile.

After a long period when there were very few registrations of new drugs for use in children, the regulatory incentives introduced in both North America and Europe should now stimulate research directed towards the identification and evaluation of new drugs in pediatric oncology.

Further reading

Bleyer WA, Dedrick RL (1977). Clinical pharmacology of intrathecal methotrexate. I. Pharmacokinetics in nontoxic patients after lumbar injection. *Cancer Treat Rep* **61**, 703–8.

Boddy AV, Ratain MJ (1997). Pharmacogenetics in cancer etiology and chemotherapy. *Clin Cancer Res* **3**, 1025–30.

Champagne MA, Capdeville R, Krailo M, et al (2004). Imatinib mesylate (STI571) for treatment of children with Philadelphia chromosome-positive leukemia: results from a Children's Oncology Group phase 1 study. *Blood* **104**, 2655–60.

Cheymol G (2000). Effects of obesity on pharmacokinetics: implications for drug therapy. *Clin Pharmacokinet* **39**, 215–31.

Cole TJ, Bellizzi MC, Flegal KM, Dietz WH (2000). Establishing a standard definition for child overweight and obesity worldwide: international survey. *BMJ* **320**, 1240–3.

Dubois D and Dubois EF (1916). A formula to estimate the approximate surface area if height and weight be known. *Arch Int Med* **17**, 863–71.

Frei E, III, Elias A, Wheeler C, Richardson P, Hryniuk W (1998). The relationship between high-dose treatment and combination chemotherapy: the concept of summation dose intensity. *Clin Cancer Res* **4**, 2027–37.

Geoerger B, Doz F, Gentet JC et al (2008). Phase I study of weekly oxaliplatin in relapsed or refractory pediatric solid malignancies. *J Clin Oncol* **26**(27), 4394–400.

Hirschfeld S, Ho PT, Smith M, Pazdur R (2003). Regulatory approvals of pediatric oncology drugs: previous experience and new initiatives. *J Clin Oncol* **21**, 1066–73.

Jacobs S, Fox E, Krailo et al (2010). Phase II trial of ixabepilone administered daily for five days in children and young adults with refractory solid tumors: a report from the children's oncology group. *Clin Cancer Res* **16**(2), 750–4.

Kaspers GJ, Zwaan CM (2007). Pediatric acute myeloid leukemia: towards high-quality cure of all patients. *Haematologica* **92**, 1519–32.

Lee DP, Skolnik JM, Adamson PC (2005). Pediatric phase I trials in oncology: an analysis of study conduct efficiency. *J Clin Oncol* **23**, 8431–41.

McLeod HL, Relling MV, Crom WR et al. (1992). Disposition of antineoplastic agents in the very young child. *Br J Cancer Suppl* **18**, S23–S29.

Meinhardt A, Burkhardt B, Zimmermann M, et al (2010). Phase II window study on rituximab in newly diagnosed pediatric mature B-cell non-Hodgkin's lymphoma and Burkitt leukemia. *J Clin Oncol* **28**, 3115–21.

Mosteller RD (1987). Simplified calculation of body-surface area. *N Engl J Med* **317**, 1098.

Panetta JC, Iacono LC, Adamson PC, Stewart CF (2003). The importance of pharmacokinetic limited sampling models for childhood cancer drug development. *Clin Cancer Res* **9**, 5068–77.

Pieters R, Appel I, Kuehnel HJ, et al (2008). Pharmacokinetics, pharmacodynamics, efficacy and safety of a new recombinant asparaginase preparation in children with previously untreated acute lymphoblastic leukemia- a randomized phase II clinical trial. *Blood* **112**, 4832–38.

Pui CH, Evans WE (2006). Treatment of acute lymphoblastic leukemia. *N Engl J Med* **354**, 166–78.

Reilly JJ, Workman P (1993). Normalisation of anti-cancer drug dosage using body weight and surface area: is it worthwhile? A review of theoretical and practical considerations. *Cancer Chemother Pharmacol* **32**, 411–8.

Schultz KR, Bowman WP, Aledo A, et al (2009). Improved early event-free survival with imatinib in Philadelphia chromosome-positive acute lymphoblastic leukemia: a children's oncology group study. *J Clin Oncol* **27**, 5175–81.

Vassal G, Tranchand B, Valteau-Couanet D et al. (2001). Pharmacodynamics of tandem high-dose melphalan with peripheral blood stem cell transplantation in children with neuroblastoma and medulloblastoma. *Bone Marrow Transplant* **27**, 471–7.

Verschuur AC, Grill J, Lelouch-Tubiana A, Couanet D, Kalifa C, Vassal G (2004). Temozolomide in paediatric high-grade glioma: a key for combination therapy? *Br J Cancer*. **91**(3):425–9.

Zwaan CM, Den Boer ML, Beverloo HB, et al (2006). Dasatinib (SPRYCEL) in Children and Adolescents with Relapsed or Refractory Leukemia: Preliminary Results of the CA180018 Phase I/II Study. *Blood*. **108**, 613a.

Zwaan CM, Kearns P, Caron H, et al (2010). The role of the 'innovative therapies for children with cancer' (ITCC) European consortium. *Cancer Treat Rev* **36**, 328–34.

Zwaan CM, Reinhardt D, Zimmerman M, et al (2010). Salvage treatment for children with refractory first or second relapse of acute myeloid leukaemia with gemtuzumab ozogamicin: results of a phase II study. *Br J Haematol* **148**, 768–76.

Chapter 5

Radiotherapy in paediatric oncology

Mark Gaze and Tom Boterberg

Introduction

Radiotherapy is a key component of treatment for many childhood cancers. The role is usually to improve local control, but in some cases it is part of a curative strategy for metastatic disease. Radiotherapy may also be used in the salvage of relapsed patients and for palliation.

The patient's pathway through radiotherapy

Treatment centres

Children should only receive radiotherapy in centres suitably equipped, staffed and experienced in paediatric radiotherapy, supported by the necessary paediatric backup facilities. This includes radiation oncologists with training and experience in paediatric radiotherapy fully integrated into the core paediatric oncology multidisciplinary team, the availability of play specialists and paediatric anaesthetic facilities, and sufficient on-site paediatric support to deal with emergencies. This may mean that some children cannot receive treatment in the radiotherapy centre closest to their homes. It will need to be explained to families that this inconvenience is offset by improved safety and quality.

Decision making

It is essential that radiation oncologists meet regularly with paediatric haematology and oncology colleagues and radiologists, pathologists, and surgeons to discuss the management of all patients in the light of full diagnostic and prognostic information.

While the decision to treat with radiotherapy is often straightforward, in many cases it is not simple, and discussion is vital. Children with cancer should be treated where possible in appropriate clinical trials, and outside trials radiotherapy should be given according to approved guidelines.

Assessment

The initial consultation will help to make it clear that radiotherapy is an important part of treatment, and confirm that the radiotherapy team is part of the overall team caring for the child. An early introduction to the radiotherapy team is important as it may prevent the family from feeling that radiotherapy is an afterthought, or has been suggested because things have not gone according to plan. A frank discussion should help to allay any misunderstandings about radiotherapy. Early familiarity with the team will reduce subsequent anxieties, and will help to prevent the problems which can arise after delayed referral.

An important part of the initial assessment is to decide whether it is likely that the child will be able to cooperate with the radiotherapy team, be able to tolerate the requirements of immobilization while awake, and feel comfortable being left alone in the treatment room. If not, arrangements will have to be made for preparations and treatment under general anaesthesia.

Informed consent

It is important that families receive accurate and complete information about the indications for, practicalities of, and likely early and late side effects of the radiotherapy required. This should be given verbally by members of the radiotherapy team, and be supplemented by written information. Children should be given relevant information in a sensitive and age-appropriate manner, which may include comics or videos. Families speaking other languages should have the services of an interpreter available at every interaction with the radiotherapy team. Children and their families should have an opportunity for their questions to be answered in full and in an unhurried manner. Often, if there are anxieties about radiotherapy, it is recommended that families have more than one opportunity to discuss the information and ask questions. Finally, the receipt of informed consent for radiotherapy treatment should be documented according to local practice.

Positioning and immobilization

It is essential for the accurate and safe delivery of radiotherapy that the patient does not move during imaging for planning, or treatment. As indicated above, this may require the use of daily general anaesthesia. For young children who are to be treated awake, the input of an experienced play specialist in the preparation can be indispensable.

To minimize movement, an immobilization device may be necessary, for example a head and neck shell fixed to a base board. This will ensure accurate reproducibility of set-up on a daily basis.

Imaging and target volume definition

The art of radiotherapy is to ensure that all areas involved by tumour get an adequate radiation dose, while uninvolved normal tissues receive as little radiation as possible, in order to minimize the risk of adverse effects.

To achieve this, a series of targets is defined on the basis of imaging which is interpreted in the light of the known pathology and likely patterns of spread, and natural barriers. Usually, prior to radiotherapy, a CT scan is performed in the radiotherapy department with the patient immobilized in the treatment position. The images obtained can be fused with other imaging for example MRI or PET scans which define the extent of tumour at critical times such as at diagnosis, following induction chemotherapy or following surgery.

The first step in target volume definition is usually to define the gross tumour volume (GTV) by contouring it slice by slice on the planning CT scan. Even if the tumour has shrunk as a result of chemotherapy, it may still be helpful to outline the original GTV on earlier scans. When this volume is then transferred to the radiotherapy planning CT scan, it indicates the area at risk of recurrence.

The GTV will then be expanded into a clinical target volume (CTV). The CTV includes the original tumour volume plus a margin to encompass any subclinical extension of disease.

The CTV is then expanded by another margin to create the planning target volume (PTV) which takes into account errors and uncertainties in planning and set-up and internal and external motion. The margin between CTV and PTV will depend on the anatomical site and accuracy of immobilization as determined by departmental audit.

It is also necessary to outline organs at risk so that dosimetrists and planning systems can limit the dose received by healthy normal tissues, especially those that are most sensitive to adverse effects from radiation.

Planning and dosimetry

Dosimetrists, working under the guidance of the responsible doctors, will prepare treatment plans, which indicate how the treatment will be delivered, and the doses received by the tumour and normal tissues. Plans should take into account the need to give homogenous irradiation to the PTV while minimizing exposure to organs at risk.

Dose volume histograms (DVH) that show the planned dose to the target volumes and relevant organs at risk should be produced. These allow the doctor to check that the target is receiving full irradiation, and that doses to organs at risk are acceptable. Sometimes achievement of these two things is not practicable. A compromise is then needed with part or all of the PTV receiving less than the ideal radiotherapy dose and/or organs at risk receiving more than is usually recommended. The doctor then approves the best plan, and the DVH document the doses received as a guide to follow-up.

Dose prescription and fractionation

The clinician will specify the total dose to the tumour and the number of fractions in the course (hence the dose per fraction), the course duration, and the type of radiation and its energy. Typically in paediatric radiotherapy a dose per fraction of 1.5 to 1.8 Gy is used. Normally treatments are given once each day, 5 days per week.

There is evidence that prolongation of the overall treatment time may compromise outcome. Compensation should therefore be made for any gap so that the overall treatment time does not exceed that intended. The simplest and best ways of doing this are to treat on days which are normally days off (for example treat on Saturdays around public holidays) or to give two treatments per day, with a minimum inter-fraction interval of 6 hours.

In some cases hyperfractionated (a larger number of smaller fractions than standard) and accelerated (given in a shorter than standard overall time) schedules are used to reduce late effects and overcome repopulation in highly proliferative tumours. This requires more than one treatment a day, and the inter-fraction interval should be at least 6 hours, preferably 8 hours for radical brain treatments. In other cases, hypofractionation (a smaller number of larger than standard fractions) is used for stereotactically guided treatment of small volumes or in palliation.

Verification of treatment accuracy

It is important that radiotherapy is delivered to the highest possible standards. Quality assurance procedures for radiotherapy delivery, particularly geometric variation for set-up errors, are essential. This is usually done with electronic portal imaging or integrated (cone beam) CT scanning. Dose verification may be done with *in vivo* dosimetry.

Supportive care

The blood count should be checked before treatment. Irradiation of anaemic children should be avoided, as anaemia is known to compromise the outcome of radiotherapy. If necessary, a blood transfusion should be given to bring the haemoglobin up to 12 g/dl. Nausea and vomiting can usually be prevented by the use of anti-emetics. Radiotherapy may cause loss of appetite, and nutrition is important, especially in children receiving daily general anaesthesia. The advice of a paediatric dietician and nutritional supplements, naso-gastric or gastrostomy feeding, or even total parenteral nutrition may be needed.

Radiotherapy can be stressful for children, their parents and other family members. This can have both a psychological and practical basis. Psychological supportive care for the family can be very beneficial. Traveling for radiotherapy, or staying away from home, can be expensive. Availability of free family accommodation in a nearby hotel or dedicated hostel for children and young people with cancer is ideal. Families should have access to support from social workers, or other appropriate healthcare professionals who can advise on benefits and other practical issues.

Documentation

It is important that there is a summary of radiotherapy treatment, which is accessible to treating paediatric oncologists and is also available in long term follow-up. This should include adequate patient identifiers and sufficient details of the diagnosis and other principal treatments (i.e. chemotherapy and surgery) to allow it to be read in context.

Follow up

It is important that the patient is followed up in the long term with regard to late effects as well as for local tumour control and survival. Periodic assessments of relevant normal organ function should be systematically documented. Appropriate psychosocial support should be available as the child grows up and reaches maturity to answer questions that might arise and to address proactively other survivorship issues.

Types of radiotherapy

Conventional external beam radiotherapy

The technical aspects of radiotherapy are evolving continuously, so it is difficult to define what might be considered 'conventional' or standard therapy compared with what is historic and what is innovative. Advances in diagnostic imaging and computer science have largely led this progress.

Nowadays, conventional radiotherapy usually implies the use of:

- megavoltage photons (or sometimes electrons for superficial lesions) from a linear accelerator
- target volume definition based on images acquired on a CT simulator
- three dimensional planning with two or more shaped beams in the same plane or in several planes to allow conformal treatment of an irregular volume.

Intensity modulated radiotherapy

Intensity modulated radiotherapy (IMRT) is a way of changing the dose distribution of radiation in tissue by using beams where the amount of energy varies in different parts of the beam. The aim is to achieve the best possible dose distribution, especially where the target has a complex shape and there are adjacent critical structures. This can be achieved in a number of ways of increasing complexity.

The use of additional smaller segment fields to supplement a principal field, or field-in-field boost, is a relatively straightforward method for forward-planned IMRT to reduce non-homogeneity of the delivered dose within a target volume.

Inverse-planned IMRT requires the clinical oncologist to define target volumes and organs at risk as with conventional conformal radiotherapy, and to specify the desired target dose, and constraints on the dose which an organ at risk may be allowed to receive. The planning computer used by the dosimetrist then calculates the best field arrangement to deliver this. This usually uses a larger than conventional number, often five or seven, of beam alignments which may be non-co-planar. A step and shoot approach entails movements of the linear accelerator gantry and multi-leaf collimator between the delivery of each treatment field. A more sophisticated delivery involves dynamic gantry and collimator movements with the beam on.

Whatever form of IMRT is used, the result is to better conform the shape of the high-dose volume to the shape of the target, and to diminish the volume of healthy normal tissue that is incidentally included in the high-dose volume. The price of this is usually low-dose irradiation of a much larger volume of normal tissue than is the case with conventional radiotherapy.

There have been concerns that the low-dose bath effect seen with IMRT may result in a greater number of second cancers than has been the case with conventional radiotherapy. These anxieties have limited the use of IMRT in children. However, IMRT does allow full irradiation of the tumour in some circumstances where, with conventional radiotherapy, it has been necessary to compromise the dose to the tumour in order to respect normal tissue tolerance. Also, it has been recognized that most second cancers occur in or adjacent to the high-dose volume rather than in the low dose area, so the hazards of using IMRT in children may have been overstated. As always in paediatric radiotherapy, it is important to weigh up the likely benefits and potential risks of any proposed treatment very carefully, and make a balanced judgment of what is in the child's best interests.

Stereotactic radiotherapy

Stereotactic radiotherapy has been used for quite some time to treat small intracranial lesions. Accuracy of treatment of small volumes with narrow margins is achieved with the use of a fixed headframe (for a single treatment or radiosurgery) or relocatable headframe (for fractionated courses of treatment).

More recently, interest has developed in stereotactic body radiotherapy for small lesions in, for example, the lungs or liver. As external frames would not be helpful, image guidance is used to ensure accuracy of treatment delivery. Hypofractionated or single treatments are used rather than fully fractionated courses of treatment. So far there has been only limited use of stereotactic body radiotherapy in children.

Image-guided and adaptive radiotherapy

The term image-guided radiotherapy (IGRT) is potentially misleading, as target volume definition has been based on imaging for years. IGRT refers instead to the use of imaging equipment integrated into treatment units to ensure accurate delivery of treatment. The position of the target may be indicated by implanted fiducial markers or by normal anatomy. Imaging is used with each fraction of treatment to ensure that the irradiated volume covers the target volume, which may move during (as with respiration) or between treatments.

Adaptive radiotherapy implies the ability to change the irradiated volume during a course of treatment in response to a change in the target volume. It is dependent on image guidance.

Proton beam radiotherapy

This is a form of particle radiotherapy using high-energy protons produced by a cyclotron or synchro-cyclotron. The advantage lies in the dose distribution that can be achieved with protons. Unlike photons which are exponentially attenuated as they pass through tissue, protons travel for a finite distance, and deposit most of their energy towards the end of their path, the Bragg peak. This means that it is possible to spare, completely, normal tissues beyond the target.

In the treatment of relatively radio-resistant well-defined skull base tumours, cure rates may be increased as higher doses can be delivered to the target with effective sparing of adjacent critical structures like the brainstem. In other circumstances, the dose distributions that can be achieved with protons are advantageous because the dose to normal tissues for a given target dose can be reduced, thereby limiting normal tissue toxicity.

Although proton beam therapy has a long history, there is very little level-one evidence of benefit in the patient's outcome in comparison with photon radiotherapy. Most of the case for the use of proton beam therapy has been made from theoretical predictions. The principal disadvantage of proton beam therapy currently is that the high cost of treatment units means that their availability is very limited. This is likely to change over the next decade.

Brachytherapy

Brachytherapy, with direct implantation of radioactive sources, was a valuable form of treatment decades ago. Interest waned with the introduction of the linear accelerator, which made treatment of deeply seated tumours much easier, the increasing awareness of radiation protection hazards, and the difficulties of achieving a perfect geometrical implant. With the development of machines for remote afterloading of implanted catheters, the radiation protection risks have largely been overcome. The ability to use CT-based planning with varying position and dwell times for the source has got round the need for perfect geometry. These technical advances have lead to a resurgence of interest in brachytherapy in paediatric oncology. In some childhood cancers, brachytherapy allows conformal irradiation of small target volumes with greater sparing of normal tissues than is possible with external beam radiotherapy.

Molecular radiotherapy

This is essentially the use of radiotherapy as a drug. It is possible where a metabolic pathway can be used to allow accumulation of a radionuclide within tumour cells. For example, in patients with well-differentiated thyroid cancer of follicular cell origin, radioactive iodine can be biologically targeted into residual normal thyroid tissue and metastases. In children, lymph node and distant metastases are more common than in adults with thyroid cancer, yet thanks to the use of radioactive iodine this is a highly curable disease.

In neuroblastoma, the catecholamine analogue meta-iodobenzylguanidine (mIBG) can be used for diagnostic scintigraphy (^{123}I-mIBG) and for therapy (^{131}I-mIBG). Therapeutic mIBG is recognized as an established palliative treatment, and it may also have value if used intensively in patients with refractory disease as part of a multi-modality strategy for cure.

Side effects of treatment

Factors affecting radiation injury to normal tissues

The incidence and severity of adverse reactions to radiotherapy among children treated for cancer are related to several factors, knowledge of which allows for new strategies to be devised that may reduce adverse effects without compromising the chances of cure. These factors include: whether or not radiotherapy is used at all; the total dose used; the dose per fraction; the volume and type of tissue irradiated; the type of radiation used; the use of concomitant chemotherapy; and, not least, the age of the patient at the time of treatment.

Early side effects

Early or acute side effects occur during, or in the first weeks after, radiotherapy. They are the result of the depletion of stem cells in the healthy tissue surrounding the tumour area to be irradiated. In most cases they subside with time or supportive therapy only, although some of them may be life threatening and require early interruption of therapy.

The most common early side effects are skin reactions like erythema and alopecia, and mucositis-like stomatitis, oesophagitis, cystitis, and diarrhoea, all depending of the site of the body to be treated. Nausea and vomiting may occur in case of abdominal irradiation. Fatigue is a general and frequently encountered early effect which may take several months to resolve. Many of these side effects can also be aggravated by the concurrent use of chemotherapy, especially actinomycin and anthracyclines. Chemotherapy may even mimic side effects of radiotherapy at sites where no radiation is given, requiring appropriate care and explanation to the parents.

Late side effects

Late side effects are defined as toxicity occurring or persisting from three months onwards after radiotherapy. They are usually irreversible and sometimes worsen with time. Therefore, all care should be given to prevent this type of side effect. On the other hand, some of these side effects are very difficult to prevent and should be considered as 'the price to be paid' for cure. Finding the right balance is a huge challenge for doctors, patients, and their parents.

Late central nervous system side effects

Although the number of neurons usually does not increase after birth, the brain matures by the development and branching of axons and the formation of new synapses. This process mostly takes place within the first 3 years of life and is almost complete by the age of 6, although it continues at a much lower rate till the end of puberty. Radiotherapy may affect this process by killing astrocytes and oligodendrocytes, thus causing demyelinization. Radiotherapy also affects vascular endothelial cells. Mostly these effects are irreversible, although sometimes a transient somnolence syndrome is seen. This is characterized by drowsiness, apathy and irritability and usually occurs 1 to 2 months after the end of treatment. It is self-limiting within 12 weeks of its onset.

Even at rather low doses, whole brain irradiation may lead to functional disturbances in the brain, although no obvious structural changes can be observed. The most common side effects are neurocognitive deficits: lower IQ, worse short-term memory, lower speed of processing new information, and concentration difficulties. In medulloblastoma, safe replacement of craniospinal irradiation by chemotherapy has proved challenging. Despite its risk for late central nervous systems (CNS) side effects, craniospinal irradiation is still standard treatment for older children and parents should be well informed about this. Chemotherapy can be used to allow postponing radiotherapy until a more suitable age of the child to receive radiotherapy to the brain. However, it should be noted that the neurocognitive deficits are usually limited if small volumes are treated, even at high doses and in small children.

High doses or re-irradiation may lead to brain necrosis. This may develop years after treatment and may even mimic tumour recurrence. Steroids are commonly used for treatment, and in some cases resection may be necessary to stop the process. Concurrent radiosensitizing chemotherapy increases the risk to develop brain necrosis.

Necrosis of the spinal cord is a very serious complication leading to irreversible paralysis. Fortunately it is only very rarely encountered as great care is taken to keep the dose to the spinal cord within safe limits.

Radiotherapy may damage blood vessels, and this in turn can lead to neurotoxicity. Patients with neurofibromatosis type 1 are at increased risk. Moya moya may lead to strokes. Cavernous haemangiomas or cavernomas are being recognized increasingly commonly after brain radiotherapy. Usually these are incidental finding on surveillance MRI scans. Sometimes a cavernoma may bleed into the brain. This may be either a minor bleed without overt brain damage, or rarely a catastrophic haemorrhage with resulting neurodisability or death.

Late renal side effects

Acute renal side effects are usually rare, but long-term effects may be important and include chronic renal failure, hypertension, and anaemia. The development of these conditions is insidious and takes several years after treatment. Careful follow-up of patients who received abdominal radiotherapy is therefore very important. Concurrent chemotherapy like cisplatin or previous surgery to the kidney may necessitate lowering the dose, at least to part of the kidney. In patients who have undergone nephrectomy, special attention is needed to spare the contralateral kidney as much as possible, not only to preserve its function *per se*, but also not to hinder the compensatory hypertrophy.

Late musculoskeletal and soft tissue side effects

In adults, muscles and bones are very radioresistant. In children, muscles and bones are in full development and these dividing tissues are therefore very sensitive to radiation, especially the epiphyseal growth plates. A dose around 12–15 Gy will impair the chondroblast function and have an adverse effect on bone growth. Avascular necrosis is also possible and the risk is higher if concurrent steroids are to be given. The effect on growth is usually greatest following the onset of puberty, when the growth spurt starts. Disproportion between body parts may not only have functional implications, but also leads to psychological and social problems.

Spinal irradiation will result in shorter height, but may also be accompanied by deformities. Even if all care has been taken to uniformly irradiate the involved vertebrae, flank surgery and radiation-induced hypoplasia of the unilateral paraspinal and abdominal muscles may contribute to the development of scoliosis. Partial irradiation of the head and neck region can lead to facial bone hypoplasia and consequent asymmetry of the face. When growth is complete, plastic surgery may sometimes be used to improve cosmetic appearances. Radiation-induced impaired dental development may be aggravated by an increased risk of dental caries if xerostomia develops after irradiation of the salivary glands.

Thoracic irradiation including the breast bud, or the developing breast in pubertal girls, may lead to hypoplasia. Plastic surgery for breast augmentation to restore symmetry may be considered once growth is complete. Irradiation of the developing breast raises the risk of breast cancer developing subsequently. Patients at risk should have screening performed as part of their long term follow-up from an earlier age than is standard for breast cancer screening.

Late pulmonary side effects

Radiation pneumonitis usually develops between 3 and 6 months after radiotherapy. Cough and dyspnoea are the most common symptoms and diffuse infiltrates can be seen on imaging. If no spontaneous remission occurs, steroid treatment may be needed. In some cases, pneumonitis will lead to lung fibrosis, although fibrosis can also be seen without preceding pneumonitis. Whole lung irradiation to doses of 15 Gy is considered safe and without clinically important consequences, although lung function tests usually reveal some degree of restrictive disease at adult age. Bleomycin, actinomycin and busulfan are radiosensitizing chemotherapeutic agents and should be avoided or only used with great care in combination with radiotherapy on the lungs. Anaesthetists should be aware of oxygen toxicity in patients treated with bleomycin and radiotherapy. Obviously, smoking should be firmly discouraged, but especially following lung radiotherapy.

Late cardiac side effects

Severe cardiac damage has been seen in the past, including cardiomyopathy, valvular disease, and myocardial infarction. However, it should be noted that these patients had large volumes (often nearly the whole heart) treated with high doses, up to 45 Gy or higher. Currently, the use of radiotherapy has been reduced, as have volume and dose. The main reason for cardiac toxicity nowadays is probably not the dose to the ventricles (which may in part support doses of 50 Gy or more), but to the valves and coronary arteries. Patients treated with radiotherapy on the heart should be encouraged to have a healthy life style with enough physical exercise, regular blood pressure checks and without smoking or excessive intake of fatty food. Finally, the use of anthracyclines also plays a role in the development of cardiomyopathy.

Late endocrine side effects

Most endocrine deficiencies result from irradiation of the hypothalamic–hypophyseal axis. They may develop very insidiously and years after radiotherapy, so close follow-up is necessary. Doses of as low as 18 Gy can be sufficient to impair growth hormone secretion after a period of 18 months or 2 years. Above 36 Gy, growth hormone secretion may be totally stopped and at doses above 40 Gy other hormones like ACTH, TRH, and the gonadotrophins may be affected. Hyperprolactinaemia and early puberty may also develop. Hormone replacement therapy should be started as soon as it is judged safe.

Radiotherapy above about 20 Gy to the thyroid gland increases the risk of primary hypothyroidism. In patients treated with doses around 40 Gy, the risk of developing hypothyroidism is as high as 50%. Even compensated hypothyroidism, where the thyroid-stimulating hormone (TSH) is elevated but the T3 and T4 are within the normal range, should be treated with thyroid hormone replacement therapy to reduce the risk of a raised TSH level over a prolonged period stimulating the development of thyroid cancer.

Late side effects on fertility

Spermatogenesis is especially radiosensitive. A dose as low as 15 cGy (0.15 Gy) is enough to result in a reversible reduction of the sperm count and permanent sterilization has been observed at cumulative doses of 1–2 Gy. Small fractionated doses seem to be more toxic than a single fraction dose. Therefore adequate shielding of the testicles from radiation, for example during pelvic radiotherapy, should be undertaken if possible. A dose above 10 Gy usually results in permanent azoospermia. If possible and indicated, semen cryopreservation or testicle biopsy cryopreservation should be organized in post-pubertal boys before any radiotherapy starts. Testosterone production by the Leydig cells is usually not affected by doses below 20 Gy.

In girls, permanent sterility can be seen at an ovarian dose of 8 Gy or higher. Hormonal deficit develops from 12 Gy onwards and is usually permanent above 20 Gy. Until some years ago, avoiding irradiation of the ovaries or oophoropexy (surgical relocation of the ovary outside the irradiated volume) were the only possibilities to protect the ovarian function in girls who needed radiotherapy to the pelvic region. Partial ovarian cryopreservation and follicle cryopreservation are new techniques that allow preservation of fertility. However, even partial irradiation of the uterus results in a higher risk of intra-uterine death, stillbirth or a child with a low birth weight, due to the uterus or cervix being partially less well developed. Sometimes treatment does not lead to complete infertility, but female survivors of childhood cancer may have their reproductive period reduced by premature ovarian failure and an early menopause. This should be discussed with young women attending long-term follow up clinics.

Late ocular side effects

The radiosensitivity of the eye depends on which part is irradiated. The retina and optic pathways are rather resistant and may tolerate doses up to 54 Gy without major toxicity. Above 54 Gy, optic neuritis and permanent blindness may develop. By contrast, the lens is very radiosensitive and cataract formation may occur after doses as low as 2–6 Gy. However, lens replacement is an effective and safe treatment for these patients. Irradiation of the lacrimal gland may result in dry eye syndrome, a very painful condition that may require enucleation. The dose constraints are not very clear: 40 Gy is considered as acceptable, although less than 26 Gy to 50% of the volume is probably safer.

Late hepatic side effects

The tolerance of the liver before hepatitis and liver failure due to atrophy and the development of fibrosis, depends on the total dose, the volume, concurrent chemotherapy, and previous surgery.

A mean dose of 30 Gy to the entire liver can be safe if part of it (25%) receives a dose of 10 Gy or less and no previous surgery was performed or concurrent chemotherapy is needed. After partial hepatectomy, irradiation of the regenerating liver should be performed with great care, excluding as much liver as possible. Combined with actinomycin, the upper dose limit may need reduction to 15 Gy. Total body irradiation (TBI), or other hepatic radiotherapy combined with chemotherapy, may result in veno-occlusive disease.

Second cancers

All patients who have survived cancer are at risk of developing a second cancer. This may be due to their genetic background, epigenetic risk factors and, last but not least, previous treatment with chemotherapy and radiotherapy. All of these factors may influence each other, making it even more complicated to assess that risk and to counsel patients with regard to secondary prevention. Patients with DNA repair deficiencies like xeroderma pigmentosum are particularly sensitive to radiotherapy and the development of second tumours after radiotherapy. Girls treated at or just before puberty for mediastinal Hodgkin lymphoma are at higher risk to develop breast cancer and should therefore be screened earlier than the general population. Basal cell carcinomas are often seen on irradiated skin. Radiotherapy to the thyroid may not only result in hypothyroidism, but also in the development of thyroid cancer.

Compromising the chance of survival by omitting radiotherapy in the hope of minimizing late effects including second malignant neoplasms, is not an attractive option. Therefore, patients should receive radiotherapy where indicated. The knowledge that they are at risk of developing a second tumour or other late effects justifies their life-long follow up by a multidisciplinary team.

Further reading

Alvarez JA, Scully RE, Miller TL et al.(2007) Long-term effects of treatments for childhood cancers. *Curr Opin Pediatr* **19**, 23–31.

Bhandare N, Kennedy L, Malyapa RS, Morris CG, Mendenhall WM (2008) Hypopituitarism after radiotherapy for extracranial head and neck cancers in pediatric patients. *Am J Clin Oncol* **31**, 567–72.

Bölling T, Könemann S, Ernst I, Willich N (2008) Late effects of thoracic irradiation in children. *Strahlenther Onkol* **184**, 289–95.

Carver JR, Shapiro CL, Ng A et al. (2007) ASCO Cancer Survivorship Expert Panel. American Society of Clinical Oncology clinical evidence review on the ongoing care of adult cancer survivors: cardiac and pulmonary late effects. *J Clin Oncol* **25**, 3991–4008.

Castellino S, Muir A, Shah A et al. (2010) Hepato-biliary late effects in survivors of childhood and adolescent cancer: a report from the Children's Oncology Group. *Pediatr Blood Cancer* **54**, 663–9.

Fossati P, Ricardi U, Orecchia R (2009) Pediatric medulloblastoma: toxicity of current treatment and potential role of protontherapy. *Cancer Treat Rev* **35**, 79–96.

Hodgson DC, Hudson MM, Constine LS (2007) Pediatric Hodgkin lymphoma: maximizing efficacy and minimizing toxicity. *Semin Radiat Oncol* **17**, 230–42.

Indelicato DJ, Keole SR, Shahlaee AH, Shi W, Morris CG, Marcus RB Jr (2008) Definitive radiotherapy for Ewing tumors of extremities and pelvis: long-term disease control, limb function, and treatment toxicity. *Int J Radiat Oncol Biol Phys* **72**, 871–7.

Ness KK, Morris EB, Nolan VG et al. (2010) Physical performance limitations among adult survivors of childhood brain tumors. *Cancer* **116**, 3034–44.

Puri DR, Wexler LH, Meyers PA, La Quaglia MP, Healey JH, Wolden SL (2006) The challenging role of radiation therapy for very young children with rhabdomyosarcoma. *Int J Radiat Oncol Biol Phys* **65**, 1177–84.

Selo N, Bölling T, Ernst I et al. (2010) Acute toxicity profile of radiotherapy in 690 children and adolescents: RiSK data. *Radiother Oncol* **97**, 119–26.

Timmermann B, Schuck A, Niggli F et al. (2007) Spot-scanning proton therapy for malignant soft tissue tumors in childhood: First experiences at the Paul Scherrer Institute. *Int J Radiat Oncol Biol Phys* **67**, 497–504.

Bölling T, Ernst I, Pape H et al. (2010) Dose-Volume Analysis of Radiation Nephropathy in Children: Preliminary Report of the RiSK Consortium. *Int J Radiat Oncol Biol Phys* **80**, 840–4.

Waber DP, Turek J, Catania L et al. (2007) Neuropsychological outcomes from a randomized trial of triple intrathecal chemotherapy compared with 18 Gy cranial radiation as CNS treatment in acute lymphoblastic leukemia: findings from Dana-Farber Cancer Institute ALL Consortium Protocol 95–01. *J Clin Oncol* **25**, 4914–21.

Wright KD, Green DM, Daw NC (2009) Late effects of treatment for wilms tumor. *Pediatr Hematol Oncol* **26**, 407–13.

Chapter 6

Clinical trials in childhood cancer

Kathy Pritchard-Jones and Maria Grazia Valsecchi

Introduction

Childhood cancer was regarded as almost universally fatal until the first clinical trials performed by Sidney Farber in the late 1940s showed that it was possible to induce temporary remissions in childhood leukaemia. Over the ensuing decades, clinicians have organized themselves into national and then international co-operative groups, with the aim of conducting clinical trials to improve outcomes in these rare diseases. Such collaborative efforts have optimized the dose intensity and combinations of multi-agent conventional chemotherapy and have helped define the role of surgery and radiotherapy to achieve maximum overall survival. This means that in the early 21st century, approximately 80 per cent of children newly diagnosed with cancer, who are treated in countries where participation in clinical trials is widely available, can expect to be long-term survivors. However, these high overall survival rates present challenges for future trial design, to secure further incremental improvements in survival or to demonstrate survival equivalence from the promising targeted agents that may have reduced side effects. Recent advances in understanding cancer biology have defined even smaller subgroups of childhood cancers according to molecular signatures. This means that international recruitment is essential to conduct trials within a reasonable time frame. Such collaboration across linguistic and cultural boundaries presents not only legal and regulatory hurdles but also challenges the childhood cancer research community to reappraise their individual therapeutic preferences. The introduction of new paediatric regulations in North America and Europe should encourage manufacturers of new anti-cancer drugs to support the whole process.

This chapter will review how the conventional approaches to reliably defining the benefit of a new drug or a new treatment strategy must be adapted.

Design and implementation of clinical trials in childhood cancer

For a clinical trial to have the best chance of success, it must ask a clear question that is seen as important both to the clinicians who will implement the trial and the patients who will participate. For these reasons, early engagement with families affected by childhood cancer is key: if a trial question cannot be explained easily to those who represent the patient group, then it will be even more difficult to be understood by parents at the distressing time of initial diagnosis of cancer in their child. The issue of study design is equally crucial and, quoting Sir David R. Cox, 'a seriously defective design may be incapable of rescue even by the most ingenious of analyses; a good design may lead to conclusions so clear that simple analyses are enough'. The design of a study basically aims at answering reliably the research question by both minimizing biases (i.e. systematic errors that may deviate the estimate of interest from its 'true' unknown value) and by maximizing precision (i.e. accuracy of estimates, through control of random errors with appropriate sample size).

Background definitions

Clinical trials are traditionally classified into four phases (I–IV) following the stages of pharmacological development of new drugs for human use:

- **Phase I** is the earliest stage, carried out to investigate pharmacokinetics and safety of the new product, so as to establish the most tolerable dose
- **Phase II trials** study the safety and the activity profiles on a larger scale. They may define disease types or subgroups with better response rates and, hence, lead to
- **Phase III trials**, in which the new treatment is compared to an alternative (an established 'standard of care' or placebo). Here, the aim is to demonstrate improved efficacy or increased safety with equal efficacy
- **Phase IV trials** are performed, usually on an observational basis, after the new intervention has received regulatory approval, and aim at obtaining additional information about risks (e.g. rare but serious side effects, long-term side effects), benefits (long-term outcomes), and optimal use.

Of note, in these definitions, the new product's beneficial property is either referred to as activity or efficacy, with two different meanings. **Activity** relates to the biological activity and to disease control, while **efficacy** relates to an outcome measure that unequivocally reflects tangible benefits to patients. Examples are the impact of a drug/therapeutic strategy on response, either morphological or molecular (activity), as compared to the impact on event free survival or survival (efficacy).

This classification into Phase I–IV trials has recently been criticized because it does not provide a general terminology able to accommodate the development of medical products that do not necessarily fit that of traditional pharmaceuticals (e.g. biologically targeted agents). Piantadosi proposed a more flexible and general approach that classifies studies on the basis of their principal aim, as follows:

- **Early-development studies** (translational or treatment-mechanism testing studies)
- **Middle-development studies** (assessing treatment tolerability)
- **Late-development studies** (including comparative studies as well as expanded safety or post-marketing studies). The traditional classification is easily recognized within this new 'descriptive' one.

Early-development studies include translational trials and the name reflects their purpose: connecting laboratory findings to clinic and vice versa. A more traditional early-phase study is the one focussed on understanding the treatment mechanism and the dose-safety profile, in a context guided by a biological model. At this stage, biomarkers that are associated with the desired effect on the biological target should be developed (pharmacodynamic studies).

Assessment of the clinical outcome of the new treatment is formally introduced in Middle-development studies, where its relationship to safety and activity is studied. This stage is particularly important when various new compounds/interventions are available and it is necessary to select out the more promising ones. Phase II trials are a typical example. Given the developmental purpose, they usually involve a broader definition of activity, for instance utilizing biomarkers (e.g. tumour or host genotype or surrogate marker in peripheral blood lymphocytes associated with target inhibition) or an early response (e.g. complete remission rate in leukaemia) to better identify the patient population who may benefit. In specific circumstances, Middle-development studies can comprise a randomized question, when there are two or more new promising treatments and the primary objective is to select the one to be considered for a successive comparative trial.

Comparative trials are the most important among Late-development studies and are focussed on questions of comparison of treatment efficacy (as such they correspond to classical Phase III trials). These represent the gold standard for gathering evidence in medical research as they are designed to minimize bias through control over treatment assignment, systematic errors and ascertainment of endpoints, and are completed by predefined analysis. Replication of trials and consolidation of their results with meta-analyses further increase the credibility of conclusions. A key feature in comparative trials is equipoise, defined as the state in which any rational, informed person (patient, clinician or researcher) does not favour a treatment over the other(s) being studied. This condition of genuine uncertainty is fundamental in clinical research comprising a randomization procedure.

Overview of clinical studies in childhood cancer

Phase I trials

Phase I trials are nearly always 'first in child' studies rather than 'first in man'. In other words, a new anti-cancer drug is only offered to children with cancer when there is already some knowledge of the dose tolerated by adults and the expected side effects. This reduces the number of children who may otherwise be exposed to a potentially subtherapeutic dose and gives clinicians and families some reassurance about what toxicities to expect. However, there may be unpredictable side effects in the growing child and this approach is not applicable to the introduction of a new agent designed against a target that is unique to cancer in the paediatric age group.

A conventional phase I trial determines the maximum tolerated dose (MTD) of a drug in the patient group under investigation, gives a preliminary indication of the toxicity profile and whether the acute phase is reversible, and introduces the concept of 'dose limiting toxicity' (DLT). In adults, blood sampling for pharmacokinetic analysis is mandatory, in order to determine if the dose and schedule achieves sustained blood levels of the active agent equivalent to those required for activity in preclinical models. Dose escalation occurs between successive cohorts of patients and is based on the assumption that the greater the dose, the greater the likely anti-tumour activity but also the more likely there is to be toxicity. In the conventional '3 x 3' design, three patients are entered at each dose level and if no DLT (i.e. grade 3 or 4 toxicity) is observed, the dose is escalated to the next predetermined level. If one patient experiences a DLT, then the cohort is expanded to six patients. This cycle continues until two patients (out of three or six) experience DLT, the MTD is then specified as the previously tested dose level. Sometimes, a predetermined maximum feasible dose is specified, based on the pharmaceutical properties of the agent.

Variations to the '3 x 3' design have been proposed to accelerate patient recruitment and reduce the time periods for which a trial is suspended for observation for potential toxicity. The 'rolling 6' design permits continued enrolment of up to six patients at each dose level, pending toxicity evaluation of the first three patients enrolled. The 'continuous reassessment method' aims to enroll each patient at the current best estimate of the MTD, using all information available after the first toxicity has been observed. Other methodological adaptations have been developed to include 'time to event' in modeling the dose–toxicity relationship and summary toxicity scores that can take account of a multiplicity of organ toxicities and moderate grade events, all of which may be important considerations in testing new drugs in young children.

Phase II trials

A phase II trial is an uncontrolled trial for obtaining an initial estimate of the anti-tumour activity of an agent. The purpose is to determine with a reasonable degree of confidence whether the new anti-cancer agent has sufficient activity against a specified tumour type as to warrant its further development or evaluation in that tumour type. A further consideration is to minimize the number of patients treated with a drug of low activity. The classical study design comprises a single arm, multi-stage (usually two stage) recruitment plan with the endpoint of anti-tumour efficacy. The statistical analysis is based on testing the null hypothesis that the true response rate is less than some uninteresting level, p0 (often set at 0.20 or 20 per cent). Certain other parameters must be predefined: p1, the minimum desired response rate for the drug to be considered interesting, the type I error, alpha, which is the probability of wrongly rejecting the null hypothesis (i.e. concluding that the treatment is efficacious when the true response rate is no greater than p0), and the type II error, beta, the probability of wrongly concluding that the drug is ineffective. If p0 is set at 0.20, p1 at 0.40 and alpha and beta at 0.10, then the Simon's optimum design would stop the trial after evaluation of 17 patients if three or fewer showed a response. If more than three patients responded, then recruitment would continue to a total of 37 patients, at which evaluation more than 10 patients would need to have responded to conclude the treatment is efficacious.

Such a design presents practical problems in childhood cancer studies. First, the endpoint of response may take several weeks to manifest, leading to periods of suspension of recruitment between the first and second stage, which can present difficulties for clinicians and patients waiting to be enrolled. Second, the fortunate reality is that there are very few available patients who are eligible for early phase trials in childhood cancer, due the effectiveness of current therapies for most newly diagnosed patients. Third, many of the patients with relapsed or progressive disease do not have readily 'measurable' disease; that is, a soft tissue lesion visible on cross-sectional imaging. Instead, children with relapsed neuroblastoma and sarcomas may have only bone or bone marrow disease, reducing the number of eligible patients. Hence, a classical phase II trial testing efficacy in a single or restricted range of childhood cancers inevitably requires international collaboration in order to recruit in a reasonable time frame of 18–24 months. This presents practical and financial challenges for implementation.

Early drug development studies of targeted therapies in childhood cancer present new challenges. For example, only rare subpopulations of childhood leukaemias would theoretically benefit from tyrosine kinase inhibitors for BCR-ABL+ ALL or FLT3 inhibitors in AML (or infants with ALL) whose leukemic cells have FLT3 internal tandem duplications. These therapies open a different scenario as the dose-limiting toxicity approach is generally not appropriate and because the clinical development may be aimed primarily at assessing the combination of the target agent with standard agents. When a phase II trial does not use the new drug as a single agent, activity data become difficult to interpret because there might be an unquantifiable response due to the underlying therapy. Even if historical data are available on the adopted underlying standard therapy, these may not be fully appropriate for the patient mix on which the phase II study is conducted. These considerations stimulated the development of randomized Phase II designs such as the screening design or selection design (see Simon *et al.* 1985 in Further reading). Randomized phase II studies are smaller than phase III studies (as they look for large differences and relax the type I error rate), they tend to be quicker, as they assess activity (or early intermediate endpoints) rather then efficacy and are applied to high-risk patient populations. For these reasons they should not compromise the conduct of a definitive phase III study on the promising new drug combination on the population of newly diagnosed patients.

Phase III trials

Phase III trials in childhood cancer are generally offered to newly diagnosed patients. They are designed to be 'low risk' to participants in terms of not compromising their chance of cure, and the best interests of the child are prioritized above any research objectives. These trials usually compare the current best known treatment (the standard arm) against a modification of that treatment (the experimental arm), and are designed to test whether there is either an improvement in efficacy or the same efficacy with reduced toxicity. In designing a trial, the number of children who can potentially be recruited in order to ensure sufficient statistical power must be anticipated. For most childhood cancers, the numbers that need to be recruited into a randomized trial are large in comparison with the annual numbers of children diagnosed in an average-sized European country per year (Tables 6.1 and 6.2). Optimal sample size in clinical trials depends strongly on the target difference the trial aims to detect: the smaller the difference, the greater the number of participants that needs to be enrolled. The required sample size can easily reach thousands of patients when the study is powered to detect less than a 10 per cent absolute increase in event-free survival (EFS). Such relatively modest, yet clinically important improvements are to be expected with more efficient definition of therapeutic strategies using existing chemotherapeutic agents. Even for the high-risk cancers, where patients have a dismal prognosis and new experimental therapeutic approaches offer hope of more marked improvements, required sample sizes are in the hundreds, yet these high-risk cancers generally represent small subgroups.

Since the 1970s, many countries have developed national childhood cancer study groups, which have stimulated the development of tumour-specific committees to design and run clinical trials. High rates of participation in national clinical trials have been achieved through the active engagement of clinicians and patients in specialist treatment centres and through national consensus. However, even for the more common childhood cancers, achieving the numbers required for a robustly powered trial within a reasonable time-span (normally 5 years' recruitment) ideally requires participation from several countries. This adds to the expense and the time required to

Table 6.1 Approximate number of newly diagnosed cases/yr and expected number of deaths/yr for the commoner subgroups of childhood cancer diagnosed before age 15 years, expected in a European country, total population ~60 million

Diagnostic subgroup	Expected no. of cases/year*	Expected no. of deaths/year*
Acute lymphoblastic leukaemia	372	71
Acute myeloid leukaemia	69	26
Hodgkin lymphoma	58	<2
Non-Hodgkin lymphoma	82	16
Medulloblastoma	70	31
Astrocytomas	155	33
Neuroblastoma	89	38
Retinoblastoma	43	2
Renal tumours	81	13
Hepatoblastoma	11	3
Osteosarcoma	31	10
Ewing sarcoma	22	6
Rhabdomyosarcoma	55	17
Malignant germ cell tumours	31	2

*Estimated from population-based registration and mortality figures for Great Britain (Stiller C, 2007) and Europe (Steliarova-Foucher et al, 2006).

Table 6.2 Number of subjects needed in different scenarios of superiority and non-inferiority trials with two parallel groups of equal allocation and comparison of event-free survival (EFS) based on log-rank test (one-sided test, type I error 0.025 and 0.80 power)

Standard treatment 5-year EFS	Standard treatment Δ in 5-year EFS*	Total number of subjects (events)
25%	+20%	167 (109)
25%	+15%	280 (189)
60%	+10%	711 (249)
60%	+5%	2897 (1086)
90%	−4%	2077 (249)
90%	−3%	3554 (409)

*A positive Δ indicates the target improvement and a negative Δ indicates the target non-inferiority margin that the trial aims to detect. The number of subjects to be enrolled in each treatment group is half the total number reported in the last column.

design and implement such trials and can mean national compromise in terms of accepting what is defined as the 'standard' arm. Nonetheless, expansion of recruitment from national to international communities has been largely successful, although it has sometimes required an innovative approach. For example, a study design that prospectively used the principles of meta-analysis was adopted in an international trial on intensification of maintenance treatment in ALL.

In the rarer paediatric cancers or in specific subgroups, international cooperation is often the only way to produce solid evidence and to improve clinical practice. Thus, when the SIOPEL group of the International Society of Paediatric Oncology (SIOP) commenced clinical trials in the very rare tumour group hepatoblastoma, this led to considerable improvements in survival in participating countries (Fig. 6.1).

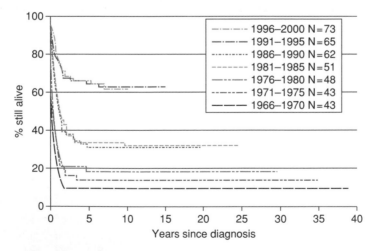

Fig. 6.1 Rapid improvement in survival of children with hepatoblastoma (average 11 cases/yr) in Great Britain following the introduction of participation in the SIOPEL clinical trials in 1991. The number of cases diagnosed per quinquennium is indicated.
Reproduced from Stiller C. (Ed). Childhood Cancer in Britain: Incidence, survival, mortality, with permission from Oxford University Press.

Very large numbers are also needed for non-inferiority trials. These are typically used when the aim is to reduce treatment burden, toxicity, and long-term side effects for patients who have a good risk profile, without compromising overall survival rates. For instance, in ALL, they are useful in patients with very good clinical outcome, at least 90–95 per cent 5-year EFS, for whom the attempt is to optimize therapy under controlled conditions, de-intensifying certain therapy elements with known short- or long-term side effects, without compromising the EFS outcome. Up to 30 per cent of children with ALL treated in current protocols in North America and Western Europe, may be candidates for this type of trial. In general, however, non-inferiority 'head-to-head' trials, where a novel drug replaces an existing one, are often viewed with suspicion as they may be used to promote drugs of less therapeutic value. Switching the objective of a trial from superiority to non-inferiority can be much more seriously misleading than the opposite switching as, for instance, a poorly conducted or an underpowered superiority trial may easily lead to a non-significant result, because treatment effect is diluted or it has wide confidence intervals.

As a final consideration, trial design requires that experts in various fields (clinical, biological, pharmacological, biostatistical) cooperate to formulate in advance, as clearly and precisely as possible, based on up-to date- knowledge, the objectives and hypothesis of the trial. Data from a trial where the results support a sound, pre-specified hypothesis is more persuasive than one where the results are 'surprising' and unplanned testing for non-inferiority in trials designed for superiority should be discouraged. Study design that incorporates both non-inferiority and superiority testing are possible, and may be useful and applicable in selected contexts.

Novel strategies for clinical trial design

The issues raised by the more precise characterisation of subgroups in paediatric oncology continue to grow in importance. Advances in understanding the molecular basis of many childhood cancers and the development of more sensitive methods for assessing response mean that even the common childhood cancers such as ALL are now being sub-divided into ever smaller subgroups with different survival profiles, such as infants or Philadelphia-chromosome positive patients, each with their own therapeutic questions. New statistical approaches to design are therefore needed to address important therapeutic questions. These include increased efficacy for those subgroups where survival is still very poor. They also include optimizing the design of phase I and II studies, given the limited number of patients available and the growing number of new drugs that must be evaluated for toxicity and activity. These kinds of questions have stimulated the development of adaptive designs. Such designs may be most useful when drug activity is evaluated in terms of early response to treatment, rather than in phase III studies, where efficacy is measured by long-term evaluation of event-free and overall survival.

A broad range of design modifications, for instance sample size re-estimation, discontinuation of treatment arms, changes in the primary measure of treatment response, is allowed by adaptive designs. Adaptive designs make use of known interim findings to modify the sampling plan and are therefore data driven. For this reason, they raise concern about the unintended consequence of introducing bias and imprecision in the estimates. In addition, the adoption of an adaptive design for a Phase III trial could be seen as contradicting the confirmatory nature of such Late-development studies, especially if these are pivotal trials aiming at approval of a new product. Adaptive approaches are justified by the need to cope with difficult experimental situations, where the paucity of available knowledge determines uncertainty about crucial aspects of the study. These difficulties must be acknowledged in advance, so that any modification of the trial design, for example sample size re-estimation, is anticipated and justified in the study protocol. Adaptive designs cannot, in fact. be used as a remedy for poor trial planning, but actually require

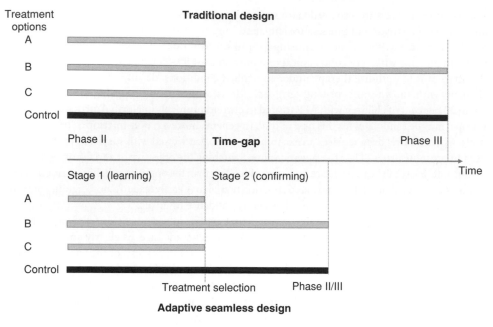

Fig. 6.2 Comparison of adaptive seamless and traditional design.

more upfront planning both statistically and in managing logistics and implementation. In short, a proper adaptive design must control potential sources of bias, first of all by ensuring that type I error is fully preserved and valid estimates and confidence intervals for the treatment effect will be available as a summary of the totality of evidence. Additional measures to be taken operationally, in order to maintain the integrity of the trial, include the careful disclosure of interim analyses. In practice, access to the available data and related results must be limited (it is recommended that clinical team be isolated from both) and communication of interim analysis decisions is to be preferred over communication of interim results.

A general concern about monitoring designs is heterogeneity in treatment effects estimated from the different stages of the trial. This may be due to random variation, but in practice it cannot be excluded that a calendar time effect might be present, for instance because of a learning process or a change in important prognostic factors occurring over time. Heterogeneity in stage results can be detected by applying a heterogeneity test, although its statistical power is generally limited. Should it indicate that a discrepancy exists, further investigation into possible causes is recommended.

An interesting example of adaptive design is the so-called adaptive 'seamless' design, in which two separate phases of drug development, that could be conducted as separate trials, are in fact combined into a single one, both operationally and inferentially. Data gathered from the first, learning stage (e.g. dose selection) are used to adapt the trial plan of the second, confirming stage and data from both are used to run the final analysis and answer study questions. This adaptive 'seamless' design does not simply select out the most promising treatment option, but actually allows continuation of the preferred arm without the need to start a new trial (see Fig. 6.2). Application of this type of study requires that the endpoint for the learning phase be immediately available for continuation with the confirming stage and that it be adopted as a primary endpoint also to answer the study question. A multi-arm, multi-stage trial design was recently proposed to compare many new therapies at once against a control treatment and reject insufficiently active therapies in a randomized pairwise comparison with the control, performed at different stages with a seamless move from one stage to the next.

Bayesian designs

Bayesian statistics is a methodology, used both in the design and in the analysis stage of a trial, that provides a coherent method for learning from evidence as it accumulates. This is performed by combining prior information with accumulating evidence through a mathematical model, and leads to the so-called 'posterior distribution' of the clinical endpoint of interest.

The Bayesian approach may be useful especially when good prior information on clinical use of a device or treatment exists, so that incorporating it in the design and analysis of the future trial may result in a smaller or shorter study. It can also be used when prior information is only partially (or not) informative, because it can provide flexible methods for interim analyses and modifications of on-going trials (e.g. changes to sample size or changes in the randomization scheme).

The Bayesian approach for trial design usually does not determine sample size in advance; instead, it may specify a particular criterion to stop the trial. Appropriate stopping criteria may be based on a specific amount of information about the clinical measure of interest (e.g. a sufficiently narrow credible interval, as defined below) or an appropriately high probability for a pre-specified hypothesis.

At any point during a Bayesian clinical trial, it is possible to update the computation of the expected additional number of observations needed to meet the stopping criterion. Because the sample size is not explicitly part of the stopping criterion, the trial can be terminated whenever enough information has been collected to answer the trial questions. When sizing a Bayesian trial, it is recommended that the minimum sample size is pre-specified according to safety and effectiveness endpoints. It is also wise to anticipate a minimum level of information from the current trial needed to verify model assumptions and appropriateness of prior information used.

Pre-specified interim analyses can be part of a Bayesian trial and various methods are available. The final analyses within the Bayesian approach include hypothesis testing and interval estimates. For Bayesian hypothesis testing, the posterior distribution can be used to calculate the probability that a particular hypothesis regarding the endpoint is true, given the observed data. Interval estimates in the Bayesian context are called credible intervals: a 95 percent credible interval is the interval with 95 per cent posterior probability of including the 'true' unknown treatment effect.

A Bayesian framework could be used to design phase II trials more efficiently by thinking of them as randomized selection trials comparing several therapies. Thus, in rare subgroups, it has been proposed to formally combine, at the design stage, the expected outcome of the new small trial being planned with the prior information on treatment effect generated by earlier studies. A Bayesian approach of this kind provides an estimate of the potential contribution to the demonstration of treatment effect of the new trial which, if seen in isolation, would be underpowered.

Regulatory agencies have recently issued guidelines on clinical trials in small populations that indicate the possibility of using non-standard designs. These guidelines propose that there are no special methods for designing, carrying out or analysing clinical trials in small populations but note that the need for statistical efficiency should be weighed against the need for clinically relevant/interpretable results, the latter being more important. This is in line with that discussed in the review paper by Cox: while frequentist formulations of analysis are typically best suited for careful assessment of the strength of evidence, Bayesian formulations may allow the insertion of additional information which may open the route to bolder speculations, sometimes providing an alternative to sensitivity analysis.

Practical considerations in conducting clinical trials in childhood cancer

The conduct of clinical trials is a highly regulated process, designed to give maximum safety to patients whilst allowing them access to innovation in a well designed, controlled scientific study that has a high chance of achieving its aims. Each country has its own legal framework for ethical review procedures and regulatory approval processes. Ensuring consistent data quality when working across national, cultural, legal and linguistic boundaries adds further to the challenges. Hence, multi-national trials require additional time to design and implement.

In Europe, the EU Clinical Trials Directive (CTD) 2001/20/EC, introduced into national law in May 2004, aimed to provide a common set of regulations and defined standards of quality of clinical studies across member states. However, it has had several undesirable impacts, including increased cost and bureaucracy for non-commercial trials conducted by universities and public research institutions. The outcome of a review of the impact of the EU CTD on such investigator-driven clinical trials is currently awaited. However, the basic requirement that each trial should have an overall sponsor who takes responsibility for obtaining a clinical trial authorization, ensures the suitability of each participating institution and investigators, and oversees pharmacovigilance, will not diminish.

Although there are many ethical considerations in undertaking clinical research on children, a 'therapeutic alliance' begins between doctors and families when a child is first diagnosed with cancer. All parents want their child to access the best treatment available and entry into a phase III trial is generally considered 'best practice' in paediatric oncology. More research is needed, however, to understand how best to present the alien concept of a randomized clinical trial at this stressful time and to understand why there are differences in randomization rates between countries participating within the same clinical trial.

Engaging families as informed partners in clinical trials is a key goal of sound practice, but achieving this is far from straightforward. One key issue concerns whether to involve a child with cancer in the decision about participating in a trial. The principle that children should be consulted, informed, and involved in decisions affecting them, but not have the final authority over decisions, is enshrined in the UN Convention of the Rights of the Child (UNCRC). The guiding principle of the UNCRC is that the 'best interests' of the child must be promoted, but differences of opinion between parents, children, and professionals about the 'best interests' of the child will sometimes need to be resolved. Involving a child in a decision about participation in a cancer trial may be especially complex in those situations where parents, struggling to come to terms with the diagnosis themselves, prefer to defer telling the child the full diagnosis and its implications, perhaps until treatment is established and the parents are better able to cope with their own emotions. Some parents may see a demand to involve the child in the decision—and by definition disclose the diagnosis—as interfering with their autonomy as parents. Further complexity arises because of varying definitions of minors and of the legal age of consent between different countries; some jurisdictions rely on the assessment of 'competence' rather than specifying a particular age of consent.

Patient 'misunderstandings' of concepts such as randomization are often assumed to arise from incomplete, badly written, or misleading information. Much attention, particularly from Research Ethics Committees, tends to focus on the detail of Patient Information Sheets (PIS). However, the role of written information in this context remains poorly understood, and parents may find discussion with staff more helpful than the consent document.

Summary

Despite the progress made in curing children with cancer, there is little room for complacency and, if progress is to be sustained, formidable challenges must be faced. These include the scientific challenge of studies in small populations, the complexities of the regulatory environment, ethical and organizational constraints, the emotional context, and the attitudes of individual families and physicians. Some of these issues may be addressed by innovative trial design and implementation, but all will require engagement with the communities of families and physicians on whom trials depend. Clinical research must include a well-designed social science and ethical evaluation of how best to inform and engage the patient community who need clinical trials to continue in order for progress to be made.

Further reading

Cox, DR (2007) Applied Statistics: a review. *The Annals of Applied Statistics* **1**, 1–16.

Estlin EJ, Cotterill S, Pratt CB, et al. (2000) Phase I trials in pediatric oncology: perceptions of pediatricians from the United Kingdom Children's Cancer Study Group and the Pediatric Oncology Group. *J Clin Oncol* **18**, 1900–5.

European Agency for the Evaluation of Medicinal Products: Committee for medicinal products for human use (2005) Guideline on clinical trials in small populations CHMP/EWP/83561/2005 http://www.emea.europa.eu/pdfs/human/ewp/8356105en.pdf.

Freedman, B (1987) Equipoise and the ethics of clinical research. *New England Journal of Medicine* **317**, 141–5.

Garattini S, Bertelè V (2007) Non-inferiority trials are unethical because they disregard patients' interests. *Lancet* **370**, 1875–7.

Kumar A, Soares H, Wells R, et al. (2005) Are experimental treatments for cancer in children superior to established treatments? Observational study of randomised controlled trials by the Children's Oncology Group. *BMJ* **331**, 1295.

Lee D P, Skolnik JM, Adamson PC (2005) Pediatric phase I trials in oncology: an analysis of study conduct efficiency. *J Clin Oncol* **23**, 8431–41.

Machin D, Campbell M, Fayers P, Pinol A (1997) *Sample Size Tables for Clinical Studies*, 2nd edition. Malden, MA: Blackwell Science.

Parmar MKB, Barthel FMS, Sydes M, et al. (2008) Speeding up the evaluation of new agents in cancer. *J Nat Can Inst* **100**, 1204–14.

Piantadosi S. (2005) *Clinical Trials: A Methodologic Perspective*, 2nd Edition. New York: Wiley.

Pritchard-Jones K, Dixon-Woods M, Naafs-Wilstra M, Valsecchi MG. (2008) Improving recruitment to clinical trials for cancer in childhood. *Lancet Oncol* **9**, 392–9.

Rubinstein L V, Korn EL, Freidlin B, et al. (2005) Design issues of randomized phase II trials and a proposal for phase II screening trials. *J Clin Oncol* **23**, 7199–206.

Simon CM, Siminoff LA, Kodish ED, Burant C. (2004) Comparison of the informed consent process for randomized clinical trials in pediatric and adult oncology. *J Clin Oncol* **22**, 2708–17.

Simon R, Wittes RE Ellenberg SS (1985) Randomised phase II clinical trials. *Cancer Treat Rep* **69**, 1375–81.

Simon R. (1989) Optimal two-stage designs for phase II clinical trials. *Control Clin Trials* **10**, 1–10.

Steliarova-Foucher E, Coebergh JW, Kaatsch P et al. (eds) (2006) Cancer in Children and Adolescents in Europe. *Eur J Cancer* Special Edition **42**, 1913–2190.

Stiller C. (ed.) (2007) *Childhood Cancer in Britain: Incidence, survival, mortality*. Oxford: Oxford University Press.

Tan SB, Dear KB, Bruzzi P, Machin D (2003) Strategy for randomised clinical trials in rare cancers. *BMJ* **327**, 47–9.

Valsecchi MG, Masera G. (1996) A new challenge in clinical research in childhood ALL: the prospective meta-analysis strategy for intergroup collaboration. *Ann Oncol* **7**, 1005–8.

Valsecchi MG, Silvestri D, Covezzoli A, De Lorenzo P. (2008) Web-based international studies in limited populations of pediatric leukemia. *Pediatr Blood Cancer* **50**, 270–3.

Chapter 7

Allogeneic stem cell and immunotherapy

Rupert Handgretinger and R. Maarten Egeler

Introduction

Allogeneic haematopoietic stem cell transplantation (HSCT) is the only currently available curative approach for a number of children with malignant and non-malignant diseases; the malignant diseases comprise mainly haematological malignancies whereas the non-malignant disorders include haemoglobinopathies, inborn disorders of the immune system and metabolism. The first paediatric HSCT was performed in 1969 in a child with leukaemia with a matched sibling donor. A few years later, HSCT was being used successfully to cure otherwise incurable leukaemias in adults. The next decades produced remarkable advances in the understanding of histocompatibility and brought the development of novel immunosuppressive drugs that allowed a more effective prophylaxis of graft-versus-host disease (GvH) disease. The advances in HLA typing strategies (see later in this chapter) and more effective prevention of GvH disease allowed the inclusion of stem cell donors beyond HLA-matched siblings. With the establishment of international bone marrow donor registries, HSCT has become a therapeutic option for an increasing number of patients with otherwise incurable haematological malignancies and other diseases. With the addition of unrelated cord blood transplantation and the possibility of including haploidentical family members with up to three HLA loci mismatches in the donor pool, a stem cell donor can nowadays be identified for almost every patient for whom an allogeneic HSCT is considered to be superior to conventional chemotherapies of for whom it is the only currently known curative approach.

The success of HSCT relies on the eradication of the underlying malignant disease and the replacement of defective or tumour-infiltrated bone marrow by the preparative regimen. However, recently it has become evident that success also depends to a large extent on the balance between the donor's alloreactive T lymphocytes against the recipient's tissues (GvH disease) and the favourable reaction of the donor's T lymphocytes towards the malignant cells [graft-versus tumour (GvT) effect]. More recently, convincing evidence has accumulated that the transplanted innate donor immune system also contributes to the eradication of residual malignant cell. In this context, natural killer (NK) cells as key members of the innate immune system seem to play a major role in preventing relapses and also infectious complications after HSCT.

This chapter reviews practical aspects of HSCT, its application to children and young adults, and approaches to exploiting the anti-tumour effects of HSCT as well as additional post-transplant anti-tumour and anti-infectious strategies to improve the outcome of HSCT.

Donor selection for HSCT

The selection of donors for HSCT depends on the match between the prospective donor and the recipient in terms of the products of a group of genes on chromosome 6, the so-called major histocompatibility complex (MHC). The products of the MHC are referred to as human leukocyte antigens (HLA). The genes most relevant to transplantation histocompatibility are divided into class I (*HLA-A*, *-B*, and *-Cw*) and class II (*HLA-DR*, *-DQ*, and *-DP*) genes. Class I specificities are present on all nucleated cells of an individual, whereas class II genes are found primarily on cells of the immune system, such as B lymphocytes and macrophages. In contrast to previous serological methods, HLA specificities are nowadays mostly identified by DNA sequencing. A locus name is a one- or two-digit number, indicating a serological defined specificity (e.g. HLA-A2). A DNA sequence registered with the World Health Organization (WHO) is assigned a number with the first digits usually related to the closer serologic equivalent, such as HLA-A*02:01 and the following digits represent the order of sequence registration for alleles of that group (for example HLA-A*02:01:01:01). The asterisk indicates that the data are derived from DNA testing. HLA antigens present peptides derived either from cell proteins or from exogenous proteins to the T-lymphocyte receptor; an immune response is initiated if the HLA peptide complex is identified by the T-lymphocyte receptor as foreign to the host. A given HLA specificity can bind a range of peptides with specific characteristics and the polymorphism of the HLA systems allows a wide range of peptide binding in the population and has evolved to facilitate microbial immunity. The HLA system has proven to be the most polymorphic genetic region known in the human genome. Individuals inherit a set of HLA, called a haplotype, from each parent and both haplotypes are fully expressed. Therefore, the probability that a child shares both haplotypes with a full sibling is 25 per cent, the chance of sharing one haplotype is 50 per cent and the chance of sharing neither haplotype is 25 per cent. The HLA genes are closely linked and the recombination rate is therefore limited.

Classically, the optimally matched donor is a full sibling who shares the same parental haplotypes with the recipient, and approximately one-third of patients have a fully matched sibling. Alternative donors include unrelated and partially mismatched related donors. Initially, the definintions of appropriate matching emphasized HLA-A, -B, and -DR and matching levels were referred to as 6/6 or 5/6, and so on. Studies on additional transplant antigens, such as HLA-C or HLA-DQB, suggested a better clinical outcome with higher levels of matching, so that most transplant centers would prefer a match of all HLAs (10/10 match). Unfortunately, the likelihood of identifying an unrelated donor decreases with the degree of matching. Besides the degree of matching, the direction of mismatching is important to consider in the context of graft rejection or GvH disease. The recipient's immune system can potentially generate immune responses against the grafted cells [host-versus-graft (HvG) reaction]. However, a more important consideration may be the immune responses generated by the engrafting immunocompetent cells toward recipient's tissues [graft-versus-host (GvH) reaction] and the outcome is influenced by the degree of matching and mismatching in each direction.

More recent concepts of donor selection include the determination of the donor's killer immunoglobulin-like receptor (KIR) haplotypes, especially if there are several HLA-matched donors available. A significant influence of the donor's KIR genotype on the outcome of adult patients with AML has been described after matched unrelated transplantation.

Stem cell source

In the early years of transplantation, bone marrow was exclusively used as a stem cell source for transplantation. The discovery in clinical application of granulocyte colony-stimulating growth factor (G-CSF) and granulocyte macrophage colony-stimulating growth factor (GM-CSF) led to the observation that bone marrow stem cells can be mobilized in large numbers into the peripheral blood stream and that mobilized peripheral blood stem cells (PBSCs) can completely reconstitute hematopoiesis. Bone marrow is still a major source of stem cells for matched sibling donor (MSD) and matched unrelated donor (MUD) transplants, but PBSCs are being increasingly collected from such donors. The use of growth factors such as G-CSF in paediatric donors to mobilize stem cells into the peripheral blood or to increase the number of stem cells in the bone marrow is controversial. In addition to the lack of long-term safety data for paediatric donors, no clear benefit of G-CSF-mobilized PBSCs or bone marrow over conventional bone marrow transplantation has been shown in paediatric transplantation and the use of growth factors in paediatric donors might be restricted to individual situations or to clinical research protocols. In paediatric haploi-dentical transplantations, mobilized PBSCs are often used to increase the number of transplanted stem cells, as high numbers of infused stem cells are important for safe engraftment across the HLA barrier (megadose concept). Another stem cell source is umbilical cord blood (UCB) from related donors or from unrelated donors stored in cord blood banks. However, a limiting factor of UCB is the lower number of stem cells contained in the grafts, which can lead to a delay in engraftment or in non-engraftment. To overcome this obstacle, the use of two cord blood units for one patient (double-cord) is being increasingly used to improve engraftment.

Preparative regimens

The most commonly used preparative regimens prior to allogeneic transplantation for paediatric ALL include various doses of fractionated total body irradiation (TBI) ranging from 12 Gy to 14.75 Gy in combination with additional drugs, such as cyclophosphamide, etoposide, cytarabin, thiotepa or fludarabin. Non-TBI based regimens with busulfan/cyclophosphamide with or without additional cytotoxic drugs, such as etoposide, thiotepa or fludarabin, are also used. While multiple studies indicate that TBI-based preparative regimens are associated with a lower risk of relapse compared to chemotherapy-only regimens in ALL, no larger randomized prospective and conclusive trials to support either TBI or non-TBI based regimens have been reported in children. In patients with AML, paediatric studies are limited and there seems to be no obvious difference between TBI and non-TBI-based preparative regimens and busulfan/cyclophosphamide is most commonly used.

The preparative regimen should have a cytotoxic anti-tumour effect, but should also provide adequate immunosuppression in order to ensure engraftment. Less aggressive so-called non-myeloablative stem cell transplantation regimens have been described, especially for patients who otherwise cannot tolerate a conventional myeloablative regimen or to avoid long-term side effects associated with myeloablative conditioning. Such regimens range from minimal, to facilitate engraftment (fludarabin plus low-dose TBI), to more intensive but still not myeloablative regimens (reduced-intensity conditioning or RIC, such as reduced doses of fludarabin plus busulphan). The rationale behind non-myeloablative stem cell transplantation is the induction of an optimal graft-versus-malignancy effect by donor-alloreactive effector cells. While this form of transplantation is frequently used in adult and elderly patients, the data in children remain insufficient to conclude that the reduced cytotoxic anti-leukaemic effect of the preparative regimens is counter-balanced by an increased anti-leukaemic effect of the allograft and therefore, such regimens should only be used in the context of controlled clinical trials.

Indications for transplantation

Paediatric ALL is the most common malignant disease in childhood. International studies of childhood ALL in developed countries have achieved 5-year event-free survival rates up to 90 per cent. However, despite the improvements in the therapy and survival of patients with ALL, a significant number of patients will experience a relapse and the goal of most therapeutic ALL studies is to identify patients at risk of relapse as early as possible during initial treatment and then proceed with intensified chemotherapy or even with an allogeneic HSCT. Various clinical studies have identified high-risk features of patients with ALL in CR 1 in whom an allogeneic HSCT might yield better leukaemia-free and overall survival compared to patients treated with chemotherapy only. These high-risk features include the presence of chromosomal translocations, such as t(4;11) or 11q23 (*MLL* gene rearrangements), Philadelphia chromosome t(9;22), hypodiploidy (<44 chromosomes), and poor response to induction, such as induction failure (5 per cent or more leukaemic cells) or the presence of minimal residual disease (MRD) of more than 1 per cent after 4–6 weeks of first-line therapy. Especially the levels of MRD at certain time points of the first-line therapy seem to play a major role for risk stratification and for the identification of patients for whom an allogeneic HSCT might provide a better outcome compared to chemotherapy alone.

Nevertheless, a significant number of children will relapse and relapsed ALL is the fourth most common malignant disease of childhood. Various treatment strategies for patients with relapsed ALL are investigated and the goal is to identify patients in CR 2 who would benefit from allogeneic HSCT. The majority of transplants are performed in relapsed patients in CR 2 or beyond, given the fact that the probability of leukaemia-free survival with chemotherapy alone is only in the range of 10–40 per cent. Older age at relapse (>10–15 years of age) and a short CR 1 result in lower rates of leukaemia-free survival (LFS). Patients who relapse in the bone marrow during therapy or early after treatment have a poor outcome with chemotherapy alone and allogeneic HSCT yields a better outcome for these patients. Patients with early or late relapse of T-ALL have a poor prognosis and transplantation of this subgroup is recommended. About two-thirds of patients with a late extramedullary relapse and about one-third of those with early extramedullary relapse or late non-T marrow relapse or early combined non-T relapse can be rescued by chemotherapy alone. However, the persistence of high-level MRD after relapse therapy in these patients also identifies patients at risk for subsequent relapses and an allogeneic HSCT might be indicated in these patients. The role of HSCT in infant ALL is controversial. Most of these patients have a rearrangement of the MLL gene in chromosome 11q23 and an associated poor outcome. Allogeneic HSCT with matched sibling donors does not seem to improve the prognosis for this subgroup and therefore, HSCT might be restricted to research protocols aimed at investigating new approaches for childhood ALL with rearrangement of the 11q23 chromosomal region.

The role of allogeneic HSCT in patients with acute myeloid leukaemia in CR 1 is controversial. Most patients will not benefit from an allogeneic HSCT and overall survival seems to be similar with chemotherapy alone compared to allogeneic HSCT. However, there might be subgroups in AML who might benefit from allogeneic HSCT and further research will hopefully identify subgroups in AML in which transplantation will improve the outcome of treatment. While 80–90 per cent of patients with AML will achieve a remission with contemporary treatment, 30–40 per cent of these patients will subsequently suffer recurrence, and after recurrence, the likelihood of survival is poor and the length of first remission might be a predictor of subsequent survival. Allogeneic HSCT in CR 2 is associated with improved outcome after relapse and patients with CR 1 >12 months had a better survival than patients with CR 1 <12 months.

Other indications for allogeneic HSCT in children with hematological malignancies include children with myelodysplastic syndromes, and children who will most likely benefit from HSCT are those with refractory anaemia with excessive blasts (RAEB), refractory anaemia with excessive blasts in transformation (RAEB-t), an age younger than 2 years and a haemoglobin F level of 10 per cent or higher. For patients with juvenile myelomonocytic leukaemia (JMML), conventional chemotherapy is unlikely to eradicate the stem cell abnormality and HSCT offers the greatest likelihood for cure. Therapy-related myelodysplastic syndromes and acute myeloid leukaemia

(AML) are defined as clonal malignant disorders that arise after exposure to cytotoxic agents and HSCT seems to be a potential curative treatment for these patients.

For adult patients with chronic myeloid leukaemia (CML), imatinib is currently considered as the best upfront treatment and should also be offered to children. However, allogeneic HSCT is still the only known approach to eliminate the clonal disease. Children are mostly treated with imatinib until the best response is achieved followed by HSCT from an optimal selected donor, which might be within 2 years after diagnosis in patients with a low risk score.

Allogeneic HSCT for solid tumours

Only few data on allogeneic HSCT for solid tumours of childhood are available. Various case reports in different tumour entities suggest an allogeneic graft-versus-tumour effect in some patients. Previous reports in neuroblastoma did not show differences in the progression-free survival. However, with the advent of RIC regimens, the reduced transplant-related mortality (TRM) and more insight into the biology of allogeneic HSCT, prospective clinical trials should clarify the role of allogeneic transplantation in children with solid tumours.

The anti-malignancy effect in allogeneic HSCT

Graft-versus-host and graft-versus-Leukaemia

Although the patient's preparative regimen itself has a considerable anti-tumour effect, it is only one of the pillar of successful eradication of a patient's malignant disease. The other pillar is the elimination of residual malignant cells through immunological anti-tumour effects induced by the graft. Major disparities or minor differences in donor and recipient HLA antigens are the reasons for more or less intensive alloreactive immune responses of graft-containing lymphocytes either against the recipients normal cells, resulting in GvH disease, and/or against the recipients residual tumour cells, described as GvT effect. In patients with leukaemia, the graft-versus-leukaemia (GvL) effect appears to play a more and more important role in the therapy of patients. In a large retrospective study, the effect of GvH disease on relapse was demonstrated to be significantly affected by the type of transplant (T-cell depleted or T-cell repleted graft) or the development of GvH disease. Recipients of grafts from genetically identical twins had the highest risk of relapse followed by T-cell depleted grafts and T-cell depleted grafts without the subsequent development of GvH disease. The concept that the occurrence of GvH disease is associated with GvL is further supported by clinical observations that lower relapse rates are seen in patients who developed acute and/or chronic GvH disease. Retrospective and prospective randomized trials in children with acute leukaemia demonstrated that a reduced dose of cyclosporin A (CsA) used for GvH disease prophylaxis after matched sibling transplantion is associated with a significant reduction of leukaemia relapse. Moreover, a low dose of CsA and a low level of CsA in the first 10 days after allogeneic transplantation conferred significant protection against leukaemia relapse in patients with early and advanced leukaemia. The occurrence of chronic GvH disease is also associated with a reduced relapse rate. In a large retrospective study in children with malignancies, the relapse probability rate was 16 per cent versus 39 per cent in children with or without cGvH disease, respectively. The potential anti-leukaemic effect of GvH disease is also supported by anecdotal case reports in children. The existence of GvL is further corroborated by the successful infusion of viable donor lymphocytes (DLI) for the post-transplant treatment of relapses. A more recently described approach is the prospective preemptive alloimmune intervention in high-risk paediatric acute leukaemia guided by the levels of MRD before stem cell transplantation. This intervention extended the length of remission post transplant, but relapses occurred at extramedullary sites less susceptible for cellular anti-leukaemic strategies.

Graft-versus-host and graft-versus-solid tumour

While the graft-versus-leukaemia effect has mainly been studied in children with hematological malignancies, allogeneic HSCT has rarely been used in paediatric patients with solid tumours. One of the reasons is the rather disappointing outcome of earlier clinical studies in which allogeneic bone marrow grafts were not superior to autologous marrow grafts in patients with neuroblastoma. In this study, myeloablative regimens similar to the conditioning regimens used in hematological malignancies were applied with considerable risk of GvH disease and TRM. Another case-controlled study of children with neuroblastoma comparing 17 allogeneic and 34 autologous transplants found no difference in progression-free survival (35 per cent and 41 per cent at 2 years, respectively. In adults patients, a GvT and GvL was found incidentially in a patient with concurrent breast cancer and AML. A clinical study in a group of women with metastatic breast cancer also demonstrated suggestive evidence of a GvT against breast cancer. A clear graft-versus-solid-tumour effect was described in adult patients with metastatic renal cell using non-myeloablative preparative regimen. Only few other reports exist describing a GVT in adult patients with colon carcinoma, ovarian carcinoma, and prostate cancer.

For paediatric patients with solid tumours, a graft-versus-solid-tumour effect has only been reported in single patients or in small studies. Using RIC regimens, few case reports exist indicating that there might be a role for a GvT effect in paediatric solid tumours. An impressive graft-versus-solid-tumour effect and long-term remission was described in a patient with relapse of a metastatic Ewing sarcoma. In this patient, the tumour response was clearly correlated with the occurrence of GvH disease. This patient is now in complete remission for more than 11 years (own unpublished observation). In a small study of five patients with relapsed/refractory neuroblastoma, two achieved a long-term remission after haploidentical stem cell transplantation followed by DLI.

The advent of RIC regimens and the reduction of TRM over the last decades will allow prospective clinical trials in paediatric patients in order to detect whether these approaches will harness graft-versus-solid-tumour effects in patients with otherwise noncurable relapsed/refractory solid tumours. Further research is necessary to integrate cellular therapeutic strategies into conventional therapies. Based on the available data obtained so far in children, clinical controlled studies of allogeneic transplantation using RIC regimens are warranted.

Graft-versus-tumour effects mediated by natural killer (NK) cells

The concept of alloreactive NK cells

The development and function of NK cells are controlled by NK cell receptors that recognize HLA class I alleles. Among the NK cell recepors are the polymorphic activatory or inhibitory killer-cell immunoglobulin-like receptors (KIR) that recognize polymorphic epitopes of HLA-A, -B and -C, also called KIR ligands. The concept of alloreactive NK cells is based on the observation that NK cells attack lympho-hematopoietic target cells that express HLA class I molecules for which they do not express the corresponding inhibitory receptor. NK cells are in a permanent activated state due to binding of natural cytotoxicity receptors (NCRs) to unknown ligands expressed on normal or malignant hematopoietic cells (Fig. 7.1). In the presence of a corresponding ligand for the inhibitory receptor (e.g. self HLA-Cw alleles, -Bw4 alleles and some HLA-A alleles), the cytotoxic function of NK cells is inhibited and the target cells are resistant to NK-mediated lysis (Fig. 7.1a). In contrast, if the target cell does not express the corresponding inhibitory ligand for the KIR, NK cells lyse their target cells. This situation is often encountered in HLA-mismatched, but also in HLA-matched allogeneic stem cell transplantion due to the disparity of the donor's KIR repertoire and the HLA class I type of the recipients (Fig. 7.1b). The term alloreactive NK cells is used to

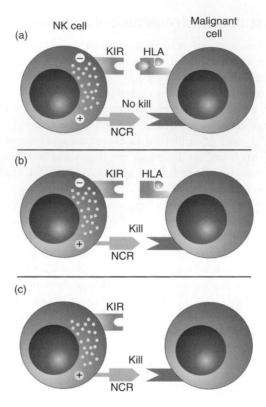

Fig. 7.1 The expression of inhibitory receptors (KIR) on NK cells and the expression of KIR-binding or KIR-nonbinding HLA class I molecules on malignant cells. (a) The KIR receptor finds its corresponding HLA ligand, which inhibits the cytotoxicity of the NK cells towards the target cells. (b) The HL -ligand is not recognized by the KIR receptor and is thus not inhibited, which leads to the killing of the target cell via binding of the natural cytotoxicity receptor (NCR) via yet unknown ligands. In the context of allogeneic transplantation, this situation is an NK alloreactive constellation. (c) These tumour cells do not express HLA class I alleles and thus the KIR receptors cannot be engaged, which results in NK cell activation and killing of the target cells.

describe this situation. However, based on the concept of the interaction of inhibitory receptors with HLA class I molecules, additional clinical situations can be envisioned (Fig. 7.1c). Tumour cells can have a reduced expression or complete lack of HLA class I molecules, which can be encountered in leukaemic blasts or certain tumours, such as neuroblastoma or Ewing sarcoma. This constellation leads to killing of the tumour cells and the intensity of killing is dependent on the amount of residual HLA molecules expressed on the surface of the target cells.

Graft-versus-leukaemia effects mediated by alloreactive NK cells

In the search for new donor selection criteria to augment GvL effects, alloreactive NK cells were first described in HLA three-loci-mismatched haploidentical transplantation using T-cell depleted grafts in patients with AML but not ALL. These results were confirmed in matched or partially matched unrelated, sibling and cord blood transplant settings. These studies did not consider a role for the gene variability which in its extent and functional importance is similar to that of HLA class I. KIR genes are encoded by a set of 15 loci and two pseudogenes that are closely linked and inherited as a haplotype. KIR gene content can further be organized in KIR haplotypes A and B. KIR A haplotypes have simple, fixed gene content, whereas KIR B haplotypes have variable gene content. Based on this distinction, all individuals can be assigned to either A/A genotype (i.e. homozygous for A haplotypes) or the B/x genotype (having one or two B haplotypes). In addition, KIR A and B haplotypes have distinctive centromeric (Cen) and telomeric (Tel) gene-content motifs. Because HLA and KIR segregate independently on different chromosomes, HLA-identical individuals can have completely different KIR genotypes and the KIR gene family is a second immunogenetic system. The influence of the donor KIR genotype was shown previously and the outcome of matched unrelated donor transplantation for AML was significantly better if the donors had the B/x rather than the A/A genotype; similar effects have been reported in sibling donor settings.

In a retrospective study of HLA-matched unrelated transplantation of 1086 patients with AML and 323 patients with ALL, donors were KIR genotyped and assigned to their KIR haplotype motifs. In patients with AML, but not ALL, centromeric (cen-B) and telomeric (tel-B) B motifs both contributed to relapse protection and improved survival compared to A motifs. Cen-B/B homozygosity had the strongest independent effect and with Cen-B/B homozygous donors, the cumulative incidence of relapse was 15.4 per cent compared to 36.5 per cent for Cen-A/A donors ($p<0.0001$). Overall, a significantly reduced rate of relapse was seen with donors having two or more B gene-content motifs for HLA-matched and mismatched transplants. Therefore, KIR genotyping of HLA-matched donors and selection of the 'best matched donor' should increase the frequency of transplants using unrelated donor grafts with favourable KIR gene content and could result in superior disease-free survival for adult patients transplantated for AML.

In contrast to adult patients where NK-mediated GvL effects have only been seen in AML but not ALL, NK alloreactivity has been demonstrated in studies of paediatric patients with ALL and a significant lower risk of relapse has been observed in patients with ALL after transplantation from NK-alloreactive donors compared to patients whom received a graft from NK-nonalloreactive donors.

Potential graft-versus-solid tumour effects mediated by NK cells

The concept of alloreactive NK cells might also apply for the treatment of paediatric metastatic solid tumours. It has been shown that KIR-ligand mismatched alloreactive NK cells effectively lyse primary solid tumours obtained from different cancers as well as tumour cell lines established from melanoma or renal cell carcinoma. In addition, some paediatric tumours such as neuroblastoma express only low amounts of HLA class I molecules on their surface and are therefore susceptible target cells for NK cells. Tumour cell lines obtained from rhabdomyosarcoma and Ewing sarcoma show a variable susceptibility to NK cell-mediated lysis (own unpublished observations). Based on this concept, clinical protocols using a RIC approach and haploidentical transplantation of CD3/19-depleted and NK cell-enriched stem cell grafts have been initiated in patients with advanced and refractory paediatric malignant solid tumours including neuroblastoma, rhabdomyosarcoma, and Ewing sarcoma.

Post-transplant cellular therapies

Prevention of relapse using allogeneic T lymphocytes

Allogeneic T lymphocytes can produce a strong GvL effect, but the beneficial effect is limited by GvH disease. An easier way to identify and treat patients at risk for relapse may be the frequent determination of a patient's chimerism status post-transplant. A mixed chimerism (i.e. the simultaneous presence of host- and donor-derived cells) may herald an impending relapse, especially if the proportion of donor cells is further decreasing, whereas patients with a complete donor chimerism have a better relapse-free survival. Based on these observations, strategies to either maintain a complete donor chimerism or to revert a decreasing mixed to a complete donor chimerism by either withdrawal of immunosuppression or chimerism-guided DLI have been successfully employed.

The response to DLI may vary from disease to disease. The best results have been obtained in patients with relapsed CML after transplantation followed by AML/MDS and ALL. Although the first patient successfully treated by DLI for residual disease was a child with ALL, the haematological responses to DLI are rare in patients with ALL. In order to reduce the risk of GvH disease after DLI, genetic manipulations of donor T cells with herpes simplex thymidine kinase suicide gene have been suggested. If GvH disease develops, transduced T cells can be eliminated by treatment of the patient with gancyclovir. Given the low response rates to DLI apart from CML patients, more potentially effective strategies are currently under investigation, among them the adoptive transfer of donor-derived leukaemia–specific T cells. Pioneering studies showed the feasibility of generating and expanding leukaemia-specific T cells using recipient leukaemic blasts or leukaemic dendritic cells and of inducing remissions after the post-transplant adoptive transfer into patients with relapsed CML after HSCT. Recent findings support the hypothesis that major HLA antigens are principally responsible for the GvL effects. It has been reported that the genomic loss of the mismatched HLA locus in relapsed AML blasts is a major *in vivo* escape mechanism from T-cell-mediated immune surveillance after haploidentical transplantation. Donor T cells were able to recognize the original HLA-heterozygous blasts but not the mutant blasts which lost the unshared HLA haplotype.

An alternative strategy is to generate donor-derived cytotoxic lymphocytes (CTL) specific for minor histocompatibility antigens (mHag) or CTLs that recognize leukaemia-specific antigens, such as PR3, WT1 or breakpoint cluster region (BCR)-ABL (Fig. 7.2).

Prevention of relapse using NK cells

In contrast to T lymphocytes, NK cells do not induce GvH disease and can therefore be used as anti-leukaemic effector cells in post-transplant adoptive transfer studies. Recent advances in T-cell depletion technologies from mobilized peripheral stem cells allow the co-infusion of large numbers of NK cells. This technology, in combination with RIC regimens, is associated with a much lower TRM and with the same rate of engraftments compared to the previously approach using CD34+ positively selected haploidentical stem cell grafts and fully ablative conditioning regimens. Purified alloreactive haploidentical NK cells were adoptively transferred several days after conditioning and transplantation with purified CD34+ stem cells from the same haploidentical donor. This approach resulted in a long-term remission in a patient with infant leukaemia who relapsed after a standard myelablative allogeneic transplantation and presented with refractory leukaemia at time of haploidentical second transplantation.

Prevention of infection using adoptive transfer of T cells

Viral infection and reactivation or fungal infections contribute significantly to mortality and morbidity after allogeneic HSCT. This is caused by the more or less delayed immune reconstitution encountered with various graft manipulations techniques (i.e. T-cell repleted or T-cell depleted grafts, CD34+ enriched grafts) or grafts sources (PBSCs, bone marrow or umbilical cord blood). In a retrospective study, the risk factors for the development of invasive aspergillosis were: length of neutropenia, status of underlying disease, myeloablative conditioning regimens,

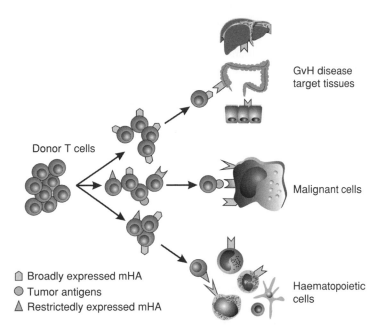

Donor T cells

GvH disease
target tissues

Malignant cells

◻ Broadly expressed mHA
◯ Tumor antigens
△ Restrictedly expressed mHA

Haematopoietic
cells

Fig. 7.2 Donor-derived T lymphocytes can proliferate and exert cytotoxicity against minor histocompatibility antigens (mHA) or against tumour antigens, which can result in GvH disease or anti-tumour response, dependent on the nature and distribution of the mHAs.

cytomegalovirus (CMV) disease, GvH disease grade II–IV, and bone marrow or cord blood as graft source compared to PBSCs. In patients at risk or patients with active disease, the adoptive transfer of functionally active *Aspergillus*-specific T cells might be a therapeutic option to restore immune effector functions rapidly and methods for the rapid and clinical large-scale generation of *Aspergillus*-specific T cells have been developed. After haploidentical transplantation, non-recipient reactive, pathogen-specific T-cell clones were adoptively transferred. While no GvH disease occurred, high-frequency T-cell responses to pathogens could be detected.

Adenovirus (ADV) and CMV infection remains a major risk factor for transplant-related morbidity and mortality in paediatric patients. In patients with chemotherapy-refractory CMV or ADV disease, the adoptive transfer of ADV hexon-specific T cells or the adoptive transfer of CMV pp-65-specific T cells proved to be safe, did not induce GvH disease and was effective in viral control and elimination in a majority of the treated patients.

The adoptive transfer of Epstein–Barr (EBV)-specific T cells selected from the donor also proved to be safe and effective. Another approach to adoptively transfer a broader donor immunity might be photodynamic purging of alloreactive T cells. With this method, alloantigen-stimulated T cells take up a dye which becomes highly cytotoxic to the alloreactive T cells through oxidative damage after exposure to visible light. With this approach, alloantigen-specific T cells are maximally reduced, whereas pathogen-specific responses to pathogens like CMV, ADV, varicella zoster virus, herpes simplex virus, *Aspergillus fumigatus*, *Candida albicans* and *Toxoplasma gondii* were mainly retained.

Cotransplanting mesenchymal stem cells

Mesenchymal stromal cells (MSC) have the capacity to differentiate into multiple lineages and also exhibit a number features which underscore their important role in allogeneic HSCT.

They secrete cytokines important for haematopoieisis, can be immunosuppressive and can promote engraftment of haematopoietic stem cells in experimental animal models. *In vitro* preparations of MSC from bone marrow are available and MSC can be rapidly expanded *in vitro* for clinical application. In paediatric patients, MSC have been successfully cotransplanted with haploidentical T-cell-depleted grafts in 32 patients. No graft failure was seen and the infusion was without any side effects. The immunosuppressive effects of MSC were first demonstrated in a child with therapy-resistant grade IV acute GvH disease of the gut and liver. Subsequently, a phase I/II multicentre trial was conducted in 30 adult and 25 paediatric patients with therapy-resistant GvH disease. No toxicities were seen after infusion of the MSC and 55 per cent of the patients showed a complete remission of their GvH disease. The overall response rate was higher in children (80 per cent) than in adults (60 per cent). MSC seem to be a promising cellular therapy in children for the prevention and treatment of GvH disease and to improve engraftment or graft dysfunctions. However, data on the long-term safety and efficacy are pending.

Summary

The safety of allogeneic HSCT in children has dramatically improved since its initial establishment 40 years ago. Better patient and donor selection, progress in supportive care, prevention of infections and less toxic conditioning regimens have contributed to lower TRM and improved overall survival. Nevertheless, the outcome is not yet satisfactory and further research into new strategies to improve the outcome is necessary. New strategies under active research by many investigators include: the expansion of the donor pool by including cord blood or haploidentical donors; the exploitation of GvL without GvH disease; the use of new donor selection criteria such as KIR genotyping to identify alloreactive donors among several HLA-matched donors to prevent relapse; the prevention or treatment of severe infections by adoptive transfer of pathogen-specific T cells; the prevention of relapse by adoptive transfer of leukaemia-specific T cells; and the cotransplantation of MSC to facilitate and improve engraftment and to prevent or treat severe acute or chronic GvH disease.

Further reading

Baker KS, Bresters D, Sande JE (2010) The burden of cure: long-term side effects following hematopoietic stem cell transplantation (HSCT) in children. *Pediatr Clin North Am* **57**, 323–42.

Ball LM, Bernardo ME, Roelofs H, et al. (2007) Cotransplantation of ex vivo expanded mesenchymal stem cells accelerates lymphocyte recovery and may reduce the risk of graft failure in haploidentical hematopoietic stem-cell transplantation. *Blood* **110**, 2764–7.

Ballen KK, Spitzer TR. (2011) The great debate: haploidentical or cord blood transplant. *Bone Marrow Transplant* **46**, 323–9.

Barrett AJ (2008) Understanding and harnessing the graft-versus-leukaemia effect. *Br J Haematol* **142**, 877–88.

Capitini CM, Cooper LJ, Egeler RM, et al. (2009) Highlights of the First International 'Immunotherapy in Pediatric Oncology: Progress and Challenges' Meeting. *J Pediatr Hematol Oncol* **31**, 227–44.

Cooley S, Weisdorf DJ, Guethlein LA, et al. (2010) Donor selection for natural killer cell receptor genes leads to superior survival after unrelated transplantation for acute myelogenous leukemia. *Blood* **116**, 2411–9.

Feuchtinger T, Opherk K, Bethge WA, et al. (2010) Adoptive transfer of pp65-specific T cells for the treatment of chemorefractory cytomegalovirus disease or reactivation after haploidentical and matched unrelated stem cell transplantation. *Blood* **116**, 4360–7.

Gyurkocza B, Rezvani A, Storb RF. (2010) Allogeneic hematopoietic cell transplantation: the state of the art. *Expert Rev Hematol* **3**, 285–99.

Handgretinger R, Kurtzberg J, Egeler RM (2008) Indications and donor selections for allogeneic stem cell transplantation in children with hematologic malignancies. *Pediatr Clin North Am* **55**, 71–96, x.

Handgretinger R, Lang P. (2008) The history and future prospective of haplo-identical stem cell transplantation. *Cytotherapy* **10**, 443–51.

Jacobsohn DA (2008) Acute graft-versus-host disease in children. *Bone Marrow Transplant* **41**, 215–21.

Kanold J, Paillard C, Tchirkov A, et al. (2008) Allogeneic or haploidentical HSCT for refractory or relapsed solid tumors in children: toward a neuroblastoma model. *Bone Marrow Transplant* **42** Suppl 2, S25–S30.

Kolb HJ (2008) Graft-versus-leukemia effects of transplantation and donor lymphocytes. *Blood* **112**, 4371–83.

Lang P, Pfeiffer M, Muller I, et al. (2006) Haploidentical stem cell transplantation in patients with pediatric solid tumors: preliminary results of a pilot study and analysis of graft versus tumor effects. *Klin Padiatr* **218**, 321–6.

Lankester AC, Ball LM, Lang P, Handgretinger R (2010) Immunotherapy in the context of hematopoietic stem cell transplantation: the emerging role of natural killer cells and mesenchymal stromal cells. *Pediatr Clin North Am* **57**, 97–121.

Le BK, Frassoni F, Ball L, et al. (2008) Mesenchymal stem cells for treatment of steroid-resistant, severe, acute graft-versus-host disease: a phase II study. *Lancet* **371**, 1579–86.

Leung W, Iyengar R, Turner V, et al. (2004) Determinants of antileukemia effects of allogeneic NK cells. *J Immunol* **172**, 644–50.

Miller JS, Warren EH, van den Brink MR, et al. (2010) NCI First International Workshop on The Biology, Prevention, and Treatment of Relapse After Allogeneic Hematopoietic Stem Cell Transplantation: Report from the Committee on the Biology Underlying Recurrence of Malignant Disease following Allogeneic HSCT: Graft-versus-Tumor/Leukemia Reaction. *Biol Blood Marrow Transplant* **16**, 565–86.

Pui CH, Campana D, Pei D, et al. (2009) Treating childhood acute lymphoblastic leukemia without cranial irradiation. *N Engl J Med* **360**, 2730–41.

Ringden O, Karlsson H, Olsson R, et al. (2009) The allogeneic graft-versus-cancer effect. *Br J Haematol* **147**, 614–33.

Rocha V, Locatelli F (2008) Searching for alternative hematopoietic stem cell donors for pediatric patients. *Bone Marrow Transplant* **41**, 207–14.

Seggewiss R, Einsele H. (2010) Immune reconstitution after allogeneic transplantation and expanding options for immunomodulation: an update. *Blood* **115**, 3861–8.

Shaw BE, Arguello R, Garcia-Sepulveda CA, Madrigal JA (2010) The impact of HLA genotyping on survival following unrelated donor haematopoietic stem cell transplantation. *Br J Haematol* **150**, 251–8.

Velardi A, Ruggeri L, Mancusi A, et al. (2009) Natural killer cell allorecognition of missing self in allogeneic hematopoietic transplantation: a tool for immunotherapy of leukemia. *Curr Opin Immunol* **21**, 525–30.

Wagner JE, Gluckman E (2010) Umbilical cord blood transplantation: the first 20 years. *Semin Hematol* **47**, 3–12.

Chapter 8

Supportive care during treatment

Julia Chisholm and Marianne van de Wetering

Introduction

Supportive care is a critical component of cancer management in children. As the intensity of primary treatment has escalated, so have side effects such as myelosuppression and infection. Improved outcomes are dependent on careful support of children through therapy and it has been important that advances in supportive care have paralleled advances in cancer therapy. In this chapter we will highlight a few key aspects.

Infection

Infection remains a common cause of hospital admission during cancer therapy and is the commonest cause of death after disease relapse/progression. Children are at increased risk of bacterial, viral, protozoal, and fungal infections and the prevention and treatment of infection are central to supportive care.

Many factors influence the frequency and severity of infection in cancer patients. These include myelo- or immunosuppression as a result of disease or therapy and disruption of natural barriers to infection. Neutropenia (absolute neutrophil count <500 cells/mm^3) is the most important risk factor, with both the depth and duration of neutropenia influencing infection risk. Death has been reported in 1–3 per cent of episodes of febrile neutropenia (FN) in children.

Around 15–20 per cent of all episodes of FN in children are associated with positive blood culture isolates. The pattern of infective pathogens has changed significantly over time. Previously Gram-negative bacteria infections predominated but Gram-positive organisms now cause up to 70 per cent of proven bloodstream infections, Gram-negative infections 28 per cent and fungal infections 2 per cent.

The commonest Gram-positive organisms are coagulase-negative *Staphylococci*, but enterococci and viridans group streptococcal species are becoming problematic because of the potential for severe disease and increasing antibiotic resistance. Among Gram-negative organisms, the most frequent are *Escherichia coli*, *Klebsiella* species, *Pseudomonas aeruginosa*, *Serratia* species and *Proteus* species. Infections with Gram-negative bacteria producing extended spectrum beta-lactamases are of increasing concern in hospital and community but are not yet widely reported in children with cancer. Infections with fungal organisms such as *Candida* species, *Aspergillus* species or other opportunistic fungi, and viruses such as cytomegalovirus (CMV), varicella zoster virus (VZV), adenovirus and infections with *Pneumocystis jirovecii* (pneumocystis pneumonia or PCP) may occur.

Prevention of infection

A number of strategies are commonly used to reduce the risk of infection although the evidence for some of these is lacking.

The environment

Neutropenic patients are at increased risk of hospital-acquired infections and the hospital environment should be avoided where possible. Children are encouraged to continue their normal lifestyle including school and hobbies. Teachers should be informed of the risks to the child with cancer and asked to alert the child's parents when there is VZV or measles in the school.

The hospital environment

If hospitalized during neutropenia, children are often cared for in single rooms although many specialist paediatric oncology units now manage neutropenic children on the open oncology ward. Careful handwashing is essential and prevents the spread of infection.

Nutrition/diet

There is no proof of the role of special measures concerning food products during neutropenia but potentially contaminated products such as unpasteurized milk or cheese, seafood and pâté should be avoided. Special dietary restrictions normally apply to patients undergoing haematopoetic stem cell transplant (HSCT).

Invasive procedures

Any procedure that can disrupt the normal mucosa or skin barriers should be avoided during neutropenic periods (e.g. dental procedures). Insertion of a central venous catheter is best done when the child is not neutropenic but if it is essential during neutropenia the catheter could be flushed after insertion with an antibiotic (vancomycin or teicoplanin) and heparin combination.

Antibiotic prophylaxis

Oral antibiotics may be used to preserve beneficial anaerobic organisms while preventing colonization of the gut by pathogenic aerobic organisms. Historically trimethoprim/sulfamethoxazole (TMP/SMZ) was used but more recently quinolones have been employed. Selective decontamination of the digestive tract (SDD) is effective in preventing bacteraemia (mainly Gram-negative bacteraemia) during neutropenic episodes and reduces deaths from infective causes. Quinolones are slightly more effective than TMP/SMZ. SDD should be considered for patients with an estimated infection risk above 10 per cent, such as patients with haematological malignancy, HSCT patients, and relapsed patients. The risk of emergence of resistant organisms as the result of routine prophylaxis has not been significant to date but requires further study.

Fungal prophylaxis

The need for fungal prophylaxis is less clear than for bacterial prophylaxis, but is recommended as standard of care in high-risk patients (i.e. HSCT patients, haematological malignancy, and relapsed patients). Early diagnosis of invasive fungal infection is expected to improve outcomes, but prevention remains the ultimate goal. Fluconazole provides effective prophylaxis against most *Candida* infections although some species such as *Candida krusei* may be resistant. *Aspergillus* prophylaxis requires itraconazole, voriconazole, posaconazole, micafungin or an intravenous amphotericin B preparation but co-administration of itraconazole and vincristine risks severe vincristine neurotoxicity. Monitoring of children at increased risk for *Aspergillus* infection is essential.

Viral prophylaxis

Aciclovir is used in patients at high risk of CMV and VZV activation, namely patients on very intensive solid tumour protocols and those undergoing HSCT. Clinical VZV (shingles) is common after viral prophylaxis is discontinued in HSCT patients and it is currently recommended to continue for up to a year post-HSCT.

Prevention of *Pneumocystis jirovecii* pneumonia

TMP/SMZ is highly effective in preventing PCP and is important for all patients undergoing treatment for leukaemia, lymphoma, HSCT and patients with solid tumours with prolonged neutropenic episodes. An alternative to TMP/SMZ prophylaxis is aerosolized or intravenous pentamidine. Dapsone can be given if patients cannot tolerate pentamidine.

Granulocyte colony-stimulating factor

Granulocyte colony-stimulating factor (G-CSF) is widely used in adult and paediatric practice to reduce the depth and duration of chemotherapy-associated neutropenia. The need for primary administration of colony-stimulating factors is usually determined by protocol, to support the administration of dose-intense chemotherapy, in patients with a greater than 20 per cent risk of experiencing FN or in the setting of progenitor cell mobilization. Secondary prophylactic G-CSF administration is allowed if previous episodes of neutropenia have led to severe infections, delay or dose-reduction of chemotherapy. The recommended G-CSF dose is 5 µg/kg/day subcutaneously or intravenously. G-CSF should be started 24–72 hours after chemotherapy and continued until the neutrophil count is >1000/mm^3 on two occasions.

Immunization in prevention of infection

Some aspects of vaccine-acquired immunity are lost during cancer therapy. Booster vaccinations are recommended for all children 6 months after completing therapy and a complete revaccination programme is recommended for children at a year or more after HSCT (Table 8.1). There is a balance between the most significant time for infection risk and the likelihood of response to therapy. Live attenuated vaccines should not be administered until at least 6 months after stopping chemotherapy but if herd immunity for measles is low, single antigen measles vaccine may be given during or soon after chemotherapy with measles vaccination repeated 6 months after stopping chemotherapy. Hepatitis B vaccination ideally is given after completing chemotherapy, but in high-risk groups or areas it can be given during chemotherapy with reduced immunogenic response. Periodic booster doses are usually necessary, with the timing determined by serologic testing at 12-month intervals. There are no data on changes in immune status or revaccination against human papilloma viruses after chemotherapy or HSCT.

Most countries recommend yearly influenza vaccination during chemotherapy and after HSCT as well as vaccination of household contacts. A Cochrane systematic review emphasized the paucity of data on this vaccine. Serological responses are lower than expected in healthy controls and antibody levels considered protective in healthy individuals may not prevent clinical infection in an immunocompromised individual. There are no data on whether vaccination of paediatric cancer patients protects against clinical infection. However, as the vaccine is well tolerated it is not contraindicated.

VZV vaccination has been given to VZV IgG negative patients during leukaemia maintenance therapy. The vaccine is immunogenic but some patients develop vaccine-related infection requiring aciclovir treatment. In addition, chemotherapy must be omitted for 1 week before and 1 week after the time of vaccination and steroids should not be given for 2 weeks after vaccination. The vaccine has not been widely studied in other groups of children with malignancy. For these reasons, geographical differences in practice exist with respect to VZV vaccination of susceptible children with cancer.

Live or attenuated vaccines such as measles, mumps, rubella (MMR) or oral polio are contraindicated during cancer therapy. Siblings or household contacts may safely receive MMR but enhanced inactivated polio vaccine (e IPV) should be given in place of oral polio vaccine (see Table 8.1).

Table 8.1 Vaccination recommendations during and after chemotherapy treatment (recommendations do not apply to children during/after autologous or allogenic bone marrow transplant)

Timing in relation to chemotherapy	Vaccination*	Recommendation
During chemotherapy	MMR	If low herd immunity, then use single-antigen measles vaccine
	OPV	Not allowed. If needed then eIPV*
	DTaP	Prefer to wait until stopping chemo
	Hepatitits B	High risk areas—Recombivax HB
After chemotherapy	DTaP/MMR/HiB	Restart schedule 6 months after stopping chemotherapy
Special considerations	Influenza vaccine	Not contraindicated during chemo
	Varicella zoster	Degree of protection uncertain
	Pneumococcal vaccine	No evidence-based recommendation
		In maintenance chemotherapy, safe and immunogenic, not registered yet for use in children with cancer. Indicated for splenic dysfunction e.g. splenectomy in Hodgkin's lymphoma, post-radiotherapy (radiation spleen)

* DTaP, Diphteria, tetanus, acellular pertussis vaccine; eIPV, enhanced inactivated polio vaccine; HiB, *Haemophilus influenzae* b conjugate vaccine; MMR, measles, mumps, rubella vaccine; OPV, oral polio vaccine.

Treatment of infection in children with cancer

Febrile neutropenia is defined as neutrophil count of <500 cells/mm^3 (or above 500 cells/mm^3 and expected to fall) and significant fever. Fever definitions vary but include a single temperature >38.5°C, or a temperature of >38°C twice in 12 hours. Management is a medical emergency because of the potential risk of overwhelming sepsis. Children who are neutropenic and significantly unwell but without fever should also be managed as for FN; occasionally Gram-negative sepsis presents with abdominal pain and diarrhoea but without fever, especially in children receiving steroid therapy.

Febrile, neutropenic children with cancer require careful assessment. Treatment is divided into empirical therapy and 'planned progressive therapy' stages.

Assessment

A careful history and thorough physical examination is needed, including emphasis on the mucosal membranes, the chest, soft tissues, central venous catheter site, and perianal area. The assessment phase is ongoing: careful and repeated evaluation for specific symptoms and signs or a focus of infection is critical but there may be minimal signs of inflammation at an infected site during neutropenia. Laboratory evaluation should include a complete blood count, liver enzymes, renal function, and blood culture. Urine culture, stool culture testing for *Clostridium* toxin, cerebrospinal fluid examination and chest X-ray should be done only if clinically indicated. Based on the patient history and initial clinical findings, patients may be assessed as at low or high risk of complications of FN although as yet there is no validated multicentre, multinational risk assessment tool in paediatric FN.

Empirical antibiotic therapy

The progression of infection in neutropenic patients can be rapid, so empirical intravenous antibiotic therapy should be started promptly. The initial goal is to provide broad spectrum cover against both Gram-negative and Gram-positive organisms. This is usually achieved by combining antibiotics such as a cephalosporin or extended spectrum beta-lactam with an aminoglycoside. Monotherapy with a carbapenem such as meropenem or imipenem is a reasonable alternative. Even patients assessed as low risk at presentation should always receive empirical intravenous therapy for at least 24–48 hours unless treated as part of a clinical trial or according to an established institutional low-risk protocol. The empirical antibiotic regimen should be reviewed regularly in each institution, taking account of changes in the spectrum of infections, antimicrobial susceptibility patterns, and the underlying aetiology of the neutropenia.

'Planned progressive' therapy

The therapeutic plan should be modified according to clinical response and microbiological findings. Children who are clinically well, lack a significant clinical focus of infection other than upper respiratory tract infection, have no positive cultures and whose fever settles quickly, can discontinue antibiotics once afebrile for 24–48 hours. Some protocols allow for step down to oral antibiotics in patients at low risk of significant complications. If the patient without a positive clinical focus or cultures has persistent fever after 3–5 days of treatment, reassess carefully, take further cultures and look for a focus. If the child is clinically well, the same antibiotics can be continued. If the child is deteriorating clinically, consider changing antibiotics and/or adding anaerobic cover. Add antifungal therapy after 4–5 days of persistent fever where there is no other explanation, and consider early CT of chest and sinuses, abdominal ultrasound scan, and opthalmological examination for retinal candidiasis.

Patients with positive blood cultures require a minimum of 7–10 days of intravenous antibiotics after eradication of the organism. If fever settles quickly, therapy for the isolated organism should be optimized but maintain broad-spectrum antibiotic cover to prevent breakthrough bacteraemia. It is not usually necessary to continue antibiotics until the neutrophils recover. Invasive fungal infection requires a prolonged course of antifungal therapy.

If fever persists in a child with a positive culture, optimize antibacterial therapy before making any other changes and consider adding antifungal therapy after 4–5 days of fever. Rarely, fever may be due to the medication but stopping antibiotics can be dangerous and should only be considered after a very careful, thorough exclusion of other causes of fever. Figure 8.1 shows an algorithm for management of FN.

Central venous catheter infections

Complications related to the long-term use of central venous catheters are minimized by recommended protocols for catheter placement and care, but there is the potential for infection of the bloodstream and/or device, the subcutaneous pocket. and the tunnel or exit site. The overall incidence of catheter-related infections is approximately 2/1000 catheter days.

Most infections are with Gram-positive organisms (mainly coagulase-negative *Staphylococcus)* but cover for Gram-negative organisms is necessary until an organism is identified. More than 80 per cent of documented catheter-related infections can be treated successfully by giving antibiotics through the catheter, but treatment failures may result from infections with multiple organisms, fungi, *Pseudomonas aeruginosae*, resistant Gram-negative organisms and tunnel infections. In *Staphylococcus. aureus* infection, antibiotics should be administered for at least 2–3 weeks if the catheter is left in place. Persistent bacterial catheter infections and most fungal (*Candida*) catheter infections require catheter removal. Catheter removal should also be considered early in the acutely unwell, septic patient whose condition is not responding rapidly to broad-spectrum antibiotics and fluid resuscitation.

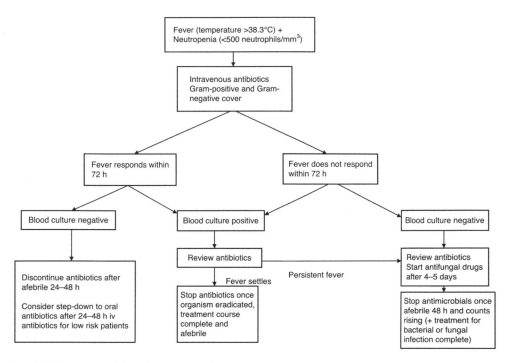

Fig. 8.1 Treatment of fever in neutropenia.

Fever without neutropenia

The non-neutropenic, febrile child should be evaluated very carefully. Laboratory evaluation includes a blood count, c-reactive protein (CRP) and blood culture from the central venous catheter and management is dictated by the clinical findings. If the child is clinically well other than fever with no clinical focus of infection, blood-culture results can be awaited before starting antibiotics. If there is a clinical focus of bacterial infection (e.g. ear, throat, skin) consider appropriate oral antibiotics such as amoxicillin, or co-amoxiclav until the blood-culture result is known. If the non-neutropenic child is unwell with fever, commence empirical antibiotics as for a neutropenic child and give appropriate supportive care, pending further results.

Viral infections

The most common viral pathogens that affect the immunocompromised child are the herpes viruses including herpes simplex virus (HSV), VZV, CMV, and Epstein–Barr virus (EBV).

Herpesviruses can result in mucosal lesions, skin lesions and neurologic symptoms. Systemic treatment with aciclovir is needed for at least 5 days. Aciclovir is not routinely indicated for chemotherapy-induced mucositis.

Primary infection with VZV results in chickenpox. In the immunocompromised child, severe complications may be seen leading to a fulminating illness with visceral dissemination of the virus. Untreated VZV pneumonitis can be fatal in up to 7 per cent of affected children. Treatment should be intravenous aciclovir or the newer oral drugs such as famciclovir or valaciclovir which show a better oral absorption than acyclovir. Children should be tested for VZV IgG at diagnosis and VZV negative patients should be given prophylaxis with varicella zoster immune globulin or aciclovir after significant contact.

CMV can result in fever, rash, hepatosplenomegaly, pneumonia, neurologic symptoms and retinitis. Treatment is with ganciclovir intravenously or foscarnet. Prolonged courses of therapy are necessary to eradicate the infection.

Blood product transfusion

Anaemia and thrombocytopenia can occur as a consequence of chemotherapy or the underlying disease.

Red cell transfusion

The haemoglobin concentration should be maintained at safe levels but normal physiological levels are not required. There is no evidence for the transfusion threshold but most centres choose a level of <6.5 g/dl. If the child is septic or has cardiopulmonary problems a level of <9.5 g/dl is used, and with radiotherapy an even higher level of 7.0–11.5 g/dl is maintained because of the need for adequate oxygenation during radiotherapy. Leukodepleted, packed red cells are given at a dose of 10–15 ml/kg over 4–6 hours. Leukodepletion reduces the chance of HLA sensitization and infection with prions and CMV. Irradiated products are not routinely required but important exceptions are before HSCT, after HSCT until lymphocytes have recovered (6 months after transplant), in severe combined immunodeficiencies, in neonates, and in Hodgkin's Lymphoma. There are insufficient data to recommend the routine use of erythropoetin in pediatric oncology.

Platelet transfusions

Platelet transfusions are indicated if a thrombocytopenic patient is actively bleeding. Prophylactic platelet transfusions are indicated in patients who are septic, have a known bleeding disorder or are undergoing an invasive procedure such as central venous catheter insertion or lumbar puncture. There is little evidence about the appropriate transfusion threshold. In patients with sepsis, platelets are usually kept >15 x 10^9/l and for invasive procedures the level is kept >50 x 10^9/l. Single donor transfusions can be used if patients develop allo-immunization which reduces the therapeutic effect of transfused platelets.

Nausea and vomiting

Nausea and vomiting remain an important concern in cancer treatment but adequate control can usually be achieved. Techniques such as relaxation, distraction, and explanation of procedures should be considered along with anti-emetic medication. Adult guidelines can not automatically be applied to children, as no adequate paediatric pharmacokinetic trials have been performed.

A validated nausea and vomiting tool such as the PENAT score (comparable with the face pain rating scale for assessment of pain) should be used to assess the severity of nausea and vomiting at regular intervals. Management is adjusted according to findings.

Chemotherapeutic agents are grouped in three classes: low emetogenicity (<10 per cent of patients experience nausea and vomiting), moderate emetogenicity (50 per cent of patients experience nausea and vomiting), and high emetogenicity (100 per cent of patients experience nausea and vomiting). Starting medication is tailored to the drug of highest emetogenicity within the chemotherapy combination (Table 8.2). In low emetogenicity chemotherapy, no anti-emetic therapy is needed. Agents such as metoclopromide, domperidone or promethazine can be used.

Table 8.2 Anti-emetic therapy in relation to different types of chemotherapy

Emetogenic potential	Drug	Anti-emetic therapy	Delayed emesis
Low	Bleomycin Busulfan oral Steroids Fludarabine Hydroxyurea Interferon Melfalan oral Mercaptopurine Methotrexate <50 mg/m^2 Thioguanine Vinblastine Vincristine	None or Domperidone 1–2 mg/kg/day in 4 doses, oral or Promethazine 0.5–0.8 mg/kg/day in 4 doses, oral or Metoclopromide 0.3–0.5 mg/kg/day in 2–4 doses, oral or rectal	None
Moderate	Asparaginase Cytarabine <1 g/m^2 Doxorubicin Etoposide Fluouracil <1000 mg/m^2 Gemcitabine Methotrexate 1 g/m^2 Thiotepa Topotecan Cyclophosphamide <750 mg/m^2 Actinomycin Epirubicin Idarubicin Mitoxantrone <15 mg/m^2	Ondansetron 15 mg/m^2/day in 2–3 doses, iv, oral or rectal and Dexamethasone 5 mg/m^2 loading dose (max. 8 mg) followed by 5 mg/m^2/day in 3 doses, iv or oral	None
High	Carboplatin Carmustine Cisplatin Cyclophosphamide >750 mg/m^2 Cytarabine >1 g/m^2 Actinomycin Doxorubicin >60 mg/m^2 Irinotecan Melfalan (iv) Methotrexate >1 g/m^2 Mitoxantrone >15 mg/m^2 Procarbazine	Ondansetron 15 mg/m^2/day in 2–3 doses, iv, oral or rectal and Dexamethasone, loading dose 10 mg/m^2 (max. 20 mg) followed by 5 mg/m^2/day in 3 doses If NK1 antagonist is considered in older children, a standard dose of 125 mg is given orally before starting chemotherapy followed by 80 mg/day in 3 doses Beware: With NK1 antagonist, use lower dose dexamethasone, (as for moderate emetogenic) group)	Continue ondansetron for 72 hours after stopping chemotherapy

In moderately emetogenic chemotherapy, a serotonin receptor antagonist is indicated, usually ondansetron; corticosteroids can be added as the drugs work synergistically. In highly emetogenic chemotherapy, the combination of a serotonin receptor antagonist plus steroids should be used. Continue one of the anti-emetics till 72 hours after stopping the chemotherapy to prevent delayed emesis. Radiotherapy can also lead to nausea and vomiting and a serotonin receptor antagonist is often given 30 minutes before treatment.

An aggressive anti-emetic plan at the start of therapy minimizes the initial experience of nausea and reduces the risk of anticipatory nausea and vomiting. If anticipatory vomiting does occur, benzodiazepines are usually effective.

New 5HT3 antagonists (palanosetron R) and NK-1 antagonists (aprepitant R) have improved difficult to manage acute and delayed emesis in adults but no randomized trials have been performed yet in children.

Nutrition support

Good nutrition is important during cancer therapy. Patients may present undernourished at diagnosis and cancer treatment may profoundly impact their nutritional status.

Children with malnutrition or at high risk of developing malnutrition should be reviewed by a paediatric dietician for advice about healthy eating and vitamin supplementation. For children requiring nutritional intervention, enteral nutrition is the management of choice if gut function is maintained. Patients may be offered nutritional supplements such as high-calorie, nutrional drinks, if able to swallow normally and tolerate such supplements. Alternatively, nasogastric tube feeding or gastrostomy feeding may be indicated. Gastrostomy feeding is particularly suited to older children or young people who wish to avoid the cosmetic associations or irritation of a nasogastric tube or to children who otherwise cannot tolerate a nasogastric tube. When gut function is poor for a prolonged period or where nasogastric feeds cannot be tolerated, intravenous total parenteral nutrition is used.

Mouth care

Good mouth care plays an important role in the prevention of infection and is essential for children developing complications such as mucositis, oral candidiasis, xerostomia or herpes simplex infections. The evidence for mouth-care interventions is incomplete but guidelines based on available evidence are now available.

At diagnosis, an assessment of the mouth and teeth is essential and children should be referred to a dentist or dental hygienist promptly. During cancer therapy, children should brush their teeth twice daily using a soft toothbrush and fluoride toothpaste or clean the mouth with oral sponges moistened with water or diluted chlorhexidine. Regular assessment of the oral mucous membranes during inpatient therapy using one of the available scoring systems will allow early detection of, and intervention for, mucositis and other problems. Children who develop mucositis need ongoing basic mouth care and adequate analgesia.

Constipation

This is a common problem in children and young people with cancer and appropriate therapeutic intervention can greatly improve quality of life. The etiology is mostly multifactorial: these patients have reduced activity, reduced oral fluid and food intake, and take medications such as opioids, vinca alkaloids, carboplatin, and ondansetron which contribute to constipation. There are no randomized controlled studies performed in this age group to inform laxative choice so management is directed towards the most likely cause of constipation in the individual child. Stool softeners and osmotic laxatives (such as lactulose and sorbitol) are most often used and bowel evacuants are rarely needed.

Tumour lysis syndrome

Tumour lysis syndrome (TLS) is a set of complications that can arise from treatment of rapidly proliferating, drug-sensitive neoplasms. These are typically haematologic malignancies (particularly Burkitt lymphoma and the acute leukaemias) but rarely also solid tumours. Chemotherapy causes rapid destruction of tumour cells leading to release of intracellular substances into the bloodstream. Metabolic disturbances include hyperuricaemia, hyperphosphatemia, hypocalcemia, and hyperkalemia. Clinical manifestations occur 12–72 hours after initial start of therapy and can include renal failure (from precipitation of uric acid crystals and calcium phosphate salts), seizures, and cardiac arrhythmias.

Prevention of TLS relies on identification of at-risk patients. Such patients should have laboratory and clinical TLS parameters monitored every 4–6 hours until stabilized. Intensive care facilities must be close. In high-risk TLS, the nephrologist should be notified early and patients should be located in a facility with ready access to dialysis.

Standard supportive care to prevent TLS consists of vigorous hyperhydration (3000 ml/m^2/day), forced diuresis, with or without diuretics (loop diuretics or osmotic diuretics), and avoidance of hyperuricemia, The primary treatment for hyperuricemia has been allopurinol (50–100 mg/m^2 every 8 hours orally, maximum 300 mg/m^2/day) combined with hyperhydration. Alkalinization of the urine with sodium bicarbonate has been used historically and may still be indicated in high-risk patients. However, the addition of rasburicase (recombinant urate oxidase dose 0.2 mg/kg iv once a day) is preferred for high-risk patients and alkalinization becomes unnecessary. Urate oxidase catalyses conversion of uric acid to water-soluble allantoin which is readily excreted in urine. It decreases uric acid levels more than allopurinol, with a rapid drop occurring within 4 hours of administration.

Management is tailored according to risk of TLS. Low-risk patients [solid tumours and AML with white blood cell count (WCC) <25 x 10^9/l] only need monitoring and hyperhydration. ALL with WCC <100 x10^9/l, AML with WCC >25 x 10^9/l and large cell anaplastic lymphoma are classified as intermediate-risk disease for which monitoring, hyperhydration, and allopurinol is given. High-risk disease (ALL WCC>100 x 10^9/l, Burkitt lymphoma and other stage IV lymphoma) should be managed in specialized pediatric oncology units where patients need careful monitoring, hyperhydration, and rasburicase.

Conclusion

This chapter highlights the most important aspects of supportive care in the child with cancer. Pain management will be discussed in Chapter 10 (End of life Care). Other aspects have not been discussed here such as the use of CAM (complementary and alternative medicine) or the role of integrative medicine (the use of CAM in conjunction with standard medical treatment). The critical importance of supportive care continues to be the relief of cancer and treatment-related symptoms, less morbidity, and reduced mortality.

Further reading

Antonarakis ES, Evans JL, Heard GF, et al. (2004) Prophylaxis of acute chemotherapy-induced nausea and vomiting in children with cancer: what is the evidence? *Pediatr Blood Cancer* **43**, 651–8.

Baskin JL, Pui CH, Reiss U, et al. (2009) Management of occlusion and thrombosis associated with long-term indwelling central venous catheters. *Lancet* **374**, 159–69.

Bow EJ, Laverdiere M, Lussier N, et al. (2002) Antifungal prophylaxis for severely neutropenic chemotherapy recipients: a meta analysis of randomized-controlled clinical trials. *Cancer* **94**, 3230–46.

Cairo MS, Coiffier B, Reiter A, Younes A (2010) Recommendations for the evaluation of risk and prophylaxis of tumour lysis syndrome (TLS) in adults and children with malignant diseases: an expert TLS panel consensus. *Br J Haematol* **149**, 578–86.

Cunningham RS, Bell R (2000) Nutrition in cancer: an overview. *Semin Oncol Nurs* **16**, 90–8.

Dupuis LL, Taddio A, Kerr EN, et al. (2006) Development and validation of the pediatric nausea assessment tool for use in children receiving antineoplastic agents. *Pharmacotherapy* **26**, 1221–31.

Gafter-Gvili A, Fraser A, Paul M, et al. (2005) Antibiotic prophylaxis for bacterial infections in afebrile neutropenic patients following chemotherapy. *Cochrane Database Syst Rev* **4**, CD004386.

Glenny AM, Gibson F, Auld E, et al. (2010) The development of evidence-based guidelines on mouth care for children, teenagers and young adults treated for cancer. *Eur J Cancer* **46**, 1399–1412.

Goossen GM, Kremer LC, van de Wetering MD (2009) Influenza vaccination in children being treated with chemotherapy for cancer. *Cochrane Database Syst Rev* **2**, CD006484.

Herrstedt J (2008) Antiemetics: an update and the MASCC guidelines applied in clinical practice. *Nat Clin Pract Oncol* **5**, 32–43.

Mendes AV, Sapolnik R, Mendonca N (2007) New guidelines for the clinical management of febrile neutropenia and sepsis in pediatric oncology patients. *J Pediatr (Rio J)* **83** (2 Suppl), S54–63.

Mermel LA, Farr BM, Sherertz RJ, et al. (2001) Guidelines for the management of intravascular catheter-related infections. *Clin Infect Dis* **32**, 1249–72.

Patel SR, Chisholm JC, Heath PT (2008) Vaccinations in children treated with standard-dose cancer therapy or hematopoietic stem cell transplantation. *Pediatr Clin North Am* **55**, 169–86, xi.

Phillips RS, Gibson F (2008) A systematic review of treatments for constipation in children and young adults undergoing cancer treatment. *J Pediatr Hematol Oncol* **30**, 829–30.

Rheingans JI (2007) A systematic review of nonpharmacologic adjunctive therapies for symptom management in children with cancer. *J Pediatr Oncol Nurs* **24**, 81–94.

Sartori AM (2004) A review of the varicella vaccine in immunocompromised individuals. *Int J Infect Dis* **8**, 259–70.

Smith TJ, Khatcheressian J, Lyman GH, et al. (2006) Update of recommendations for the use of white blood cell growth factors: an evidence-based clinical practice guideline. *J Clin Oncol* **24**, 3187–205.

Chapter 9

Psychosocial care

Martha Grootenhuis, Esther Meijer-van den Bergh,
Jantien Vrijmoet-Wiersma and Momcilo Jankovic

Introduction

The diagnosis of cancer in a child is one of the most stressful events that can happen to a family. It confronts child and parents with a range of stressors, including the most feared: the death of the child. Although treatment has greatly improved over the last decades and survival rates have increased dramatically, parents and children still face an extensive period of intensive treatment which fundamentally impacts their lives. The whole family has the difficult task to adjust to a situation dominated by the stresses of long-lasting uncertainty and uncontrollability.

Children differ from adults. From birth until adulthood children are in a process of physical, cognitive, emotional, and social development. In developing their abilities to cope with their environment, children are dependent on adults. Together they are in a child-rearing relationship, in which an important role is given to their parents. Younger children need their parents to cope with basic fears and basic desires and also with the demands of socialization. Older children need their parents in learning to cope with questions related to physical growth, development of personal identity and difficulties of functioning in peer groups. Children also differ from adults in their understanding and experience of health, illness, and medical care. Depending on the child's developmental level, special needs have to be met in the context of the family (parents, siblings) and the enlarged social environment (friends, school, health-care workers). Each phase of treatment has its own characteristics that contribute to the reactions of parents and children. In this chapter, psychosocial care in these different phases will be described, focusing on both children and parents.

Acute phase

For all children and their parents, the diagnostic phase and start of treatment is very stressful. It commences with invasive medical procedures necessary to obtain a diagnosis. The child has to endure pain and the parents have to witness their child in pain and fear. The challenge is to accomplish a realistic, and for the child an age appropriate, understanding of diagnosis and treatment implications. This is especially necessary for decisions to be made at the beginning of treatment (e.g. study randomization). Children may anxiously ask 'am I going to die?' in a phase where their parents are in emotional turmoil and experience loss of control. In the past, it was not common to communicate frankly with children about cancer, survival, and death. Fortunately, it is now argued that enabling children to assimilate information and feelings allows them to cope better. Research has shown that providing information to the child with cancer about diagnosis and prognosis is beneficial for the child's emotional experience of his situation. In this phase, parents may feel guilty about late identification of symptoms related to the disease. Parents may also be angry due to delay in referral to the hospital. Learning to cope with these feelings takes time.

Furthermore, parents have to cope with the reactions of other family members (e.g. siblings, grandparents, etc.), which sometimes can give a profound extra burden.

A second stressor at this stage is learning to deal with the effects of medical treatment. Chemotherapy usually starts shortly after diagnosis. The child rapidly comprehends what cancer treatment is about: painful medical procedures (e.g. port-a-cath, lumbar punctures, bone marrow aspirations), sickness because of chemotherapeutic agents (nausea, vomiting, mycosis), and side effects such as hair loss. As well as the chemotherapeutic treatment in the hospital, parents have to administer cancer treatment to their child at home (e.g. dexamethasone). Managing this is challenging and makes parents feel extremely responsible.

A third stressor, especially at the beginning of treatment, is to inform the social environment (other family members, school, employers). Ensuring social support is of major importance because of the long duration of treatment. It is well known that social support is a protective factor in the adaptation to the disease. Families need ongoing support and to stay in touch with every day life as much as possible. Many families receive social support (e.g. for the care of siblings, household, etc.) but it is also important for a social worker to support the family in all the emotional and practical or financial consequences of the disease and treatment (including contact with employers, or welfare insurances). Special care is needed for non-native families. Both language and cultural background can make it very difficult to communicate properly about the cancer and its treatment. Using an interpreter in breaking the bad news, but also in subsequent conversations about changes in the course of treatment, contributes to their understanding.

To help parents adjust to the circumstances after diagnosis can be demanding (e.g. administering medication, timing of routine hospital visits, learning to evaluate symptoms and decide whether or not it is necessary to go and see the doctor and maintain balance inside the family). Thus, to help parents adjust, psychological intervention programs as well as teaching them both practical and emotional problem-solving skills can be helpful.

During treatment

Modern childhood cancer treatment, in spite of tremendous improvements in supportive care, still has many unwanted side effects. Especially older children have difficulties with losing their hair and changes in their physical appearance. These can be reversible changes such as the use of a feeding tube and substantial weight loss, but also irreversible changes such as stretch marks due to rapid increase in weight because of corticosteroid medication. Adolescents typically suffer from feelings of shame and inconvenience. The child or adolescent should be given information about the side effects of medication and treatment. Good psychosocial support may include teaching the child what he or she can do to cope with pain and other negative feelings. Cognitive behavioral techniques such as relaxation, visualization, distraction, and the use of 'helping thoughts' are beneficial.

In the first months after diagnosis, many children show adjustment towards treatment and being ill, but they also start to realize the impact of the cancer experience on their daily lives. Reactions to this adjustment can involve grief and mourning over the fact that their life as it was before being diagnosed is 'lost' or the development of a negative self-image due to the changed appearance. The way a child deals with his/her illness and treatment has a major impact on psychological well-being. Most studies in this field indicate that children with cancer as a group are not very different to control groups or comparison groups in terms of adaptation or adjustment and psychopathology in all stages of the disease and treatment. However, there are children who are at risk for difficulties in adapting to the disease, such as children who react with withdrawal or social isolation or children with premorbid psychopathology. These children need intensive psychological support during and after treatment. Possible types of treatment include: contact with fellow patients (through special camps or meetings), group training or individual therapy aimed at dealing with the disease and its consequences, in order to find their way back on track in life. For younger children, play therapy is a common way to work through emotions, while older children are often treated with cognitive behavioral therapy techniques.

Children with cancer often feel anger and disappointment because of restrictions on their participation in important areas of life, such as going to school or engaging in sports and other social activities. Sometimes it is difficult to stay in touch with friends due to poor clinical conditions. Children who attend school during treatment often feel 'different', because of their changed appearance or decline in health. As a group, however, they hardly seem different from their healthy peers in terms of their classroom behavior and social acceptance. Research shows that children with cancer who receive social support from their teachers, parents and friends report fewer psychosocial problems and have higher self-esteem.

A common problem in childhood cancer treatment is the reduced immunity due to therapy. This means that parents must be especially alert for risk of infections. Guidance in the realistic management of these risks and not becoming too obsessive and frightened is one of the issues in which psychological care can make a firm contribution. Unscheduled hospital visits due to reduced immunity problems (e.g. fever) are largely disruptive for everyday family life. Daily life becomes unpredictable and difficult to plan.

Overall, parents also experience many stress reactions during treatment. Studies on parental stress indicate that both fathers and mothers, 6 and 12 months after diagnosis, report increased feelings of anxiety and depression which only return to 'normal' levels after about 20–24 months. It is important to deal with the parental stress and adaptation to the illness and treatment, because of the relationship of parental functioning with the adjustment of the child. For some parents, additional guidance is needed from either a social worker or a psychologist. Other parents turn to their own social network for help.

Parents of children in treatment for cancer may find it hard to set limits on their sick child or to be separated from their child. One reason is that the stress of parenting a child can be enhanced by the effects of certain medications, including dexamethasone, which may cause behavioral problems in the child. Furthermore, in this stage, often one of the parents needs to go back to work. This can increase the burden on the other parent. Going to school is often encouraged and promoted by the hospital staff, but often parents are reluctant, as they are scared about the risk of infections. For the cognitive and social development of children, however, it is very important to stay in touch with the school.

After treatment

The end of the treatment in paediatric oncology can be considered a tremendous transition in care and can be very stressful. Children and parents are supported during the entire treatment by the multidisciplinary team. When treatment ends, this multidisciplinary guidance quickly diminishes and families must regain their own lives. In this phase, studies show that children of different ages report problems with physical functioning as a consequence of loss of general condition and strength or ongoing tiredness. In this new phase, returning to school, picking up the 'ordinary life' and being released from hospital care are the main goals for the children, but these goals might become hampered because of these physical impairments. Next to physical functioning, adolescents often experience a sense of distance towards their peers, which sometimes makes it difficult to reintegrate. Individual counselling can help children and adolescents to express feelings of loneliness or being misunderstood and help them to bridge the gap to 'normal life'.

When chemotherapy ends, parents typically realize that cure only lasts if there is no relapse and that there are less treatment options if the disease recurs. In this period, parents have to deal with feelings of immense uncertainty and with diminishing social support, which can be very stressful. Besides the fear of relapse, parents are being informed about late effects of the cancer treatment which also can give rise to posttreatment stress. At the same time, they have to pick up their lives, or are confronted with demands of the outside world such as employers who expect parents to return to work quickly. This increases the pressure on parents at a time when they need to pay some attention to themselves after such a long and exhausting period. Parents often describe this as the first period in which they pay attention to their own functioning. Physicians should be sensitive to symptoms of severe exhaustion in parents and refer to psychologists or social workers if needed.

Long-term follow up

Almost all children and adolescents who have been successfully treated for cancer have to deal with negative health outcomes. They may develop health problems as result of treatment (e.g. second cancers, cardiac conditions, endocrine problems or infertility), but also suffer social disadvantages in terms of academic achievement, finding a job, a partner, insurance. Regular screening of survivors concerning all the important areas of functioning in so-called 'late-effects clinics' is very important. Apart from screening for late effects, prevention is another issue that needs attention in paediatric survivorship programs and should be aimed at addressing lifestyle issues such as smoking, sunbathing and diet.

Neurocognitive long-term consequences as a result of the treatment for childhood cancer can be severe and long lasting. Children treated for brain tumours and children treated with high-dose chemotherapy are especially at risk. Treatment has impact on brain development and consequently on skills that have yet to emerge. The evidence for long-term neurocognitive deficits for survivors of childhood ALL after treatment with chemotherapy only appear to be subtle. These mainly involve processes of attention and of executive functioning, while global intellectual function is relatively preserved. Younger age at diagnosis, female sex and treatment intensity emerged as risk factors for ALL survivors. With the replacement of prednisolone in many recent treatment protocols by dexamethasone, the interest in the long-term side effects of this treatment has increased. Although results about decreased cognitive functioning during the dexamethasone pulses compared to non-dexamethasone treatment periods have been reported, others could not demonstrate any differences on long-term neurocognitve functioning.

Survivors who have been treated for brain tumours are more likely to have neuropsychological and learning difficulties as well as psychosocial difficulties. Important risk factors for brain tumour patients are hydrocephalus, dose of irradiation and time since cranial irradiation, effects of multiple treatments, female sex, and also young age at diagnosis. Improvements of the understanding of the exact neurocognitive deficits that accompany both disease and treatment factors remain important goals. Prolonged intensive rehabilitation and motoring of their neurocognitive functioning is needed for this subgroup of patients to offer interventions at a timely basis.

Studies on the long-term treatment psychosocial consequences of survivors show mixed results. Several studies report a reduced quality of life in physical and social functioning. Young adult survivors of childhood cancer achieve less developmental milestones, or at a later age than their peers. They value their functioning lower in the areas of independence, social and psychosexual development. In comparison with healthy controls, survivors are less likely to be married or living together and seem to have problems finding a job that provides financial independence. Some of the survivors report mood swings or post traumatic stress disorder (PTSD), a cluster of symptoms related to trauma such as intrusions, hypervigilance, and avoidance. However the numbers of survivors with these problems are considerably fewer than for their parents.

Parents of survivors can suffer from anxiety, tension, and uncertainty. Also a large percentage of parents report PTSD symptoms, including intrusions and avoidance behavior. Sometimes these avoidance behaviors compromise the follow up of the child (they are reluctant to revisit the hospital) and can be considered a risk factor. Raising a child who has had cancer is a challenging task for parents. It is sometimes difficult to modify habits consolidated during treatment, but that now limit the child's functioning. Finding a balance in caring for and protecting the child and, at the same time, promoting a healthy development towards young adulthood is a very hard task.

End-of-life issues

Despite the increased survival and progress in treating children with cancer, about one quarter of parents and children have to face that cure is not possible. The treatment goal shifts from cure to quality of life and dying, as quoted by Veronica, aged 13:

> What really matters in life is not so much being able to value it. What really counts, is being able to 'embrace' the moment when it finishes.

What is a terminally ill child? It is not a dying person, it is a child who has arrived at a phase of life where death is close and cure is no longer possible. This phase could last for months. It does not need to be either a 'therapeutically renouncing' or 'ruthless obstinacy' in its approach. It is essential to build up the most appropriate modality to assist a child and the family in the palliative and terminal phase. The main purpose in this phase is to keep control over both physical and psychological pain and discomfort, either with medical, psychological or spiritual interventions, and to turn any experience into something positive.

Today, most children who die of cancer die at home. Psychosocial care should be focused on helping the family with their daily life, to support parents in dealing with the dying child, their own emotions and also with any siblings. The hospital psychologist can play an important role in this situation, either in an advisory or consultative role for the professionals visiting the families at home (e.g. general practitioner, palliative nursing teams, etc.), or as caregiver. This differs according to country. For some children, talking about death and the fear of death is easier with a professional than a parent. The way in which children think about death and their understanding depends on age and cognitive and psychological development. Young children do not yet have a fully developed sense of death. They are cognitively unable to grasp the sense of irreversibility and permanence of death. On the contrary, older elementary school children have greater awareness of the irreversibility of death and teenagers generally have a fully developed awareness. Teachers and classmates at the child's school should be informed about the child's impending death. In this phase, to help the teacher, the classmates and the school is important. The continuous participation of the child in school activities can be of great importance. Most children want to participate in normal life, including school, for as long as possible, and being with their peers distracts them from being sick. Siblings of the sick child need good guidance as well. Many parents struggle with whether or not they should tell their child that he/she is dying. In a large Swedish study, parents of deceased children were asked retrospectively whether or not they told their child about their impending death and how they experienced and looked back on their decision. This study included a group of 500 parents: 34% of the parents talked with their child and none of these parents had regretted it afterwards. In the other group where parents did not talk to the child, the majority (73%) also did not regret this afterwards. The main criterion was the age of the child. Most parents chose to talk in terms of 'not getting better' or used metaphors, thus creating space for the child to ask questions. This study shows that the perception and appreciation of the situation by parents themselves should be included in the guidance in these end-of-life matters. For many parents, it is confusing, after the fatal news, to see that their child wants to continue living as if nothing has changed. Children often want to go to school and play in spite of their impending death.

Communication remains the basic issue when the diagnosis of cancer has to be reported to the patient and the family. How best to do it becomes the first step in a communicative process that involves the medical team and the family, and allows for growth and change over time until the final stage. Parents most often manage what and how their children are told about cancer. Adolescents or young adults vary in their preferences as to how much information should be disclosed to them. Some adolescents and young adults with cancer prefer to be fully informed about their disease, but approximately one-third among those who survived preferred not to know.

Many parents find it difficult to talk to young children about issues as serious as the diagnosis of cancer or impending death. Without proper communication starting at diagnosis, the child's reaction to the disease, treatment and new or altered life situations can cause additional stress for the parents at any time. Parental wishes may not always be in the best interest of the child. The parents may wish to shield the child, which may only make the patient's fear worse. Also, a conflict may arise when the family wishes to continue pursuing an unrealistic possibility of cure or, on the contrary, when the family wishes to stop curative treatment prematurely. If members of the health-care team take time to try to understand and discuss the reasons for the family's wishes, the inevitably painful conflicts can usually be overcome. The continuation of curative treatment beyond the point when cure is no longer possible should be avoided, the so-called 'ruthless obstinacy' treatment. In their desperation to avoid the upcoming death, parents often look for alternative treatments. This can be interpreted as a way of dealing with what is perceived as unacceptable. Many complementary treatments give parents feelings of control and the perception that they can contribute to the quality of life of their child. Many parents experience anticipatory grief in the shape of grief, depressive reactions or anger. The identification of these feelings as normal reactions to abnormal circumstances can be helpful. Once a child is deceased, parents often seek assistance from professionals such as a psychologist or grief counsellor. Furthermore, after a child dies, that individual child's medical history should be evaluated. This evaluation should be made by the health-care team as a group. It is very important to reflect on all events, even minor ones, that occurred during the course of the child's treatment. It is critical to reflect on the choices that were made and why, in order to help the staff come to terms with their own grieving and to learn from the experience in order to help future families.

Conclusion

Even with the increased survival rates of children with cancer, uncertainties about the nature and extent of late effects remain. To achieve optimal support for children and adolescents who grow up with childhood cancer, physicians should have knowledge about their developmental trajectory and pay attention to this during treatment and follow up. Therefore, periodical evaluation of their ongoing psychosocial, educational, and vocational needs during their developmental process should be an integral component of the comprehensive care of children and adolescents with cancer.

Further reading

Barakat LP, Kazak AE, Meadows AT, et al. (1997) Families surviving childhood cancer: a comparison of posttraumatic stress symptoms with families of healthy children. *J Pediatr Psychol* **22**, 843–59.

Butler RW, Haser JK (2006) Neurocognitive effects of treatment for childhood cancer. *Ment Retard Dev Disabil Res Rev* **12**, 184–91.

Eiser C, Hill JJ, Vance YH (2000) Examining the psychological consequences of surviving childhood cancer: systematic review as a research method in pediatric psychology. *J Pediatr Psychol* **25**, 449–60.

Geenen MM, Cardous-Ubbink MC, Kremer LC, et al. (2007) Medical assessment of adverse health outcomes in long-term survivors of childhood cancer. *JAMA* **297**, 2705–15.

Hinds PS, Hockenberry MJ, Gattuso JS, et al. (2007) Dexamethasone alters sleep and fatigue in pediatric patients with acute lymphoblastic leukemia. *Cancer* **110**, 2321–30.

Hoekstra-Weebers JE, Jaspers JP, Kamps WA, Klip EC (2001) Psychological adaptation and social support of parents of pediatric cancer patients: a prospective longitudinal study. *J Pediatr Psychol* **26**, 225–35.

Jankovic M, Brouwers P, Valsecchi MG, et al. (1994) Association of 1800 cGy cranial irradiation with intellectual function in children with acute lymphoblastic leukaemia. ISPACC. International Study Group on Psychosocial Aspects of Childhood Cancer. *Lancet* **344**, 224–7.

Kars MC, Grypdonck MH, Beishuizen A, et al. (2010) Factors influencing parental readiness to let their child with cancer die. *Pediatr Blood Cancer* **54**, 1000–8.

Kazak AE, Kassam-Adams N, Schneider S, et al. (2006) An integrative model of pediatric medical traumatic stress. *J Pediatr Psychol* **31**, 343–55.

Kreicbergs UC, Lannen P, Onelov E, Wolfe J (2007) Parental grief after losing a child to cancer: impact of professional and social support on long-term outcomes. *J Clin Oncol* **25**, 3307–12.

Landolt MA, Vollrath M, Ribi K, et al. (2003) Incidence and associations of parental and child posttraumatic stress symptoms in pediatric patients. *J Child Psychol Psychiatry* **44**, 1199–207.

Langeveld NE, Stam H, Grootenhuis MA, Last BF (2002) Quality of life in young adult survivors of childhood cancer. *Support Care Cancer* **10**, 579–600.

Last BF, Stam H, Onland-van Nieuwenhuizen AM, Grootenhuis MA (2007) Positive effects of a psycho-educational group intervention for children with a chronic disease: first results. *Patient Educ Couns* **65**, 101–12.

Martel D, Bussières JF, Théorêt Y, et al. (2005) Use of alternative and complementary therapies in children with cancer. *Pediatr Blood Cancer* **44**, 660–8.

Moore BD, III (2005) Neurocognitive outcomes in survivors of childhood cancer. *J.Pediatr Psychol* **30**, 51–63.

Patenaude AF, Kupst MJ (2005) Psychosocial functioning in pediatric cancer. *J Pediatr Psychol* **30**, 9–27.

Sahler OJ, Fairclough DL, Phipps S, et al. (2005) Using problem-solving skills training to reduce negative affectivity in mothers of children with newly diagnosed cancer: report of a multisite randomized trial. *J Consult Clin Psychol* **73**, 272–83.

Skinner R, Wallace WH, Levitt G (2007) Long-term follow-up of children treated for cancer: why is it necessary, by whom, where and how? *Arch Dis Child* **92**, 257–60.

Stam H, Grootenhuis MA, Last BF (2005). The course of life of survivors of childhood cancer. *Psychooncology*, Mar; **14**[3]: 227–38

Stam H, Grootenhuis MA, Last BF (2001). Social and emotional adjustment in young survivors of childhood cancer. *Support Care Cancer*, Oct; **9**[7]: 489–513 Review.

Temming P, Jenney ME (2010) The neurodevelopmental sequelae of childhood leukaemia and its treatment. *Arch Dis Child* **95**, 936–40.

Trask PC, Paterson AG, Trask CL, et al. (2003).Parent and adolescent adjustment to pediatric cancer: associations with coping, social support, and family function. *J Pediatr Oncol Nurs* **20**, 36–47.

Varni JW, Katz ER, Colegrove R **Jr**, Dolgin M (1994) Perceived social support and adjustment of children with newly diagnosed cancer. *J Dev Behav Pediatr* **15**, 20–6.

Vrijmoet-Wiersma CM, van Klink JM, Kolk AM, et al. (2008) Assessment of parental psychological stress in pediatric cancer: a review. *J Pediatr Psychol* **33**, 694–706.

Zebrack BJ, Zeltzer LK, Whitton J, et al. (2002) Psychological outcomes in long-term survivors of childhood leukemia, Hodgkin's disease, and non-Hodgkin's lymphoma: a report from the Childhood Cancer Survivor Study. *Pediatrics* **110**, 42–52.

Chapter 10

Palliative care for children with advanced cancer

Michelle Koh, Finella Craig and Joanne Wolfe

Introduction

The treatment of childhood cancer is one of the success stories of the 20th century. Nonetheless, for some children, prognosis remains uncertain and approximately 20 per cent of children with cancer will die of their disease. It is essential that for children with advanced cancer, disease-directed care is blended with care aimed at the psychosocial, physical, and spiritual needs of the child and family. Management demands a holistic and collaborative approach between the patient, family, and professionals.

World Health Organization (WHO): Principles of palliative care

The WHO defines palliative care for children as 'the active, total care of the child's body, mind and spirit, and also involves giving support to the family' and recommends:

- It begins when illness is diagnosed, and continues regardless of whether or not a child receives treatment directed at the disease
- The child's physical, psychological, and social distress should be addressed
- It requires an interdisciplinary approach, includes the family and utilizes available community resources
- It can be provided in tertiary care facilities, in community settings (school, respite care, primary care) and in the child's home.

Where dedicated palliative care teams exist, they should be introduced to the family at diagnosis of the malignancy, so the child and family benefit from the supportive care alongside intensive disease-directed therapy.

In this context, the palliative care team can be involved in symptom management and provide outreach home support for the family. The level of support provided by the service should be flexible, according to the child and family's requirements, which, to some extent, depends on the child's diagnosis, treatment, and prognosis. At times of crises (such as relapse) or when cure is no longer possible, the palliative care team may take a more active lead in the child's care and management, as a seamless continuation of the care they have already been receiving.

Communication and decision making: maintaining hope and preparing for death when prognosis is poor

When a child with cancer relapses, the family fluctuates between hoping for a cure and contemplating death as they face the uncertainty that surrounds their child's prognosis. This uncertainty impacts the child and family's experience, their decision making on how intensively to pursue cancer-directed therapy, consideration of palliative treatment, care planning, and prognostic communications. Acknowledging the uncertainty of prognosis and developing an awareness of the child and family's hopes and fears may lead to a greater understanding of the challenges faced and promote more open and honest communications at this critical period.

For many families, maintaining their belief that there might be a 'miracle round the corner' is crucial, yet it can co-exist alongside emotional and practical preparation for their child's death. The parents and child may talk about their plans for the future whilst, bringing forward a birthday or Christmas celebration. Professionals must not deny them the opportunity to sustain hope, alongside supporting them in preparing for and managing their child's deterioration.

Health-care professionals tend to view hope as primarily related to a positive outcome, many finding it difficult to maintain hope in the face of a poor prognosis. Parents were more likely to report that physician communication always made them feel hopeful when they were receiving more prognostic information and high-quality communication. Therefore, contrary to how many professionals may feel, disclosure of prognosis can support hope, even when the prognosis is poor.

Decision making about cancer-directed therapies

Bluebond-Langner et al. (see Further reading) studied parental decision making regarding further cancer-directed treatments for children when standard cancer treatment was unsuccessful. Parents brought to these discussions both the knowledge they acquired throughout their child's illness as well as their emotions as parents. They sought meetings with the oncologist regarding further investigative procedures and about half the parents looked for options beyond what was offered. No parent initiated discontinuation of cancer-directed, or symptom-directed therapies. The conclusion is that parents do not see cancer-directed therapy and symptom-directed care as mutually exclusive. Physicians and parents negotiate care throughout the child's treatment, whether it is directed at a curative or palliative intent.

Advanced care planning

End-of-life care planning requires effective communication to guide parents through clarifying the goals of care and establishing agreement on what treatments are appropriate to achieve these goals, including resuscitative and palliative measures. Providing choice for the place of end-of-life care is crucial and may impact on family decisions about hospital-based interventions. Bluebond-Langner's work showed that among families who felt they had time to plan where their child would die, an overwhelming majority preferred to have their child die at home.

Advanced care planning requires time and often needs to be done in stages, with discussions around the appropriate level of cardio-pulmonary resuscitation, life-sustaining treatment and intensive care, the child and family's preferred place of care and place of death. This should be accompanied by assurance that symptom management and supportive care will be pro-active in whichever setting they choose.

There should be an understanding and acknowledgement of the past experiences as well as their cultural values and social set-up of the child and family. There must be clarity on the practicalities of what the different options of home, hospice or hospital care entail so that the families have realistic expectations to inform their decision making.

The care plan must be communicated to the wider multi-disciplinary team, including out-of-hours services and the ambulance service. Patient-held records of discussions, decisions, and contacts are useful communication tools.

Palliative oncological treatments

The purpose of palliative oncological treatments is to improve the quality of life, relieve symptoms and prolong the symptom-free period (Table 10.1). As a principle, side effects and toxicities must be minimal and manageable, but long-term toxicity is unlikely to be an issue. Decisions around these treatments are taken by the oncologist, in conjunction with the palliative care team, child and family.

Common and difficult symptoms

Many studies have shown that children with advanced cancer experience substantial suffering from symptoms amenable to palliation (Table 10.2). Increased availability of palliative care services,

Table 10.1 Features of palliative oncological treatments

Chemotherapy

◆ Low toxicity oral, intravenous or intrathecal chemotherapy to halt or slow disease progression and manage symptoms of disseminated disease
◆ Examples:
  • Oral etoposide in children with metastatic solid tumours, or oral temozolamide in children with relapsed brain cancers
  • Intrathecal methotraxate for symptoms due to CNS leukaemia

Monitor the efficacy of treatment closely as treatment needs to be re-considered or stopped if symptoms progress or side effects outweigh potential benefits for quality of life

Radiotherapy

◆ Useful for controlling distressing symptoms from a focal site and can prophylactically treat sites of disease before they cause symptoms, e.g. radiation to bulky bony disease before the bone fractures
◆ Given as hypofractionated regimens, i.e. fewer fractions with bigger doses per fraction
◆ Symptomatic gain should be greater than the burden of any side effects or negative impact on quality of life, e.g. attending hospital, need for anaesthetic
◆ Examples:
  • Pain caused by bulky disease, nerve compression, bone pain
  • Obstruction of any hollow passage or viscus, e.g. spinal cord compression, SVC or airway obstruction
  • Bleeding from rupture or breakdown of tumour: haemoptysis, vaginal or gastrointestinal bleeding, haematuria
  • Fungating or disfiguring tumours, which can cause immense distress by their appearance and discharge. Tumour volume reduction can help the surrounding skin and soft tissues to heal

Surgery

◆ Considered early in situations where symptoms can be anticipated, as the child needs to be well enough to tolerate surgery
◆ Examples:
  • Debulking of tumour can help with pain control
  • Drains for effusions/ascites
  • Decompression, e.g. for spinal cord compression, relief of bowel obstruction
  • Stenting of intraluminal lesions, can often be done endoscopically, e.g. biliary stents, nephrostomy stents or urinary catheterization
  • Stablization of fractures, prophylactically or post-fracture

Table 10.2 Principles of symptom management

◆ Symptom management should be planned in advance
◆ It requires a holistic approach, not just drug management
◆ Parents and patients should be empowered to have some control over the situation. They should:
  • Know what to expect
  • Know how to deal with it
  • Know who to call for help
◆ Assessment should include the use of developmentally appropriate instruments when available. Uncontrolled distressing symptoms constitute a medical emergency and should be managed aggressively

---

however, is associated with improvement in symptom control. The approach to symptom management involves:

◆ Assessment of the child's symptoms
◆ Evaluation of potentially reversible causes of the symptoms
◆ Planning and initiation of treatment
◆ Reassessment following intervention.

This is an on-going process as the disease progresses and symptoms change over time.

Although the parents often provide vital information regarding the child's symptoms, it is important to focus on what the child may be able to communicate as well as clinical signs. This is crucial for managing subjective symptoms such as pain, nausea, and breathlessness. It validates the child's symptom experience, and builds trust between the child, family, and professionals.

The child's symptom experience is affected by the pathophysiological processes, other biological and psychosocial factors.

Pain

It is crucial to assess what the mechanism of pain might be and treat any underlying causes of the child's pain.

As much information as possible should be derived directly from the child. Self-reporting using pain scales remains the 'gold standard' in measuring pain, but the child needs to be competent in using these. Parents and familiar carers can be good surrogates as they know the child's normal baseline behaviour and will be familiar with the child's pain behaviour. However, there is a risk that they may under-report pain, for fear of acknowledging a symptom that suggests disease progression. Physiological changes such as heart rate and blood pressure may help in identifying pain, but in a dying child these are likely to be affected by many confounding factors.

The WHO analgesic ladder recommends a step-wise approach of escalating analgesics for management of pain:

Step 1—mild pain, pain score <3 on a numerical scale: Paracetamol and if appropriate, non-steroidal anti-inflammatory drugs (NSAIDs). NSAIDs (e.g. ibuprofen, diclofenac) have analgesic, antipyretic, and anti-inflammatory properties. They are especially useful for musculoskeletal and liver pain. NSAIDs may cause gastric irritation, their regular use should be accompanied by gut protection (e.g. ranitidine, omeprazole). As they cause platelet dysfunction, their potential benefit must be balanced against the child's risk of bleeding.

Step 2—mild to moderate pain, pain score 3–6: Paracetamol +/− NSAIDs + weak opiate. Although the WHO guidelines suggest codeine be used as the weak opioid at step 2, a significant proportion of children are unable effectively to convert codeine to its active metabolites, other children are hypermetabolizers. Furthermore, codeine has a high toxicity-to-efficacy ratio, children experience substantial side effects even at very low doses. Many practitioners only use codeine on a short-term basis, if at all. It is preferred to initiate lower doses of more effective opioids, such as morphine and titrate as appropriate.

Step 3—moderate to severe pain, pain score 6 and above: Paracetamol +/– NSAIDs + strong opioid.

Morphine/fentanyl/oxycodone/methadone

Morphine is currently the first-line opioid of choice and it is usually appropriate to start the patient using the short-acting preparation on an 'as needed' basis, then proceeding to the twice-daily long-acting preparation once the patient's daily requirement is established. It is important to continue the use of short-acting morphine as needed, to manage any breakthrough pain.

Fentanyl is an alternative to morphine in patients with renal failure as it metabolizes to inactive metabolites in the liver and it has a shorter half-life.

Oxycodone has similar properties to morphine and has been reported to cause less vomiting and fewer hallucinations.

Methadone is an opioid with N-methyl-D-aspartate (NMDA) antagonistic properties and therefore effective in difficult pain with neuropathic qualities. Methadone has a very long half-life and should be titrated slowly due to the risk of accumulation and toxicity. Methadone is a long-acting opioid widely available as a liquid and as such can be very useful in countries where liquid long-acting morphine is not available.

Routes of administration

Medications should always be given by the most acceptable route for the child. Practical considerations, such as place of care and ease of administration, may also influence route of administration and, as a consequence of this, drug of preference.

Oral medications. This is the route of choice as long as the child is able to take and tolerate it. Enteral medications can often be continued throughout the child's terminal phase, particularly if they already have a nasogastric or gastrostomy tube.

Transdermal opioid patches are appropriate for use in patients who are unable to take or comply with oral medications and who have stable pain. They are unsuitable for patients with escalating pain, as the onset of effect of a higher dose patch is too slow.

Continuous intravenous infusion may be the preferred route of choice for a child who already has a central line and cannot manage oral medications.

Continuous subcutaneous infusion (CSCI). This route should be considered in preference to intravenous medication if the child does not have pre-existing venous access.

Buccal/sublingual. These preparations are useful in children who cannot manage oral medications, particularly for breakthrough symptoms. Most, however, will have a short duration of action, so is not an ideal route for sustained symptom relief.

Neuropathic pain

When nerves are invaded or compressed by tumour, normal pain transmission is altered, causing neuropathic pain. Often, there is considerable overlap between neuropathic and nociceptive pain. Some children report sharp pain associated with tingling and numbness or a burning sensation or a deep ache. Others may not be able to articulate this type of pain clearly. Knowledge of the disease pathology, location and invasive nature should alert physicians to the potential for neuropathic pain. A poorer than expected response to opioids may provide additional clues.

As neuropathic pain is mostly mediated through NMDA receptors, a single class of analgesic is not usually adequate; a combination of opioids and adjunct analgesics benefit patients most.

Adjunct analgesics

Adjunct analgesics can be opioid sparing and important to consider if the child's pain is likely to be neuropathic in origin, or if it is not responding to escalating opioid therapy. The most commonly used adjunct neuropathic analgesics are:

◆ Anti-depressants: amitriptylline

◆ Anti-convulsants: gabapentin, carbamazepine

◆ NMDA antagonists: ketamine, methadone.

Other agents may also be helpful for specific situations, such as bisphosphonates in the management of pain associated with metastatic bone disease.

Any patient with intractable pain despite optimal management of systemic analgesia should be discussed with an anaesthetics team, for consideration of an appropriate intervention such as epidural analgesia or a nerve block. Patients most likely to benefit include those with significant locally advanced disease, neuropathic pain or marked movement-related pain.

Breathlessness

Breathlessness may be secondary to disease causing airway obstruction, pulmonary metastases, pleural effusion or infection and pooling of secretions. This may be compounded if there is bone marrow disease causing anaemia.

Breathlessness is a subjective symptom—its severity is what the patient says it is. It can be frightening. Some general measures can help: reassurance, optimizing the child's position and, in older children, relaxation techniques. A stream of cool air on the face (e.g. by opening a window or having a fan on) stimulates the trigeminal nerve and can reduce the perception of breathlessness.

As the child becomes less conscious, he/she becomes less able to clear his secretions effectively. Glycopyrronium or a hyoscine hydrobromide patch can be used to make secretions less copious, but they can also make them thicker, and cause anti-cholinergic side effects e.g. dry mouth or eyes. They should be used judiciously, with appropriate suctioning, gentle chest physiotherapy, and mouth care.

Opioids reduce the sensation of breathlessness by reducing the ventilatory response to hypercapnoea and hypoxia. Oral morphine preparations can be tried in the first instance, although some patients respond better to a continuous infusion of morphine. A benzodiazepine can be used in conjunction as an anxiolytic.

Nausea and vomiting

Simple, practical measures can often improve nausea significantly:

◆ The child should only be given small amounts of food they enjoy, at the time they feel most able to eat. Several small meals are preferable to three large meals a day

◆ Strong smells should be avoided, such as cooking smells and perfumes

◆ Constipation must be actively managed

◆ The number of medications and drug volumes should be reduced as much as possible. Medication should be timed, so large amounts are not being given together.

The key to successful management of nausea and vomiting is to elicit the causes, as this informs the anti-emetic choice (Table 10.3).

Table 10.3 Choice of anti-emetics for different causes of vomiting

Cause (site of action)	Drug	Class/action
Raised intracranial pressure (vomiting centre)	Cyclizine	Antihistamine
	Hyoscine	Anti-muscurinic
	Levomepromazine	$5HT_2$-antagonist
Decreased intestinal motility or dysmotility	Metoclopramide	D_2-antagonist
	Domperidone	D_2-antagonist
	Erythromycin	Motilin-receptor agonist
Metabolic or drug-induced (chemoreceptor trigger zone)	Haloperidol	D_2-antagonist
	Metoclopramide	D_2-antagonist
Chemotherapy induced (gut wall/chemoreceptor trigger zone)	Ondansetron	$5HT_3$-antagonist
Broad-spectrum agent for resistant nausea (vomiting centre)	Levomepromazine	$5HT_2$-antagonist

Constipation

Constipation in children advanced cancer may be secondary to decreased mobility and oral intake or as a side effect of opioids or anti-cholinergic drugs. As a general rule, a laxative should be prescribed when prescribing any opioid for a patient. Constipation should be proactively prevented as it is often difficult to manage once established.

Three main types of laxatives are commonly used:

◆ Osmotic laxatives (macrogols)

◆ Softening agents (lactulose, docusate sodium)

◆ Stimulant agents (senna; sodium picosulphate; bisacodyl).

Rectal enemas (phosphate enemas) and suppositories (glycerine suppositories) can be tried if laxatives are ineffective but may only empty the rectum and can cause significant pain if the stool is not softened. Further, their use should be limited in children with profound neutropenia.

Fatigue

Fatigue is the most common symptom experienced by children with terminal cancer and is often under-recognized and under-treated. It is an overwhelming tiredness, out of proportion to activity and exertion, not adequately relieved by rest. It is important to address underlying aetiologies (e.g. pain, nutrition, anaemia, etc.) including psychological symptoms such as depression and anxiety. Increasingly, methylphenidate or dextroamphetamine is recommended for symptomatic relief of fatigue, regardless of the suspected aetiology. Physiotherapy and gentle exercise may be effective in relieving fatigue for children, even near the end of life.

Agitation

Agitation and restlessness are common at the end of life and can be distressing for parents and carers.

Symptomatic causes of agitation, such as pain or vomiting, should be assessed and treated. Fear and unaddressed anxieties can be a major factor and early, open discussion with the child, allowing them to express their fears and concerns may reduce agitation as death approaches. Calm reassurance is crucial and other measures, such as careful attention to lighting, particularly at night or if a child's vision is failing, as well as relaxation techniques, may be helpful. If medication is necessary, a short-acting benzodiazepine such as buccal midazolam or sublingual lorazepam is often effective. For more severe agitation, haloperidol can be very effective.

Gastrointestinal complications: malignant ascites/intestinal obstruction

These complications are less common in children than adults, but tend to happen late and close to end-of-life, and can be very difficult to manage.

Malignant ascites most commonly occurs in patients with liver involvement or peritoneal disease. Although, in children, draining ascites will usually require sedation or a general anaesthetic, it is an effective way to relieve the pain and distension. Importantly, the ascites is likely to recur, requiring repeated procedures unless a catheter is left *in situ*. The risk of hypoalbuminaemia and hypovolaemia from the draining of the peritoneal fluid also needs to be considered.

Intestinal obstruction can be caused by intraluminal, intramural or extramural obstruction, motility disorders or severe constipation. Surgery should only be considered if there is clear benefit. Medical management with antisecretory and anti-emetic medication should aim to control nausea and reduce the frequency and severity of vomiting to an acceptable level. The route of drug delivery will need to be parenteral and a nasogastric tube would only be recommended if there is faeculant vomiting or gastric outlet obstruction.

Broad-spectrum anti-emetics should be used; cyclizine as the first-line with haloperidol or levomepromazine added in if required. Laxatives (combination of senna and docusate) should be used to maintain a comfortable stool without colic; octreotide can be effective in reducing the amount of gastrointestinal secretions in children with severe outlet obstruction.

Parenteral hyoscine butylbromide can be rapidly effective for colic. If the coeliac or superior mesenteric plexus is involved, there may be severe neuropathic pain that will require opioids and an anti-neuropathic pain agent.

Bone marrow failure

Decisions surrounding the appropriate use of transfusions need to be addressed sensitively as families who have been through intensive oncological treatments will be used to having anaemia or thrombocytopenia managed aggressively. Continued transfusions are usually warranted when the child with advanced cancer remains active.

In the context of end-of-life care, transfusions should be recommended only if the child's symptoms are likely to be ameliorated by the transfusion. The burden of transferring the child and spending several hours in hospital must be considered, as well as the potential fluid shifts the transfusion will cause.

Bleeding is a major distressing symptom of bone marrow failure. The child may bleed from fungating tumours, nose and gums, and pressure areas.

Management includes:

◆ Preparing the family adequately; dark towels and sheets can help moderate the anxiety of the child and witnesses

◆ Positioning of the child. For example, in acute haemoptysis or a severe nose-bleed, lie them on their bleeding side, or upright/reclined with head tilted forward

◆ Topical of application of adrenaline 1-in-1000 or tranexamic acid intravenous preparation, soaked in gauze, applied to bleeding point. A mouthwash preparation of tranexamic acid is also available

◆ An anxiolytic such as buccal midazolam can help calm the distressed child.

Anxiety and depression

Anxiety and depression are common emotions in children with life-limiting conditions. It is important to assess if the symptoms are appropriate reactions to the difficult situation, or more severe and entrenched emotions that require intervention.

The child psychiatry team should be consulted on the medical management of psychological symptoms. Serotonin-reuptake inhibitors such as citalopram can be effective, however require several weeks to achieve maximum benefit. Thus, when indicated, such medications should be started early on. Psychostimulants (dextroamphetamine and methylphenidate) deserve special consideration in treating depression near the end of life, because they take effect quickly. Non-medical interventions, such as counselling, cognitive behavioural therapy, drama, art or play therapy, are also important.

Acute anxiety can be managed with a short-acting benzodiazepine such as buccal midazolam.

Issues around feeding at the end-of-life

Loss of appetite and loss of interest in food is common in children who are dying. Fluid and caloric requirements decrease as their underlying illness deteriorates and activity levels decrease.

Artificial hydration and feeds need to be given judiciously. If the child is already on artificial hydration, reassess the child's likely fluid requirement and reduce the amount given appropriately. If the child had previously been orally feeding, it is not usually beneficial to start artificial hydration. Close attention should also be paid to mouth care and care of pressure areas.

At the end-of-life, artificial hydration could alleviate signs of dehydration, but worsen peripheral oedema, ascites, pleural effusions, respiratory distress, and frequency of urination. The potential benefits of artificial hydration therapy need to be considered against the distress of worsening fluid retention.

Spiritual distress

Health-care professionals often feel uncomfortable and inadequate in addressing the spiritual needs of the dying child and family. It is important to access the spiritual and faith leaders in the interdisciplinary team or in the child's community. Often, a multi-faith chaplain will be expert in exploring spiritual distress in a non-religious context with families who may not have a specific religious belief.

The main spiritual need described by parents is maintaining connection with their child. Parents maintain connection at the time of death by physical presence and after the death through memories, mementos, memorials, altruistic acts such as organ donation. and charitable work. The other spiritual needs include the need for truth, compassion, prayer and ritual; connection with others; bereavement support; meaning and purpose; anger, blame and dignity. Professionals can support parents by ensuring that the child and family remain a unit at the time of death, encouraging the family to create memories, fostering an honest relationship and being a trusted partner in their child's care.

Based on his study, interviewing children with cancer, Bearison explains, 'When they are trying to come to grips with the fear of dying and, sometimes, with the inevitability of impending death, many children find solace in putting themselves in the hands of God'.

Family support and bereavement care

The child and family face a series of losses even before the child approaches the terminal stages of the illness. These range from the physical loss of skills and abilities; social losses such as social isolation, pressure on parents' marriage; financial losses as parents often have to reduce or give up their jobs to care for the child in addition to the financial cost of care; emotional loss of their hopes and dreams for their child.

Families need to be allowed to grieve and adapt to these changes at their own pace. Siblings have to cope with different relationships with their parents and the unwell child; grandparents grieve not only for their grandchild, but also the heartbreak that their child is enduring.

Support for the children may be available through schools and hospices, music, drama or play therapy; voluntary sector organizations provide sibling support; adults and older children may find pre-bereavement counselling valuable, with therapy continuing through and after their bereavement.

Social work input is invaluable in helping the family obtain their financial entitlements and funding for extra care or home adaptations. In many countries there are voluntary organizations that provide practical help such as help with household chores or care of the other children.

The sick child should be encouraged to maintain their interests and have things to look forward to. This is often includes continuing an appropriate level of educational input, play and social interaction with their peers. It is often useful, with the family's permission, to provide relevant information for the school.

After the child's death, the family may need to be supported through the activities of mourning, be given information about the sources of support, referred to specialist bereavement counselling if needed.

Health-care professionals

Whilst caring for a dying child is challenging, to do this well can be hugely rewarding. Creating a safe environment in which to address the emotional challenges faced by health-care professionals is essential. It is often necessary to provide several different mechanisms for this: group discussion, one-to-one peer support and individual psychological support. This support should be routinely available and not just provided at times of crises or after a particularly difficult death.

Further reading

Bearison DJ (1991) God and prayer, in Bearison DJ *'They Never Want to Tell You' Children Talk About Cancer*, pp.129–31. Cambridge (MA): Harvard University Press.

Bennett M (2010) Palliative medications: drugs for neuropathic pain. *Euro J Palliat Care* **17**, 167–9.

Bluebond-Langner M, Belasco JB, Goldman A, Belasco C (2007) Understanding parents' approaches to care and treatment of children with cancer when standard therapy has failed. *J Clin Oncol* **25**, 2414–9.

Bruera E, Driver L, Barnes EA, et al. (2003) Patient-controlled methylphenidate for the management of fatigue in patients with advanced cancer: a preliminary report. *J Clin Oncol* **21**, 4439–43.

De Graves S, Aranda S (2008) Living with hope and fear—the uncertainty of childhood cancer after relapse. *Cancer Nurs* **31**, 292–301.

Dimeo FC, Stieglitz RD, Novelli-Fischer U, et al. (1999) Effects of physical activity on the fatigue and psychologic status of cancer patients during chemotherapy. *Cancer* **85**, 2273–7.

Dussel V, Kreicbergs U, Joanne HM, et al. (2009) Looking beyond where children die: Determinants and effects of planning a child's location of death. *J Pain Symptom Manage* **37**, 33–43.

Goldman A (1998). ABC of palliative care: Special problems of children. *Br Med J* **316**, 49–52.

Jalmsell L, Kreicbergs U, Onelov E, et al. (2006) Symptoms affecting children with malignancies during the last month of life: a nationwide follow-up. *Pediatrics* **117**, 1314–20.

Jennings A (2010) Palliation of breathlessness: a combined approach is needed. *Euro J Palliat Care* **17**, 162–6.

Kreicbergs UC, Lannen P, Onelov E, Wolfe J (2007) Parental grief after losing a child to cancer: impact of professional and social support on long-term outcomes. *J Clin Oncol* **25**, 3307–12.

Meert KL, Thurston CS, Briller S (2005) The spiritual needs of parents at the time of their child's death in the pediatric intensive care unit and during bereavement: a qualitative study. *Pediatr Crit Care* **6**, 420–7.

Ripamonti C, Mercadante S, Groff L, et al. (2000) Role of octreotide, scopolamine butylbromide, and hydration in symptom control of patients with inoperable bowel obstruction and nasogastric tubes: a prospective randomized trial. *J Pain Symptom Manage* **19**, 23–34.

Thompson A, MacDonald A, Holden C (2006) Feeding in Palliative Care in Goldman A, Hain R, Liben S (eds) *Oxford Textbook of Palliative Care for Children*, pp.374–86. Oxford: Oxford University Press.

Twycross R, Wilcock A (2007) Anti-emetics, in Twycross R (ed) *Palliative Care Formulary*, 3rd ed, pp.175–79. Nottingham: Palliativedrugs.com Limited.

Ullrich CK, Dussel V, Hilden JM (2010) Fatigue in children with cancer at the end of life. *J Pain Symptom Manage* **40**, 483–94.

Wolfe J, Hammel JF, Edwards KE (2008) Easing of Suffering in Children With Cancer at the End of Life: Is Care Changing? *J Clin Oncol* **26**, 1717–23.

Wolfe J, Klar N, Grier HE, et al. (2000) Understanding of prognosis among parents of children who died of cancer: impact on treatment goals and integration of palliative care. *JAMA* **284**, 2469–75.

World Health Organization (1990) *Cancer pain relief and palliative care, WHO technical report series 804*. Geneva: World Health Organization.

Yee JD, Berde CB (1994) Dextroamphetamine or methylphenidate as adjuvants to opioid analgesia for adolescents with cancer. *J Pain Symptom Manage* **9**,122–5.

Chapter 11

Cancer treatment in low- and middle-income countries

Elizabeth Molyneux and Scott C. Howard

Introduction

The World Bank divides economies according to their 2009 gross national income per capita in US dollars into low income ($995 or less), lower middle income ($996–$3945), upper middle income ($3946–$12 195), and high income ($12 196 or more), calculated using the World Bank Atlas method (http://data.worldbank.org/about/country-classifications/world-bank-atlas-method). Cancer treatment in low- and lower middle-income countries, referred to hereafter as LMIC, differs substantially from that in high-income countries (HIC), and these differences are the focus of this chapter.

Health-care disparities between LMIC and HIC

Cure rates for children with cancer differ greatly between LMIC and HIC. Cancer cure depends on a series of steps which can be conceptualized as links in the chain of care, from suspicion by the patient and family to primary care, secondary care, tertiary care, and finally correct diagnosis and treatment (Fig. 11.1). The cure rate is the product of access to diagnosis, treatment, and event-free survival, each of which can be problematic in LMIC. Late diagnosis and misdiagnosis are common in health-care systems with inadequate infrastructure for early referral, inadequate pathology laboratories that often lack even basic tools like immunohistochemistry, and high costs of cancer diagnosis and staging. These and other obstacles decrease access to diagnosis in many LMIC (Table 11.1). For example, in Mali and Malawi, the reported incidence of acute leukaemia is less than 10 per cent of the incidence in HIC (Fig. 11.2). Poverty and inadequate public health infrastructure prevent or delay access to even primary care for many of the world's children, and many LMIC have few or no paediatric cancer units so that patients must sometimes travel long distances for cancer care. For example, only an estimated 44 per cent of children with cancer in Guatemala are referred to the National Pediatric Oncology Unit (the only paediatric cancer unit in the country). However, all patients who reach the PCU in Guatemala City have access to treatment, since the costs of care are paid by a non-profit foundation Ayúdame a Vivir (Help Me to Live, www.ayuvi.org.gt). In China, India, and many other countries, the greatest barrier to cure is the lack of access to treatment, because families must cover the costs of diagnosis, staging, treatment, and follow up in addition to the non-medical costs associated with missed work, travel, and lodging.

Even patients who attain access to diagnosis and treatment may not survive, since socioeconomic and cultural factors in LMIC make abandonment of treatment a common occurrence and death rates due to the toxicity of chemotherapy are frequently high. For example, in the 1980s in Recife, Brazil, 8.4 per cent of children with acute lymphoblastic leukaemia (ALL) died of toxicity

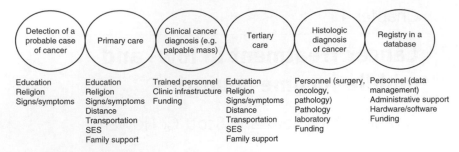

Fig. 11.1 Links in the chain of care for children with cancer. SES, socioeconomic status. Reproduced from Howard SC, et al.[1] with permission.

and 16 per cent abandoned treatment, versus 1.5 per cent toxic death and no abandonment with the same chemotherapy regimen in Memphis, USA. Similarly, in Honduras a decade ago, 21 per cent of children with ALL died of toxicity and 23 per cent abandoned treatment. Government spending on health care per capita is the strongest predictor of childhood cancer survival, because it is associated with health-care infrastructure at all levels (Fig. 11.3), and correlates strongly with access to diagnosis, treatment, and event-free survival because well-funded health systems are more likely to have tertiary care centres equiped with immunohistochemistry and flow cytometry, access to necessary chemotherapy and supportive care, and to be staffed with trained pathologists, surgeons, oncologists, radiation therapists, and nurses. Unfortunately, most paediatric oncologists have little influence over public health infrastructure, so the focus of their efforts must be to establish functional paediatric cancer units (PCUs) and to progressively develop them into centres of excellence, as discussed in the next section.

Importance of paediatric cancer units

A PCU is a centre at which children with cancer can receive services necessary to make a correct diagnosis of cancer, perform a staging evaluation, and deliver protocol-based therapy. Establishing a unit with its own physical space, dedicated personnel, and self-contained administrative structure allows the multidisciplinary team of doctors, nurses, pharmacists, social workers, psychologists, physical therapists, and data managers to work together to improve all aspects of patient care.

Table 11.1 Determinants of cure for children with cancer: estimated access to diagnosis, treatment, and event-free survival in selected regions and countries[*]

Country or region	Approximate rate of access to diagnosis	Approximate rate of access to treatment	Approximate event-free survival of treated patients	Estimated cure rate
High-income countries	100%	100%	80%	80%
Upper middle-income countries	95%	95%	70%	63%
Guatemala	44%	100%	43%	19%
China[**]	95%	10%	70%	7%
Malawi	20%	30%	40%	2%

[*] Used with permission of St Jude Children's Research Hospital (www.Cure4Kids.org).

[**] As this chapter went to press, dramatic changes in access to treatment are in progress in several regions of China, including implementation of social insurance plans to cover the costs of catastrophic illness. In affected regions, access to treatment has increased to almost 100 per cent, so the cure rate should improve substantially in the near future.

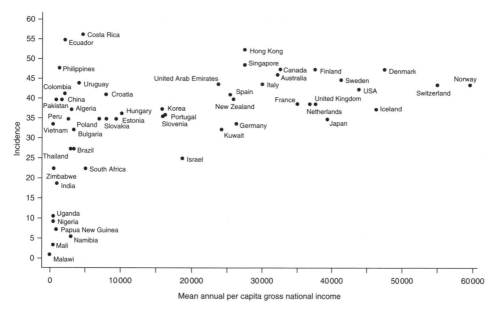

Fig. 11.2 Underdiagnosis of acute leukaemia in certain low-income countries. The reported incidence of acute leukaemia in Malawi and Mali is less than 10 per cent of that in middle- and high-income countries. Per capita gross national income and other economic indicators are available at http://data.worldbank.org/data-catalog.
Reproduced from Howard SC, et al.[1] with permission.

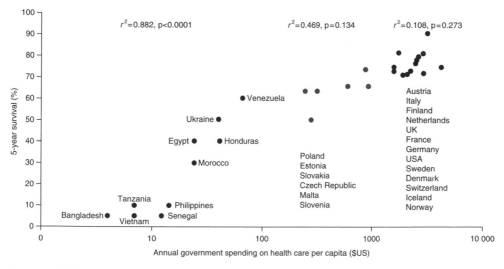

Fig. 11.3 Childhood cancer survival and government annual health-care spending per capita in ten low- and lower middle-income countries versus high- and upper middle-income countries.
The World Bank divides economies according to their 2009 gross national income per capita, calculated using the World Bank Atlas method (http://data.worldbank.org/about/country-classifications/world-bank-atlas-method).
Reproduced from Ribeiro RC, et al.[14] with permission from Elsevier.

Recruitment, training, and retention of personnel

Delivery of anti-cancer therapy requires trained personnel, but health-care providers with expertise in paediatric oncology in LMIC are far fewer per capita than in HIC. In some cases, no paediatric oncologist is available and medical oncologists with little paediatric experience or paediatricians with little oncology experience manage children with cancer. Oncology nurses in LMIC are rare, and in many hospitals nurses are required to rotate among all the hospital services, such that none gains expertise in oncology nursing and the effect of training programs is limited. Even if trained personnel are recruited, they must have a stable salary in the PCU to develop professionally and feel they have a future career path.

Education and training of health-care professionals at all levels is paramout to developing and improving a PCU, and many professional organizations have made educational materials and training scholarships available on their web sites (e.g. International Society of Pediatric Oncology www.siop.nl, American Society of Pediatric Hematology/Oncology www.ASPHO.org, International Network for Cancer Treatment and Research www.inctr.org, American Society of Hematology www.hematology.org). Online meetings can provide not only education, but also a forum to discuss individual patients, adapted protocols, and quality improvement initiatives with local, regional, and global collaborators. Cure4Kids (www.Cure4Kids.org), provides web-based conferencing tools to its 25,000 site members at no cost, and also allows for downloading of 1600 educational seminars, oncology nursing courses, and other materials of particular relevance to LMIC.

Continuous quality improvement

The process of continuous quality improvement requires a data management programme, which consists of a data manager, a database, and data analysis. Training for data managers and their supervising doctors is available at regular online meetings on www.Cure4Kids.org, and daily discussion between the data manager and the supervising doctor can improve collegiality, data quality, and the utility of data collection for improving patient care. Many free software tools are available, including spreadsheets, (www.OpenOffice.org) and EpiInfo (www.cdc.gov/epiinfo/), which allow the user to quickly configure databases with any type of data for any purpose. EpiInfo includes security features, double data entry to improve accuracy, and analytic tools. Both are easy to use and ideal for single-centre research. For centres with reliable Internet access that work within multi-centre groups, the Pediatric Oncology Networked Database (www.POND4Kids. org) is available at no cost. It has the data fields of interest defined for the 30 most common childhood cancers, customizable data entry forms and reports, anonymized data sharing among sites that choose to do so, high-level security, and automated off-site back-ups every 5 minutes. It also has a large base of existing users with whom new users can collaborate.

Data analysis to improve patient care is the most important component of any data management program, whose utility depends far more on the quality of the data collected, regular and critical analysis of results, and the quality improvement strategies implemented than on the software tool selected. The top priority in LMIC is to prevent toxic deaths, reduce abandonment, and monitor compliance with therapy and thus reduce relapse. This clinical research is best undertaken with the support and encouragement of regional colleagues in the context of regional and global networks, as discussed in the next section.

Development of PCUs and national paediatric oncology programs

Some PCUs began as pilot projects whose goal was to simply demonstrate that some children with cancer can be cured with simple therapy that can be delivered locally, like the simplified Burkitt lymphoma treatment used in Malawi. A successful pilot project can lead to development of a

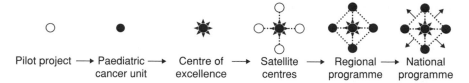

Fig. 11.4 Phases of development of paediatric oncology and the central role of paediatric cancer units. Reproduced with permission of St Jude Children's Research Hospital (www.Cure4Kids.org).

PCU, which can be further developed into a centre of excellence, eventually with its own satellite centres for shared care, and finally into a regional or national network of PCUs (Fig. 11.4). For example, the Pediatric Oncology Unit of Guatemala is developing plans to provide national coverage using satellite centres and to improve event-free survival by promoting early diagnosis and referral for locally adapted protocol-based care. Implementing such care is discussed in the next section.

Protocol-based care

Protocol-based care standardizes treatment regimens and improves results for every cancer in which its effect has been measured. However, clinicians who apply protocols in LMIC face uncertainties about disease stage and risk classification, medication shortages, excess toxicity from comorbid illnesses, and preventable deaths due to poor transportation or other social factors. Furthermore, doctors in LMIC manage large numbers of patients with little time, rarely have the luxury of specializing in a subset of childhood cancers, and often lack access to experts.

Graduated regimens and clinical research

Protocols that work well in HIC may cause disastrous toxicity in LMIC, as occurred when a regimen developed at St Jude Children's Research Hospital in Memphis, USA, was adopted in El Salvador without modification. Regimens must be adapted for use in LMIC, and the rate of toxic death monitored to determine whether the supportive care in the hospital is adequate to support the proposed treatment regimens and to identify preventable causes of treatment failure. If toxic death occurs too frequently, the regimen must be further adapted pending improvements in supportive care and hospital infrastructure. Practical research to address causes of treatment failure in the local setting is best conducted with colleagues who practise in similar circumstances. For example, centres in Central America (AHOPCA) and Latin America (MISPHO) have shared protocols and compared results for the past decade, with great benefits to all. Collaborating centres in French-speaking Africa, India, and elsewhere have also developed adapted treatment regimens and locally feasible supportive care guidelines. In addition to local adaptation and implementation of protocol-based care, graduated intensity regimens have been developed for childhood ALL. The regimens establish a backbone of therapy with low toxicity and cost that will cure a large proportion of children with ALL while minimizing toxic death. If there are less than two toxic deaths among the first 25 patients, the PCU is ready to 'step up' to a more intense treatment regimen to try to reduce the rate of relapse. If two or more patients die of toxicity, the PCU can 'step down' to a safer, less intense regimen and work to improve supportive care. Rational movement from step one to step two to step three requires monitoring of patient outcomes in real time, so a data management programme is prerequisite to successful implementation of a graduated regimen strategy.

Regional and global networks

Twinning partnerships between centres in HIC and LMIC can greatly speed the development of PCUs and centres of excellence, but such partnerships are even more effective when associated with other PCUs in the same region. Interaction with colleagues who practise in a similar setting and face similar problems affords an opportunity to learn from each other's mistakes, share guidelines, and optimize adapted treatment regimens for particular LMIC. In this regard, cooperating centres in Argentina, Brazil, India, Colombia, and many other LMIC have developed shared protocols and joint advocacy programs to improve outcomes at the national and regional level.

Improving outcomes for children with cancer by developing and improving PCUs has proven effective all over the world, and regional and global networks of collaborators have kept the momentum by sharing protocols, projects, funding sources, and supportive care guidelines. Online meetings via www.Cure4Kids.org have transformed twinning programmes and regional collaborations. For example, since 2005 professionals from centres in Morocco, St Jude Children's Research Hospital, and guests from several continents meet weekly to discuss patients, review supportive care issues, and develop and implement treatment protocols adapted to local conditions.

Treatment challenges in LMIC

Toxicity of treatment

Chemotherapy is especially toxic in malnourished children with advanced disease. In HIC, more intense and toxic therapies, matched by intense and costly supportive therapy, have achieved good outcomes. In LMIC children present with advanced cancers and large tumour loads. For example, in children with Burkitt lymphoma in Africa, the tumour burden is high with frequent kidney involvement and high risk of tumour lysis syndrome even with modest chemotherapeutic regimens. The risk to the patient is increased even more by lack of rasburicase and inadequate access to laboratory testing to follow potassium levels and prevent cardiac dysrhythmias. Malnutrition and underlying infections must also be managed prior to starting chemotherapy (to the extent possible) to minimize treatment toxicity. HIV- infected children can be expected to have more episodes of fever, neutropenia, and treatment delays.

Malnutrition has been shown to be associated with more chemotherapy-induced neutropenia and fever episodes with consequent delays in therapy, but few PCUs in LIC can provide parenteral feeding, which is unacceptable to many parents who equate it with death. Nausea and vomiting and especially mucositis become difficult to manage when oral feeding is required. Pre-treatment fluids (oral or intravenous) and allopurinol (in children with hematologic cancers) should be given, as well as an anti-emetic such as metoclopromide, which is inexpensive and widely available. Enriched milk (F100) or ready-to-use therapeutic foods such as Plumpynut or Chiponde can rapidly improve nutritional status.

Nursing staff should be empowered to act quickly and independently to initiate a fever protocol and start antibiotics as soon as fever is recorded and malaria (in malaria-endemic areas) is ruled out. Treatment should be modified to suit local facilities and expertise, to use doses and drugs that can be safely given to achieve the best outcome possible. As experience is gained with protocols and as local health provision improves, the protocols can be intensified in a step-wise fashion.

Abandonment of treatment

When treatment is initiated but not completed, it is described as abandonment. In children with cancer, abandonment significantly decreases the probability of cure. The reasons for abandonment of treatment are various and individual, but there is an overarching pattern of causes reported from LMIC. The most commonly cited reason for abandonment is financial. Families from LMIC cannot afford transportation to a distant care centre. The long stays in the hospital drain family funds and keep them away from any gainful employment they had previously. In Recife, Brazil, a social support program for children with ALL and their families included transportation, accommodation, financial support, and job training. This reduced the number who abandoned treatment from 16 per cent to 1.5 per cent. While a good outcome depends on full and adequate therapy, occasionally there is disbelief that more treatment is really necessary. It is vital that parents understand this and are helped to achieve it. Keeping an open ward or providing accommodation for those who live far away and cannot easily get to and from home between courses of chemotherapy is necessary.

Assisting on the ward with extra food and basic necessities such as soap and laundry detergent helps prevent abandonment. The hospital is a bewildering place to people new to the city, so a system to welcome newcomers and provide amenities such as washing lines and cooking facilities is essential. In Blantyre, Malawi, the mothers are given a small amount of money to spend in the market every weekend on simple foodstuffs and firewood so that they can cook in a shelter close to the ward. This program improves nutritional status, and also bonds the women together in a shared and enjoyable task. Other reasons for abandonment of therapy include an extended family's reluctance or inability to help with home chores while the mother is absent in the hospital with one child; death or illness in other close relatives; anxiety about leaving the remaining children in inadequate care at home; and concerns about the fidelity of a spouse during long absences at the hospital.

Palliative care

Sometimes pragmatic decisions must be made. Surgical options may be unavailable, and if chemotherapy does not improve the patient's disease, palliative care may be needed. Palliative care offers symptom control and emotional and spiritual support. One of the most significant recent advances in LMIC is the recognition that pain control is a fundamental human right and that oral morphine must be made available for children with cancer who experience pain.

Advocacy

Given the rarity of cancer in children compared to infectious diseases and other health problems, it is not surprising that cancer is not a priority for health systems in LMIC. Therefore, other ways must be found to support cancer care. Twinning between PCUs in HIC and LMIC has been very successful. The gain is bilateral. Funds, expertise, drugs, and specialized diagnostic tests flow from high-income to low-income centres, while experience, thinking outside the box, valuing what is possible and using what is available are lessons learned by those who work in HIC centres.

Charitable organizations and professional organizations can support PCUs in LMIC with expert advice, assistance with modifying protocols, and moral support. World Child Cancer (WCC, www.worldchildcancer.org) was formed to channel support to cancer units in low-income countries. WWC offers long-term support to PCUs to help them get established and gradually develop their own support networks. The International Society of Pediatric Oncology (SIOP), with its regional organizations in Africa, Southeast Asia, and the Mediterranean, provides professional support and expertise. The Children's Oncology Group (COG, www.childrensoncologygroup.org) collaborates with South American centres for training and shared protocols, and the Groupe Franco-Africaine d'Oncologie Pediatrique (GFAOP, www.igr.fr/gfaop), has a long tradition of international collaboration between PCUs in France and those in Africa.

Table 11.2 Eleven points of the World Cancer Declaration of 2008

◆ Availability of cancer-control plans in all countries

◆ Substantial improvements in measurement of global cancer burden

◆ Substantive decrease in tobacco consumption, obesity and alcohol intake

◆ Universal vaccination in areas affected by human papilloma virus and hepatitis B

◆ Misconceptions about cancer dispelled

◆ Substantial improvements in early detection programmes

◆ Worldwide improvement in diagnosis and access to cancer treatment, including palliative care

◆ Effective pain control universally available

◆ Greatly improved training opportunities in oncology

◆ Substantial decrease in migration of health workers

◆ Major improvement in cancer survival in all countries

The World Health Organization (WHO) has developed an essential drug list for paediatric cancer treatment (http://www.who.int/selection_medicines/committees/expert/17/second_children_list_en.pdf) and the International Union against Cancer developed the World Cancer Declaration which spells out 11 essential steps in the prevention and improved care for people with cancer (Table 11.2, www.sciencedaily.com/releases/2008/09/080902122854.htm). Paediatric oncologists met in Ponte di Legno in 2004 and stated that 'all children in the world have a right to full access to essential treatment for acute lymphoblastic leukaemia and other cancers' and called upon authorities to recognize and support all measures that promote the possibility for cure. Parent support organizations can provide a strong voice to influence political decisions and raise the profile of cancer in LMIC. Mary Robinson, former UN commissioner for human rights and chair of the 2008 World Cancer summit, said '*Ultimately, it is a question of human rights and above all, it is a question of human dignity*'. (www.sciencedaily.com/releases/2008/09/080902122854.htm). Wherever we work and however meagre our tools, there is always something that we can do to improve the lives of children with cancer.

Further reading

Arora RS, Eden T, Pizer B (2007) The problem of treatment abandonment in children from developing countries with cancer. *Pediatr Blood Cancer* **49**, 941–6.

Arya LS, Kotikanyadanam SP, Bhargava M, et al. (2010) Pattern of relapse in childhood ALL: challenges and lessons from a uniform treatment protocol. *J Pediatr Hematol Oncol* **32**, 370–5.

Cavalli F (2008) The World Cancer Declaration: a roadmap for change. *Lancet Oncol* **9**, 810–811.

Gupta S, Bonilla M, Fuentes SL, et al. (2009) Incidence and predictors of treatment-related mortality in paediatric acute leukaemia in El Salvador. *Br J Cancer* **100**, 1026–31.

Harif M, Barsaoui S, Benchekroun S, et al. (2008) Treatment of B-cell lymphoma with LMB modified protocols in Africa—report of the French-African Pediatric Oncology Group (GFAOP). *Pediatr Blood Cancer* **50**, 1138–42.

Hesseling P, Broadhead R, Mansvelt E, et al. (2005) The 2000 Burkitt lymphoma trial in Malawi. *Pediatr Blood Cancer* **44**, 245–50.

Hesseling P, Molyneux E, Kamiza S, et al. (2009) Endemic Burkitt lymphoma: a 28-day treatment schedule with cyclophosphamide and intrathecal methotrexate. *Ann Trop Paediatr* **29**, 29–34.

Howard SC, Marinoni M, Castillo L, et al. (2007) Improving outcomes for children with cancer in low-income countries in Latin America: a report on the recent meetings of the Monza International School of Pediatric Hematology/Oncology (MISPHO)-Part I. *Pediatr Blood Cancer* **48**, 364–9.

Howard SC, Metzger ML, Wilimas JA, et al. (2008) Childhood cancer epidemiology in low-income countries. *Cancer* **112**, 461–72.

Howard SC, Pedrosa M, Lins M, et al. (2004) Establishment of a pediatric oncology program and outcomes of childhood acute lymphoblastic leukemia in a resource-poor area. *JAMA* **291**, 2471–5.

Hunger SP, Sung L, Howard SC (2009) Treatment strategies and regimens of graduated intensity for childhood acute lymphoblastic leukemia in low-income countries: A proposal. *Pediatr Blood Cancer* **52**, 559–65.

Israels T, Chirambo C, Caron H, et al. (2008) The guardians' perspective on paediatric cancer treatment in Malawi and factors affecting adherence. *Pediatr Blood Cancer* **51**, 639–42.

Israels T, Ribeiro RC, Molyneux EM. (2010) Strategies to improve care for children with cancer in Sub-Saharan Africa. *Eur J Cancer* **46**, 1960–6.

Israels T, van de Wetering MD, Hesseling P, et al. (2009) Malnutrition and neutropenia in children treated for Burkitt lymphoma in Malawi. *Pediatr Blood Cancer* **53**, 47–52.

Leander C, Fu LC, Peña A, et al. (2007) Impact of an education program on late diagnosis of retinoblastoma in Honduras. *Pediatr Blood Cancer* **49**, 817–9.

Magrath I, Shanta V, Advani S, et al. (2005) Treatment of acute lymphoblastic leukaemia in countries with limited resources; lessons from use of a single protocol in India over a twenty year period. *Eur J Cancer* **41**, 1570–83.

Masera G (2009) Bridging the childhood cancer mortality gap between economically developed and low-income countries. *J Pediatr Hematol Oncol* **31**, 710–12.

Masera G, Baez F, Biondi A, et al. (1998) North-South twinning in paediatric haemato-oncology: the La Mascota programme, Nicaragua. *Lancet* **352**, 1923–6.

Metzger ML, Howard SC, Fu LC, et al. (2003) Outcome of childhood acute lymphoblastic leukaemia in resource-poor countries. *Lancet* **362**, 706–8.

Mostert S, Sitaresmi MN, Gundy CM, et al. (2010) Comparing childhood leukaemia treatment before and after the introduction of a parental education programme in Indonesia. *Arch Dis Child* **95**, 20–5.

Norman K, Pichard C, Lochs H, Pirlich M. (2008) Prognostic impact of disease-related malnutrition. *Clin Nutr* **27**, 5–15.

Ribeiro RC, Steliarova-Foucher E, Magrath I, et al. (2008) Baseline status of paediatric oncology care in ten low-income or mid-income countries receiving My Child Matters support: a descriptive study. *Lancet Oncol* **9**, 721–9.

Sinfield RL, Molyneux EM, Banda K, et al. (2007) Spectrum and presentation of pediatric malignancies in the HIV era: experience from Blantyre, Malawi, 1998–2003. *Pediatr Blood Cancer* **48**, 515–20.

Sitaresmi MN, Mostert S, Schook RM, et al. (2010) Treatment refusal and abandonment in childhood acute lymphoblastic leukemia in Indonesia: an analysis of causes and consequences. *Psychooncology* **19**, 361–7.

Chapter 12

Late effects of therapy and survivorship issues

Lars Hjorth, Riccardo Haupt and Rod Skinner

Introduction

The high survival rate in children and adolescents with malignancy is accompanied by a substantial risk of late adverse events (LAEs). Treatment may interfere with physiological growth and development in children and adolescents and have an important impact on health status later in life, whilst some late toxicities may cause premature death.

The Childhood Cancer Survivor Study (CCSS) reveals that 62 per cent of adult survivors of childhood malignancy have at least one treatment-induced chronic health condition (and 38 per cent two or more), whilst 28 per cent have a severe or life-threatening problem. Similar data were reported in a Dutch study. Survivors of central nervous system tumours or haemopoietic stem cell transplantation (HSCT) are at particularly high risk.

In general, the more frequently recognized risk factors include patient age at treatment, cumulative treatment dose, and the treatment schedule of radiotherapy or chemotherapy. In addition, the patient's pre-existing clinical status and previous or concurrent exposure to other toxic treatments may predispose to greater late toxicity.

The importance of moving from cure at any cost to cure at least cost is now well recognized, especially for patients with high cure rates. For all patients, higher cure rates and the risk of late complications make long-term follow up (LTFU) a vital component of care (Fig. 12.1).

Epidemiology

Recent estimates from several western countries put the proportion of long-term childhood cancer survivors (CCS) between 0.1 and 0.15 per cent of the general population, implying that one in every 650–1000 persons is a CCS. It has been estimated that there are now ≥300 000 CCS in the USA, and 300 000–500 000 in Europe. Based on a conservative estimate that 75 per cent treated on current protocols for childhood cancer will become long-term survivors (>5 years), each year about 8000 new CCS are added to each of the US and European populations. Although their median age is estimated at 21 years, some are already >50 years and >20 per cent have already survived >30 years since cancer diagnosis. These data demonstrate the need for adult physicians to be interested in the care of CCS.

Late mortality

Cumulative mortality rates continue to rise amongst CCS as the duration of their follow up extends into adult life. During the first 15 years after diagnosis, excess mortality is mainly due to the primary cancer but beyond this point there is increasing mortality from second malignant neoplasm (SMN) and circulatory disease (Fig. 12.2).

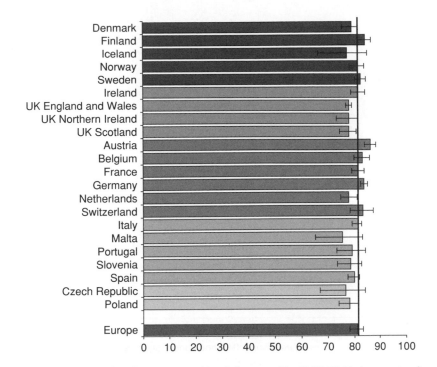

Fig. 12.1 Five-year survival for all cancers combined diagnosed in 1995–2002, by country, in European children (0–14 years) of both sexes. The data are adjusted by age, sex, case mix and period of diagnosis using a Cox proportional hazards model.
Reproduced from Gatta G. et al. *Eur J Cancer.* 2009 **45**(6): page 997, with permission from Elsevier.

There is good evidence that exposures to radiotherapy, alkylating agents or epipodophyllotoxins carry the greatest relative risks (RRs) for late mortality from SMN. The risk factors for long-term circulatory and cardiovascular risk have been less well determined but a recent French and UK study (Tukenova et al. 2010, see Further reading) evaluated this in the context of data on both chemotherapy exposure and radiation dose to the heart. The overall standardized mortality ratio (SMR) for survivors was 8.3-fold higher in relation to the general populations in France and the United Kingdom and there was a five fold increase in death from cardiovascular disease. The risk of dying was significantly higher in individuals who had received a cumulative anthracycline dose greater than 360 mg/m2 and in individuals who received an average cardiac radiation dose that exceeded 5 Gy.

These findings highlight the need for adult health care providers to understand the risks confronting CCS and for strategies to detect complications early in an attempt to prevent excess late deaths.

Secondary malignant neoplasms

Several studies have shown that CCS have an increased risk of developing secondary malignant neoplasms (SMNs). The RR is high (5–10), but in absolute numbers the individual risk is low, ranging from 1–3 additional cancers per 1000 person-years. After 20 years follow up, the cumulative risk is 3–7 per cent. The most common SMNs are breast cancer, MDS/AML, bone and soft tissue sarcoma, CNS tumours (e.g. meningiomas), and thyroid cancer. The latency period varies greatly with

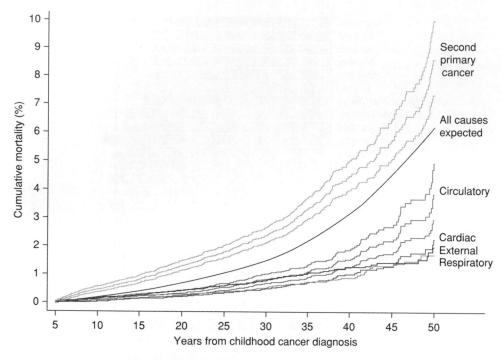

Fig. 12.2 Cumulative mortality of causes of death among survivors of childhood cancer. Reproduced from Reulen et al. *JAMA* 2010 **304**(2): page 177, with permission. Copyright © 2010 American Medical Association. All rights reserved.

an average of 12 years between first and second malignancies. Patients with a genetic tumour predisposition have an increased risk of developing a SMN. Radiotherapy is the main risk factor for developing SMNs even at doses <1 Gy, whilst alkylating agents and epipodophyllotoxins are the most commonly implicated cytotoxic drugs. Measures to decrease the risk of developing SMNs include avoidance of tobacco smoking and protection from excessive exposure to sunlight.

Neurology and nueropsychology

Long-term neurological toxicity is the commonest LAE reported in the CCSS, occurring in 27 per cent of survivors, with RR of 3.3 compared to the sibling control group. Survivors of CNS tumours are at the highest risk, followed by survivors of Hodgkin lymphoma or acute leukaemia.

There are several manifestations of CNS toxicity, including leucoencephalopathy, vasculopathy (from stenosis or occlusion), radiation necrosis, myelopathy and secondary CNS tumours, with a wide variety of clinical sequelae threatening life or greatly impairing the survivor's quality of life. In contrast, peripheral nervous system toxicity has fewer manifestations, usually presenting as peripheral neuropathy.

Leucoencephalopathy may present with focal motor signs, spasticity, seizures, and ataxia. There may also be neuropsychological dysfunction manifest by functional motor disabilities and cognitive impairment, with considerable adverse impact on intelligence, attention and learning skills, memory, verbal, and visual–spatial skills. Vasculopathy may cause seizures, stroke and dementia.

Radiation necrosis may result in neurocognitive and/or neuropsychological dysfunction, whilst myelopathy may lead to para- or quadriplegia, as well as sphincter dysfunction. A variety of secondary

CNS tumours are reported including malignant gliomas, neuroectodermal tumours, and meningiomas.

Most neurological/neuropsychological toxicity is related to CNS radiotherapy and/or CNS-directed chemotherapy (i.e. intrathecal chemotherapy, or some chemotherapy regimens such as high-dose methotrexate or cytarabine). Leucoencephalopathy and neuropsychological toxicity occur predominantly in survivors of CNS tumours or acute leukaemia treated with CNS radiotherapy or CNS-directed chemotherapy, and are commoner and more severe in patients treated at a younger age. Other aspects of neurotoxicity are related more to other treatment components, for example vasculopathy and radiation necrosis are associated with previous CNS radiotherapy, myelopathy with spinal radiotherapy and peripheral neuropathy with cisplatin or vincristine chemotherapy.

The management of neurotoxicity comprises both general and specific measures. Physiotherapy and/or occupational therapy assessment is very important in survivors with physical disabilities, whilst children with leucoencephalopathy and neuropsychological toxicity benefit from careful educational and neuropsychological assessment with provision of extra support at school and subsequent employment guidance. Surgery may be considered in selected cases of vasculopathy, and drug treatment for painful neuropathy.

Endocrine complications

Endocrine complications are the second commonest group of chronic conditions in CCS, occurring in 20–50 per cent of survivors followed into adulthood. They include: hypothalamo-pituitary, thyroid, and gonadal dysfunction; bone disease; and metabolic disorders.

Sequelae may be associated both with the tumour type and location, and with treatment. In addition to the effects of surgery or direct endocrine gland involvement by the malignancy [e.g. gonadal tumours, CNS tumours involving the hypothalamic pituitary axis (HPA)], both radiotherapy or chemotherapy may increase the risk of endocrine complications. Survivors treated with radiotherapy to the head, neck or pelvis, those treated with total body irradiation (TBI) or with alkylating agents, are at increased risk.

Hypothalamo-pituitary dysfunction

The total dose of cranial radiotherapy (CRT) is the strongest risk factor for anterior pituitary dysfunction. However, the threshold dose for specific endocrine dysfunction varies for different pituitary hormones.

Growth hormone

Growth hormone (GH) deficiency is the most common anterior pituitary deficiency observed after CRT. It may become manifest after a standard CRT dose ≥18 Gy; after >24 Gy the deficiency usually becomes manifest within 5 years, while for doses in the range of 18–24 Gy the deficiency may become manifest after 10–15 years. The risk should be considered lifelong.

Patients treated for brain tumours, sarcomas or ALL, and recipients of TBI, are at higher risk of GH deficiency. The number of new CCS with GH deficiency has been falling since leukaemic patients treated with contemporary protocols are less likely to be receiving CRT.

Growth and pubertal development should be monitored closely in children at risk of GH deficiency, to facilitate early diagnosis and treatment. Untreated GH deficiency will impair growth velocity and eventually final height. Other factors such as spinal radiotherapy, age at treatment and timing of puberty contribute to the individual's final height. Importantly, precocious puberty may mask GH deficiency which then becomes evident only after cessation of the growth spurt.

Careful examination of such individuals may maximize their potential to achieve adequate final height.

The most sensitive and specific test to diagnose GH deficiency is the insulin tolerance test (ITT). If abnormal, another stimulation test (either with GNRH-arginine or glucagon) should be performed to confirm the diagnosis. Measurement of insulin-like growth factor (IGF-1) and IGFBP-3 alone is not a good predictor of GH deficiency.

If GH deficiency is confirmed, GH replacement therapy should be considered. Concerns have arisen about the potential impact of GH treatment on tumour recurrence, but the available data do not demonstrate a significantly increased risk of tumour relapse in children treated with GH compared to those with the same type of tumour not treated with GH. Although a small but significant increased risk of second malignant tumours seems to exist for survivors under GH treatment, the second tumours are the same as those seen in CCS in general.

Gonadotrophins

Timely and appropriate gonadotrophin release from the HPA triggers hormonal release from the testis or ovary. This allows a linear growth spurt, development of secondary sexual characteristics, fertility and maintenance of gonadal function during adulthood. Except in a few cases of CNS tumours directly affecting the HPA, CRT is the main risk factor for altered gonadotrophin release. In these cases gonadotrophins may be secreted either earlier or later (precocious or delayed puberty, respectively) than the usual physiological timing.

Precocious puberty has been associated with radiation doses to the HPA as low as those given for CNS prophylactic treatment in ALL (range 18–24 Gy), in particular in females treated at a younger age. Although precocious puberty may mask GH deficiency, delayed puberty is commoner. The risk of developing gonadotrophin deficiency is dose related, especially with CRT doses >30 Gy.

Patients at risk should be closely monitored during the peripubertal years (from 9 years in females and 10 years in males). Growth and pubertal status should be assessed by Tanner scoring, and FSH/LH and 17β-oestradiol or testosterone monitored at least yearly until completion of puberty. This allows identification of hypo- or hypergonadotrophic hypogonadism, or precocious puberty, and the commencement of appropriate replacement (delayed puberty) or antagonist (precocious puberty) treatment.

Other hypothalamic tropins

Both TSH and ACTH deficiency may occur after radiotherapy doses to the brain >30 Gy in up to 10 per cent of patients at risk. Hyperprolactinaemia is rare and usually subclinical, occurring only in women treated with high-dose radiotherapy.

Gonads

Pubertal growth and reproductive function are controlled by hormones secreted by the testis or ovary. The main difference between males and females is that in males two distinct testicular cell types control sexual development (Leydig cells) and fertility (Sertoli cells), while in females the oocyte controls both pubertal development and fertility.

Ovary

Germ cell failure and loss of ovarian endocrine function occur concomitantly in females. They may be due either to pelvic, abdominal or spinal radiotherapy, TBI, or alkylating agent chemotherapy. Age at treatment is important in predicting ovarian failure since females treated at a younger age are less likely to develop ovarian failure, probably because of higher number of primordial follicles at the time of treatment.

The clinical picture depends on the age at onset and severity of the ovarian damage. Delay or absence of pubertal onset or amenorrhea, irregular menses or premature menopause may occur. Laboratory testing demonstrates elevated gonadotrophins and reduced or absent 17β-oestradiol. Replacement oestro-progestogen therapy should be considered in order to induce puberty in females without onset and/or maintenance of regular menses. Ovarian insufficiency may be permanent or transient. Replacement treatment should be discontinued at intervals to determine if spontaneous menses occur. Most of these females are infertile or at high risk of premature menopause, but if spontaneous menses occur, appropriate counseling for family planning should be given.

Uterine morphology (dimensions and structure, e.g. fibrosis or reduced endometrial thickness) should be evaluated in females treated with pelvic or abdominal radiotherapy to assess the likelihood of embryonal implantation or completion of fetal development.

Testis

The testis is sensitive both to chemotherapy and radiotherapy. Among chemotherapeutic agents, cumulative doses of alkylating agents and timing of treatment influence the risk of oligo/azoospermia. Damage to germinal epithelium is estimated to occur after a testicular dose <1.2 Gy either as direct testicular radiotherapy or during abdominal or spinal radiotherapy or an inverted Y field for Hodgkin lymphoma treatment. Leydig cells are much more radioresistant and only doses >20 Gy (prepubertal patients) or >30 Gy (postpubertal individuals) may result in complete primary hypogonadism. In contrast to females, age at treatment has minimal impact on testicular function.

The clinical picture of testicular insufficiency depends on the severity of damage. Low testosterone levels with high gonadotrophins indicate decreased Leydig cell function, resulting in delayed or absent pubertal onset, or clinical symptoms of testosterone deficiency such as reduced muscle strength, irritability and decreased libido.

Replacement testosterone therapy should be given for delayed or absent pubertal onset, or in adults with documented testosterone deficiency (<250 ng/dl <8.7 nmol/l) with or without symptoms.

Damage to the Sertoli cells is more frequent and it is always irreversible. A definitive diagnosis of male infertility may only be made after semen analysis.

Thyroid

The thyroid gland is sensitive to radiotherapy given either externally to the neck (as in Hodgkin lymphoma treatment, CRT or TBI) or targeted via thyroid metabolism (MIBG treatment in neuroblastoma). The functional changes after external beam radiotherapy often occur by 6 months after treatment, but may only become evident up to 20 years later, and comprise clinical or subclinical hypothyroidism with a combined incidence of 20–30 per cent. Hyperthyroidism and autoimmune manifestations (Hashimoto thyroiditis) have been described in a smaller proportion. The morphological changes consist of benign lesions, primarily adenomas, and malignant lesions with an average 6-fold increased risk compared to the normal population.

The effect of radiotherapy on the thyroid gland is dose and age dependent with younger children at higher risk. A linear relationship with radiotherapy doses and thyroid late complications has been observed, but after doses > 30 Gy the cancer risk decreases, probably because of a cell-killing effect.

Thyroid hormones and thyroid-stimulating hormone (TSH) should be measured routinely in at-risk patients. Frank hypothyroidism results in low thyroid hormone values, whilst subclinical hypothyroidism leads to high TSH levels. Replacement therapy should be considered in manifest hypothyroidism or in persistent compensated hypothyroidism, and multinodular goitre. Careful clinical examination of the neck to detect nodules or lumps should be performed regularly, and some units augment this with ultrasound imaging. Needle biopsy may be considered for suspicious abnormalities.

Metabolic syndrome

Metabolic syndrome (MS) is characterized by a clustering of hypertension, dyslipidaemia (low HDL cholesterol, hypertriglyceridaemia, hypercholesterolaemia), type 2 diabetes or preclinical conditions (insulin resistance, or glucose intolerance), and obesity. This condition is associated with hypertension, and a pro-inflammatory and pro-thrombotic state that may lead to atherogenic dyslipidaemia. There is evidence that survivors exposed to CRT, prolonged steroid treatment, total body or abdominal irradiation, and those with hypogonadism or limitations in physical performance are at increased risk of glucose intolerance and MS.

Diagnosis of MS in adults is defined (International Diabetes Federation) by the presence of central obesity (waist circumference ≥94 cm in males, ≥80 cm in females), and at least two of the following:

1) Raised blood pressure >130/85 mmHg

2) Raised triglycerides >150 mg/dl (1.7 mmol/l)

3) Reduced HDL cholesterol <40 mg/dl (1.03 mmol/l) in males, or <50 mg/dl (1.29 mmol/l) in females

4) Raised fasting glucose ≥100 mg/ml (5.6 mmol/l).

The International Diabetes Federation does not recommend the diagnosis of MS in children under 10 years but the criteria for the diagnosis of MS in children from 10 to 16 years of age are broadly similar to that used in adults. Survivors with predisposing or treatment-related risk factors for MS should be monitored and counselled about appropriate diet and/or physical activity and avoidance of smoking.

Heart disease

Survivors of childhood cancer are 5–15 times more likely to experience heart disease than their siblings. The major risk factors are treatment with anthracyclines and/or radiotherapy to the heart, although vinca alkaloids and alkylating agents have also been implicated in cardiovascular complications. Other risk factors are young age at treatment, female gender and length of follow up. Tukenova et al. reported a 5.8-fold increased risk of dying from cardiac disease compared to the general population. In the CCSS, anthracycline doses ≥250 mg/m² carried a 2–5-fold increased risk for congestive heart failure, pericardial disease, and valvular abnormalities.

Radiotherapy to the heart is a major risk factor for cardiovascular disease in the form of coronary artery disease, myocardial infarction, pericardial disease, and valvular abnormalities. At doses ≥15 Gy, the CCSS found a 2–6-fold increased risk for the above complications in CCS compared to healthy siblings.

There is, as yet, no sure way of alleviating these problems except for primary prevention by eliminating cardiotoxic treatment where possible. Treatment with dexrazoxane, an iron chelator used to reduce oxidative stress and thereby prevent myocyte damage, has been shown to be effective in breast cancer patients, but it has not found a generally accepted place in paediatric oncology and there has been an unconfirmed suggestion that it may be related to the development of second cancers [e.g. AML/myelodysplastic syndrome (MDS)]. Treatment with ACE inhibitors has managed to postpone but not prevent cardiac disease. Monitoring of markers of cardiac damage (e.g. NT-proBNP and troponin-T) has not yet found a place in monitoring cardiac disease in CCS. There is as yet no common protocol for how often to monitor CCS with a risk of developing cardiac disease. A general recommendation is to avoid excessive strain on the heart, such as weight lifting, and that women need careful monitoring during pregnancy and possibly their babies should be delivered by caesarean section. Even subclinical signs of cardiac dysfunction should lead to a referral to a cardiologist.

Some new treatment options such as antibodies and small molecules have also been reported to cause cardiac toxicities necessitating careful follow-up. It is very important to consider other causes of cardiac/cardiovascular problems, such as hormonal disturbances, metabolic problems, smoking, and alcohol whilst undertaking long-term follow up in at-risk patients.

Lung disease

Chronic pulmonary health conditions were reported in 11.8 per cent (RR 2.8) of survivors in the CCSS. Both restrictive and obstructive lung disease may occur, whilst bronchiectasis may result from previous infections of the lower respiratory tract. Restrictive pulmonary disease may be subclinical, manifest only by abnormalities in pulmonary function tests (PFTs), or may present with progressive dyspnoea and respiratory failure due to pulmonary fibrosis, and is usually a consequence of either chemotherapy (particularly busulfan, carmustine or lomustine) or radiotherapy to a field that includes the lungs. Obstructive lung disease occurs most commonly in survivors of HSCT and is associated with chronic graft-versus-host (GvH) disease. Previous thoracic surgery may also impair lung function. PFTs should be performed at the completion of treatment in at-risk patients and at regular intervals thereafter in symptomatic patients or those with abnormal test results. It is advisable to recommend pneumococcal and annual influenza immunization in patients with established lung disease.

Kidney disease

Nephrotoxicity may be due to glomerular or tubular damage, or both. Renal failure or the requirement for dialysis is an uncommon but serious late complication, occurring in 0.5 per cent of survivors in the CCSS (RR 8.9). Glomerular toxicity is commonly subclinical and revealed only by a high serum creatinine concentration, but may occasionally lead to chronic or rarely end-stage renal failure. Likewise, tubular damage may be subclinical, but clinically overt proximal tubulopathy may occur in 25–30 per cent of children. Chronic tubular toxicity after ifosfamide may result in hypophosphataemia and even hypophosphataemic rickets (HR), whilst cisplatin (and less commonly carboplatin) nephrotoxicity may cause hypomagnesaemia, which when severe may lead to convulsions, tetany or cardiac arrhythmias. Ifosfamide may also rarely cause nephrogenic diabetes insipidus (NDI) due to distal tubular damage, or proximal or distal renal tubular acidosis (RTA). Renal damage may also cause hypertension and proteinuria in CCS.

The main risk factors for nephrotoxicity are the specific chemotherapy drugs received, radiotherapy to a field including renal tissue and previous nephrectomy, whilst tumour-related urinary tract obstruction or pre-existing renal dysfunction may exacerbate renal impairment. Ifosfamide nephrotoxicity is commoner in patients treated with a cumulative dose $>80\,g/m^2$. The increased frequency and severity of ifosfamide nephrotoxicity in children <5 years old at treatment reported in several studies is not a universal finding especially with longer follow up. Platinum nephrotoxicity is commoner in children treated with a higher cisplatin dose rate ($>40\,mg/m^2/day$) or higher cumulative carboplatin doses, and those treated at an older age. Other cytotoxic drugs that may cause or contribute to nephrotoxicity in children include melphalan, high-dose methotrexate and the nitrosoureas (carmustine, lomustine, semustine), whilst supportive care drugs including aminoglycoside antibiotics and amphotericin, or immunosuppressive agents such as ciclosporin may contribute to or represent primary cause of renal damage.

Patients with suspected or established nephrotoxicity should undergo regular surveillance including measurement of blood pressure and growth, urinalysis for proteinuria and biochemical monitoring. Electrolyte supplementation or specific treatment of HR, RTA and NDI may be required.

Lower urinary tract

Chronic lower urinary tract toxicity may manifest as haemorrhagic cystitis (HC) which may follow either radiotherapy or oxazaphosphorine (cyclophosphamide or ifosfamide) chemotherapy. Although most acute episodes of HC resolve fully, a few patients suffer from persistent or recurrent urinary symptoms, including frequency, dysuria, irritability and/or urgency, incontinence and occasionally retention due to bladder fibrosis and dysfunction. Bladder damage due to the original malignancy or its treatment (with surgery or radiotherapy) may result in a small volume bladder or sometimes a urethral stricture. Bladder malignancy is an uncommon but well recognized late complication of HC. Urinary tract symptoms in CCS should be evaluated by urinalysis, microscopy and culture, and referral to a urologist may be required for cytoscopy or urodynamic studies. Regular urine cytology should be performed in patients with a history of previous severe HC.

Visual toxicity

A wide variety of late ocular and visual toxicities may occur, ranging from dry eyes due to impaired lacrimal gland tear production, which predisposes to corneal ulceration and scarring, to visual impairment due to posterior subcapsular cataracts. Severe visual impairment was reported in 3 per cent of survivors in the CCSS (RR 5.8) and may also be a consequence of the underlying disease in survivors of CNS tumours, 13 per cent of whom reported legal blindness in one or both eyes in another CCSS study. Rarer adverse effects include keratitis, uveitis, chorioretinopathy, and optic neuritis. Lacrimal gland dysfunction and cataracts are related to radiotherapy to fields including the eye, including the use of TBI in children with haematological malignancies, up to a third of whom may develop later cataracts. Prolonged steroid treatment may occasionally lead to cataract formation even in the absence of radiotherapy. Very rarely, chemotherapy may cause severe visual toxicity, e.g. visual loss related to high-dose fludarabine. Treatment of ocular/visual toxicities includes artificial tear replacement for dry eyes and surgical removal of cataracts (with insertion of a lens implant), but established visual loss is usually irreversible.

Hearing problems

Chronic hearing loss not corrected by a hearing aid was noted in 2 per cent of CCSS survivors (RR 6.3), and any hearing impairment in 12 per cent of CNS tumour survivors. The consequences of deafness in children include delayed speech development and impaired educational/social functioning, especially in younger children. The major cause of deafness in survivors of childhood malignancy is platinum chemotherapy, particularly cisplatin and less commonly high-dose carboplatin. Both higher cumulative cisplatin dose and younger age at treatment predict a higher risk of deafness, with a total dose >400 mg/m^2 and age <5 years associated with development of bilateral sensorineural hearing loss in 40 per cent of children. High-dose radiotherapy to a field including the middle ear may cause mixed sensorineural and conductive hearing loss, but clinically significant deafness is uncommon in children who have not also received platinum treatment.

Hearing loss may also be exacerbated or caused by other ototoxic treatment (e.g. aminoglycosides). Children with hearing loss should be assessed by pure tone audiography, or by behavioural audiometry or otoacoustic emissions (or occasionally auditory brainstem responses) in younger children, and referred for ENT or audiometric/speech therapy assessment if symptomatic hearing loss is identified. Education and Community Paediatric services should be alerted in children with significant hearing impairment. Early evaluation, even before confirmation of hearing loss, is important in infants treated with cisplatin or high-dose carboplatin.

Craniofacial and dental complications

Craniofacial and dental complications are more prevalent in patients treated at a young age. The most important risk factor is radiotherapy to the face or brain, although chemotherapy may be an added risk factor. Radiotherapy to the growing skull and face will lead to hypoplasia of the irradiated area; the younger the child and the higher the radiotherapy dose, the more pronounced the growth impairment. As normal growth occurs, the deformity becomes progressively more pronounced. Correction of skeletal complications may be problematic due to the nature of the irradiated bone which can make surgery difficult. Damage to rudimentary teeth may result in the absence of permanent teeth, whilst that occurring later in dental development may result in small, brittle teeth. Damage to dental roots may lead to tooth loss and caries is accelerated by xerostomia from radiation effect on salivary glands. Due to these potential problems, preventive measures are very important when receiving radiotherapy and/or chemotherapy and guidelines for this have recently been published.

Gastointestinal and liver problems

Surgery and radiotherapy to the gastrointestinal tract may cause late complications such as strictures and malabsorption. Large radiotherapy fields and/or high doses are associated with a higher incidence of gastrointestinal problems. Hepatitis due to viral infection after blood transfusion remains a problem although the frequency is now lower due to better blood product surveillance. Long-term follow up should include liver function tests and examination for signs of liver disease, such as hepatosplenomegaly or jaundice.

Skin complications

Late skin complications after treatment for childhood cancer include non-melanomatous skin cancer (NMSC) (most commonly basal cell carcinoma but also squamous cell carcinoma), melanoma, alopecia and sparse/patchy hair, scarring, atrophy, and pigmentation disorders. Although rarely fatal, NMSC can cause substantial cosmetic problems if not treated in timely fashion. These tumours also occur at a much younger age in CCS than in the rest of the population, sometimes even below the age of 10. Radiotherapy is the main culprit (RR 4–6). Ninety per cent of these tumours occur within the radiation field and young age at treatment confers increased risk. Higher radiotherapy dose is a risk factor for malignant melanoma, as is treatment with alkylating agents and spindle inhibitors. Chemotherapy may also increase the frequency of pigmented naevi which may be precursors to a more malignant transformation. Avoiding excess UV radiation and careful examination of irradiated areas is of vital importance in the follow up.

Skeletal abnormalities

Bone growth involves both linear growth and increase in width and density. The process is controlled by a complex interaction between many endocrine signals including GH, IGF-1, thyroid hormone, oestrogens, androgen glucocorticoids, parathyroid hormone, and vitamin D, and other factors such as nutrition and physical activity. In cancer patients, disease itself or reduced physical activity or inadequate nutrition, as well as radiotherapy or chemotherapy, may interfere with normal bone metabolism.

The most evident effect on linear growth is that of radiotherapy when given before bone maturation has completed. Bone irradiation >20 Gy, especially when long bone growth plates are included in the radiation field, leads to reduced bone growth and potentially asymmetric limb growth. If the spine is involved in the radiation field, vertebral bodies will display impaired growth leading to a reduced final height with disproportion between standing and sitting height. Scoliosis may result from soft tissue fibrosis secondary to radiotherapy to paravertebral tissues/organs. Finally, facial asymmetry may result from radiotherapy including the facial bones.

It is vital to maximize the peak bone mineral density (BMD), which normally occurs on completion of puberty, with subsequent physiological decay over decades. Dual X ray absorptiometry (DEXA) is used to assess BMD.

CRT may indirectly affect BMD by interfering with GH and sex hormone secretion; in addition, prolonged steroid treatment and antimetabolites may affect BMD with a dose-dependant effect. Survivors of HSCT are at increased risk of skeletal late complications due to the multiple effects of TBI and high-dose chemotherapy on the neuroendocrine and gonadal systems, and the effects of impaired physical activity. After treatment discontinuation, recovery usually occurs but cumulative prednisone equivalent doses >9 g/m^2 or methotrexate dose >40 g/m^2 are associated with a higher risk of failure to regain normal BMD. Finally, bone metabolism may be indirectly affected in case of urinary calcium and/or phosphate wasting in patients with ifosfamide tubulopathy secondary to ifosfamide.

DEXA examination should be performed two years after treatment completion and at the end of puberty in at risk survivors. Vitamin D supplementation and appropriate dietary calcium intake should be advised. After puberty, and in severe cases, treatment with bisphosphonates may also be considered.

Avascular necrosis of bone may occur either during or after therapy, particularly with radiotherapy and/or prolonged steroid treatment, and usually affects joints in long bones causing pain and functional impairment.

Immunological function

Immunological function usually recovers satisfactorily within 6–12 months of standard chemotherapy but is slower after HSCT and may require ≥18 months after mismatched or unrelated donor allogeneic transplants, especially in the presence of chronic GvH disease.

Patients who have undergone splenectomy or received high-dose splenic radiotherapy (>40Gy), and survivors of HSCT (especially those with functional hyposplenism following conditioning with TBI), are at increased lifelong risk of potentially life-threatening encapsulated bacterial infections (*Haemophilus influenzae*, meningococcal or pneumococcal). These individuals should be immunized with conjugate Haemophilus influenzae type b (Hib), meningococcal C and pneumococcal vaccines, and given antibiotic prophylaxis with phenoxymethylpenicillin or amoxicillin.

Survivors of HSCT

Survivors of HSCT are at particularly high risk of late adverse complications, with >90 per cent suffering from at least one and >70 per cent from at least three. Patients conditioned with TBI are at the highest risk of late toxicity and high-dose conditioning chemotherapy is an additional potent risk factor. Additive and potentially synergistic damage results from numerous other factors, including previous treatment given before transplant, the development of other serious complications after HSCT, potentially toxic supportive care drugs, and especially chronic GvH disease which may affect any organ, tissue or body system. It is important to undertake regular and detailed surveillance in view of the wide range, frequency, and severity of potential complications. For example, second malignancies are reported in up to 10–15 per cent of HSCT survivors 15 years post-HSCT (skin, oral, thyroid and CNS tumours and post-transplant lymphoproliferative disease being amongst the commonest diagnoses), whilst reproductive toxicity with germ cell failure (leading to azoospermia in males and ovarian failure in females) is virtually inevitable after TBI and occurs in at least 90 per cent after busulfan/cyclophosphamide. Chronic GvH disease occurs in up to 30 per cent of HSCT patients, with multiple potential sequelae including organ and tissue damage (e.g. pulmonary, gastrointestinal, hepatic, renal, musculoskeletal, skin, serosal effusion), as well as functional impairment (e.g. immune-mediated cytopenias, delayed immune reconstitution) and the potential adverse effects of immunosuppressive drugs.

Surgical complications

Surgical complications and late physical effects may be obvious, and although the quality of life of these patients in domains other than physical functioning may be rated as high as that in controls, there is a lifelong need for many patients to have continued contact with health services, for example for prosthetic reasons or for post-surgical complications. Other complications are varied in location and subtle, depending on the anatomy and physiology of the affected part of the body. Spinal and neurological surgery may lead to complications affecting both the central and peripheral nervous system. Thoracic surgery may affect cardiac and pulmonary function. Abdominal surgery may affect the gastrointestinal system, liver or kidneys. Surgery to the head and neck may lead to facial deformities and thyroid disease. Although surgeons always try to avoid mutilating or functional damage, for some diagnoses and tumour locations this may be unavoidable when cure is the ultimate aim.

Survivorship

Besides medical complications as discussed above, CCS may also suffer psychological or social consequences that interfere with their quality of life (QoL), comprising elements of physical, functional, social, and psychological health.

Survivors may go through contrasting experiences: on the one hand, enhancing their appreciation of life (post-traumatic growth) by promoting maturity and resilience, while at the same time increasing vulnerability because of the previous cancer history or the presence of chronic health conditions (post-traumatic stress). Different aspects of QoL have been addressed by focusing either on social, emotional or psychological aspects, or on other lifestyle indicators such as school performance, employment or marriage. Many studies have highlighted difficulties of selected groups of survivors in schooling, relationships, self-esteem, employment, and marriage. These survivors may need medical, psychological, and social care. The term 'Damocles syndrome' has been used to illustrate their psychological condition of aiming to achieve full integration as active members of the society whilst living with the fear that possible treatment complications may interfere with their aspirations.

Quality of life may also be affected by the level of integration into society, as measured by the survivors' probability (compared to age and sex-matched general population peers), of securing employment, health insurance, or of marrying. It is important that the general public recognizes and accepts the reality of cure of childhood cancer, and ensures that survivors have equal access to education, jobs, insurance, and medical care.

The future

Long-term follow (LTFU) up of CCS is essential to increase knowledge about specific groups at higher risk of long-term morbidity and mortality, identify unrecognized late adverse effects (LAEs) and improve patient care. A major concern is that chronic LAEs may increase in frequency and severity with time, and interact adversely with the normal ageing process, resulting in increasing and clinically significant impairment of vital organ systems during adulthood at a younger age than normal, and an increased risk of premature major illness or death. This highlights the important need to develop effective models of LTFU care which will optimize efficient use of health service resources to deliver maximal benefit to survivors. LTFU should be life long and transition programs should be organized for the critical entry into adult health care. LTFU care should also be tailored to each survivor, based on type and dosage of treatment received, age at treatment and at follow up. Survivors should be able to decide if, when and where they would like their follow up to be conducted and the treating centre should be able to respond to any queries that may arise over time.

Increased understanding of the pathogenesis of LAEs of treatment should ultimately reduce their frequency and severity. In particular, it should inform the design of newer and less toxic agents or protocols and facilitate the development of protective drugs to reduce or prevent damage to normal tissues. Genetic risk factors may be identified that predict a higher risk for the development of LAEs in individual patients, hence explaining why some patients develop severe LAEs whilst others with apparently similar clinical risk factors do not.

Finally, newer agents may have as yet unknown LAEs, so clinical research is vital to document the nature of and risk factors for such toxicities. In particular, it is important that phase III randomized trials should evaluate LAEs of treatment. The knowledge gained from LTFU of CCS should be used not only to facilitate design of new treatment protocols but also to provide important information for survivors and their families to enable them to become advocates for their own health. Each CCS should be provided with a paper or electronic document providing information on the cancer-related medical history, including treatment received, and offering risk-adapted suggestions for LTFU.

Further reading

Armstrong GT, Liu Q, Yasui Y, et al. (2009) Late mortality among 5-year survivors of childhood cancer: a summary from the Childhood Cancer Survivor Study. *J Clin Oncol* **27**, 2328–38.

Bhatia S, Sather HN, Pabustan OB, et al. (2002) Low incidence of second neoplasms among children diagnosed with acute lymphoblastic leukemia after 1983. *Blood* **99**, 4257–64.

Diller L, Chow EJ, Gurney JG, et al. (2009) Chronic disease in the Childhood Cancer Survivor Study cohort: a review of published findings. *J Clin Oncol* **27**, 2339–55.

Ergun-Longmire B, Mertens AC, Mitby P, et al. (2006) Growth hormone treatment and risk of second neoplasms in the childhood cancer survivor. *J Clin Endocrinol Metab* **91**, 3494–8.

Friedman DL, Whitton J, Leisenring W, et al. (2010) Subsequent neoplasms in 5-year survivors of childhood cancer: the Childhood Cancer Survivor Study. *J Natl Cancer Inst* **102**, 1083–95.

Geenen MM, Cardous-Ubbink MC, Kremer LCM, et al. (2007) Medical assessment of adverse health outcomes in long-term survivors of childhood cancer. *JAMA* **297**, 2705–15.

Glenny AM, Gibson F, Auld E, et al. (2010) The development of evidence-based guidelines on mouth care for children, teenagers and young adults treated for cancer. *Eur J Cancer* **46**, 1399–412.

Langeveld NE, Grootenhuis MA, Voute PA, et al. (2004) Quality of life, self-esteem and worries in young adult survivors of childhood cancer. *Psychooncology* **13**, 867–81.

Li Y, Womer RB, Silber JH. (2004) Predicting cisplatin ototoxicity in children: the influence of age and the cumulative dose. *Eur J Cancer* **40**, 2445–51.

Lipshultz SE, Lipsitz SR, Sallan SE, et al. (2002) Long-term enalapril therapy for left ventricular dysfunction in doxorubicin-treated survivors of childhood cancer. *J Clin Oncol* **20**, 4517–22.

Massimino M, Gandola L, Mattavelli F, et al. (2009) Radiation-induced thyroid changes: a retrospective and a prospective view. *Eur J Cancer* **45**, 2546–51.

Moller TR, Garwicz S, Perfekt R, et al. (2004) Late mortality among five-year survivors of cancer in childhood and adolescence. *Acta Oncol* **43**, 711–8.

Mulder RL, Kremer LC, van Santen HM, et al. (2009) Prevalence and risk factors of radiation-induced growth hormone deficiency in childhood cancer survivors: a systematic review. *Cancer Treat Rev* **35**, 616–32.

Mulrooney DA, Yeazel MW, Kawashima T, et al. (2009) Cardiac outcomes in a cohort of adult survivors of childhood and adolescent cancer: retrospective analysis of the Childhood Cancer Survivor Study cohort. *BMJ* **339**, b4606.

Oeffinger KC, Mertens AC, Sklar CA, et al. (2006) Chronic health conditions in adult survivors of childhood cancer. *N Engl J Med* **355**, 1572–82.

Olsen JH, Moller T, Anderson H, et al. (2009) Lifelong cancer incidence in 47,697 patients treated for childhood cancer in the Nordic countries. *J Natl Cancer Inst* **101**, 806–13.

Packer RJ, Gurney JG, Punyko JA, et al. (2003) Long-term neurologic and neurosensory sequelae in adult survivors of a childhood brain tumor: childhood cancer survivor study. *J Clin Oncol* **21**. 3255–61.

Reulen RC, Taylor AJ, Winter DL, et al. (2008) Long-term population-based risks of breast cancer after childhood cancer. *Intl J Cancer* **123**, 2156–63.

Reulen RC, Winter DL, Frobisher C, et al. (2010) Long-term cause-specific mortality among survivors of childhood cancer. *JAMA* **304**, 172–9.

Ridola V, Fawaz O, Aubier F, et al. (2009) Testicular function of survivors of childhood cancer: a comparative study between ifosfamide- and cyclophosphamide-based regimens. *Eur J Cancer* **45**, 814–8.

Siviero-Miachon AA, Spinola-Castro AM, Guerra-Junior G. (2008) Detection of metabolic syndrome features among childhood cancer survivors: a target to prevent disease. *Vasc Health Risk Manag* **4**, 825–36.

Skinner R, Leiper AD. (2004) Bone marrow transplantation. In: Wallace WHB, Green DM, (eds) *Late Effects of Childhood Cancer*. pp 304–20 London: Arnold.

Skinner R. (2011) Nephrotoxicity—what do we know and what don't we know? *J Pediatr Hematol Oncol* **33**, 128–34.

Sklar CA, Mertens AC, Mitby P, et al. (2006) Premature menopause in survivors of childhood cancer: a report from the childhood cancer survivor study. *J Natl Cancer Inst* **98**, 890–6.

Tukenova M, Guibout C, Oberlin O, et al. (2010) Role of cancer treatment in long-term overall and cardiovascular mortality after childhood cancer. *J Clin Oncol* **28**, 1308–15.

Chapter 13

Evidence-based paediatric oncology

Leontien Kremer and Robert S. Phillips

History

The term evidence-based medicine was introduced by a research group led by David Sackett and Gordon Guyatt from the McMaster Medical School in Canada in 1992, with one of the first publications about evidence based medicine published in the Journal of the American Medical Association. The work built on strong foundations, particularly a book published in 1972 by a Scottish epidemiologist called Archie Cochrane: *Effectiveness and Efficiency: Random Reflections on Health Services* which outlined the concepts of evidence-based practice. The Cochrane Collaboration (based on these ideas) was founded in 1993 and continues to grow. It is dedicated to making up-to-date, accurate information about the effects of health care readily available worldwide. The practice of evidence-based medicine is very important in delivering optimal patient care and the terms evidence-based medicine, or evidence-based practice, are used all around the world. The *BMJ* listed evidence-based medicine as one of the 15 most important medical advances since the year 1840.

What is evidence-based medicine?

Evidence-based medicine (EBM) is 'the integration of best research evidence with clinical expertise and patient values and use a process of systematically finding, appraising, and using contemporaneous research findings as the basis for clinical decisions' (see Fig. 13.1). It has been strikingly defined as 'the conscientious, explicit, and judicious use of current best evidence in making decisions about the care of individual patients'. It describes a philosophy of care which integrates the highest quality scientific research, the treating clinician's expertise, and the child's specific medical, psychological and social condition. It is a heuristic—a way of thinking—not a recipe or set of instructions.

The practical output of this philosophy can be viewed as a four-step process:

1. Ask a structured clinical question
2. Acquire relevant research
3. Appraise the studies for their validity, importance, and applicability
4. Apply the results in practice.

Evidence-based medicine in paediatric oncology

There is a daily need for valid information about therapy, diagnosis, prognosis, aetiology, and prevention for children with cancer. There is far too much information, though this information is rarely summarized and the conclusions may be conflicting. The scale of this problem has been estimated that a physician would need to read 17 journal articles a day in order to keep up to date of all research relevant to a particular area of clinical practice. In this chapter, we will give an

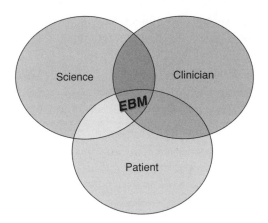

Fig. 13.1 The integration of the triad of patients, physicians, and publications.

overview how EBM can be used in daily practice of care for children with cancer and which tools are available for paediatric oncologists.

Three different 'modes' of practice of EBM in have been proposed: Replicator, User and Doer.

The 'replicator' mode describes the doctor who copies, knowingly or unconsciously, the actions and practices of a trusted colleague. This is hopefully a mentor whose work is centred on the delivery of EBM.

The 'user' mode is the commonest practice of taking evidence-grounded resources such as randomized controlled clinical trials (RCTs), systematic reviews or evidence-based guidelines and using them, without extensive appraisal, to guide clinical problem solving. When the resources that the doctor is using are solidly based on the best quality evidence that exists, this is an extremely efficient way of practicing EBM. This is the most practical and widely used way of putting evidence-based paediatric oncology into action, and the majority of this chapter will focus on how to learn to become a skilled 'user' of EBM.

The 'doer' mode refers to when the full four-step model is performed in detail; full expression of the structured question, broad search and detailed appraisal of the evidence identified, followed by a careful implementation plan. This is infrequently undertaken by a paediatric oncologist in daily clinical practice, but more common when the doctor is undertaking development of local policies, systematic reviews or guidelines. It's the most time-consuming and technically demanding of the three modes and learning this one requires detail well beyond this chapter.

Steps in EBM paediatric oncology

The first step: ask . . . and it might be given unto you

Asking an answerable question can prove terribly difficult, but when good questions are dissected the physiology becomes clear. The first step in deconstructing the anatomy of inquiry is to ask 'what sort of question is being asked?'. Clinical questions can be grossly categorized as 'foreground' and 'background'.

Background questions are generally broad, and can be caricatured as those asked by a medical student. They are often of the 'what is' or 'what causes' type: 'what is a pilomyxoid astrocytoma?', 'what causes leukaemia in childhood?'.

Foreground questions are specific, have intent, and can be asked in the domains of therapy (efficacy or harm), diagnosis, prognosis, etiology, or prevention. They frequently have three or four components summarized in a PICO:

P: Patient, problem or population (the group to which the question applies)

I: Intervention (or diagnostic test, or prognostic marker . . .)

C: Comparison (not always necessary)

O: Outcome(s) of interest (which should include patient-relevant, adverse and beneficial measures).

An example might be 'In metastatic rhabdomyosarcoma [problem], does high-dose therapy with stem cell rescue [intervention] compared with intensive conventional chemotherapy [comparison] produce higher 5-year overall survival [outcome]?' Questions of therapy can usually fit quite easily into this PICO frame.

As a final aside in the description of structured clinical questions, it is worth reflecting on how to choose which outcomes to look at. Do doctors really know what outcome their patients and families want, or do physicians presume? If the question is highly particular to one patient and their family, it may be pertinent to ask the patients and their families directly, to frame the PICO to actually answer their question.

Second step: acquisition is not a vice

Timely supply of useful evidence from the scientific medical literature is essential for the optimal care of children with cancer and professionals have a responsibility to keep up to date with research findings to ensure that their practice remains effective. These needs can be characterized by those of keeping up to date ('just in case' information) and answering day-to-day clinical questions ('just in time' information).

The use of summary or alerting systems can be used usefully to keep abreast of new information. 'EvidenceUpdates', a service from BMJ and McMaster University, alerts subscribers by email to new studies (http://plus.mcmaster.ca/evidenceupdates/). EvidenceUpdates uses research staff to select papers based on methodological quality from over 120 premier clinical journals. At least three members of a worldwide panel of practicing physicians then rate the papers for clinical relevance and interest, and often leave contextual comments which can be really useful to practicing clinicians. Further examples of paediatric resources dedicated to updating evidence include *Evidence based Child health; A Cochrane review Journal.*,[9] in which summaries and commentaries are presented of existing Cochrane systematic reviews in children.

A widely described structure of information resources to address this 'just in time' problem is that of the '5S' pyramid (Fig. 13.2). This describes how information would best be used if it were

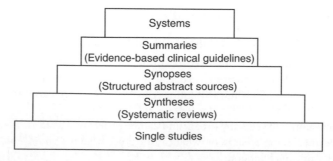

Fig. 13.2 The '5S' pyramid.

integrated into the systems of everyday working, ideally in an electronic care pathway. If this is not available, then information in a guideline or protocol could deliver the right answers in an evidence-based fashion. If these can't be found, then specific questions can be effectively answered if others provide a resource that finds, appraises and summarizes the key evidence related to a specific topic. These synopses can be incredibly useful to both answer specific questions and to try to keep up to date with the new knowledge that is flooding out of health sciences research. Without these, then a systematic review can provide a summary of the breadth of the best evidence to answer specific questions, and only rarely should we need to rely on looking at single, individual studies to answer our common queries.

We highlight examples of the 5S pyramid in the text below and in Table 13.1.

Table 13.1 Examples for the '5S' evolution of information services for evidence-based healthcare decisions

5S	Examples	Websites
Systems	TRIPdatabase	www.tripdatabase.com
	SUMsearch	www.sumsearch.org
Summaries	*General (examples)*	
Clinical Practice Guidelines	US National Clearinghouse	www.guidelines.gov
	Guidelines International Network	www.g-i-n.net
	UK National Institute for Health and Clinical Excellence	www.nice.org.uk
	Scottish Intercollegiate Guidelines Network:	www.sign.ac.uk
	New Zealand Guidelines Group	www.nzgg.org.nz
	National Health and Medical Research Council (Australië):	www.health.gov.au/nhmrc
	Agency for Healthcare Research and Quality	www.ahrq.gov
	World Health Organization	www.who.int
	Evidence based guidelines	www.ebm-guidelines.com
	Paediatric oncology (examples)	
	SIOP (Society of Paediatric Oncology)	www.siop.nl
	Children's Oncology Group	www.childrensoncologygroup.org
Synopsis	ACP Journal Club	www.acpjc.org
Structured abstract sources	Bandolier	www.medicine.ox.ac.uk/bandolier
	BMJ Clinical Evidence	www.clinicalevidence.bmj.com
	EBM-Journal (EBM Online)	www.ebm.bmj.com
	'Evidence based Child health; A Cochrane review journal'	www.onlinelibrary.wiley.com
	'Archimedes' 'Picket' Archives of Diseases of Childhood	www.adc.bmj.com
	UpToDate	www.uptodate.com
Synthesis	The Cochrane Library; (Cochrane database of systematic and Dare; non Cochrane reviews)	www.cochranelibrary.com
Systematic reviews		www.ncbi.nlm.nih.gov/pubmed
	Pubmed	
Single studies	Pubmed	www.ncbi.nlm.nih.gov/pubmed
	Embase	www.embase.com
	The Cochrane Library (trials)	www.cochranelibrary.com

Systems: computerized decision support, care pathways and search sites

There are few opportunities in paediatric oncology to use computerized decision support systems where evidence-based guidelines are included in computer systems for daily practice. But the idea of having a 'pathway' of care, based on the best available evidence, is not new to paediatric oncologists. Every treatment protocol we use has, built into it, a plan of investigation, treatment, response assessment and follow-up. The use of care pathways has been demonstrated to have good improvements in patient-related outcomes in a number of adult and paediatric specialty areas, although no direct evidence exists for children with malignancies.

In order to undertake the most efficient searches for rapidly available information, then search sites such as 'TRIPdatabase' and 'SUMsearch' may be very helpful.

Summaries: evidence-based clinical practice guidelines

Clinical guidelines are defined as 'systematically developed statements to assist practitioner and patient decisions about appropriate health care for specific clinical circumstances'. Guidelines are frequently produced by multidisciplinary, multiprofessional teams which include health-care professionals of different types, guideline methodologists, health economists and patient/carer partners. A guideline includes a systematic search for literature relevant to the intended key clinical questions, and summaries of the selected evidence according to a set of validity criteria. In a second step, the guideline developers formulate their recommendations for clinical practice by combining these evidence summaries with existing clinical knowledge and the weighting of ethical, cultural, and patient values.

Guidelines can have pitfalls, as can all forms of research. For example, the high number of topics to be covered by a guideline in a limited time may mean the evidence summaries are suboptimal, and guidelines may become 'stale' as it is difficult to refresh them frequently and keep the knowledge up to date. The term 'evidence based' guidelines is usually used if the structured process of EBM has been followed; starting with clinical questions, extensive search of literature, quality assessment, data extraction. and summary of the evidence. After this, recommendations will be formulated and the reasons why specific choices have been made will be explicitly described. The term 'evidence based' does not only apply to those recommendations where strong evidence supports the choice for a clinical decision but refers to the whole process of performing evidence-based summaries and formulating the recommendations.

Some useful sites to find guidelines related to paediatric oncology are in Table 13.1.

Synopses: evidence-based journals, structured abstracts and other summaries

Several journals present evidence-based summaries of the knowledge in health care. Examples are *ACP Journal Club*, *Bandolier*, *BMJ Clinical Evidence* and *EBM-Journal* (*EBM Online*). These journals focus on a general medical audience, sometimes with paediatric issues being included.

A further resource is UpToDate (www.uptodate.com). This is an internet-based electronic textbook that offers a clinical decision support system using current evidence to answer clinical questions. All topics are peer reviewed. However, all the steps of EBM are not clearly described which makes the influence of bias is difficult to judge. UpToDate covers around 8000 topics but only a few topics important for the care of children with cancer are included.

Syntheses: systematic reviews in childhood cancer

The synthesized evidence in systematic reviews can help health-care professionals to keep up to date. In a systematic review, the three first steps of EBM are included—formulating a clinical relevant question, performing an extensive search for literature and assessing the methodological quality of the selected studies—furthermore a meta-analysis can be included. A systematic review aims to minimize the occurrence of bias through a systematic search, selection and assessment of methodological quality and to reduce random error by using quantitative methods (i.e. meta-analysis) where appropriate. In paediatric oncology, 117 systematic reviews, including 18 Cochrane reviews, had been published between 1988 and November 2006. Unfortunately the methodological quality of most of the systematic reviews in paediatric oncology seemed to have serious methodological flaws, leading to a high risk of bias. The largest single provider of systematic reviews for health care is the Cochrane Collaboration with approximately 6000 systematic reviews included in the Cochrane Library. The Cochrane Collaboration developed standardized methods to perform systematic reviews and since 2006 the Cochrane Childhood Cancer Group has been registered within The Cochrane Collaboration. (www.ccg.cochrane.org) The aim of the Cochrane Childhood Cancer Group is to conduct and maintain systematic reviews on interventions and diagnosis for cancer in children and young adults with respect to prevention, treatment, supportive care, psychosocial care, palliative and terminal care, nursing care. and late effects of treatment. As of 2010, 30 author groups from all around the world are preparing and updating Cochrane systematic reviews in collaboration with the Cochrane Childhood Cancer Group. Those who prepare systematic reviews for the CCG are mostly volunteers.

Studies

If no other sources are available, the only option to get scientific information is to identify as many single studies as are relevant to the question in PubMed or similar bibliographic databases. Each question, for example therapy (efficacy or harm), diagnosis, prognosis, etiology, or prevention, is best answered by a different study design. For example, for treatment questions a RCT is the most optimal design, but for questions about prognosis a well-designed cohort study design is needed. These issues are captured in the levels of evidence of the new Centre for Evidence-based Medicine in Oxford (http://www.cebm.net).

Third step: appraisals are more than criticism

The process of critical appraisal is to examine in detail a study, in order to determine if it provides a valid, important and applicable answer to a specific clinical question. It is not the process of finding flaws and destroying research: it is evaluating strengths and weaknesses and coming to a conclusion in clear sight.

There are a wide range of structured checklists, but we favour the 'JAMA Users' Guides', now available in online and published text formats (www.jamaevidence.com). These checklists are very helpful when undertaking formal assessment of individual studies, guidelines, evidence summaries and systematic reviews.

The core parts of the appraisal for synthesized evidence (like systematic reviews or guidelines) can be captured in FAST, a rapid appraisal mnemonic. Further appraisal should be undertaken if these quick questions do not give clear answers.

F: Find all studies?

The central tenet of systematic reviewing is to find all eligible studies to minimize the risk of chance leading to an incorrect conclusion. Reviewers should detail the exhaustive extent to which they tried to find all relevant studies.

A: Appraise them correctly?

Studies should be included which give the best chance of answering the question truthfully. For questions of therapy, this will typically be randomized controlled trials. For prognosis, it may be large cohorts. For diagnostics, it should have groups of patients given both the test under study and the reference standard to really 'make' or 'exclude' the diagnosis. The reviewer should have clearly stated what criteria they used to appraise studies, and reported their appraisal results.

S: Synthesis (and look at heterogeneity)

Examine how the review has drawn all the information together. If the reviewers have undertaken meta-analysis, were the studies clinically similar enough to make this sensible? Were their results similar enough to compare?

This second part is often assessed with a heterogeneity measure, such as the I^2 statistic, which ranges from 0 to 100 per cent, with larger values representing greater statistical heterogeneity. As a rule of thumb, an I^2 above 50 per cent suggests important heterogeneity. It should be that any observed heterogeneity has an attempt at explanation, perhaps by analysing the groups in different drug doses, or by the different quality of trials, in order to explain the inconsistencies. If there are no detectable explanations though, the best result that can be offered may be based on a random-effect model.

Finally, it's worth looking to see if the information was examined for publication bias and other biases? How might these biases have affected the result?

T: Transferability

This is the step of considering how the review might actually be used in practice, and will be commented more upon in the next section. Clinical guidelines also require appraisal before use in a local health care environment. An excellent checklist is the AGREE instrument (http://www. agreecollaboration. org).

Fourth step: apply the results in practice

After the first three steps of EBM, a decision should be made how to apply the results in practice or how to formulate recommendation for (a group of) patients.

For only 20 per cent of the interventions in clinical practice do we know that the treatment is beneficial or we know that there is a trade-off between benefits and harms. (www.clinicalevidence. bmj.com). Even in these cases, a weighting of the science, clinical expertise, patients, and socio-cultural values will be essential. When the evidence is uncertain, making these decisions and tradeoffs explicit becomes even more important. Furthermore, the costs incurred or saved should be taken into account.

In the world of paediatric oncology, there are frequently times when the rarity of the condition makes 'gold standard' evidence unobtainable. For these sorts of situations, Jeremy Howick, Paul Glazsiou and Jeffrey Aronson have captured a concept for evaluating evidence on treatment issues. They have then revisited the Revised Bradford-Hill Guidelines for Causation and developed the concept of parachutes of evidence: a trio of the main 'chute (direct evidence), and two subsidiary 'chutes (mechanistic and parallel evidence).

Direct evidence is the data we rely on most securely. This is when the RCT gives results of some therapy being effective, or when an exceptionally effective intervention is enormously better than all others (like when insulin was first used in diabetic ketoacidosis).

Parallel evidence is the stuff we use in paediatrics a lot: where similarities exist between the direct evidence in other populations and the ones we treat, and by replication of results across different areas.

Mechanistic evidence is still the shakiest: coherence with other theories of how things work, and a plausible biological explanation.

Another reason why evidence could be difficult to translate directly to practice is when, for example, the results of a systematic review are focused on concepts. As an example a systematic review of anti-emetics to prevent nausea and vomiting after chemotherapy tells you 'anti-emetics work'. But you can't just prescribe 'anti-emetics', so how can you transfer the review result into clinical practice? A couple of suggestions have been offered, and both have clinical common sense:

(1) go for the strategy of the largest trial (it has the most weight in the review, so has the 'most' evidence)

(2) go for the most often used dose/drug/approach (it was shown to be feasible the most often).

This clear conceptualization of how the various guises that evidence exists in can link to help us work out what works, what works best, and what's likely to work for this patient. There are systems under development that help to give a consistent shorthand to these balances: the GRADE methodology is an important new development, particularly for assessing the results of studies of interventions (www.gradeworkinggroup.org).

In conclusion, for each clinical decision the science, values of patients, cultural values, clinical expertise, and the amount of costs, should be taken into account.

Common criticisms of evidence-based medicine

Since the introduction of EBM, criticisms to this paradigm shift have been described which can be divided into 'limitations universal to the practice of medicine', 'misperceptions of evidence-based medicine' and 'genuine limitations of evidence-based medicine'.

Within the first section, 'limitations universal to the practice of medicine,' fall criticisms such as 'There is a shortage of coherent, consistent scientific evidence' or 'There is no evidence available', along with complaints stating 'It is difficult to translate evidence to the care of individual patient'. In instances like this, the methods of evidence based medicine can be used to make these general limitations of health care more explicit.

The second group of criticisms of EBM are based on misperceptions. For example the criticism that evidence-based medicine 'denigrates clinical expertise', or 'ignores patients' values' or 'promotes "cookbook" medicine' arise through a failure to include all the important steps of EBM. A further example of misperception is that 'only randomized trials or systematic reviews' constitute the 'evidence' in EBM. This is not true and several sources of best available evidence may inform clinical decision-making.

Finally, some of the criticisms of EBM are genuine limitations of the process: there is a need to develop new skills and apply the process during limited time and with limited resources. To overcome this barrier, we believe an increasing number of prepared evidence-based products and training programmes will be available in the future.

The way forward

To take paediatric oncology further forward, in developing its evidence base and the implementation of that evidence, we need to continue doing lots of what we are doing:

◆ We need to work as international collaborators, focussed on the cure and support of children with malignancies by engaging in high quality research, including our patients, their families and our colleagues in other specialities.

◆ We need to continue to collaborate in developing high quality trials in paediatric oncology. As previously stated in the *Lancet*: 'Participation in protocol-driven clinical research is clearly better than the ad hoc patterns of non-protocol treatments, paediatric cancer trials offer a paradigm for paediatric clinical research'.

◆ We need to collaborate in summarizing the evidence. The Cochrane Childhood Cancer Group offers the unique possibility to collaborate worldwide in preparing scientific summaries of evidence.

◆ We need to collaborate in performing evidence-based guidelines. An example is the recently started world-wide collaboration in developing evidence-based guidelines for survivors of childhood cancer. Within the development of guidelines it will be important to collaborate in performing the evidence summaries and in discussing the overlap in recommendations country-specific recommendations.

◆ We need to develop new systems and strategies to implement up-to-date high quality knowledge form science in daily practice.

◆ We need to develop training for researchers and clinicians in clinical epidemiology.

In conclusion, we need interventions to bridge the gap between science and practice in paediatric oncology worldwide and make our practice as evidence-based as possible.

Further reading

Caldwell PH, Murphy SB, Butow PN, Craig JC (2004) Clinical trials in children. *Lancet* **364**, 803–11.

Coulthard MG, Phillips B, Wacogne I (2010) What are we Picketing and why? *Arch Dis Child* **95**, 575.

Davidoff F, Haynes B, Sackett D, Smith R (1995) Evidence based medicine. *BMJ* **310**, 1085–6.

Evidence-based medicine working group (1992) Evidence-based medicine. A new approach to teaching the practice of medicine. *JAMA* **268**, 2420–5.

Field MJ, Lohr KN (1990) Clinical Practice Guidelines. Directions for a New Program. Committee to Advice the Public Health Service on Clinical Practice Guidelines. Washington DC: National Academy Press.

Godlee F (2007) Milestones on the long road to knowledge. *BMJ* **334** (suppl 1), s2–s3.

Haynes RB (2006) Of studies, syntheses, synopses, summaries, and systems: the '5S' evolution of information services for evidence-based healthcare decisions. *Evid Based Med* **11**, 162–4.

Howick J, Glasziou P, Aronson JK (2009) The evolution of evidence hierarchies: what can Bradford Hill's 'guidelines for causation' contribute? *J R Soc Med* **102**, 186–94.

Klassen T, Offringa M (2006) Editor's introduction. *Evidence-Based Child Health: A Cochrane Review Journal* **1**, 1–2.

Lundh A, Knijnenburg SL, Jørgensen AW, et al. (2009) *Quality of systematic reviews in pediatric oncology—a systematic review*. Cancer Treat Rev **35**, 645–52.

Phillips B (2010) FAST appraisal Archives of Disease in Childhood. **95**, 560.

Phillips B. Towards evidence based medicine for paediatricians. *Arch Dis Child.* 2003;**88**(1):82–3.

Phillips R, Glasziou P (2008) Evidence based practice: the practicalities of keeping abreast of clinical evidence while in training. *Postgrad Med J* **84**, 450–3.

Rotter T, Kinsman L, James E, et al. (2010) Clinical pathways: effects on professional practice, patient outcomes, length of stay and hospital costs. *Cochrane Database Syst Rev* **17**, CD006632. Review.

Sackett DL, Rosenberg WM, Gray JA, et al. (1996) Evidence based medicine: what it is and what it isn't. *BMJ* **312**, 71–2.

Straus SE, McAlister FA (2000) Evidence-based medicine: a commentary on common criticisms. *CMAJ* **163**, 837–41.

Ten Bruggencate MJ, Kremer LC, Caron HN, et al. (2009) Pediatr Blood Cancer **52**, 231–6.

Chapter 14

Acute lymphoblastic leukaemia

Rob Pieters and Martin Schrappe

Epidemiology

Acute lymphoblastic leukaemia (ALL) is the most common type of cancer in childhood. It accounts for 20–25 per cent of all childhood cancers. The peak incidence is at 2–5 years of age which is mainly due to a peak of ALL cases with hyperdiploid ALL and TEL/AML1 gene rearranged ALL. The incidence rate is higher in high-income countries and is higher in Hispanic children and lower in black children as compared to white children. Males are affected more often than females except in infants.

The etiology of ALL is characterized by the fact that immature lymphoid cells acquire different consecutive genetic lesions of which the first lesion often occurs already before birth. For example, the most common translocation that occurs in childhood ALL, the TEL/AML1 translocation, can be traced back in the Guthrie cards of the patients taken at the time of birth. However, only few children who are born with this translocation will develop ALL, proving that this lesion is a pre-leukaemic event and that leukaemogenesis is multifactorial and depends on multiple consecutive genetic events. Not more than a few per cent of children with ALL cases have an underlying predisposing genetic syndrome which is almost entirely accounted for by Down syndrome.

Clinical presentation

Most symptoms at diagnosis are secondary to leukaemic infiltration of the bone marrow: pallor, fatigue, fever, petechiae,haematomas. Bone pain and rejection to walk in young children are alarm symptoms. Physical examination may show enlargement of liver, spleen, and lymph nodes. In rare cases, dyspnea or signs of the vena cava superior syndrome can be due to enlargement of mediastinal lymph nodes. Other rare symptoms are one-sided testicular enlargement or focal neurological abnormalities due to leukaemic involvement of the testes or the nervous system, respectively.

Diagnosis

The blood cell counts often show anaemia and/or thrombocytopenia and granulocytopenia. The leukocyte count is increased to $>10\ ^9/l$ in only half of cases. Even leucopenia may occur. The differential count of the peripheral blood shows leukaemic cells in the majority but not all cases. Nowadays, the diagnosis of ALL is made by a combination of morphology, immunophenotyping and cytogenetic and molecular genetic techniques examining the bone marrow and peripheral blood. Although these latter techniques have become very important, classic cytomorphology still plays an important role, especially when differential diagnosis with other diseases such as myelodysplastic syndrome, aplastic anaemia or pancytopenias due to infections is difficult and when low numbers of leukaemia cells are obtained by punctures. Although most protocols still require the classic cut-off level of 25 per cent malignant blast cells in the bone marrow for the diagnosis of leukaemia, lower percentages of blast cells will be accepted for the diagnosis if this is confirmed by immunophenotyping and genetic abnormalities that are typical for ALL. In morphology, myeloperoxidase (MPO) staining is used for the discrimination of lymphatic leukaemia (MPO–) from myeloid leukaemia that is in most but not all cases MPO positive. Immunophenotyping is used to determine the type of ALL (B-lineage or T-lineage) and the differentiation stage of the leukaemic cells. Genetic techniques are used for the detection of recurrent chromosomal or molecular abnormalities. The combination of the three methods leads not only to the diagnosis of ALL but also to the classification of ALL into prognostic risk groups, with consequences for the treatment to be delivered.

Central nervous system (CNS) involvement is diagnosed in case of >5 leucocytes/µl with identifiable leukaemic cells (so-called CNS3 status) or in case of neurological symptoms based upon leukaemic infiltration. CNS2 status refers to the presence of leukaemic cells but no leucocytosis (<5 cells/µl) in the spinal fluid. CNS1 means no leukaemic cells and no leucocytosis in the spinal fluid. TLP+ and TLP– refer to the fact whether a traumatic lumbar punctures was done or not. TLP+ with leukaemic cells in the spinal fluid is not defined as CNS involvement although in some protocols extra intrathecal chemotherapy is administered in case of TLP+.

Prognostic factors and risk classification

Many clinical and biological factors predict clinical outcome. However, many factors such as age, gender, immunophenotype, genetic abnormalities, and white blood cell count are related to each other. Thus, large series and proper analyses that take this fact into account need to be done to establish the independent and quantitative value of each prognostic factor. Moreover, therapy is often adjusted based upon these factors, thereby influencing the contribution of a factor to outcome.

In most protocols, early response to therapy that reflects many of these factors is also used for therapy stratification. Many European protocols use the response in the peripheral blood to one week of systemic prednisone and one dose of intrathecal methotrexate (MTX). Others use the response in the bone marrow after 2 weeks of therapy. A classic parameter still used in all protocols is whether or not complete morphological response is obtained after induction therapy which is defined as <5 per cent blasts in the bone marrow and the absence of other evidence of leukaemia. Measurement of so-called minimal residual disease (MRD) is incorporated in many protocols. MRD is measured by flow cytometry during or at the end of induction or by polymerase chain reaction (PCR) at the end of induction and in the first months of therapy.

Finally, it is also important to keep in mind not only how strong a prognostic factor is but also how large the group is that it recognizes. Table 14.1 presents the most important prognostic factors currently used for therapy stratification.

Treatment

The backbone of each ALL treatment protocol consists of four phases: induction, consolidation, intensification or re-induction, and maintenance or continuation therapy (Table 14.2). The different phases contain elements that aim to treat the CNS. Only few patients receive CNS irradiation or allogenic haematopoietic stem cell transplantation (HSCT) in addition to chemotherapy. Current treatment protocols results in 5-year event-free survival (EFS) rates up to 85 per cent and 5-year survival rates of up to 90 per cent. However, relapses and secondary tumours may also occur more than 5 years after diagnosis. This accounts even more for the occurrence of death later than 5 years after diagnosis because relapsed patients may be salvaged for a significant

Table 14.1 Most important prognostic factors currently used for therapy stratification

Clinical and biological factors	Favourable (prevalence in %)	Less favourable (prevalence in %)
Gender	Female (~45%)	Male (~55%)
White blood cell count	Low (e.g. <50 ^{9}/l) (~80%)	High (e.g. >50 ^{9}/l) (~20%)
Age	1–10 yr (~75%)	<1 (~4%)
		15–18 yr (~7%)
Central nervous system	CNS1 (~75%)	CNS3 (~3%)
	TLP– (~90%)	TLP+ (~10%)
Immunophenotype	Common/preB ALL (~80%)	proB ALL (~4%)
		T-ALL (~15%)
Genetic abnormalities	TEL/AML1 (~25%)	MLL translocations (~5%)
	Hyperdiploidy (~25%)	BCR–ABL (~3%)
	E2A/PBX (~3%)	Hypodiploidy (1%)
Early response to therapy		
Day 8 prednisone response	<1 x 10 ^{9}/l (~90%)	≥1 x 10 ^{9}/l (~10%)
Day 15 bone marrow response	M1 marrow: <5% blasts (~60%)	M3 marrow: >25% blasts (~15%)
Morphological complete remission after induction therapy	Yes (~98%)	No (~2%)
Bone marrow minimal residual disease by PCR	$<10^{-4}$ after 5 weeks (~25–40%)	$>10^{-3}$ after 12 weeks (~5%)

number of years before they ultir... ...ore the final EFS and survival rate are lower than the 5-years figures that are ...

Induction

The goal of induction therap... ...logical remission and restore normalhaematopoiesis. This i... ...herapy in ~98 per cent of all children. Almost all protocol... ...xamethasone), vincristine and L-asparaginase as a so-ca... ...otherapy for this course.

Table 14.2 backbone of chem... ...rape...

Induction	Consolidation	...on	Maintenance
Prednisone/ dexamethasone	(high-dose) Methotrexate	...thasone	(low-dose) Methotrexate
Vincristine	6-Mercaptopurine		6-Mercaptopurine
Asparaginase	Intrathecal therapy	As...ginase	(Prednisone/ dexamethasone)
(Anthracycline)	(Cyclofosfamide)	(Anthracycline)	(Vincristine)
Intrathecal therapy	(Cytosine arabinoside)	Intrathecal therapy	Intrathecal therapy
	(L-Asparaginase)	(Cyclofosfamide)	
		(Cytosine arabinoside)	

The addition of an anthracycline as fourth systemic drug is matter of debate, especially for certain low-risk groups. Some studies have made clear that at least ~50 per cent of children can be cured without the use of anthracyclines but the important question is how to define these patients at diagnosis. Berlin, Frankfurt, Münster (BFM) protocols use prednisone as single systemic drug in the first week of treatment which has been shown to be of predictive value and which is an easy way to reduce tumour load in a controlled way to avoid tumour lysis syndrome.

About 2 per cent of patients do not achieve remission after induction therapy, which may be due to early death which is most often caused by infection or bleeding or which may be due to chemotherapy-resistant leukaemic cells. The long-term outcome of this latter group is not as poor as was thought previously; about 30–40 per cent of these children are long-term survivors with intensive treatment.

Consolidation and intensification

Consolidation and intensification courses aim to eradicate the residual leukaemic cells. BFM protocols use a post-induction course consisting of low-dose araC, 6-mercaptopurine (6-MP) and cyclofosfamide which reduces the MRD load significantly. Other groups use different combinations of drugs which will also reduce MRD in this phase. Many study groups use high-dose MTX and 6-MP in combination with frequent intrathecal therapy in the consolidation phase. The use of high-dose MTX significantly reduces the risk of bone marrow relapse.

Drugs used in the intensification or re-induction course are the same as used in the induction. Several randomized studies have proven the value of the intensification. Intensified and double delayed intensification improves outcome for patients with a slow initial response to treatment. In patients with a rapid early response, a more intensive but not a longer intensification treatment was of benefit. Omission of the intensification led to a significant rise in the relapse rate although the same study made clear that about 50 per cent of patients was cured without the use of this intensification.

Dexamethasone or prednisone?

Several but not all randomized studies have shown that the use of dexamethasone at a dose of $6 \, mg/m^2$ results in a lower rate of bone marrow and CNS relapses than prednisone at a dose of $40 \, mg/m^2$ (Table 14.3). This benefit of dexamethasone might be due to higher free plasma levels and a better CNS penetration or to the fact that the used doses of dexamethasone and prednisone are not really equivalent as some *in vitro* studies suggest. The counterpart is that dexamethasone also leads to more side effects.

Which dose of which L-asparaginase?

Several studies have shown that intensification of L-asparaginase in induction and intensification has improved outcome or that suboptimal use of L-asparaginase leads to an unfavourable outcome. (Table 14.4) It is important to recognize the differences in pharmacokinetics and pharmacodynamics between the different L-asparaginase preparations to prevent mistakes in administration of these drugs. L-asparaginase derived from *Escherichia coli* has a longer half-life than the preparation described from *Erwinia chrysanthemi* (Erwinase), which results in differences in serum asparagine depletion. Two randomized studies comparing these two drugs at the same dose schedule resulted therefore in lower relapse rates, more side effects and higher survival rates when using the *E. coli* preparation. If Erwinase would have been given at the right dose–intensity schedule, this difference probably would not have occurred. These studies also illustrate that the dose-intensity of L-asparaginase is an important contributor of outcome in childhood ALL. In line with this, intolerance to L-asparaginase or inactivation of L-asparaginase due to neutralizing antibodies also

Table 14.3 Studies comparing prednisolone with dexamethasone

Study group [reference]	Years	Study design and study population	Dose of glucocorticoid	Dexa vs Pred* in induction	Dexa vs pred administered in other parts of treatment	Outcome result
CALGB 7111 [Jones B, et al. (1991) Med Pediatr Oncol 19, 269–75]	1971–1974	Randomized; All risk groups (n=646)	Pred 40 mg/m²/day vs. dexa 6 mg/m²/day	Days 1–28 or days 1–21 or days 11–31	7-day pulses in maintenance	Isolated CNS relapse rates: pred 25.5%; dexa 14.3%
DCSLG ALL VI [Veerman AJ, et al. (1996) J Clin Oncol 14, 911–8]	1984–1988	Historical control Non-HR patients (n=190)	Dexa 6 mg/m²/day. Historical control DCLSG ALL V (n=240) had similar eligibility criteria and used pred 40 mg/m²/day in induction, less intrathecal therapy and no medium high-dose methotrexate (2 g/m²), but cranial irradiation at age-dependent doses of 15 to 25 Gy	Days 1–28	14-day pulses in maintenance	EFS at 10 years on DCLSG ALL VI (82±3) was almost 30% better compared to ALL V. Isolated CNS relapse rates: ALL VI 1.1%; ALL V 12.9%
DFCI 91–01 [Silverman LB, et al. (2001) Blood 97, 1211–8]	1991–1995	Historical control All risk groups (n=377)	SR patients: dexa 6 mg/m²/day. HR patients: dexa 18 mg/m²/day. Historical control DFCI 87–01 used pred 40 mg/m²/day in SR and pred 120 mg/m²/day in HR patients, less asparaginase in intensification (20 instead of 30 weeks), and not all patients received high-dose methotrexate and it was randomized to low dose	-	5-day pulses in intensification and maintenance	EFS at 5 years DFCI 91–01 83±2%; DFCI 87–01 78±2%. Isolated CNS relapse rates: DFCI 91–01 1.1%; DFCI 87–01 4.1%

(continued)

Table 14.3 (continued)

Study group [reference]	Years	Study design and study population	Dose of glucocorticoid	Dexa vs Pred* in induction	Dexa vs pred administered in other parts of treatment	Outcome result
CCG 1922 [Bostrom BC, et al. (2003) Blood 101, 3809–17]	1993–1995	Randomized SR patients (n=1060)	Pred 40 mg/m²/day vs. Dexa 6 mg/m²/day	Days 1–28	5-day pulses in consolidation and maintenance	EFS at 6 years pred 77±2%; dexa 85±2% Isolated CNS relapse rates: pred 7.1%; dexa 3.7% Excess of myopathy and hyperglycemia with dexa; behavioural problems and tendency towards pancreatic toxicity with dexa.
UK MRC ALL97 and ALL97/99 [Mitchell CD. et al. (2005) Br J Haematol 129, 734–45]	1997–2002	Randomized all risk groups (n=1603)	Pred 40 mg/m²/day vs. dexa 6.5 mg/m²/day	Days 1–28 in ALL97 and days 1–29 in ALL97/99	5-days pulses in interim maintenance and maintenance	EFS at 5 years Pred 76±3%; dexa 84±3% Isolated CNS relapse rates: pred 5.0%; dexa 2.5%. Excess of behavioural problems, myopathy, osteopenia and weight gain with dexa
TCCSG L95–14 [Igarashi S. et al. (2005) J Clin Oncol 23, 6489–98]	1995–1999	Randomized only SR and IR patients (n=359)	Pred 60 mg/m²/day vs. Dexa 8 mg/m²/day; During intensification reduced to Pred 40 mg/m²/day vs. Dexa 6 mg/m²/day	Days 1–31	Days 1–14 in four intensification elements for SR and three elements for IR patients	No differences in EFS at 8 years; no statistically significant difference with regard to site of relapse or toxicity; a tendency towards less CNS relapses with dexa was set off by an increase in bone marrow relapses in SR; tendency towards higher incidence of complications with dexa.

*Pred, prednisolone; dexa, dexamethasone.

Table 14.4 Comparative studies on the dose-intensity of L-asparaginase

Comparison	Less intensive dose schedule	More intensive dose schedule		Reference
Non-equivalent dose schedules of asparaginase in ALL	60% EFS	73% EFS	significant	Duval M, et al. (2002) Blood 99, 2734–9
Non-equivalent dose schedules of asparaginase in ALL	78% EFS	89% EFS	significant	Moghrabi A, et al. (2007) Blood 109, 896–904
20 extra weeks of asparaginase in risk group ALL	79% EFS	88% EFS	significant	Pession A, et al. (2005) J Clin Oncol 23, 7161–7
20 extra weeks of asparaginase in intermediate risk group ALL	72% EFS	76% EFS	not significant	Rizzari C, et al (2001) J Clin Oncol 19, 1297–303
20 extra weeks of asparaginase in T-ALL	55% EFS	68% EFS	significant	Amylon MD, et al. (1999) Leukemia 13, 335–42
20 extra weeks of asparaginase in T-NHL	64% EFS	78% EFS	significant	Amylon MD, et al. (1999) Leukemia 13, 335–42
<25 weeks versus >25 weeks of asparaginase in ALL	71% EFS	90% EFS	significant	Silverman LB, et al. (2001) Blood 97, 1211–8

predicts an inferior outcome if this leads to discontinuation of L-asparaginase without proper replacement by alternative L-asparaginase preparations. PEGylated L-asparaginase (PEG-asparaginase) is less immunogenic and leads less frequently to antibody formation and many study groups will therefore use PEG-asparaginase in their current or upcoming treatment protocols. PEG-asparaginase has a much longer half life than the other preparations and this drug has to be administered once every 2–4 weeks instead of once every 2–3 days for the other preparations to ensure complete and continuous asparagine depletion in the serum.

Maintenance

The aim of maintenance treatment is to further reduce minimal residual cells that are not detectable with current techniques at this stage in the far majority of cases and to suppress the outgrowth of these cells. The importance of the maintenance therapy is illustrated by the fact that outcome depends on the intensity and duration of maintenance given. Most protocols continue the maintenance up to the time point of 2 years after diagnosis or after achievement of morphological remission. Other protocols include a time period of 2 years maintenance treatment for girls and 3 years for boys. A meta-analysis showed that longer maintenance leads to lower relapse rates but also increased toxic death rates. Reduction of the duration of maintenance to less than 2 years led to an increased relapse risk but also showed that a significant proportion of patients survive without 2 years of maintenance. Again, like with the omittance of anthracyclines, the question is how to recognize these patients. It can be hypothesized that a long maintenance is more likely to be of benefit for the more 'smouldering' types of ALL such as TEL/AML1 rearranged ALL and hyperdiploid ALL, whereas the more aggressive leukaemias such as MLL rearranged ALL, T-ALL and BCR-ABL rearranged ALL that are characterized by very early relapses have less benefit of maintenance therapy.

The backbone of every maintenance course is weekly (oral or intravenous) methotrexate and daily oral 6-MP. Doses of these drugs are usually adapted according to leucocyte count or to lymphocytes, neutrophil, and platelet count. At an international expert meeting, consensus was reached to use a target leucocyte count of $1.5-3 \times 10^9/l$. Starting doses may differ between protocols but most often $50 \, \text{mg/m}^2$ MTX and $20-30 \, \text{mg/m}^2$ 6-MP are used at the start of maintenance. There are large intra- and inter-individual differences in the doses that are tolerated or that are needed to achieve the target leucocyte count. Intra-individual differences reflect intercurrent factors such as viral infections. Inter-individual differences reflect underlying pharmacogenetic host factors such as polymorphisms in the thiopurine methyltransferase gene which encodes an enzyme that inactivated thiopurines. Maintaining the highest dose of 6-MP and MTX leads to a better outcome. Treatment adherence and compliance of both doctors and patients (especially adolescents) may therefore also have impact on outcome. Administration of 6-MP in the evening leads to a better outcome for unknown reasons. 6-MP should not be given with milk products since these contain xanthine oxidase which decreases its bioavailability. Two of three randomized studies show that the even-free survival is the same when 6-thioguanine (6-TG) or 6-MP is used in maintenance; one study showed less relapses in the 6-TG arm but the liver toxicity with features of veno-occlusive disease was much higher with 6-TG. Therefore, 6-MP remains the thiopurine of choice in maintenance.

Intensification of the maintenance by adding pulses with prednisone/dexamethasone and vincristine is a matter of debate. A large recent randomized study did not show a benefit of these pulses although a smaller but comparable study did show a benefit with a very comparable background of treatment. Two meta-analyses showed that the use of pulses led to an improved outcome in the past; however, the most recent meta-analysis showed no benefit for pulses against the background of several contemporary treatment protocols. So, for the whole ALL population, the use of pulses is probably not beneficial. However, pulses may contribute to a better outcome for specific risk groups or for patients treated on a protocol of low intensity such as the recently published DCOG-ALL9 study that lacked an intensification course for a large part of patients.

Central nervous system-directed therapy

CNS-directed therapy is a prerequisite for successful treatment of ALL. In the 1960s, more than half of patients suffered from CNS relapses. Several treatment elements were effective in reducing this high CNS recurrence rate. First, cranial or craniospinal irradiation is very effective in preventing CNS relapses but it has two very major side effects. Neurocognitive disturbances occur especially in young children and secondary brain tumours and carcinomas occur. Because the secondary tumours occur very late (up to 20–30 years after radiation) and at a relatively high rate, it is important to study very long follow up to compare the outcome after the use of radiation with other CNS-directed therapies. These other therapies are intrathecal chemotherapy and systemic application of drugs that penetrate the CNS such as high-dose MTX, dexamethasone and high-dose cytosine arabinoside.

A meta-analysis published in 2003 showed that the use of intensive intrathecal therapy and radiation lead to comparable EFS rates. Also comparable EFS rates were found when using high dose MTX but detailed analysis showed that high dose MTX resulted in a higher CNS relapse rate but a lower bone marrow relapse rate than radiation. So. Although the majority of CNS relapses can be prevented by adequate systemic and intrathecal chemotherapy, this does not exclude the possibility that specific high-risk groups may benefit from radiation and this is a matter of debate at this moment. Most clinical protocols still use radiation for a small minority of high-risk patients such as patients with a CNS3 status at diagnosis and T-ALL patients with a high tumour burden at diagnosis. Elimination of cranial radiation in the latter group led to an increase in systemic but not CNS relapses. Studies from the UK, The Netherlands and St Jude showed very low CNS relapse rates using protocols that did not contain radiation at all. It is unclear whether the use of intrathecal triple therapy (MTX, araC, hydrocortisone) has benefits over the use of intrathecal MTX as single drug. One randomized study showed a lower CNS relapse rate with triple therapy but a remarkable higher bone marrow relapse rate. Most protocols advise extra intrathecal injections for patients with a CNS3 or CNS2 status or in case of a traumatic lumbar puncture at diagnosis. Other severe late effects such as growth impairment, avascular necrosis of the bones, and obesity have to be taken into account when CNS treatment without radiotherapy is discussed.

Allogenic haematopoietic stem cell transplantation

Autologous HSCT is not effective and should not be used in treatment of ALL. The strong improvements of chemotherapeutic regimens has reduced the need for allogenic HSCT (alloHSCT) in childhood ALL. In addition, only few studies have proven the efficacy of alloHSCT in specific high-risk groups and there is a serious lack of studies that aim to elucidate the role of alloHSCT in ALL. A collaborative study analysing the data of many study groups showed that BCR–ABL-positive ALL cases benefit from alloHSCT after having received intensive chemotherapy courses. However, even in this patient group, the role of alloHSCT has been debated since the introduction of abl tyrosine kinase inhibitors. Another collaborative analysis showed that alloHSCT was of no benefit for children with MLL-rearranged ALL. A very recent publication made clear that only a quarter of infant MLL-rearranged ALL cases, namely those that carry two other high risk features (age <6 months at diagnosis and WBC > 300×10^9/l or poor prednisone response) may benefit from alloHSCT. Whether T-ALL cases with very high WBC benefit from alloHSCT is matter of debate. Part of patients who do not achieve morphological complete remission after induction therapy may have a better outcome with alloHSCT. Given these facts and given the serious acute and late effects of alloHSCT, its role in first line treatment for childhood ALL is limited and in practice, about 5 per cent of cases will undergo alloHSCT.

Specific patient groups

Adolescents

Studies in four different countries show that outcome for adolescents with ALL is better when these patients are treated on a pediatric rather than an adult protocol. The 5-year EFS was approximately 30 per cent higher when treated according to a pediatric protocol (Table 14.5). This was not explained by differences in patient characteristics or by differences in immunophenotype and genetic abnormalities, but by differences in the dose intensity of the treatments. The pediatric protocols contained more glucocorticoids, vincristine, L-asparaginase, MTX, and 6-MP. Longer delays between courses in adolescents treated according to the adult protocols might also have played a role. Finally, it is possible that haematologists treating adults have a different attitude in managing toxicities because they generally treat older patients who do not tolerate intensive therapy well. The toxicity caused by HSCT is accepted as part of standard therapy, whereas they are less used to glucocorticoid- and asparaginase-induced toxicities. In the Dutch study for instance, use of the adult ALL treatment protocol resulted in both a significant higher relapse rate and in a significant higher toxic death rate for adolescents.

Infants

Infants have an inferior outcome mainly due to the fact that ~80 per cent of them have a very aggressive type of ALL characterized by the presence of a MLL rearrangement. Several specific

Table 14.5 Outcome of adolescents treated on a pediatric or adult lymphoblastic protocol

Study group [Reference]	Patient number	Age category (years)	5-year EFS (%)
United States [Deangelo DJ (2005) Hematology Am Soc Hematol Educ Program, 123–30]			
Paediatric	196	16–21	64
Adult	103	16–21	38
Dutch [de Bont JM, et al. (2004) Leukemia 18, 2032–5]			
Pediatric	47	15–18	69
Adult	44	15–18	34
French [Boissel N, et al. (2003) J Clin Oncol 21, 774–80]			
Pediatric	77	15–20	67
Adult	100	15–20	41
United Kingdom [Ramanujachar R, et al. (2007) Pediatr Blood Cancer 48, 254–61]			
Pediatric	61	15–17	65
Adult	67	15–17	49

collaborative treatment protocols are used by the Children's Oncology Group (COG), Japan and the Interfant collaborative Study Group consisting of many European and non-European study groups. The survival rate with current treatment is 50–60 per cent. Infant ALL cells have been shown to be relatively resistant to glucocorticoids and L-asparaginase but highly sensitive to araC, which is therefore more intensively used in protocols for treatment of infant ALL. Within infant ALL, all types of MLL rearrangement are associated with the same poor prognosis; the younger the infant, the worse the outcome. The survival rate of congenital ALL is only 20 per cent. The role of alloHSCT in infant ALL goes together with many late side effects and its efficacy is limited to a small very high-risk group of infant ALL as indicated above.

BCR–ABL-positive ALL

The translocation t(9;22) fuses the BCR gene on chromosome 22 to the ABL gene on chromosome 9, causing an abnormal abl tyrosine kinase activity. The incidence of BCR/ABL increases with age and is seen in ~3 per cent of children with ALL but in >25 per cent of adults with ALL. Overall, children with BCR/ABL ALL have a survival rate of about 60 per cent with intensive chemotherapy and alloHSCT but initial good responders to therapy have a better outcome and initial poor responders a worse outcome. In the last decade, targeted therapy of the abl tyrosine kinase with inhibitors such as imatinib, dasatinib, and nilotinib have become available. Recent data from the COG suggest that intensive use of such tyrosine kinase inhibitor on top on intensive chemotherapy strongly improves outcome. In the near future, it will be clear how these inhibitors should be incorporated in therapy and whether this will lead to a further reduction in the use of alloHSCT in these patients.

Relapse

Treatment outcome for relapsed patients mainly depends on time and site of relapse and on biological characteristics of the leukaemia. Poor prognostic features are a short duration of initial remission, bone marrow involvement at relapse, T-cell phenotype, the presence of t(9;22) or MLL abnormalities in infancy, and of course the tumour load measured as MRD level after the first courses of chemotherapy for relapse. Overall, about one third of patients with relapsed ALL will be cured. Patients with favourable characteristics (e.g. late relapse or isolated CNS relapse) can be cured without alloHSCT; some patients with unfavourable characteristics benefit from alloHSCT.

Toxicity and late effects

Almost all side effects of treatment are temporary. The most important cause of toxic death is infections: 0.5–1.5 per cent of patients die from infections during induction therapy, and between 1 and 3 per cent while in complete remission. The most frequent drug-specific toxicities include: neuropathy and constipation caused by vincristine; mucositis caused by MTX; diabetes, behaviour disturbances, Cushingoid appearance, osteoporosis, and avascular necrosis of bone caused by glucocorticoids; allergic reactions and thrombosis caused by Asparaginase. Older patients (e.g. >10 years) experience more toxicity than younger patients, for example avascular necrosis of bone, hyperglycemia, thromboembolic complications, and liver function disturbances. Late effects include cardiomyopathy due to antracyclines, neurocognitive deficits and secondary brain tumours due to cranial radiation and avascular necrosis of bone (although often reversible) due to glucocorticoids.

Perspectives

Improvements in therapy are still being made by studying dose schedules of the known drugs especially glucocorticoids and L-asparaginase. Many study groups study reductions (e.g. anthracycline dose) in specific risk groups (e.g. TEL/AML rearranged ALL) and, on the other hand, intensification of L-asparaginase and dexamethasone.

Recent genome-wide screening techniques and subsequent additional molecular analyses have revealed new genetic abnormalities with prognostic relevance. Examples are the discovery of the BCR-ABL like genetic subtype, IKZF1 abnormalities and CRLF2 overexpression that predict a poor outcome. The coming years will learn how to use these newly discovered abnormalities for stratification. The same techniques will lead to more knowledge on the host characteristics which may lead to better recognition of patients at risk of specific side effects.

There is hope that after the use of tyrosine kinases, the genomic studies will not only identify new targets of therapy but will also lead to the clinical application of new targeted drugs. Besides kinase inhibitors, several monoclonal antibodies are very promising in this respect. With the current survival rates, it will be a challenge to investigate how these new drugs can be incorporated in existing pediatric treatment regimens.

Further reading

Arico M, Schrappe M, Hunger SP, et al. (2010) Clinical outcome of children with newly diagnosed Philadelphia chromosome-positive acute lymphoblastic leukemia treated between 1995 and 2005. *J Clin Oncol* **28**, 4755–61.

Balduzzi A, Valsecchi MG, Uderzo C, et al. (2005) Chemotherapy versus allogeneic transplantation for very-high-risk childhood acute lymphoblastic leukaemia in first complete remission: comparison by genetic randomisation in an international prospective study. *Lancet* **366**, 635–42.

Basso G, Veltroni M, Valsecchi MG, et al. (2009) Risk of relapse of childhood acute lymphoblastic leukemia is predicted by flow cytometric measurement of residual disease on day 15 bone marrow. *J Clin Oncol* **27**, 5168–74.

Childhood Acute Lymphoblastic Leukaemia Collaborative Group (CALLCG).(2009) Beneficial and harmful effects of anthracyclines in the treatment of childhood acute lymphoblastic leukaemia: a systematic review and meta-analysis. *Br J Haematol* **145**, 376–88.

Childhood ALL Collaborative Group (1996) Duration and intensity of maintenance chemotherapy in acute lymphoblastic leukaemia: overview of 42 trials involving 12 000 randomised children *Lancet* **347**, 1783–8.

Clarke M, Gaynon P, Hann I, et al. (2003) CNS-directed therapy for childhood acute lymphoblastic leukemia: Childhood ALL Collaborative Group overview of 43 randomized trials. *J Clin Oncol* **21**, 1798–809.

Conter V, Valsecchi MG, Silvestri D, et al. (2007) Pulses of vincristine and dexamethasone in addition to intensive chemotherapy for children with intermediate-risk acute lymphoblastic leukaemia: a multicentre randomised trial. *Lancet* **369**, 123–31.

Den Boer ML, van Slegtenhorst M, De Menezes RX, et al. (2009) A subtype of childhood acute lymphoblastic leukaemia with poor treatment outcome: a genome-wide classification study. *Lancet Oncol* **10**, 125–34.

Eden TO, Pieters R, Richards S, et al. (2010) Systematic review of the addition of vincristine plus steroid pulses in maintenance treatment for childhood acute lymphoblastic leukaemia - an individual patient data meta-analysis involving 5,659 children. *Br J Haematol* **149**, 722–33.

Greaves M (2006) Infection, immune responses and the aetiology of childhood leukaemia. *Nat Rev Cancer* **6**, 193–203.

Mody R, Li S, Dover DC, et al. (2008) Twenty-five-year follow-up among survivors of childhood acute lymphoblastic leukemia: a report from the Childhood Cancer Survivor Study. *Blood* **111**, 5515–23.

Moghrabi A, Levy DE, Asselin B, et al. (2007) Results of the Dana-Farber Cancer Institute ALL Consortium Protocol 95–01 for children with acute lymphoblastic leukemia. *Blood* **109**, 896–904.

Mullighan CG, Su X, Zhang J, et al. (2009) Deletion of IKZF1 and prognosis in acute lymphoblastic leukemia. *N Engl J Med* **360**, 470–80.

Nachman JB, Sather HN, Sensel MG, et al. (1998) Augmented post-induction therapy for children with high-risk acute lymphoblastic leukemia and a slow response to initial therapy. *N Engl J Med* **338**, 1663–71.

Pieters R, Hunger SP, Boos J, et al. (2010) L-asparaginase treatment in acute lymphoblastic leukemia: a focus on Erwinia asparaginase. *Cancer* **117**, 238–49.

Pieters R, Schrappe M, De Lorenzo P, et al. (2007) A treatment protocol for infants younger than 1 year with acute lymphoblastic leukaemia (Interfant-99): an observational study and a multicentre randomised trial. *Lancet* **370**, 240–50.

Pui CH, Campana D, Pei D, et al. (2009) Treating childhood acute lymphoblastic leukemia without cranial irradiation. *N Engl J Med* **360**, 2730–41.

Reiter A, Schrappe M, Ludwig WD, et al. (1994) Chemotherapy in 998 unselected childhood acute lymphoblastic leukemia patients. Results and conclusions of the multicenter trial ALL-BFM 86. *Blood* **84**, 3122–33.

Relling MV, Hancock ML, Boyett JM, et al. (1999) Prognostic importance of 6-mercaptopurine dose intensity in acute lymphoblastic leukemia. *Blood* **93**, 2817–23.

Schrappe M, et al., (2000) Improved outcome in childhood acute lymphoblastic leukemia despite reduced use of anthracyclines and cranial radiotherapy: results of trial ALL-BFM 90. German-Austrian-Swiss ALL-BFM Study Group. *Blood* **95**, 3310–22.

Schultz KR, Bowman WP, Aledo A, et al. (2009) Improved early event-free survival with imatinib in Philadelphia chromosome-positive acute lymphoblastic leukemia: a children's oncology group study. *J Clin Oncol* **27**, 5175–81.

Seibel, NL, Steinherz PG, Sather HN, et al. (2008) Early postinduction intensification therapy improves survival for children and adolescents with high-risk acute lymphoblastic leukemia: a report from the Children's Oncology Group. *Blood* **111**, 2548–55.

Tubergen DG, Gilchrist GS, O'Brien RT, et al. (1993) Improved outcome with delayed intensification for children with acute lymphoblastic leukemia and intermediate presenting features: a Childrens Cancer Group phase III trial. *J Clin Oncol* **11**, 527–37.

van Dongen JJ, Seriu T, Panzer-Grümayer ER, et al. (1998) Prognostic value of minimal residual disease in acute lymphoblastic leukaemia in childhood. *Lancet* **352**, 1731–8.

Veerman AJ, Kamps WA, van den Berg H, et al. (2009) Dexamethasone-based therapy for childhood acute lymphoblastic leukaemia: results of the prospective Dutch Childhood Oncology Group (DCOG) protocol ALL-9 (1997–2004). *Lancet Oncol* **10**, 957–66.

Chapter 15

Acute myeloid leukaemia

Gertjan Kaspers and Dirk Reinhardt

Introduction

Acute myeloid leukaemia (AML) is the second most frequent type of leukaemia in children, after acute lymphoblastic leukaemia (ALL). AML encompasses the myeloid leukaemias, but also acute eythroblastic and acute megakaryoblastic leukaemia. Therefore, the term acute non-lymphoblastic leukaemia as used in the past formally is better, but AML is being used in clinical practice. Improvement in the prognosis of AML in children came somewhat later than for ALL, but has definitely occurred. Applying contemporary chemotherapy, 60–70 per cent of children with AML are cured in high-income countries. In contrast to ALL, treatment is relatively short and usually consists of four or five courses of very intensive combination chemotherapy given over 3–6 months. Experience with such treatment and high-quality supportive care is of utmost importance in this setting. Therefore, the treatment of childhood AML should be centralized in a limited number of paediatric oncology centres.

Epidemiology and etiology

The incidence of AML in children is about 7.6 per million children per year and it accounts for about 20 per cent of acute leukaemias in this age group and for about 5 per cent of all types of childhood cancer. An increased frequency of AML, especially of acute monoblastic and megakaryoblastic leukaemia, occurs within the first 2 years of life (1.5/100 000). The incidence remains relatively low during childhood (0.5/100 000) and starts to increase during adolescence and in young adults (0.9/100 000). There is a very high concordance rate for leukaemia in monozygous twins, probably the result of a common prezygotic or intrauterine genetic event or transplacental passage of a single leukaemic clone. The incidence of AML seems rather similar all over the world, with one clear exception, which is acute promyelocytic leukaemia (APL). APL is a subtype of AML, and occurs more frequently among the Hispanic and Mediterranean populations, and genetic susceptibility seems to play a role. Occasionally it is suggested that AML is more frequent in certain Asian countries, but underreporting of other types of cancer such as ALL as an explanation cannot be excluded yet.

It seems that the incidence of some types of childhood cancer is increasing, albeit by only 1 per cent per year. This is also true for acute leukaemias, but the cause of this rising incidence is unknown. A partial explanation could be the improved survival rates in childhood malignancies. This positive development might be responsible for an increasing incidence of treatment-related AML (tAML) during the last decades. AML is the most frequent secondary malignancy in children treated for ALL, lymphomas or other solid tumors, induced by intensified therapy with exposure to alkylating agents such as cyclophosphamide, ifosfamide or melphalan and to topoisomersase II inhibitors.

The cause of AML is unclear in most cases. Unlike ALL, there is no indication that infections play a role in the development of AML. In a minority of cases, a predisposing condition to develop AML is present, such as a chromosal breakage syndrome (e.g. Fanconi anemia), a stem cell disease

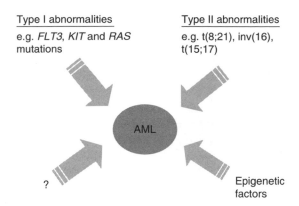

Type I abnormalities
e.g. *FLT3*, *KIT* and *RAS*
mutations

Type II abnormalities
e.g. t(8;21), inv(16),
t(15;17)

AML

?

Epigenetic
factors

Fig. 15.1 A model for leukaemogenesis in acute myeloid leukaemia, involving type I abnormalities that lead to increased self-renewal capacity and proliferation, and type II abnormalities, that result in impaired differentiation, and other partly unknown factors.
(Adapted from Kelly LM, Gilliland DG (2002). Genetics of myeloid leukemias. *Annu Rev Genomics Hum Genet.* **3**:179–98).

(congenital neutropenia, also known as Kostmann syndrome), and most frequently Down syndrome. In even fewer cases nowadays a causative factor is clear, such as ionizing irradiation, previous chemotherapy, and certain chemicals.

Although the etiology usually is unknown, the pathophysiology of AML is becoming more and more clear. AML is a clonal disorder of haematopoietic stem cells, common myeloid-lymphoid or early myeloid progenitors. The hierarchical differentiation of AML in part resembles normal haematopoiesis. Like normal haematopoietic stem cells (HSC), the leukaemic stem cell (LSC) is characterized by the capacity of self-renewal, proliferation, remnant differentiation programs, and maturation. Several stages of leukaemic blast differentiation could be defined.

One model for AML development describes the coincidence of type II and type I mutations as indispensable (Fig. 15.1). The type II (or class II) mutations are typically recurrent translocations [(t(8;21), inv(16), t(15;17), etc.] which are involved in an impaired differentiation and maturation of early haematopoietic progenitors. The isolated occurrence in a cell clone does not cause overt leukaemia directly, however it may define a pre-leukaemic stem cell. Only if a second activating mutation (type I) occurs as an additional event, does the uncontrolled proliferation and decreased rate of apoptosis cause the survival advantage of the leukaemic blasts, displace normal haematopoiesis and result in a frank leukaemia. Type I mutations are typically related to cytokine receptors or other factors in signal transduction pathways such as FLT3-receptor, c-kit-receptor, *ras*, PTPN11, and WT1.

Although these events seem to be sufficient to cause leukaemia in some combinations, in most subtypes additional events, specific conditions of the bone marrow microenvironment or dysfunctions of the immunological system might contribute to the probability of leukaemia. These molecular abnormalities become more important in this era of targeted therapy, but they also provide opportunities for monitoring minimal residual disease during and after treatment. Figure 15.2 illustrates current knowledge on chromosomal and molecular abnormalities in paediatric AML.

Symptoms and signs: clinical presentation

The presentation of a child with AML is not fundamentally different from a child with ALL, although children with AML tend be older, on average 7–8 years of age. The children usually have

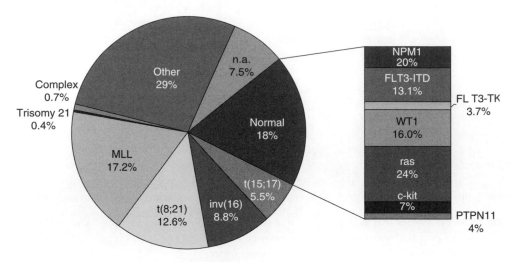

Fig. 15.2 Percentages of AML karyotypes; frequency of type I mutations.

malaise and often weight loss. Major symptoms are caused by the leukaemic infiltration of the bone marrow, resulting in reduced normal haematopoiesis. This translates into anaemia—resulting in paleness, fatigue, and headache—and to thrombocytopenia—resulting in skin bleeding, epistaxis, and sometimes other signs of increased bleeding tendency. Fever is a frequent symptom, either reflecting the inflammation caused by leukaemia or an infection as a consequence of the insufficient number of normal white blood cells. The bone marrow infiltration often gives bone pain, which can be very severe. Enlargement of liver and/or spleen has been reported in about 50 per cent of patients, and so is lymphadenopathy. A well-known extramedullary localization of AML is the central nervous system (CNS), most typically presenting as asymptomatic disease detected at routine examination of the cerebrospinal fluid. However, CNS involvement can also present with, for example, headache, intracerebral bleeding, and seizures.

Certain subtypes of AML (discussed later) have characteristic clinical problems. In acute promyelocytic and acute monoblastic leukaemia, bleeding tendency is often more severe than expected as based on the platelet count. This is caused by diffuse intravascular coagulation. Acute myeloblastic leukaemia with the so-called t(8;21) often is associated with chloromas. Also called granulocytic or myeloid sarcomas, chloromas are extramedullary manifestations of AML presenting as solid masses. Acute myelomonocytic leukaemia in general, and especially the patient group with eosinophilia and the chromosal abnormality inv(16) in their AML cells, has a very high frequency of extramedullary involvement, in up to 60 per cent of patients. Finally, acute monoblastic leukaemia often is characterized by skin involvement and gingival swelling, and sometimes with eye involvement.

A significantly increased white blood cell (WBC) count may result in so-called sludging, with hyperviscosity of the blood and leukostasis. This can give rise to, for example, dyspnoe and to confusion.

Diagnosis and biology of AML

A correct and rapid diagnosis of AML is of utmost importance for optimal treatment. First, the presence of AML should be established without doubt, which occasionally is difficult when it resembles ALL or, for example, in case of a low blast count. Next, the extent of the disease should be determined, as especially CNS disease has therapeutic consequences. Examinations required to determine the extension of AML are a chest X-ray, lumbar puncture for investigation of the cerebrospinal fluid, and an ultrasound of the abdomen. The chest X-ray should be done the same day a leukaemia is suspected, because of the possibility of mediastinal enlargement and compression on the trachea and upper airways. If that is the case, depending on the severity, general anaesthesia may be contraindicated and so might be investigations for which the patient must lie down flat. It also should lead to prompt treatment. A diagnostic lumbar puncture should only be done when there is no significant risk of bleeding and thereby introduction of peripheral leukaemic cells into the cerebrospinal fluid. If necessary, platelets should be transfused first. In case of APL, a lumbar puncture should be postponed because of the very high risk of bleeding complications. Another reason to withhold a lumbar puncture is when localized CNS disease is suspected with the risk of herniation. The abdominal ultrasound should look for hepatosplenomegaly and lymphadenopathy, but also for renal enlargement caused by leukaemic infiltration. The latter should make the clinician aware of the risk of renal dysfunction in the first days of treatment.

Of course, the diagnosis of leukaemia requires laboratory investigations. However, the importance of a detailed history and physical examination cannot be underestimated. For example, the history may reveal the suspicion of a preceding myelodysplastic syndrome. Physical examination is important to detect features compatible with syndromes such as Down syndrome and Fanconi anemia, but also to correctly determine extramedullary disease. For example, testicular involvement, gingival hyperplasia, and leukaemia cutis will only be detected at physical examination. Physical examination may also reveal serious bleeding tendency, and a compromised circulation because of anaemia or sludging, which should result in immediate and appropriate supportive care and antileukaemic treatment.

For the diagnosis of leukaemia, bone marrow aspiration is always attempted. Abnormal cells may also be present in sufficient number in the peripheral blood. However, if this is not the case and if a bone marrow aspiration does not provide enough cells ('dry tap'), a bone biopsy should be done and smears should be made, 'rolling' the biopsy over the slide. Normally, enough abnormal cells from bone marrow and peripheral blood are available for extensive characterization. First, this is done by morphological examination of the smears after staining. Additional enzymatic stainings are also helpful to diagnose AML (Table 15.1). It requires experience to distinguish leukaemic cells from normal precursors and, for example, from non-malignant blasts in case of an infection, to identify a low percentage of leukaemic cells, and to distinguish AML from ALL. Similarly, experience is required for diagnosing the correct FAB type according to the French-American-British (FAB) classification, described in Table 15.2. Although the most recent World Health Organization (WHO) classification (Table 15.3) relies more on chromosomal abnormalities than on morphology, a correct morphological diagnosis remains the basis and is essential for correct initial treatment. This can be simply illustrated by two examples. First, it is essential to quickly distinguish AML from ALL in case of a high WBC count and the need to install antileukaemic treatment immediately. A glucocorticoid such as prednisone or dexamethasone is indicated in case of ALL, but is contraindicated in AML because it may actually increase the WBC count. Second, the early morphological recognition of AML FAB type M3 (acute promyelocytic leukaemia, APL) directs therapy. The diagnosis APL or even the suspicion of APL should prompt the clinicians to start all-trans retinoic acid (ATRA) immediately. ATRA is essential in the initial treatment of APL because it quickly reduces the risk of bleeding complications. Early bleeding is life threatening in patients with APL and fatal in 5–10 per cent of children with APL. In addition, continued use of ATRA makes a very important contribution to the cure of most children with APL with contemporary treatment. Finally, sometimes additional investigations for immunophenotypical and chromosomal abnormalities fail or are not available. In these cases, morphology may indicate the presence of a specific chromosomal abnormality that is associated

Table 15.1 The usefulness of enzymatic staining in the diagnosis of AML

	M0	M1–M3	M4	M5	M6	M7	ALL
MPO	–	+	+	–	–	–	–
ANAE	–	–	+	+	–	+/–	–
SB-B	–	+	+	–	–	–	–
PAS	–	–	+/–	+/–	+	–	+

MPO = myeloperoxidase, ANAE = acid alpha-naphthyl acetate esterase, SB-B = Sudan-Black B, PAS = Periodic Acid Schiff positive.

with a better prognosis. This is especially the case for AML FAB type M2 with auer rods, which is associated with t(8;21), and for AML FAB type M4 with eosinophilia, which is associated with inv(16). The other example, AML FAB type M3 or APL which is associated with t(15;17), was described above.

In conclusion, paediatric haemato-oncologists and those in training for that speciality, should be capable of diagnosing AML based on morphological examination of bone marrow or peripheral blood smears. The official WHO classification requires at least 20 per cent of leukaemic cells in the bone marrow for the diagnosis of AML. In the past, this was 30 per cent with the FAB classification. In addition, the presence of specific recurrent chromosomal abnormalities, independent from the percentage of leukaemic cells, already leads to the diagnosis of AML in the WHO classification, such as for t(8;21), inv(16) and t(15;17). It seems that many paediatric collaborative groups do not follow the WHO classification completely. Especially, in case of 20–30 per cent leukaemic cells in the bone marrow, additional features such as organ involvement and extramedullary disease are taken into account before the diagnosis of AML or as alternative myelodysplastic syndome (MDS) is established (Fig. 15.3). If no additional features are present and doubt remains about the diagnosis being AML or MDS, a bone marrow aspiration and biopsy should be repeated after several weeks, to look for progressive disease resulting in clear AML. However, the presence

Table 15.2 Different types of AML according to the French-American-British (FAB) classification, with percentage of the total number of cases per FAB type, and the relation with karyotypic abnormalities

FAB Subtype	Full name (% of total number of cases)	Associated chromosomal abnormalities
M0	Acute myeloblastic leukaemia with minimal differentiation (3%)	
M1	Acute myeloblastic leukaemia without maturation (10–15%)	
M2	Acute myeloblastic leukaemia with maturation (25–30%)	t(6;9)
M2au+	AML M2 with auer rods	t(8;21)(q22;q22)
M3	Acute promyelocytic leukaemia (5–10%)	t(15;17)
M4	Acute myelomonocytic leukaemia (5–15%)	inv(16); del(16q)
M4Eo	Acute myelomonocytic leukaemia with abnormal eosinophils (5–15%)	inv(16); t(16;16)
M5	Acute monocytic leukaemia (15–25%)	t(9;11); t(11;19); del(11q)
M6	Acute erythroid leukaemia (1–3%)	
M7	Acute megakaryocytic leukaemia (5–10%)	t(1;22)

Adapted from Bennett JM, Catovsky D, Daniel MT et al. (1991). Proposal for the recognition of minimally differentiated acute myeloid leukaemia (AML-M0). *Br J Haematol* **78**, 325–29.

Table 15.3 Novel classification of acute myeloid leukaemia based on the WHO guidelines

WHO Classification of AML
AML with recurrent genetic abnormalities
AML with t(8;21)(q22;q22), AML1(CBF-alpha)/ETO
Acute promyelocytic leukaemia (AML with t(15;17)(q22;q11-q12) and variants), PML/RAR-alpha
AML with abnormal bone marrow eosinophils: inv(16)(p13;q22) or t(16;16)(p13;q22), CBFß/MYH11 (=PEBP2β)
AML with 11q23 (MLL gene) abnormalities
AML with t(6;9), t(1;22) or inv(3)/t(3;3)
Provisionally: AML with mutated NPM1 or CEBPA
AML with multilineage dysplasia
With prior myelodysplastic syndrome
Without prior myelodysplastic syndrome
AML and myelodysplastic syndromes, therapy related
Alkylating agent-related
Epipodophyllotoxin-related
Other types
AML not otherwise categorized
AML minimally differentiated
AML without maturation
AML with maturation
Acute myelomonocytic leukaemia
Acute monocytic leukaemia
Acute erythroid leukaemia
Acute megakaryocytic leukaemia
Acute basophilic leukaemia
Acute panmyelosis with myelofbrosis
Chloroma or myeloid sarcoma
Myeloid proliferations related to Down syndrome
Transient abnormal myeloproliferation/transient myelo-proliferative disease
Myeloid leukaemia of Down syndrome

of specific cytogenetic abnormalities such as mentioned above leads to the diagnosis of AML independent from the blast percentage, also in children.

Additional characterization of AML is based on immunophenotype and chromosomal abnormalities. Immunophenotyping is nowadays done with multi-colour flow cytometry in high-income countries, but can be done on slides if such facilities are lacking. Immunophenotyping may profit from the asynchronous or aberrant antigen expression on the leukaemic blasts. Asynchronous expression is the simultaneous expression of stem cell antigens (CD34/CD117) and antigens indicating myeloid differentiation [CD13, CD14, CD15, CD33, myeloperoxidase (MPO)]. Aberrant expression includes the simultaneous expression of myeloid antigen and lymphoid or natural killer cell antigens (CD2, CD7, CD19, CD56). Typical antigens indicative for

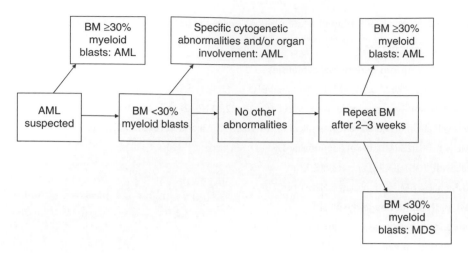

Fig. 15.3 A systematic approach for dissecting acute myeloid leukaemia (AML) from myelodysplastic syndrome (MDS).

AML are CD33, CD13, CD14, CDw41, CD15, CD11b, CD36, and CD61. In the diagnostic setting, immunophenotyping is especially important for the diagnosis of acute undifferentiated leukaemia (FAB type M0; no expression of MPO but reactivity with CD13 and/or CD33) and acute megakary-oblastic leukaemia (FAB type M7, expression of CD36, Cd41, Cd42b or CD61)), because these subtypes are notably difficult to recognize and distinguish morphologically. Specific immu-nophenotypes could also be defined for acute erythoid leukaemia (FAB M6, expression of CD235a/glycophorin) and for acute monoblastic leukaemia (AML FAB M5; CD33/CD56/CD36). Some immunophenotypes are associated with genetic aberration, such as the combination of CD33/CD19/CD56 positivity that is indicative of t(8;21). Immunophenotype is also instrumental in measurement of minimal residual disease by the detection of leukaemic cells with a leukaemia-aberrant immunophenotype (see later).

Chromosomal abnormalities can be detected with a number of techniques. Conventionally, karyotyping is being used, but more and more fluorescent *in situ* hybridization (FISH) is routinely applied as well, while polymerase chain reaction (PCR) techniques are being used in addition to detect molecular abnormalities. In case of karyotyping, at least 20 metaphases are needed in order to reliably exclude an abnormal karyotype. If karyotyping and other techniques looking for chro-mosomal abnormalities fail, another attempt to obtain leukaemic cells should be considered, in view of the clinical relevance of these investigations. FISH is a reliable and robust technique to detect, for example, gene rearrangements. PCR techniques and other assays such as the multiplex ligation polymerase assay are useful for the detection of somatic molecular abnormalities, occurring in the leukaemic cells exclusively.

There is a wide range of other techniques that are being used to characterise leukaemic cells, such as microarrays, comparative genomic hybridization, and proteomics. However, the results are not being applied in clinical practice yet and are therefore not discussed here except for the detection of molecular abnormalities. The latter abnormalities are being detected mainly with PCR techniques, and were already mentioned as involved in leukaemogenesis. Often these molec-ular abnormalities are distinguished in type I and type II aberrations. Type I aberrations lead to increased self-renewal and increased proliferative capacity, and well-known examples are muta-tions in the *RAS*, *KIT*, *FLT3*, *WT1* and *PTPN11* genes. Type II aberrations cause a differentiation arrest, and often concern chromosomal rearrangements of transcription factors, including *PML-RARα* [t(15;17)(q22;q21)], *AML1-ETO* [t(8;21)(q22;q22)], *CBFB-MYH11* [inv(16)(p13q22)],

MLL-rearrangements or mutations in *NPM1* or *CEBPA*. Independent from being involved in leukaemogenesis or not, molecular abnormalities have other potential clinical applications. This includes a prognostic significance, as discussed below. In addition, molecular abnormalities can be used for the detection of minimal residual disease. Perhaps most importantly, they have the potential to provide leukaemia-specific treatment targets.

Prognostic factors

The above described characterization of AML and its extension has prognostic relevance. Chromosomal abnormalities dominate clinical features, such as age, sex, and WBC count, disease extension and morphology of the AML cells, as prognostic factors. In addition, early clinical response as determined by either morphological examination of bone marrow 1, 2 or 4 weeks after start of treatment, or by more sophisticated minimal residual disease measurements, are important predictors of long-term outcome.

Clinically, a high WBC count remains an adverse prognostic factor. Otherwise, extramedullary involvement does not seem to impact prognosis with current intensive therapy, including high-dose cytarabine. If information on chromosomal abnormalities is lacking, morphological subtypes can be used to predict outcome. Favourable are FAB type M2 with auer rods, FAB type M3 (APL), and FAB type M4, especially (but not exclusively) if associated with eosinophilia. Moreover, myeloid leukaemia of Down syndrome (usually FAB type M7, occasionally M6) has a favourable prognosis and will be described later as a separate disease entity. Immunophenotype is not of significant prognostic relevance in AML. More and more, cytogenetic abnormalities are being used as prognostic factor, and most groups agree with three cytogenetic risk groups. The low-risk group has core-binding factor AML, i.e. either inv(16), t(16;16) or t(8;21), or has APL with t(15;17). Patients with these low-risk cytogenetic features, but a less than favourable early treatment response, most likely should remain low-risk patients. Patients with other molecular abnormalities, such as mutations in CEPBA and NPM1, and with t(1;11), may also qualify for the low-risk group, but there is no consensus on that yet. The intermediate (i.e. standard) risk group has no specific cytogenetic abnormalities as defined for low- or high-risk groups. The high-risk group includes patients with AML cells that harbour FLT3-ITD in association with mutated WT1, monosomy 7, an abnormal chromosome 5 (monosomy 5, 5q-), t(6;9), t(9;22), t(6;11), t(10;11), abnormalities of 12p, or a complex karyotype with 4 or more cytogenetic aberrations.

The use of prognostic factors for risk-group adapted therapy is described below.

Risk classification

According to the WHO classification, AML subgroups are defined by the history of the disease—a preceding myelodysplastic syndrome or treatment for a malignancy, by recurrent cytogenetic abnormalities such as t(8;21), inv(16), t(15;17), and MLL rearrangements, and by the lack of such features (not otherwise characterized). This last category largely reflects the former FAB classification, which is based on morphology and cytochemistry.

AML is a heterogeneous disease, and the prognosis of the subtypes varies widely. In addition, the prognostic relevance of an identified factor does not only depend on the biological characteristics but also on the applied therapy. The occurrence of balanced translocations—t(8;21)/ inv(16)—affecting core-binding factors (CBF-AML) is associated with a relatively good prognosis. This has been shown in both children and adults. The event-free and overall survival in this particular group of children is more than 70 per cent and 85 per cent, respectively. Even in case of relapse, these karyotypes remain a favourable prognostic factor, and these patients have achieved an overall survival of more than 60 per cent from relapse.

Further, APL can be treated successfully in most cases, if the frequently occurring early compli-cations such as severe bleedings or infections can be treated or better, prevented. Especially the introduction of ATRA therapy has prevented early deaths and enables survival rates of about 90 per cent in APL.

Nucleophosmin-1 (NPM1), occurring in about 8 per cent of childhood AML, seems to be associated with a favourable prognosis. In the subgroup of AML with a normal karyotype, the incidence is up to 20 per cent. Interestingly, in children the non-type A mutations are more frequent than in adults. Further, a correlation with increasing age was observed.

A special entity is myeloid leukaemia of Down syndrome (ML-DS). If adapted treatment is applied, the prognosis is good. The intensity of the treatment schedule should be significantly reduced as compared to standard protocols. By contrast to other AML subtypes, the immediate continuation of treatment is not time-sensitive; a treatment element should be started only if the child is in a good general condition.

In the past, MLL rearrangements were generally recognized as a poor prognostic factor; however, at least two studies in children found the t(9;11) as a favourable marker . These results, based on a relatively low number of patients, have not been confirmed by larger study groups. The prognosis of childhood AML with t(9;11) seems to be insignificantly better than in other MLL-positive leukaemia; however was still within the range of intermediate- and high-risk patients.

Several aberrations that are associated with a very poor prognosis in adults do not discriminate in children. For example, a complex karyotype (more than three aberrations) or 7q– do not predict a particularly poor outcome in children. However, isolated monosomy 7 is associated with an impaired complete remission (CR) rate and a poor outcome.

Several additional molecular events, mostly type I mutations, have been identified as a prognostic marker in childhood AML. Most data are available about the poor prognostic value of internal tandem duplications in the *FLT3* gene (FLT3-ITDs). Especially in children with normal karyotype, FLT3-ITD is associated with poor prognosis. While FLT3-ITD and NPM1 are frequently associated with AML with normal karyotype, the relevance of other aberrations such as *RAS* or *c-KIT* mutations remains unclear. Recently, *WT1* mutations have been identified as a poor prognostic factor in childhood AML.

Interestingly, there are recent reports that described a possible prognostic relevance of certain polymorphisms in AML, however probably depending on age and treatment regimen.

A lot of other prognostic factors have been proposed. These include the WBC count at diagno-sis, age, the occurrence of extramedullary leukaemia or the immunophenotype, however the prognostic relevance seems to be associated to intensity and schedule of therapy.

Apart from genetic characteristics, treatment response is an important prognostic factor. Assessed by bone marrow morphology, complete remission—defined as less than 5 per cent blasts and sufficient haematological regeneration (neutrophils higher than 1000/μl; platelets higher 80.000/μl)—is a strong predictor for outcome. More difficult is the measurement of early response. Morphology is impeded by a low sensitivity and specificity, but has been successfully used at day 14 or 15 and/or day 28 after first induction to stratify patients to risk groups.

Minimal residual disease

Several attempts have been made to establish more sensitive methods to measure response and minimal residual disease (MRD). Quantitative reverse transcription PCR (RT-PCR) allows the sensitive detection and quantification of known fusion genes such as *AML1/ETO* or *CBF/MYH11*. As the frequency of these aberrations is about 30 per cent, only a minority of children can be monitored based on these leukaemia-specific abnormalities. More critical is the fact that a relevant portion of patients remains 'MRD-positive' throughout the complete course of the disease, with persisting cells with the fusion gene. Up to 40 per cent of the children show detectable *AML/ETO1* even after intensive therapy without predicting relapse. By contrast, the monitoring of *PML/ RARα* in APL has generally shown to be very predictive and is used to stratify treatment intensity. This even includes the recommendation to act upon molecular refractory disease and to treat a molecular relapse.

In *MLL*-gene rearranged AML the situation is even more complicated. Persistence of the rearranged *MLL* gene is clearly associated with a very high risk of relapse, however, in most cases the *MLL* arrangement is not detectable after the first or second chemotherapy induction course, which does not exclude relapse. Further, re-occurrence of the *MLL* rearrangement is strongly associated with relapse with 2 to 4 weeks. Whether this very short pre-warning phase has any clinical meaning is unclear.

Another approach to monitor MRD is immunophenotyping. In almost all cases of AML, a leu-kaemia-associated immunophenotype (LAIP) can be defined based on an asynchronous expression of differential, stage-dependent antigens (simultaneous expression of stem cell antigens and antigens of myeloid maturation) or based on lineage-aberrant antigen expression. Although some studies demonstrated the possibility to monitor the treatment response, the independent value of the MRD diagnostic is so far hampered by the limited specificity. First, the LAIP of the bulk of leukaemic blasts could differ from the immunophenotype of the leukaemic stem cell, second, the expression pattern of leukaemic blasts changes during treatment and at relapse. Third, especially in a regen-erating bone marrow, the leukaemic blasts may not be distinguishable from normal progenitors. The discovery of a leukaemic stem cell-specific antigen (CLL-1) within the CD34+/CD38– com-partment might improve the specificity of immunophenotyping and provide a more reliable method in the future. This also might be achieved by improved techniques (8 color-flow) and bet-ter methods of analysis.

Treatment and prognosis

Over the last three decades, the prognosis of childhood AML has markedly improved (Fig. 15.4). In children, the first approaches with intensive chemotherapy were initiated in the 1970s. These protocols were adapted from ALL treatment schedules. In the 1980s, the benefit of intensified elements including cytarabine and anthracyclines became obvious. Several other drugs such as etoposide (a topoisomerase II inhibitor), amsacrine, thioguanine or cyclophosphamide have been combined. The mechanism of action of these drugs has been described elsewhere.

Most of the treatment protocols recommend four or five elements of intensive chemotherapy. At least with regard to children with favorable cytogenetics, the results of the United Kingdom MRC group and the AML-BFM group did not provide strong evidence that a fifth intensive element improves outcome. However, the subgroup of AML with t(8;21) might benefit from high dose cytarabine during induction and/or consolidation.

In spite of different treatment regimens of several study groups, the final results of different study groups for disease-free (DFS) and overall survival (OS) have been within similar ranges. The most relevant treatment differences concern the cumulative dose of anthracyclines and the per-centage of patients that undergoes allogeneic haematopoietic stem cell transplantation (alloHSCT). Table IV summarizes the EFS and OS of several large clinical trials in paediatric AML.

Induction

Anthracycline- and cytarabine-based regimens are generally accepted to induce remission in AML. Sequential studies proved the efficacy of intensive, high-dose chemotherapy. Double induction

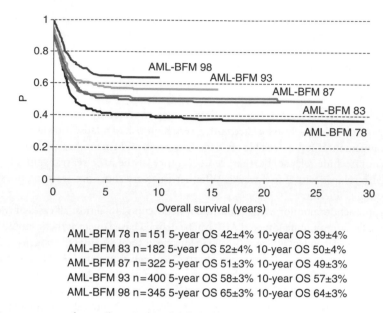

AML-BFM 78 n=151 5-year OS 42±4% 10-year OS 39±4%
AML-BFM 83 n=182 5-year OS 52±4% 10-year OS 50±4%
AML-BFM 87 n=322 5-year OS 51±3% 10-year OS 49±3%
AML-BFM 93 n=400 5-year OS 58±3% 10-year OS 57±3%
AML-BFM 98 n=345 5-year OS 65±3% 10-year OS 64±3%

Fig. 15.4 Improvement of overall survival in childhood AML: example AML-BFM Studies 78 to 98.

schedules are widely in use. Today, 80 to 90 per cent of the children with AML achieve CR after induction depending on the risk group.

Cytarabine is used in different dose regimens. Whereas in first induction frequently 3 x 60mg/m^2 daunorubicin is administered combined with lower-dose cytarabine (and often etoposide), in second induction, several studies schedule high-dose cytarabine with 1, 2 or 3g/m^2 as mono-therapy or combined with mitoxantrone or an anthracycline. Newer analogs of cytarabine such as fludarabine, cladribine or clofarabine are frequently used in re-induction in relapsed AML, but are rarely included in frontline protocols so far. The addition of chlor or fluor to the basic cytosine-arabinoside impairs the intracellular degradation by purine nucleoside phosphorylase or hydrolysis. The latest development in this field is clofarabine, which might combine the advantages of fludarabine and cladribine and which showed promising results in relapsed AML. However, a randomized comparison to the already used drugs is still lacking.

Post remission

In most studies, post-remission treatment includes intensive chemotherapy such as high-dose cytarabine-based regimens, and additionally an anthracycline or etoposide. After two courses of induction, between two to six intensive post-remission courses have been scheduled in paediatric

Table 15.4 Results from paediatric AML studies

Study	5-year event-free survival	5-year overall survival	Percentage of alloHSCT in first CR
MRC 12	56%	66%	8%
BFM 98	40%	62%	8%
LAME91	48%	62%	30%
NOPHO	50%	66%	25%
CCG 2961	42%	52%	25%

AML studies. In high-risk AML, although not uniformly defined, at least three treatment elements are given.

Stem cell transplantation

The value of alloHSCT in first CR is controversial. Whereas some groups still recommend alloHSCT for all AML subgroups (except for APL) if a matched sibling donor (MSD) is available, other groups recently tend to restrict HSCT to intermediate- or high-risk AML patients. The CCG (Children's Cancer Group, now part of the Children's Oncology Group) studies, which previously recommended alloHSCT, could not prove the advantage of alloHSCT in patients with favourable or unfavourable cytogenetics.

Although, as confirmed in a recent meta-analysis, the relapse rate of intermediate- and high-risk AML could be lowered by allo-SCT in most studies, the higher treatment related mortality counterbalanced this advantage. The currently declining relevance of alloHSCT in first CR is mainly due to the improvements in chemotherapy and supportive care . New approaches like intensity-reduced conditioning regimens should be evaluated to make possible advantages of alloHSCT such as a graft-versus-leukaemia effect available. New specific prognostic factors need to be identified to define those patients who will benefit from alloHSCT. These must not necessarily include the very high-risk patients, who seem to be resistant to any therapy including alloHSCT.

By contrast, there is a clear indication to perform alloHSCT in refractory or relapsed AML. Even more experimental approaches, such as haploidentical SCT or cord blood SCT, may be indicated in these cases, if a matched donor is lacking. Interestingly, recent data suggest that children with very late relapse and favorable prognostic features can also be rescued by chemotherapy only.

Maintenance

With the exception of APL, there is no evidence of a benefit of maintenance therapy in childhood AML. Only the AML-BFM group applies a low-dose maintenance therapy adapted from adult AML studies, because the combination of thioguanine and cytarabine showed improved results in some adult groups. However, this has not been prospectively proven in children.

Side effects and late effects

Side effects

Each treatment option in childhood AML had considerable acute and long-term adverse effects and almost all organ systems are involved. Of the acute side effects and toxicities, expected myelosuppression and the consecutive high risk of severe infections and septicemia are the most relevant since infections are responsible for most treatment-related deaths.

Improved supportive care and intensive care can reduce early deaths by infections or leukaemia to less than 5 per cent. This includes guidelines for supportive care including prophylactic and preemptive antibiotic and antifungal therapy, recent development of effective and orally applicable antifungal drugs, and the availability of antiviral compounds. Improved intensive care has also enabled the management of severe complications and continuation of the treatment.

The most impressive effect has been achieved by the introduction of ATRA into the initial treatment of APL, which reduced the early deaths in this particular subgroup substantially.

Efforts to reduce the duration of myelosuppression by administering the granulocyte growth factor G-CSF resulted in a limited shortening of neutropenia but did not change the rate of severe infections or the probability of survival. In fact, there is increased incidence of relapse in children with favorable cytogenetics and an increased expression of the G-CSF receptor isoform IV, who had been treated with G-CSF. In conclusion, G-CSF should not routinely be administered to children with AML. Other options such as application of supportive granulocyte infusions are controversial and efficacy has not been proven.

Another open question concerns the management of hyperleukocytosis. It is undisputed that rasburicase and antiproliferative therapy should be started immediately; however, because of the risk of tumor lysis, the best starting dose cannot easily be defined. Children with severe hyperleukocytosis (>100 000 leukocytes/ μl blood; APL > 10 000 leukocytes/μl) should be treated on an intensive care unit, especially if they show any additional abnormal parameter such as related to coagulation, blood-gas analysis, renal parameters, and increased lactate.

If tumor lysis is expected, the first dose of cytostatics probably should be low (i.e. cytarabine 20mg/m^2). If no tumor lysis is induced, doses should be quickly increased to 40mg/m^2. When the WBC has decreased to less than 50 000 WBC/μl blood, the full-dose schedule should start. By contrast, if there is even an increase of WBC, the dosage of cytarabine should be increased immediately (i.e. 100mg/m^2/day continuous infusion). In case of insufficient decrease of blast, an early introduction of antracyclines should be considered.

Another option that should be considered in case of a critically ill child due to hyperleukocytosis, is an exchange transfusion or leukapheresis, although the efficacy of this procedure is not proven.

Late toxicity

Late sequelae of therapy (see also Chapter 12) can be attributed to the initial disease and to the complications of its treatment. The literature offers a range of perspectives on the incidence of significant late effects in survivors of AML. In one retrospective study from the AML-BFM study group only about 5 per cent of all long-term survivors were reported to experience severe late toxicities (such as blindness/cataracts, severe osteonecrosis, cardiomyopathy or secondary malignancies). In comparison to reports from other studies, this incidence is relatively low and there is much greater morbidity in patients who undergo allogenic HSCT. The importance of anthracycline drugs in schedules for the treatment of AML raises particular concern about the risk of cardiotoxicity.

Challenges and perspectives

Prognosis of paediatric AML has improved significantly to even above 70 per cent long-term survival in some recent unpublished clinical studies. The biggest challenge is to further improve outcome to a cure rate of well above 90 per cent with reasonable side effects and limited late effects of treatment. Current conventional chemotherapy cannot be intensified further, because of toxicity. Some novel but conventional (non-targeted) drugs, such as liposomal daunorubicin and clofarabine will likely make an improvement, but main steps forward are more likely to be achieved with really novel drugs. These agents usually are targeted, which has the implication that they will be used only in patients whose AML cells harbour the treatment target. An example is tyrosine kinase inhibitors, for example targeting mutated *FLT3* or *c-KIT*. Another example is monoclonal antibodies that either alone or by being linked to a cytotoxic agent exert an antileukaemic effect. A good example of the latter is gemtuzumab ozogamicin, which concerns an anti-CD33 antibody linked to the highly toxic calcheamicin. Studies on such novel agents in subgroups of paediatric AML will require international collaboration, because of the rarity of these subgroups. An important challenge in such international collaborative studies is that ideally a common chemotherapeutic backbone is being used. Although most paediatric groups worldwide are now using four to five courses of intensive chemotherapy, there still are many differences in drugs, doses and schedules. Another main challenge is the performance of clinical trials under the EU directive and good clinical practice guidelines. Although this directive has a positive effect on the number of clinical studies on new agents in children with cancer, it has become a very complicated process in which unfortunately not all countries apply the EU directive similarly. Investigator-initiated studies have become much more cumbersome and there is a risk that such studies will be done less often. That would be a major problem, because company-driven studies are still rare in children with cancer including AML.

Despite these challenges, the paediatric community has always been able to improve the treatment and outcome of all types of malignancies. Techniques are rapidly improving to identify subgroups that should be treated differently. More and more novel drugs emerge that could be used in different subgroups. Therefore it seems realistic to expect long-term survival in more than 90 per cent of paediatric AML patients, with an acceptable quality of life during treatment and with limited late effects.

Further reading

Bonnet D, Dick JE (1997) Human acute myeloid leukemia is organized as a hierarchy that originates from a primitive hematopoietic cell. *Nat Med* **3**, 730–7.

Creutzig U, Diekamp S, Zimmermann M, Reinhardt D (2007) Longitudinal evaluation of early and late anthracycline cardiotoxicity in children with AML. *Pediatr Blood Cancer* **48**, 651–62.

Creutzig U, Zimmermann M, Lehrnbecher T, et al. (2006) Less toxicity by optimizing chemotherapy, but not by addition of granulocyte colony-stimulating factor in children and adolescents with acute myeloid leukemia: results of AML-BFM 98. *J Clin Oncol* **24**, 4499–506.

Ehlers S, Herbst C, Zimmermann M, et al. (2010) Granulocyte colony-stimulating factor (G-CSF) treatment of childhood acute myeloid leukemias that overexpress the differentiation-defective G-CSF receptor isoform IV is associated with a higher incidence of relapse. *J Clin Oncol* **28**, 2591–7.

Gibson BE, Wheatley K, Hann IM, et al. (2005) Treatment strategy and long-term results in paediatric patients treated in consecutive UK AML trials. *Leukemia* **19**, 2130–8.

Gilliland DG (2001) Hematologic malignancies. *Curr Opin Hematol* **8**, 189–91.

Greaves MF, Wiemels J (2003) Origins of chromosome translocations in childhood leukaemia. *Nat Rev Cancer* **3**, 639–49.

Harrison CJ, Hills RK, Moorman AV, et al. (2010) Cytogenetics of childhood acute myeloid leukemia: United Kingdom Medical Research Council Treatment trials AML 10 and 12. *J Clin Oncol* **28**, 2674–81.

Hasle H, Alonzo TA, Auvrignon A, et al. (2007) Monosomy 7 and deletion 7q in children and adolescents with acute myeloid leukemia: an international retrospective study. *Blood* **109**, 4641–7.

Jeha S, Gandhi V, Chan KW, et al. (2004) Clofarabine, a novel nucleoside analog, is active in pediatric patients with advanced leukemia. *Blood* **103**, 784–9.

Kaspers GJ, Zwaan CM. (2007) Pediatric acute myeloid leukemia: towards high-quality cure of all patients. *Haematologica* **92**, 1519–32.

Langebrake C, Creutzig U, Dworzak M, et al. (2006) Residual disease monitoring in childhood acute myeloid leukemia by multiparameter flow cytometry: the MRD-AML-BFM Study Group. *J Clin Oncol* **24**, 3686–92.

Lehrnbecher T, Zimmermann M, Reinhardt D, et al. (2007) Prophylactic human granulocyte colony-stimulating factor after induction therapy in pediatric acute myeloid leukemia. *Blood* **109**, 936–43.

Leung W, Hudson MM, Strickland DK, et al. (2000) Late effects of treatment in survivors of childhood acute myeloid leukemia. *J Clin Oncol* **18**, 3273–9.

Lipshultz SE, Lipsitz SR, Mone SM, et al. (1995) Female sex and drug dose as risk factors for late cardiotoxic effects of doxorubicin therapy for childhood cancer. *N Engl J Med* **332**, 1738–43.

Mann G, Reinhardt D, Ritter J, et al. (2001) Treatment with all-trans retinoic acid in acute promyelocytic leukemia reduces early deaths in children. *Ann Hematol* **80**, 417–22.

Perel Y, Auvrignon A, Leblanc T, et al. (2002) Impact of Addition of Maintenance Therapy to Intensive Induction and Consolidation Chemotherapy for Childhood Acute Myeloblastic Leukemia: Results of a Prospective Randomized Trial, LAME 89/91 for the Group LAME of the French Society of Pediatric Hematology and Immunology. *J Clin Oncol* **20**, 2774–82.

Rubnitz JE, Raimondi SC, Tong X, et al. (2002) Favorable impact of the t(9;11) in childhood acute myeloid leukemlia. *J Clin Oncol* **20**, 2302–9.

Testi AM, Biondi A, Lo CF, et al. (2005) GIMEMA-AIEOPAIDA protocol for the treatment of newly diagnosed acute promyelocytic leukemia (APL) in children. *Blood* **106**, 447–53.

Zwaan CM, Meshinchi S, Radich JP, et al. (2003) FLT3 internal tandem duplication in 234 children with acute myeloid leukemia: prognostic significance and relation to cellular drug resistance. *Blood* **102**, 2387–94.

Zwaan CM, Reinhardt D, Zimmerman M, et al. (2010) Salvage treatment for children with refractory first or second relapse of acute myeloid leukaemia with gemtuzumab ozogamicin: results of a phase II study. *Br J Haematol* **148**, 768–76.

Chapter 16

Myelodysplastic syndrome, myeloid leukaemia of Down syndrome, and juvenile myelomonocytic leukaemia

Henrik Hasle and Charlotte Niemeyer

Introduction

Myeloid malignancies in children are subdivided into four main groups; acute myeloid leukaemia (AML), myelodysplastic syndrome (MDS), juvenile myelomonocytic leukaemia (JMML), and the myeloid leukaemias of Down syndrome (ML-DS). Acute myeloid leukaemia is dealt with in Chapter 15.

The rarity of MDS in children and the lack of definite morphologic and cytogenetic markers have contributed to the paucity of MDS in the paediatric literature. Most protocol-based studies on MDS and JMML have been performed by the European Working Group of MDS in childhood (EWOG-MDS; www.ewog-mds.org).

Classification of myelodysplastic syndrome (MDS)

The French-American-British (FAB) group classification, has since 1982, divided MDS into five subgroups based upon experience in adult patients: refractory anaemia (RA), RA with ringed sideroblasts (RARS), RA with excess of blasts (RAEB), RAEB in transformation (RAEB-T), and chronic myelomonocytic leukaemia (CMML). The FAB classification had prognostic impact in children but did not address the specific diseases and morphological features in children and the frequent occurrence of associated anomalies.

A paediatric approach to the WHO classification separated myelodysplastic and myeloproliferative disorders in children into three main groups; JMML, MDS, and ML-DS. MDS was further subdivided into refractory cytopenia (RC), RAEB and RAEB-T. The change in nomenclature from RA to RC reflects that anaemia is not a prerequisite for the diagnosis. The revised WHO classification from 2008 recognizes ML-DS as a unique group and describes refractory cytopenia of childhood (RCC) as a new entity (Table 16.1).

Epidemiology

Incidence, sex, age and subtype distribution

Combined population based data from Denmark and British Columbia in Canada showed an annual incidence of MDS of 1.8 and of JMML of 1.2 per million children corresponding to a total of 6 per cent of all haematological malignancies in children, although data from the UK suggest a lower incidence of MDS of 0.8 per million. The UK study excluded secondary MDS partly explaining the lower incidence. The male/female distribution in paediatric MDS is equal with a median age

Table 16.1 Diagnostic categories of myelodysplastic and myeloproliferative diseases in children according to the paediatric approach to the WHO classification and the revised WHO classification

Myelodysplastic/myeloproliferative disease
◆ Juvenile myelomonocytic leukaemia (JMML)
Myeloid proliferations related to Down syndrome (DS)
◆ Transient abnormal myelopoiesis (TAM)
◆ Myeloid leukaemia of Down syndrome (ML-DS)
Myelodysplastic syndrome (MDS)
◆ Refractory cytopenia (RCC) (PB blasts <2% and BM blasts <5%)
◆ Refractory anaemia with excess blasts (RAEB) (PB blasts 2–19% or BM blasts 5–19%)
◆ RAEB in transformation (RAEB-T) (PB or BM blasts 20–29%)/AML with myelodysplasia-related changes (PB or BM blasts >20%)

at presentation of 6.8 years. The exclusion of Down syndrome from patient series of MDS has decreased the number of cases diagnosed as RAEB or RAEB-T by approximately 50 per cent.

Associated abnormalities

MDS has been reported in a number of constitutional cytogenetic abnormalities other than Down syndrome, but there is only solid evidence for an association between trisomy 8 mosaicism and MDS. Trisomy 8 in leukaemic cells may be due to constitutional trisomy 8 in 15–20 per cent of the cases. Reports of MDS and AML in patients with Klinefelter and Turner syndrome have appeared sporadically but no increased risk has been documented in larger cohort studies.

Inherited bone marrow failure disorder

All inherited bone marrow failure disorders have to be considered as having an increased risk of MDS/AML. The risk varies greatly and is highest in Fanconi anaemia and severe congenital neutropeni (SCN). In Fanconi anaemia, myeloid neoplasia develops in a large fraction of patients during childhood or early adult life. The risk varies according to genetic subgroup and associated abnormalities. Diagnosing low grade MDS in a patient with Fanconi anaemia is a challenge because cytopenia and dysplasia may be part of the bone marrow failure and cytogenetic aberrations may be temporary or reappear as new clones.

Studies from the SCN International Register show a 15-year cumulated risk of MDS of 15 per cent. Partial or complete loss of chromosome 7 is found in more than half the patients who develop MDS. There is no direct cause-and-effect relationship between the development of MDS and growth factor therapy using G-CSF but the risk of MDS is highest in patients with a poor response to G-CSF.

MDS/AML develops in approximately 30 per cent of those with Shwachman-Diamond syndrome (SDS) and is often associated with chromosome 7 abnormalities of which isochromosome 7q may represent a separate entity with a long stable clinical course and a low risk of MDS. Most SDS patients can be diagnosed by clinical features: screening for *SBDS* gene mutations in children diagnosed with primary hypoplastic RCC identifis only very few SDS patients (<1 per cent).

Patients with dyskeratosis congenita (DC) carry mutations in genes encoding components of the telomerase complex like *DKC1*, *TERC* or *TERT*. These mutations impair telomerase activity, causing excessive telomere shortening and eventually inducing cellular senescence and apoptosis.

The cumulative incidence of MDS/AML in DC may be similar to what has been reported in Fanconi anaemia.

A considerable portion of patients with DC cannot be diagnosed by clinical features alone. Screening of a large cohort of patients with RCC for mutations in the genes of the telomerase complex gave rise to the assumption that up to 5 per cent of children with RCC will have undiagnosed DC with unrecognized *TERC* mutations in about 1–2 per cent.

MDS/AML has been described in familial platelet disorder and occasionally in Diamond-Blackfan anaemia and congenital amegakaryocytic thrombocytopenia but no reliable estimates of the excess risk is available.

Acquired aplastic anaemia

MDS develops in 10–15 per cent of those patients with aplastic anaemia not treated with HSCT. The risk of MDS is higher among those diagnosed as non-severe aplastic anaemia, suggesting that some cases of RCC are misdiagnosed at initial presentation. Prolonged treatment with the combination of G-CSF and cyclosporine may be associated with development of MDS; a high risk of MDS is especially noted in those with a poor response to G-CSF.

Familial MDS

Families with several members affected with MDS often show monosomy 7 or deletion 7q. There are no conspicuous clinical characteristics of the familial cases. Germline mutations in *RUNX1* and *CEBPA* may cause familial MDS/AML but the genetic cause remains obscure in most reported pedigrees.

Pathophysiology

MDS is a clonal disease arising in a stem or progenitor cell giving rise to myelopoiesis, erythropoiesis and megakaryopoiesis. The initiating events of MDS have remained obscure, in children like in adults, however, a tumour-suppressor gene, *TET2*, may be mutated as an early genetic event in about 20 per cent of adult patients with various myeloid disorders including MDS but no *TET2* mutations have so far been found in pediatric MDS and JMML.

Congenital disorders with DNA repair defects like Fanconi anaemia or acquired mutations in genes maintaining genetic stability may result in a mutator phenotype predisposing to MDS. Subsequent events, e.g. mutations in proto-oncogenes like *RAS*, *TP53*, or *WT1*, and karyotypic changes like monosomy 7, may be part of a final common pathway of disease progression.

Clinical and laboratory features

The presenting features in MDS are those of pancytopenia. Single lineage cytopenia may occasionally be the predominant characteristic. A few patients have been diagnosed during evaluation as possible sibling stem cell donors. Fetal haemoglobin (HbF) is frequently moderately elevated, WBC is low to normal, and leukocytosis is generally not a feature of MDS. Some patients present with moderate hepatosplenomegaly but most have no organomegaly. Extramedullary myeloid tumour may be the presenting feature of MDS but blasts in the cerebrospinal fluid is not.

Bone marrow features

The bone marrow may be hypocellular (most cases of RCC), normocellular, or hypercellular (most cases of RAEB). Both peripheral blood and bone marrow display characteristic dysplastic

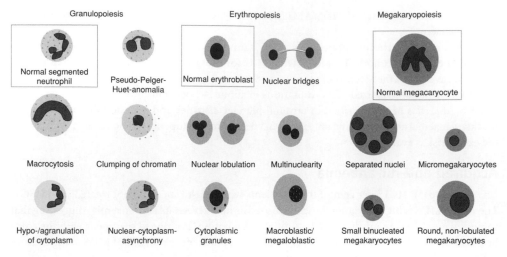

Fig. 16.1 Cytological features of myelodysplasia. Courtesy of Irith Baumann.

features with megaloblastic erythropoiesis, bizarre small or unusual large megakaryocytes, and dysgranulopoiesis (Fig. 16.1). These characteristic dysplastic features are suggestive of MDS but not diagnostic.

Cytogenetics

An abnormal karyotype is found in 55 per cent of children with advanced primary MDS and in 76 per cent with secondary advances MDS. The numerical abnormalities dominate and structural abnormalities are frequently part of a complex karyotype with numerical abnormalities. This is in contrast to AML where structural abnormalities are by far the most frequent findings.

Monosomy 7 is the most common cytogenetic abnormality in childhood MDS seen in 25 per cent of the patients. Trisomy 8 and trisomy 21 are the most common numerical abnormalities after monosomy 7. Constitutional trisomy 21 is clinically obvious when present, whereas constitutional trisomy 8 mosaicism may be clinically silent and should be tested for when trisomy 8 is found in the bone marrow.

Monosomy 7 is associated with a shorter time to progression in children with RCC but otherwise not an unfavourable feature in childhood MDS. AML specific translocations, e.g. t(8;21)(q22; q22), t(15;17)(q22; q12), or inv(16)(p13q22) should be considered as AML regardless of the blast count.

Immunophenotype

Flow cytometry immunophenotyping has not the same diagnostic yield in MDS as in acute leukaemia, but may be of value in the quantitative and qualitative assessment of immature progenitor cells especially when bone marrow smears are of suboptimal quality. Little data on immunophenotype characteristics of MDS in children have been reported and there is no consensus on uniformly used standard protocols and techniques available.

Differential diagnosis

The two main diagnostic challenges are: (i) to distinguish RCC from aplastic anaemia and other non-clonal disorders including inherited bone marrow failure syndromes; and (ii) to differentiate

MDS with excess of blasts from *de novo* AML. The traditional classification has been based on pure morphology but a number of additional factors need to be considered.

MDS versus non-clonal disorders

Bone marrow dysplasia may be present in a variety of disorders of very different aetiologies, for example infection, drug therapy, and chronic disease. RCC is a diagnosis of exclusion after ruling out infectious diseases like parvovirus, herpes virus 6, HIV, and visceral leishmaniasis. Vitamin B12 deficiency, copper deficiency, drug therapy, rheumatoid arthritis, and metabolic disorders may also cause cytopenia and dysplasia. RARS is extremely rare in children and the finding of sideroblastic anaemia should prompt investigation for possible inherited mitochondrial cytopathy or disorders of haeme synthesis; mitochondrial disorders like Pearson syndrome should not be considered MDS.

Although dysplasia is essential for the diagnosis it constitutes only one aspect of the morphological diagnosis and may be discrete. Since haematopoiesis is often dysplastic in patients with inherited bone marrow failure disorders, MDS should only be diagnosed if the BM blast count is increased, a persistent clonal chromosomal abnormality is present, or the bone marrow becomes hypercellular in the presence of persistent PB cytopenia.

Refractory cytopenia of childhood versus aplastic anaemia

As bone marrow cellularity is decreased in most cases of RCC, a trephine biopsy is fundamental for the evaluation of a child with suspected aplastic anaemia or MDS. In contrast to aplastic anaemia, hypoplastic RCC shows scarcely scattered granulopoiesis, patchy islands of immature erythropoiesis and micromegakaryocytes or absent megakaryopoiesis. Of note, the morphological picture of recovering aplastic anaemia (e.g. under immunosuppressive therapy) cannot be distinguished from RCC.

Separating MDS from AML

The major differential diagnosis of advanced MDS is AML. There are significant differences between MDS and AML in clinical features, cytogenetics and in response to therapy. The latter reflect fundamental biologic differences, thus making the morphologically based classification a surrogate marker for the distinction between biological entities (Table 16.2). The morphologically defined RAEB-T group is heterogeneous and blast count in a single specimen is insufficient to differentiate MDS from AML. Biological features rather than any arbitrary cut-off in blast count may be more important in distinguishing MDS from (chemosensitive) AML. An algorithm

Table 16.2 Major differences between MDS and AML in children

MDS		AML
WBC	low-normal	low-normal-high
Hepatomegaly	infrequent	common
Cytogenetic aberrations	numerical (-7)	structural
Dysplasia	multilineage	infrequent
Haematopoiesis	clonal (including CR)	non-clonal
Cell of origin	stem cell	lineage-restricted
Response to chemotherapy	poor	moderate
Iatrogenic model	alkylating agents	epipodophyllotoxins

to facilitate the distinction between MDS and AML is presented in Chapter 15. Monosomy 7 is strongly suggestive of MDS and patients presenting with monosomy 7 and a blast count above 30 per cent may share many features with MDS rather than with true *de novo* AML.

In borderline cases, with bone marrow blasts around 20 per cent and no cytogenetic clues to the diagnosis, the bone marrow examination should be repeated after about 2 weeks. The major diagnostic pitfall may be associated with undue haste in starting therapy. Significant organomegaly or increased WBC is suggestive of a diagnosis of AML. It should be emphasized that most children with myeloid malignancies have clear-cut AML, some have MDS with low blast count and only a few percentages have borderline features.

Prognosis and natural course

Children with RCC and RAEB or even RAEB-T may show a long and stable clinical course without treatment. Blood transfusions may only be required infrequently and severe infections are rarely seen. The condition may smoulder with unchanged cytopenia for months or even years. In a series of 67 children with primary RCC; four died from complications of pancytopenia prior to therapy or progression and 20 progressed to more advanced MDS at a median of 1.7 years from presentation. RCC with monosomy 7 is associated with a higher risk of progression, once progression has occurred the outcome is inferior even after HSCT.

The International Prognostic Scoring System (IPSS) for MDS weighted data on bone marrow blasts count, cytopenia and cytogenetics and separated patients into four prognostic groups. Only thrombocytopenia and bone marrow blasts greater than 5 per cent correlate with poor survival in children. Overall the IPSS provides little diagnostic information in children but identifies a very small group of the patients with low-risk disease and a very favourable outcome. Adolescence and complex cytogenetics are associated with a poorer outcome.

Spontaneous regression of MDS has occasionally been reported in the literature. The frequency of spontaneous remission is unknown, but estimated to occur in well below 5 per cent of the patients.

Treatment

MDS is a clonal disorder of an early stem or progenitor cell with limited residual non-clonal stem cells. Therefore, haematopoietic stem cell transplantation (HSCT) is the main curative therapy approach for children with all types of MDS. A diversity of therapy strategies like haematopoietic growth factors, differentiating agents, amifostine, anti-angiogenic drugs, immune modulation, low dose cytotoxic drugs, have been investigated in adults and in the elderly who are not candidates for HSCT. DNA methyltransferase inhibitors have shown clinical efficacy in adults with MDS. Hypermethylation may occur at a similar frequency in children and adults, thus making children potential candidates for epigenetic therapy, but so far treatment results from larger paediatric studies are lacking.

Immunosuppressive therapy with antithymocyte globulin and cyclosporine has been reported in small series of children with hypoplastic RCC from EWOG-MDS and from Japan. Complete or partial response was noted in 70 per cent and the overall and failure-free survival rates at 3 years were 90 per cent and 60 per cent, respectively. The long-term outcome of immunosuppressive therapy in MDS is not known.

AML-type chemotherapy

Conventional intensive chemotherapy without HSCT is unlikely to eradicate the primitive pluripotent cells involved in MDS, rendering the therapy non-curative in most patients.

Induction chemotherapy is associated with significant morbidity and mortality with a complete remission rate less than 60 per cent, treatment-related mortality rate 10–30 per cent, many relapses, and overall survival less than 30 per cent. Children with monosomy 7 diagnosed as AML have a poor response to induction chemotherapy as in MDS patients but, in contrast to MDS, those who responded well to chemotherapy had an outcome similar to AML patients. The EWOG-MDS experiences showed poor response to chemotherapy in RAEB-T and no benefit from chemotherapy before HSCT.

Haematopoietic allogeneic stem cell transplantation

Myeloablative busulfan-based regimen (e.g. with busulfan, cyclophosphamide and melphalan) have cured more than half of children with advanced MDS and increased blast count both after matched family donor (MFD) and matched unrelated donor (MUD) HSCT. Total body irradiation (TBI) can generally be omitted since it has no superior anti-leukaemic effect compared with busulfan and is associated with more long-term effects in children. It remains unknown whether AML-type induction chemotherapy prior to HSCT for advanced MDS can reduce relapse and thus improve DFS. Data from EWOG-MDS on children with primary advanced MDS showed no benefit of intensive AML-type therapy preceding HSCT. Considering the significant morbidity and mortality of induction chemotherapy and the high rate of transport-related mortality (TRM) following HSCT, highest in adolescents, most children with MDS may benefit from HSCT as first-line therapy sparing the toxicity related to induction chemotherapy. Relapse following HSCT for advanced MDS is associated with a very grave outcome. Successful donor leukocyte infusions have occasionally been reported. Especially early relapse detected by increasing mixed chimerism may benefit from withdrawal of immunosuppressive therapy and donor leukocyte infusion. Close analyses of chimerism status post-HSCT may allow initiation of pre-emptive immunotherapy.

In contrast to advanced MDS, relapse following HSCT is rare in RCC. HSCT early in the course of the disease has therefore been recommended for all children and adolescents with MDS. However, in children with RCC and absence of profound cytopenia, postponement of HSCT with a watch and wait strategy may be justified especially in patients with a normal karyotype. Following a myeloablative preparative regimen in RCC, EWOG-MDS reported a 5-year DFS of 78 per cent and 76 per cent for children receiving a MFD-HSCT or MUD-HSCT, respectively. A fludarabine based reduced-intensity conditioning regimen has been piloted in a few children with RCC and normal karyotype resulting in survival comparable to those of patients treated with myeloablative HSCT.

Secondary MDS

Children with MDS secondary to chemotherapy or radiation therapy generally have a poor survival. AML-type therapy may induce remission but very few patients remain in remission and even HSCT has been reported to offer cure to only 20–30 per cent of patients. The frequency of severe treatment-related toxicity is high while the risk of relapse may be similar to that observed for patients with primary MDS.

The few published data on HSCT in MDS arising from inherited bone marrow failure disorders indicate a poor outcome for this heterogeneous group of patients. Early HSCT before neoplastic transformation or during less advanced MDS may be associated with improved survival. Cooperative studies are needed to provide further information on the appropriate timing, preparative regimen and prophylaxis of graft versus host (GvH) disease for the different subtypes of MDS in childhood.

Myeloid leukaemia and Down syndrome

Individuals with Down syndrome (DS) have a strongly age-related increased risk of leukaemia with a more than 150-fold increased risk of myeloid leukaemia during the first 5 years of life. Myeloid leukaemia develops in 1 per cent of the children with DS, corresponding to an annual incidence of 0.6–1.0 per million children. The age distribution is very unusual with 49 per cent being 1 year of age at diagnosis, 34 per cent 2 years of age, and only 2 per cent more than 4 years of age. Only very few presented before 1 year of age. There appears to be no age overlap between myeloid leukaemia of DS and transient abnormal myelopoiesis.

Transient abnormal myelopoiesis

Increased WBC and circulating blasts with cell surface antigens characteristic of megakaryoblasts often accompanied by anaemia and thrombocytopenia may be seen in up to 10 per cent of newborns with DS. The percentage of blasts is often higher in blood than in bone marrow and a bone marrow aspiration is in most cases of limited additional diagnostic value. Clonal abnormalities are observed in 35 per cent. The condition is referred to as transient abnormal myelopoiesis (TAM), transient leukaemic reaction, or transient myeloproliferative disorder. The presentation is indistinguishable from leukaemia and some have therefore favoured the name transient leukaemia. TAM involves selectively the trisomic cells in individuals with DS mosaic.

Life-threatening complications, mainly progressive hepatic dysfunction, may occur in 10–20 per cent of the patients with TAM, but spontaneous remission appears in the majority within 1–3 months. Generally, no chemotherapy is indicated in TAM, however, in those with progressive hepatic or pulmonary problems a short course of low-dose cytarabine may be very effective. Myeloid leukaemia develops 1–3 years later in about 25 per cent of the children who have recovered from TAM.

Myeloid leukaemia of Down syndrome

Myeloid leukaemia in DS has been classified as MDS or AML. The bone marrow in myeloid leukaemia in DS children is often fibrotic and assessment of the blast count may be difficult. In contrast to non-DS children, there are no biological or therapeutic differences between MDS and AML in DS. The recent recognition of the unique biological features of *GATA1* mutated disease has resulted in consensus about the term myeloid leukaemia of Down syndrome (ML-DS). ML-DS is preferred to acute megakaryoblastic leukaemia because other phenotypes in DS are observed sharing the same biologic and clinical characteristics. It is no longer appropriate to use the terms MDS or AML (AKML) in young children with DS and leukaemia. Only in the rare case of a DS patient older than 4 years of age without *GATA1* mutation may MDS still be considered. Cases of AML in older DS children (4 years or older) tend to be *GATA1* negative and implicate a worse prognosis.

Pathobiology

Leukaemia in children with trisomy 21 mosaicism selectively involves the trisomic cells, pointing at the etiological role of the additional chromosome 21 as the first hit in the multistep process leading to leukaemia. Patients with the typical ML-DS have an acquired mutation in the *GATA1* gene. The mutation is not found in AML-M7 in non-DS or in other AML patients. The *GATA1* mutation is also found in patients with TAM. The *GATA1* gene encodes a transcription factor essential for the normal erythroid and megakaryocytic differentiation in accordance with the selective involvement of these two lineages in ML-DS.

A model of the pathogenic steps in myeloid leukaemia of DS is presented in Fig. 16.2. Trisomy 21 is the first event that may predispose the cells to a proliferative advantage or further mutations.

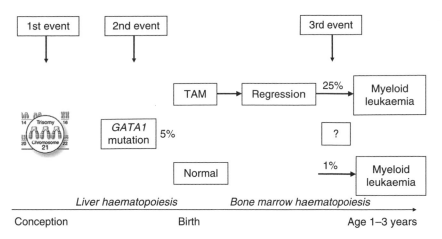

Fig. 16.2 Pathogenetic model for myeloid leukaemia of Down syndrome.

GATA1 mutation is found in TAM and may be present in 3–4 per cent of newborns with DS and normal haematology. The mechanisms of the spontaneous regression of TAM remain unexplained but may be associated with the natural switch of haematopoiesis from foetal liver to bone marrow. A large proportion of those with TAM and about 1 per cent (> 100-fold increased risk) of DS without abnormal haematology in the newborn period develop myeloid leukaemia.

Clinical and laboratory features

Isolated thrombocytopenia is often the presenting feature of ML-DS. At diagnosis, both platelet count and WBC are lower than in non-DS patients and in contrast to the very high WBC seen in TAM. The blast cells have in most cases morphologic and antigen features of megakaryoblasts, although other morphological variants may occur. Many patients have a relatively indolent course, characterized by a period of thrombocytopenia and dysplasia with relatively few blasts in the bone marrow.

Cytogenetics

Numerical aberrations, mainly trisomy 8 and an extra chromosome 21 (tetrasomy 21), are the most common acquired cytogenetic abnormalities. The recurrent structural aberrations seen in AML are not seen in ML-DS. Karyotype is not known to be a prognostic factor in DS.

Treatment

In contrast to TAM, ML-DS is fatal if untreated. The prognosis of ML-DS was considered very poor before 1990 when reports from the Nordic Society of Paediatric Haematology and Oncology (NOPHO) and the Paediatric Oncology Group (POG) showed a surprisingly high survival rate for DS patients receiving AML treatment. In fact, ML-DS responds well to AML treatment. Several groups have since reported long-term survival in DS patients well above 80 per cent. However, intensive timing of induction is associated with an increased mortality. DS children are at a low risk for relapse, due to the high risk for treatment-related toxicity they benefit from less time-intensive therapy allowing recovery prior to initiation of the next chemotherapeutic course. HSCT in first remission is clearly not indicated in children with ML-DS, and is generally associated with excess toxicity.

DS myeloblasts are 10-fold more sensitive to cytarabine *in vitro* than non-DS cells. The increased sensitivity of DS blasts may be related to the expression of chromosome 21 localized genes like cystathionine-β-synthetase and superoxide dismutase. Further studies of the molecular mechanism of the increased sensitivity to chemotherapy in DS may lead to new approaches in the treatment of AML.

Juvenile myelomonocytic leukaemia (JMML)

JMML is a unique paediatric disorder previously named chronic myelomonocytic leukaemia (CMML) in childhood or juvenile chronic myeloid leukaemia (JCML), recognizing the distinction from CML occurring in older children and adults. JMML is considered a separate bridging disorder between MDS and myeloproliferative disorders in the WHO classification.

Epidemiology

Incidence studies from Denmark and British Columbia showed a similar JMML incidence of 1.2 in million children per year corresponding to 2.4 per cent of all haematological malignancies. However, an incidence of only 0.6 in million was reported from UK. The median age at presentation is 1.8 years, 35 per cent are below 1 year of age at presentation and only 4 per cent more than 5 years of age. JMML displays a male predominance with a male : female ratio of 2:1.

Clinical and haematological features

Patients present with pallor, fever, infection, bleeding or symptoms from the hepatomegaly, splenomegaly or generalized lymphadenopathy. A macular-papular skin rash is seen in 35 per cent of the patients. An elevated WBC with absolute monocytosis, anaemia, and thrombocytopenia is almost universal. WBC at presentation exceeds $50 \times 10^9/l$ in 30 per cent of cases and is above $100 \times 10^9/l$ in 7 per cent. Blood film appearance with immature myeloid and/or erythroid precursors as well as monocytosis is characteristic, while bone marrow monocytosis may be discrete. Blast count in the bone marrow is generally less than 20 per cent. Increased foetal haemoglobin (HbF) is one of the main characteristics of JMML with the notable exception of those with monosomy 7 generally have a normal HbF for age.

Cytogenetics

Monosomy 7 (mostly as the sole abnormality) is present in about 25 per cent of JMML, 10 per cent have other aberrations, and 65 per cent have a normal karyotype. Data from the EWOG-MDS did not show any major clinical differences between JMML in patients with and without monosomy 7.

Molecular diagnostics and pathophysiology

JMML is a clonal disorder that arises from a pluripotent stem cell. The pathophysiology is characterized by hyperactivation of the Ras/MAPK signal transduction pathway resulting in hypersensitivity of leukaemic progenitors to growth factors, particularly GM-CSF. Germline and somatic mutations that deregulate Ras signalling are implicated as key initiating events in JMML.

Ras

Members of the Ras family of signalling proteins regulate cellular proliferation by cycling between an active guanosine triphosphate bound state (Ras-GTP) and an inactive guanosine diphosphate bound state (Ras-GDP). Somatic point mutations in codons 12, 13 and 61 of *NRAS* or *KRAS*, impairing the intrinsic GTPase activity of RAS and thereby causing high constitutive Ras-GTP levels, are noted in leukaemic cells of about 25 per cent of JMML patients.

In rare cases, a developmental disorder with germline *KRAS* or *NRAS* mutations are accompanied by a myeloproliferative disorder clinically indistinguishable from JMML which, however, spontaneously regresses. Interestingly, a few cases of JMML associated with acquired somatic *NRAS* mutations have also been reported to regress spontaneously over time.

Neurofibromatosis

Neurofibromatosis (NF1) is associated with a more than 200-fold increased risk of JMML. A clinical diagnosis of NF1 is made in 10–15 per cent of children with JMML. NF1 is caused by mutations of the *NF1* tumour suppressor gene, which encodes the Ras-GTPase activating protein (Ras-GAP) neurofibromin. Loss of the normal *NF1* allele is common in JMML cells from children with NF1. Recent studies showed that a common mechanism of *NF1* inactivation is uniparental disomy, resulting in duplication of the mutant *NF1* allele.

SHP-2

Somatic mutations in *PTPN11*, the gene encoding for the non-receptor tyrosine phosphatase SHP-2, are noted in about 35 per cent of children with JMML. SHP-2 relays growth signals from activated growth factor receptors to other signalling molecules, including Ras. Most *PTPN11* mutations are predicted to disrupt the auto-inhibition of the catalytic phosphatase (PTPase) domain by the N-terminal src-homology 2 (N-SH2) domain, thereby promoting the active conformation of the protein.

A JMML-like disorder is occasionally diagnosed in young infants with Noonan syndrome (NS). NS is an autosomal dominant disorder characterized by short stature, distinct facial anomalies, a typical spectrum of congenital heart defects and developmental delays. Approximately 50 per cent of patients with NS carry germline mutations of *PTPN11*. The acquired *PTPN11* mutations found in JMML have a stronger SHP-2 activation than the germline mutations in NS, whereas the germline mutations in NS with myeloproliferation have an intermediate gain of function effect. It is presumed that the strong activation resulting from the *PTPN11* mutation in JMML is incompatible with life when occurring as a germline mutation. In contrast to JMML with somatic mutations in *PTPN11* or *RAS* or in children with NF1, most cases of JMML in NS resolve spontaneously. Normalization of myeloproliferation may take several months or even years especially the monocytosis and splenomegaly which may persist for more than 10 years. Fatal progressive disease has only been reported in a few patients with NS.

CBL

CBL is an E3 ligase which promotes ubiquitylation and thereby degradation of a large number of tyrosine kinases. *CBL* mutations are acquired somatically in adults with myeloproliferative disorders. In JMML, 10–15 per cent of the children have a developmental germline disorder with heterozygous *CBL* mutations and an unexpectedly high percentage of developmental delay, cryptorchidism, and impaired growth. *CBL* appears to function as a classic tumour suppressor with loss of heterozygosity in leukaemic cells. Clinical data reveals that some patients may experience spontaneous resolution of JMML but later develop clinical features consistent with vasculitis and other autoimmune phenomena. Of note, among the patients treated for JMML with HSCT, there is a high rate of conversion to stable mixed chimerism.

Differential diagnoses

JMML may mimic infections like Epstein-Barr virus, cytomegalovirus, herpes virus-6, and parvovirus, or immunodeficiencies like Wiskott-Aldrich syndrome and leukocyte adhesion defect.

However, since more than 80 per cent of children with JMML can be diagnosed by a typical clinical picture and molecular markers, the diagnosis has become greatly facilitated. Culture studies demonstrating GM-CSF hypersensitivity of myeloid precursors are only warranted when JMML is suspected in the absence of one of the known genetic lesions.

Natural course and prognostic factors

For patients carrying somatic *RAS* and *PTPN11* mutations or NF1, JMML is a rapidly fatal disorder if left untreated. Blastic transformation is infrequent with JMML and most untreated patients die from organ failure due to infiltration of the leukaemic cells. Low platelet count, age above 2 years, and high HbF at diagnosis are the main factors predicting a short survival. Non-transplanted children presenting with a platelet count below 33 x 10^9/l have an almost 100 per cent mortality within the first year from diagnosis. Gene expression studies and aberrant DNA methylation may separate JMML into subgroups with distinct prognosis.

Patients with germline mutations in *PTPN11*, *NRAS*, *KRAS* or *CBL* (with or without syndromic features like NS) often show spontaneous regression of their JMML-like myeloproliferation. Therefore, mutational studies have to be carried out in haematopoietic and non-haematopoietic tissue (fibroblasts or cells from buccal swabs).

Treatment

Intensive chemotherapy is mostly unsuccessful in JMML resulting in long-term survival less than 10 per cent. Isoretinoin (13-cis retinoic acid) may induce temporary remission in at least a portion of JMML patients. Purine analogs, etoposide, and cytarabine as single agents are associated with the best clinical response rates. The potential for demethylating therapy in JMML is currently being studied.

Allogeneic HSCT is the only curative approach for children with JMML and somatic mutations in *RAS* and *PTPN11*, or NF1. It results in an overall survival in more than half the patients after both matched family and matched unrelated donor HSCT or cord blood transplantation. Busulfan-based myeloablative therapy offers a similar or greater anti-leukaemic efficacy than total body irradiation, which is to be avoided because of deleterious radiation-induced late effects in these young patients. The current EWOG-MDS study uses a preparative regimen with busulfan, cyclophosphamide, and melphalan and has shown event-free survival (EFS) of around 50 per cent with no difference between related and unrelated donors. Splenectomy before HSCT, as well as spleen size at time of the allograft, did not appear to have an impact on posttransplantation outcome. Monosomy 7 is associated with an outcome comparable to or even better than that of patients with normal karyotype.

Disease recurrence generally within the first year remains the main cause of treatment failure. Age above 4 years is the major significant risk factor for failure in multivariate analysis. Reduced intensity and duration of GvH disease prophylaxis may significantly contribute to successful leukaemia control and both acute and chronic GvH disease is associated with a lower risk of relapse. Early detection of donor cells by increasing mixed chimerism may be successfully eradicated by reducing ongoing immunosuppressive therapy. Donor lymphocyte infusion (DLI) in JMML relapse is largely unsuccessful but a second or even a third transplantation gives a relatively high chance of long-term survival.

Further reading

Abildgaard L, Ellebæk E, Gustafsson G, et al. (2006) Optimal treatment intensity in children with Down syndrome and myeloid leukaemia: data from 56 children treated on NOPHO-AML protocols and a review of the literature. *Annals Hematol* **85**, 275–80.

Alter BP, Giri N, Savage SA, et al. (2010) Malignancies and survival patterns in the National Cancer Institute inherited bone marrow failure syndromes cohort study. *Br J Haematol* **150**, 179–88.

Bergstraesser E, Hasle H, Rogge T, et al. (2007) Non-hematopoietic stem cell transplantation treatment of juvenile myelomonocytic leukemia: a retrospective analysis and definition of response criteria. *Pediatr Blood Cancer* **49**, 629–33.

Cantù-Rajnoldi A, Fenu S, Kerndrup G, et al. (2005) Evaluation of dysplastic features in myelodysplastic syndromes: experience from the morphology group of the European Working Group of MDS in Childhood (EWOG-MDS). *Ann Hematol* **84**, 429–33.

Chan RJ, Cooper T, Kratz CP, et al. (2009) Juvenile myelomonocytic leukemia: a report from the 2nd International JMML Symposium. *Leuk Res* **33**, 355–62.

Forestier E, Izraeli S, Beverloo B, et al. (2008) Cytogenetic features of acute lymphoblastic and myeloid leukemias in pediatric patients with Down syndrome—an iBFM-SG study. *Blood* **111**, 1575–83.

Gohring G, Michalova K, Beverloo HB, et al. (2010) Complex karyotype newly defined: the strongest prognostic factor in advanced childhood myelodysplastic syndrome. *Blood* **116**, 3766–99.

Hasle H (2009) Malignant diseases in Noonan syndrome and related disorders. *Hormone Res* **72** Suppl 2, 8–14.

Hasle H, Abrahamsson J, Arola M, et al. (2008) Myeloid leukemia in children 4 years or older with Down syndrome often lacks GATA1 mutation and cytogenetics and risk of relapse are more akin to sporadic AML. *Leukemia* **22**, 1428–30.

Hasle H, Baumann I, Bergsträsser E, et al. (2004) The International Prognostic Scoring System (IPSS) for childhood myelodysplastic syndrome (MDS) and juvenile myelomonocytic leukemia (JMML). *Leukemia* **18**, 2008–2014.

Hasle H, Niemeyer CM (2011) Advances in the prognostication and management of advanced MDS in children. *Br J Haematol* **154**, 185–95.

Hasle H, Niemeyer CM, Chessells JM, et al. (2003) A pediatric approach to the WHO classification of myelodysplastic and myeloproliferative diseases. *Leukemia* **17**, 277–82.

Kardos G, Baumann I, Passmore SJ, et al. (2003) Refractory anemia in childhood: a retrospective analysis of 67 patients with particular reference to monosomy 7. *Blood* **102**, 1997–2003.

Klusmann JH, Creutzig U, Zimmermann M, et al. (2008) Treatment and prognostic impact of transient leukemia in neonates with Down syndrome. *Blood* **111**, 2991–98.

Kratz CP, Schubbert S, Bollag G, et al. (2006) Germline mutations in components of the ras signaling pathway in Noonan syndrome and related disorders. *Cell Cycle* **5**, 1607–11.

Locatelli F, Nollke P, Zecca M, et al. (2005) Hematopoietic stem cell transplantation (HSCT) in children with juvenile myelomonocytic leukemia (JMML): results of the EWOG-MDS/EBMT trial. *Blood* **105**, 410–19.

Niemeyer CM, Kang MW, Shin DH, et al. (2010) Germline CBL mutations cause developmental abnormalities and predispose to juvenile myelomonocytic leukemia. *Nat Genet* **42**, 794–800.

Niemeyer CM, Kratz CP (2008) Paediatric myelodysplastic syndromes and juvenile myelomonocytic leukaemia: molecular classification and treatment options. *Br J Haematol* **140**, 610–24.

Owen C, Barnett M, Fitzgibbon J (2008) Familial myelodysplasia and acute myeloid leukaemia—a review. *Br J Haematol* **140**, 123–32.

Passmore SJ, Chessells JM, Kempski H, et al. (2003) Paediatric MDS and JMML in the UK: a population based study of incidence and survival. *Br J Haematol* **121**, 758–67.

Rao A, Hills RK, Stiller C, et al. (2006) Treatment for myeloid leukaemia of Down syndrome: population-based experience in the UK and results from the Medical Research Council AML 10 and AML 12 trials. *Brit J Haematol* **132**, 576–83.

Rosenberg PS, Zeidler C, Bolyard AA, et al. (2010) Stable long-term risk of leukaemia in patients with severe congenital neutropenia maintained on G-CSF therapy. *Br J Haematol* **150**, 196–99.

Strahm B, Nollke P, Zecca M, et al. (2011) Hematopoietic stem cell transplantation for advanced MDS in children: results of the EWOG-MDS98 study. *Leukemia* **25**, 455–62.

Swerdlow SH, Campo E, Harris NL, et al. (2008) *WHO classification of tumours of haematopoietic and lymphoid tissues.* Lyon: IARC.

Yoshimi A, Baumann I, Fuhrer M, et al. (2007) Immunosuppressive therapy with anti-thymocyte globulin and cyclosporine A in selected children with hypoplastic refractory cytopenia. *Haematologica* **92**, 397–400.

Zwaan CM, Reinhardt D, Hitzler J, Vyas P (2010) Acute leukemias in children with Down syndrome. *Hematol Oncol Clin North Am* **24**, 19–34.

Chapter 17

Malignant non-Hodgkin lymphomas in children

Angelo Rosolen and Thomas Gross

Introduction

Non-Hodgkin lymphoma (NHL) is a category of haematologic malignancies that includes diseases distinct from Hodgkin lymphoma (HL), with clinical features that in part resemble those of acute leukemias, but with some characteristics of solid tumours. Although frequently the relevant symptoms and signs at presentation are consequences of the tumour mass, NHL tends to spread following the pattern of lymphoid cell distribution.

The NHL classification currently in use has included some of the most recent developments in the field of immunohistochemistry, biology and genetics, leading to a more rational identification of the different disease subtypes. Of note, the histological subtypes represented in childhood and adolescence are limited compared to the adult counterparts and mostly belong to the high-grade, clinically aggressive NHL category.

In the 1970s, using leukemia-based treatments, cure rates for children with NHL were not good; but at present over 80 per cent of children and adolescents in affluent countries survive their disease. The progress in outcome is the consequnce of a more accurate diagnostic process, of better risk-adapted chemotherapy approaches, and of the ability to prevent and control life-threatening treatment-related toxicities. Conversely, the outcome of patients with NHL treated in countries with limited resources fare worse, depending on the unavailability of certain anti-cancer medicines or from suboptimal diagnostic and therapeutic management of patients.

The increased knowledge in the field of biology of paediatric NHL will improve outcome through the use of more efficient multiagent therapies and the introduction of novel agents, including targeted therapies. Nevertheless, conditions that allow the application of standard treatments on a global or international scale are needed, to provide a better chance of cure in less priviledged areas of the world. These challenges will represent the new frontiers in paediatric NHL for the next decades.

Incidence and epidemiology

The incidence of lymphoma in children varies by age and varies considerably in different world regions. In developed countries, malignant lymphoma (including NHL and HL) comprise the third most common group of malignancies in children after leukemias and brain tumours and account for 15 per cent of all childhood malignancies in children younger than 20 years. NHL is more common than HL in children younger than 10 years. There is a marked male predominance, particularly in children younger than 15 years in whom 75 per cent of the cases occur in males. NHL is uncommon in children younger than 5 years, and the incidence of NHL increases steadily throughout life. The incidence of NHL varies according to the histologic subtype of NHL.

Burkitt lymphoma (BL) is more common in children between the ages of 5 and 15 years, whereas the incidence of lymphoblastic lymphoma (LL) is reasonably constant across all paediatric age groups. Large cell lymphoma, diffuse large B-cell lymphoma (DLBCL) and anaplastic large cell lymphoma (ALCL) occur more frequently in older children and adolescents, demonstrating a steady increase in incidence throughout childhood and peaking in adolescents. Both the incidence and relative frequency of the different subtypes of NHL vary considerably in different parts of the world; in equatorial Africa, lymphomas account for almost one half of the childhood cancers, reflecting the very high incidence of BL but a relative paucity of LL in this region. In adults, the overall incidence of NHL has increased over time, a trend that is also noted in those aged 15–19-years and in young adults older than 20; however, the incidence has remained relatively stable in younger children.

The etiology of NHL is largely unknown. Epidemiologic studies evaluating prenatal and post-natal exposures have not been fruitful for the most part, and exposures studied to date have not been associated with increased risk of lymphoma. Therapy-related secondary NHL in children is rare and is primarily LL or DLBCL. Immunodeficiency, whether inherited or acquired, is clearly related to the development of NHL, increasing the incidence of NHL more than 100 fold.

The relationship between Epstein-Barr virus (EBV) and the pathogenesis of NHL began with the elegant investigations by Denis Burkitt in the late 1950s. Dr Burkitt demonstrated that the disease was associated with climate and rainfall—in short, the regions where malaria is holoendemic. This observation lead to a collaboration with Anthony Epstein and resulted in the discovery of a herpes-virus from cultures of endemic BL tissue, the first human tumour-associated virus.

Pathology and biology

Paediatric NHL are represented by few major histological subtypes, including BL, DLBCL, LL, and ALCL, although other entities can occasionally be found in children (Table 17.1). Indolent lymphomas, which account for approximately 60–70 per cent of adult NHL, are less than 5 per cent of the total of childhood NHL. The rare follicular lymphoma (FL) and the nodal marginal zone lymphoma (NMZL) described in children appear disctinct from the adult counterpart both

Table 17.1 Main subtypes of paediatric NHL (2008 WHO Classification)

Subtype of lymphoma	Frequency
Precursor lymphoid neoplasms	
T-lymphoblastic lymphoma	15–20%
B-lymphoblastic lymphoma	3%
Mature B-cell neoplasms	
Burkitt lymphoma	35–40%
Diffuse large B-cell lymphoma	15–20%
Primary mediastinal B-cell lymphoma	1–2%
Paediatric follicular lymphoma	rare
Paediatric nodal marginal zone lymphoma	rare
Mature T-cell neoplasms	
Anaplastic large cell lymphoma, ALK positive	15–20%
Peripheral T-cell lymphoma (NOS)	rare

clinically and histologically and are reported as distinct entities in the most recent World Health Organization (WHO) classifcation. While adult NHL are of B-cell phenotype in about 80 per cent of the cases, in paediatric NHL approximately 55 per cent of all cases are of B-cell phenotype.

An accurate and complete diagnosis depends on adequacy of tumour tissue for morphological, immunophenotypic, and molecular analyses and requires ideally fresh tissue from an open biopsy. In selected cases, flow cytometric analysis of cytologic preparations may be sufficient to make a diagnosis and this should be the approach of choice in case of intracavitary effusions in patients in critical clinical conditions.

Precursor cell or lymphoblastic lymphoma

Precursor cell or lymphopblastic lymphoma (LL) accounts for 15–20 per cent of paediatric NHL (Table 17.1). Conventionally, LL is distinguished from acute lymphoblastic leukemia (ALL) based on the extent of bone marrow involvement (ALL is defined when BM blasts are >25 per cent). The current WHO classification identifies the diagnostic category of lymphoblastic leukemia/ lymphoma based on clinical and pathologic similarities between LL and ALL, but recent gene expression and genetic studies would suggest that they may differ biologically.

Morphologically, the malignant cells of LL appear indistinguishable from ALL, being of small or intermediate size, with high nuclear: cytoplasm ratio and finely disperse chromatin. Nucleoli may be evident and occasionally blasts may have cytoplasmic vacuoles morphologically resembling L3 blasts (a feature that is not exclusive of BL). LL blasts in the lymph nodes show high mitotic rate and cause diffuse effacement of nodal architecture, with occasionally spared reactive follicles. A 'starry sky' appearance similar to that typically found in BL may be caused by the presence of numerous macrophages.

Immunophenotypically, LL blasts do not express surface immunoglobulin (SIg) but characteristically are positive for TdT (terminal deoxynucleotidyl transferase) in more than 95 per cent of the cases and often for CD99, independently of their T- or B-cell lineage. T-LL express, in different combination, T-cell markers typical of middle to late stages of thymocyte differentiation, including CD1a, CD2, CD5, CD7, CD4, and/or CD8. T-cell receptor antigens are frequently not expressed and CD3 is more often detected in the cytoplasm than on cell surface. Approximately 10–15 per cent of LL cases display precursor B-cell markers, including CD19, CD10 and variable expression of HLA-DR and CD20, but not SIg (Table 17.2).

Although specific data on LL are scarce, chromosomal translocations described in ALL have been reported also in LL. Recently, deletions in chromosome 6q [del(6q)] have been reported in LL, similarly to ALL and other malignancies, but differently from ALL del(6q) appear to have a negative prognostic impact in LL. Translocations often involve rearrangements of T-cell receptor (TCR) or Ig gene rearrangements with proto-oncogenes, resulting in the juxtaposition of promoter and enhancer elements of TCR or Ig genes and transcription factor genes including *HOX11*, *TAL1* and *LYL1*. T-LL displays early TCR gene rearragements that can be detected by molecular assays, whereas B-cell precursor LL shows Ig gene rearrangements. They represent a unique marker that can be exploited through the use of molecular assays to determine clonality, thus assisting in the differential diagnosis between LL and atypical or reactive lymphadenopathy.

Burkitt lymphoma

Burkitt lymphoma (BL) is the most frequent histological subtype of NHL diagnosed in children. Morphologically it is characterized by cells of intermediate size with nuclei containing prominent nucleoli and limited amount of basophilic cytoplasm in which vacuoles are almost invariably present. These features are typical of the L3 morphology. BL has a very high mitotic activity and

Table 17.2 Summary features of childhood non Hodgkin lymphomas

Histology	Immunology	Clinical features	Cytogenetics	Genes involved
Burkitt and Burkitt-like	B cell (sIg+)	Abdominal masses, gastrointestinal tract tumours, involvement of Waldeyer's ring	t(8;14)(q24;q32)	*IgH-cMYC*
			t(2;8)(p11;q24)	*Igk-cMYC*
			t(8;22)(q24;q11)	*Igλ-cMYC*
Diffuse large B-cell	B cells of germinal center or post germinal center	Abdominal masses, gastrointestinal tract tumours, involvement of Waldeyer's ring		
Mediastinal large B-cell	B cells of medullary thymus	Mediastinum		
Anaplastic large cell	T cell (mostly), null cell or NK cell (CD30+)	Skin, nodes, bone	t(2;5)(p23;q35)	*NPM-ALK*
			t(1;2)(q21;p23)	*TPM3-ALK*
			t(2;3)(p23;q21)	*TFG-ALK*
			t(2;17)(p23;q23)	*CLTC-ALK*
			t(X;2)(q11-12;p23)	*MSN-ALK*
			inv 2(p23;q35)	*ATIC-ALK*
Precursor T lymphoblastic	T cell (thymocyte phenotype)	Anterior mediastinal mass with upper torso adenopathy	t(1;14)(p32;q11)	*TCRad-TAL1*
			t(11;14)(p13;q11)	*TCRad-RHOMB2*
			t(11;14)(p15;q11)	*TCRad-RHOMB1*
			t(10;14)(q24;q11)	*TCRad-HOX11*
			t(7;19)(q35;p13)	*TCRb-LYL1*
			t(8;14)(q24;q11)	*TCRad-MYC*
			t(1;7)(p34;q34)	*TCRb-LCK*
Precursor B lymphoblastic	B-cell precursors	Cutaneous masses, isolated lymph node masses, primary bone lymphoma		

tissue section often show the 'starry-sky' morphology resulting from clear macrophages scattered among the rather intensely stained population of blasts. Although not exclusive of BL, the 'starry-sky' pattern is characteristic of BL.

The current revised WHO classification of lymphoid malignancies includes under the term BL also the subtypes previously defined as Burkitt-like and atypical Burkitt lymphomas, since it is not possible to differentiate them based solely on morphology. Those tumours which present with features intermediate between BL and DLBCL are now placed into the category of unclassifiable B-cell lymphoma.

Immunophenotypic studies of BL demonstrate mature malignant B-cells expressing CD19, CD20, CD22, CD10, CD79, and monoclonal SIg. Because BL is a very highly proliferating human malignancy, with doubling time of less than 24 hours, analysis of proliferation markers such as Ki-67 or MIB-1 will show reactivity in more than 95 per cent of the cells and this is one of the features defining BL in the WHO classification.

BL cells harbor characteristic chromosomal translocations involving the MYC oncogene locus on chromosome 8q24 (Table 17.2). The most common translocation, t(8;14)(q24;q32), which involves the IgH gene locus, occurs in 80 per cent of cases. The consequence of MYC rearrangements in BL is the deregulation of MYC expression, which promotes cell cycle progression and cell transformation. The remaining 20 per cent of BL have either a t(2;8)(p12;q24) or, less frequently, a t(8;22)(q24;q11) involving MYC and either the kappa or lambda immunoglobulin light chain gene loci, respectively on chromosomes 2 or 22. While MYC is involved in both sporadic and endemic BL, the breakpoints within the *MYC* gene and in the IgH loci differ between the two BL subtypes. The most common translocation, t(8;14)(q24;q32), can be detected by long-distance polymerase chain reaction (LD-PCR) assay. Based on this approach the MYC-IgH rearrangements can be used as makers to analyze minimal BM infiltration at diagnosis and its response to chemotherapy with a sensitivity of 1/10,000.

Diffuse large B-cell lymphoma

Similarly to BL, DLBCL is characterized by a mature B-cell phenotype but cells display varying morphologic and cytologic appearances. Centroblastic, immunoblastic, anaplastic, and T-cell rich B-cell lymphoma are histological subtypes of DLBCL encountered in childhood. Malignant cells are rather large in size and show more abundant cytoplasm compared to BL cells. Paediatric DLBCL have a high proliferation rate, although lower that BL, as determined by Ki-67 or MIB-1, i.e. <90 per cent. They express cell SIg and a number of B-cell markers, including CD19, CD20, CD22, CD79, and PAX5. CD30 can be detecetd in some DLBCL and this creates the need to differentiate it from HL, particularly the lymphocyte predominant subtype, and from ALCL. Expression of CD15 and lack of expression of CD45 and most B-cell markers, such as CD79 and PAX5, suggest the diagnosis of HL, whereas differential diagnosis of ALCL may rely on the presence of ALK and T-cell markers.

In contrast to adult DLBCL, paediatric cases are less frequently positive for BCL2, but can express high levels of the germinal center markers CD10 and BCL6. No consistent cytogenetic abnormalities have been associated with DLBCL of children and adolescents, but more complex karyotypes than BL have been reported. Chromosomal translocations involving the *MYC* oncogene are more frequent in paediatric compared to adult DLBCL, whereas BCL2 translocations are rarely seen in paediatric cases. Recent gene expression profile studies, together with specific immunostaining using markers of germinal center, have demonstrated that more than 80 per cent of the paediatric DLBCL belong to the germinal center B-cell-like subgroup, suggesting that DLBCL of children and adolescents are biologically more similar to BL than to DLBCL seen in older patients.

A rare (1–2 per cent of all paediatric NHL) and clinically distinct entity among large B-cell lymphoma is primary mediastinal large B-cell lymphoma (PMBL). It originates from thymic B cells and is characterized by diffuse proliferation of large cells and evident sclerosis. PMBL both for the almost exclusive mediastinal localization and for the morphologic appearance may be difficult to distinguish from HL. Cell surface markers in PMBL are similar to those seen in DLBCL and include CD19, CD20, CD22, CD79, and PAX5, but very often only cytoplasmic Ig and not SIg are present. CD30 is commonly expressed. Studies of gene expression show overlap of gene expression profiles between PMBL and HL suggesting that biologically PMBL is more similar to HL than DLBCL.

Anaplastic large cell lymphoma

Anaplastic large cell lymphoma (ALCL) is composed of large cells with significant anaplasia and high levels of CD30 expression on the cell surface. The majority of ALCL express T-cell markers, but as many as 15–20 per cent of ALCL have neither T- nor B-cell markers and are defined null-cell ALCL. Characteristically ALCL cells are large, pleomorphic, multinucleated or horse-shoe shaped cells (hallmark cells). They are present in differing proportion in the various morphologic subtypes of ALCL. The most frequent morphologic subtype (more than 70 per cent of cases) is the 'common type' in which typical anaplastic and hallmark cells predominate. The lymphohistiocytic and the small cell variants account for about 20 per cent of cases and appear to be clinically more aggressive. A histological feature of ALCL is the propensity of the tumour cells to invade the lymph-node sinuses and partial involvement of the lymph node. Cells consistently express CD30 and typically are positve for the epithelial membrane antigen (EMA). CD3 is often expressed and TCR gene rearrangements can be detected by molecular assays in the vast majority of the cases. Other T-cell markers (CD2, CD4, CD5, CD7, CD8) and expression of perforin and granzyme (positive in the majority of ALCL) can be used in the diagnosis of ALCL, whereas B-cell markers are negative.

More than 90 per cent of systemic ALCL in children and adolescents express the anaplastic lymphoma kinase (ALK) originated from chromosomal translocations. Most often paediatric ALCL harbor the chromosomal translocation t(2;5)(p23;q35) which juxtaposes the nucleophosmin (*NPM*) and the *ALK* genes, giving rise to the fusion gene *NPMALK* (Table 17.2). The NPM–ALK protein retains the kinase activity of wild-type ALK (a cell surface receptor normally expressed only in the nervous system). The NPM-ALK fusion protein is detectable in more than 90 per cent of ALCL cases in the cytoplasm and in the nucleus of malignant cells by immunohistochemistry, and its transcript can be identified by reverse transcriptase polymerase chain reaction (RT-PCR), a highly sensitive and specific method for the identification of ALK rearrangements at RNA level. Detection of NPM–ALK transcript is increasingly applied in the diagnosis of ALCL but, most importantly, is exploited in the assessment of minimal disseminated disease that has been shown to be one of the most relevant prognostic parameters in ALK-positive ALCL of childhood. A number of variant partners of ALK have been reported in the *ALK* gene rearrangements and they are characterized often by specific pattern of cellular ALK expression as detecetd by anti-ALK antibodies.

Rare NHL in paediatrics

Follicular lymphoma (FL) is rarely seen in children, but represent almost one third of NHL in adults. Paediatric FL is histologically indistinguishable from adult FL. FL is characterized by alterations of lymph-node architetcture due to proliferation of small neoplastic lymphocytes, reproducing a follicular or a mixed (follicular and diffuse) growth pattern. A large cell, or Grade III, component is more frequently observed in paediatric cases. Immunophenotype shows reactivity for B-cell markers (CD20, CD79a, CD445RA, CD22, PAX5). However, BCL2 expression and t(14 ;18)(q32;q21) rearrangements which are found in 80–90 per cent of adult FL, are rarely found in paediatric cases. Paediatric FL can be distinguished from reactive lymphadenopathy based on clonality detected by Ig rearrangements, since they may express identical phenotypes.

Based on the peculiarities of paediatric FL, in the current WHO classification it is considered as a separate entity from adult FL.

Other rare B-cell lymphomas are nodal and extranodal (mucosa-associated) marginal zone lymphoma (MZL). These entities histologically overlap the adult lymphomas and may be difficult to differentiate from reactive lymphocytic proliferations.

Another rare group of paediatric NHL represented in the WHO classification are the peripheral T-cell lymphomas (PTCL). Morphologically they have variable appearances with medium to large size neoplastic cells, with irregular nuclei and basophylic cytoplasm, infltrating the lymph node. Cells show aberrant expression of T-cell markers (CD2,CD3, CD5 or CD7) and may co-express or lack both CD4 and CD8. TCR rearrangements are almost invariably detectable.

Clinical presentation

Childhood NHL may present very heterogeneously. The classic clinical manifestations of the different subtypes are summarized in Table 17.2.

Precursor cell/lymphoblastic lymphoma

The majority (50-70 per cent) of children with precursor T-cell LL present with rapidly enlarging neck and mediastinal lymphadenopathy, although subdiaphragmatic nodal presentations are occasionally seen (Table 17.2). Symptoms often include cough, wheezing, shortness of breath, and orthopnea, though swelling of the neck, face, and upper extremities from superior vena cava (SVC) obstruction can occur. Haemodynamic compromise due to pericardial effusions may also occur. Subdiaphragmatic disease is often present and may include hepatosplenomegaly, kidney infiltration, and retroperitoneal nodal disease. Fewer than 2 per cent of males will have overt testicular disease, manifest as painless enlargement of one or both testes.

In contrast to the clinical features associated with precursor T-cell LL, children and adolescents with precursor B-cell LL tend to have limited disease in sites including skin, bone, testes, and peripheral lymph nodes (Table 17.2). The cutaneous lesions are typically in the scalp and appear as enlarging, discoloured masses. Morphologically detectable bone marrow involvement is uncommon at presentation.

Burkitt lymphoma/leukemia

Burkitt lymphoma/leukemia (BL) accounts for about 40 per cent of childhood NHL. The predominant sites of involvement and patterns of spread are different in patients with sporadic compared to endemic BL (Table 17.3). Jaw involvement is the most common site of disease in endemic BL. In endemic cases of BL, lesions in multiple quadrants of the jaw or orbital tumours with or without maxillary disease are observed in the majority of children, especially those younger than 5 years. Abdominal disease is also very common. In contrast to sporadic BL, bone marrow infiltration at diagnosis and at relapse is uncommon, but CNS disease occurs in almost one third of patients. CNS disease may present as headache and increased intracranial pressure from meningeal infiltration, cranial nerve palsies, or an isolated epidural tumour and paraplegia.

The most common site of disease in sporadic cases of BL is the abdomen. Abdominal disease may present with pain or distention, nausea and vomiting, gastrointestinal bleeding, or rarely intestinal perforation. Approximately 25–30 per cent of children present with a right lower quadrant mass or acute abdominal pain caused by an ileocecal intussusception, which is often confused with acute appendicitis. The majority of patients with abdominal BL have massive disease involving the mesentery, retroperitoneum, kidneys, ovaries, and peritoneal surfaces (often associated with malignant ascites). Therefore, surgical debulking is neither feasible nor appropriate in these patients.

Table 17.3 Comparison of endemic and sporadic Burkitt lymphoma

Feature	Endemic	Sporadic
Clinical features	5–10 years	6–12 years
	Males >Females	Males >Females
Most common distribution of disease	Equatorial Africa, New Guinea, Amazonian Brazil, Turkey	North America, Europe most common
Annual incidence	10 in 100 000	0.2 in 100 000
Common tumour sites	Jaw, abdomen, central nervous system, cerebrospinal fluid	Abdomen, marrow, lymph nodes, ovaries
Histopathologic features	Diffuse growth pattern, monomorphic intermediate-sized cell, starry-sky pattern	Same
Immunologic features	CD20+, usually IgM, κ or λ CD10+, BCL2–	CD10+, usually IgM, κ or λ CD10+, BCL2–
Presence of Epstein-Barr virus DNA in tumour cells	95%	15%
Presence of t(8;14), t(2;8), or t(8;22)	Yes	Yes
Chromosome 8 breakpoints	Upstream of cMYC	Within cMYC

The head and neck region is the second most common site of disease in sporadic BL but, in contrast to patients with endemic BL, jaw involvement is observed in fewer than 10 per cent of cases of sporadic disease. Bone marrow involvement occurs in approximately 20 per cent of cases of sporadic BL. Almost 20 per cent of patients present without lymphomatous masses but with fever, pallor, and/or bleeding secondary to pancytopenia from extensive marrow replacement by tumour cells (>25 per cent blasts). These children may also have peripheral lymphadenopathy and hepatosplenomegaly; however, mediastinal primaries are more rarely seen than in other paediatric NHL. BL can involve almost any organ including testes, breasts, thyroid gland, skin, epidural space, bone, or pancreas.

Diffuse large B-cell lymphoma

Children with DLBCL have a more heterogeneous range of clinical presentations compared to patients with BL. In contrast to BL, the bone marrow and CNS are unusual sites of disease. DLBCL usually presents with nodal disease, though bone (single or multiple sites) is relatively common. In immunocompromised individuals, extranodal disease is common and primary DLBCL of the brain is not uncommon. Primary mediastinal B-cell lymphoma is a distinct entity. It is typically diagnosed in young adult females in the third to fourth decades of life. The tumour is locally invasive (e.g. pericardial and lung extension), often associated with the SVC syndrome, and extrathoracic involvement often includes the kidney.

Anaplastic large cell lymphoma

ALCL tends to present in lymph nodes and extranodal sites, especially the skin, soft tissues, and bone (Table 17.2). ALCL includes primary cutaneous (C-ALCL) and systemic ALCL. Primary cutaneous ALCL can be difficult to distinguish from lymphoid papulosis (LyP), and both are quite rare in children. LyP is defined as a chronic, recurrent, self-healing papulonecrotic or papulonodular skin disease. The lesions are usually smaller than 2 cm and are red-brown papules and nodules that may develop central haemorrhage, necrosis, crusting, and subsequently disappear spontaneously within 3–8 weeks. In primary cutaneous ALCL, the nodules are usually larger than 2 cm and may be single or multiple and show ulceration. This entity is distinguishable from the systemic form of ALCL because the neoplastic cells in C-ALCL do not express EMA or ALK.

The clinical presenting features of systemic ALCL in children are quite variable but often include constitutional symptoms of fever and weight loss. About two thirds of cases present with disseminated disease. The most frequent sites of involvement in systemic ALCL are: peripheral nodes; mediastinal adenopathy; and extranodal sites including skin, soft tissue, and bone. Skin involvement is much more frequent than in other childhood lymphomas and is a most common site of extranodal disease in ALCL. Spontaneous regression or waxing and waning of skin disease has been observed in systemic ALCL, albeit less frequently than in primary cutaneous ALCL. Bone disease is also common and it is multifocal in as many as 10 per cent of patients. The CNS and bone marrow are occasionally involved, and in several cases a leukemic presentation has been described. Diagnosis of bone marrow involvement may be difficult and require immunostaining with CD30 and/or ALK to identify rare tumour cells.

Rare NHL in paediatrics

Indolent mature B-cell NHL in children are rare but include follicular lymphoma (FL) which tend to present with nodal (often cervical), cutaneous and testicular involvement. Nodal marginal zone lymphoma (NMZL) is an indolent B-cell lymphoma and can present as nodal or extranodal disease mucosa-associated tissue lymphoma (MALT).

Mature (peripheral) T-cell and NK-cell lymphomas are a heterogeneous group of aggressive lymphomas. Among these, the NK-cell lymphoma and NK-like T-cell lymphomas usually involve the upper aerodigestive tract (midline lethal granuloma, angiocentric T-cell lymphoma) but also can present in the skin. Approximately 4-5 per cent of cases of mycosis fungoides (MF) are diagnosed in patients younger than 20 years. MF in paediatrics is most commonly misdiagnosed as refractory eczema, but misdiagnosis of psoriasis, tinea corporis, pityriasis, and vitiligo is also common. The time from onset of symptoms to diagnosis is often years. Disseminated disease is rarely been observed in paediatric MF. Subcutaneous panniculitic T-cell lymphoma (SPTL) typical presents as subcutaneous nodules on the trunk and lower extremities but occasionally on the face. The most common differential diagnoses include erythema nodosum and cellulitis.

Diagnosis and staging

The most expeditious and least invasive procedure should be used to establish the diagnosis, and the staging evaluation should be expedited because many children with NHL have rapidly growing tumour masses that can cause life-threatening complications. Essentially all types of paediatric NHL may present as an anterior mediastinal mass, which may result in significant respiratory distress or SVC syndrome. Due to the risk of respiratory failure and difficulties to intubate these children, sedation should be avoided in any child with an anterior mediastinal mass. The prebiopsy use of irradiation or steroids for respiratory distress may result in rapid shrinkage of the mediastinal mass but may jeopardize establishing a tissue diagnosis. However, up to 48 hours of prednisone (40–60 mg/m^2/day) have been given in this situation with rapid clinical improvement and preservation of diagnostic tissue. However, the use of steroids can make it difficult to determine if CNS disease was present at diagnosis.

A close examination of the peripheral blood and a bone marrow aspirate/biopsy should be undertaken in all patients. A bone marrow or pleural fluid examination may be diagnostic in the evaluation of a child with a mediastinal mass without anesthesia. Similarly, examination of bone marrow or ascites may provide a diagnosis in a child with unresectable abdominal tumour. The lack of anemia, neutropenia, or thrombocytopenia does not rule out bone marrow involvement.

Radiologic studies should include computed tomography (CT) or magnetic resonance imaging (MRI) of the primary site. The role of routine bone scans is controversial. Functional imaging—gallium scans or positron emission tomography (PET) scans—are usually performed at diagnostic work-up. PET may be more sensitive than gallium. At present, there is no data that upstaging a patient based solely on PET scanning is prognostic in childhood NHL. There is very limited data using PET scanning to assess rapidity of response for prognosis, and numerous studies have demonstrated that PET scanning has poor predictive value for detecting recurrence for paediatric lymphoma. The remainder of the work-up should include a complete serum metabolic profile and a lumbar puncture with examination of a cytocentrifuged specimen of cerebrospinal fluid.

The goal of staging studies should be to assess rapidly the extent of disease to determine prognosis and to assign appropriate therapy. The Ann Arbor staging classification does not adequately reflect prognosis in childhood NHL for several reasons. The progression of disease in childhood NHL does not follow an orderly and predictable pattern of lymphatic spread, as in HL. Extensive extranodal disease is more common in children with NHL than adults with NHL. Therefore, the clinical staging system proposed at the St Jude Children's Research Hospital (Table 17.4) has been widely accepted. It relies on noninvasive procedures that can be carried out expeditiously. Like the Ann Arbor staging system, the St Jude staging system takes into account primary site as well

Table 17.4 St Jude staging system for non-Hodgkin lymphoma

Stage I
A single tumour (extranodal) or single anatomic area (nodal) with the exclusion of thoracic or abdomen
Stage II
A single tumour (extranodal) with regional node involvement
Two or more nodal areas on the same side of the diaphragm
Two single (extranodal) tumours with or without regional node involvement on the same side of the diaphragm
A primary gastrointestinal tract tumour that is resectable, usually in the ileocecal area, with or without involvement of associated mesenteric nodes
Stage III
Two single tumours (extranodal) on opposite sides of the diaphragm
Two or more nodal areas above and below the diaphragm
All the primary intrathoracic tumours (mediastinal, pleural, and thymic)
All extensive primary intraabdominal diseasea
All paraspinal or epidural tumours, regardless of other tumour site(s)
Stage IV
Any of the above with initial central nervous system and/or bone marrow involvement

Note: >25% blasts in the marrow is considered leukemic disease. Any identifiable tumour cell in the CSF constitutes CNS disease.

Modified from Murphy SB (1980) Classification, staging and end results of treatment of childhood non-Hodgkin's lymphomas: dissimilarities from lymphomas in adults. *Semin Oncol* **7**, 332–9.

as disease extent in assigning clinical stage. The primary differences between St Jude staging system and the Ann Arbor staging system are as follows:

In the St Jude Stage I disease, localized thoracic and abdominal disease are excluded, other localized extranodal disease, however, is considered Stage I.

In St Jude Stage II disease, localized (resected) abdominal disease is included, and again any thoracic disease is excluded.

St Jude Stage III disease includes any thoracic disease, paraspinal disease or facial nerve palsy in addition to disease on both sides of the diaphragm.

The only disease involvement considered Stage IV in St Jude system is marrow or central nervous system (CNS) disease.

Using the St Jude staging system, almost 40 per cent of children with NHL present with stage I and II and the remainder with more advanced stage III and IV disease. The distinction between lymphoma and leukemia is arbitrary and is based simply on the percentage of a bone marrow aspirate that is infiltrated by malignant cells. If the bone marrow has more than 25 per cent blasts or malignant cells, the patient is considered to have acute leukemia rather than NHL. Children with between 5 per cent and 25 per cent bone marrow involvement are considered to have stage IV NHL, whereas fewer than 5 per cent blasts in the bone marrow is considered to not have tumour involved. As opposed to many leukemia criteria, any identifiable tumour cell in the CSF constitutes CNS disease.

Treatment

Therapy of NHL is one of the most successful endeavours in paediatric oncology. Before the 1970s, only a small percentage of children with NHL could be cured of their disease by radiotherapy and surgery, limiting the cure to localized disease. Introduction of multiagent chemotherapy used in ALL, based on morphologic similarities between ALL and NHL, which invariably progress to a leukemic state if not treated, improved significantly NHL results. Presently, the role of surgery is limited to few selected cases of localized NHL where a complete excision of the tumour is possible upfront and to obtain good quality diagnostic material from a tissue biopsy. For extensive disease, debulking surgery is not recommended because it cannot be curative in most instances and likely delays the start of chemotherapy.

Radiotherapy has also a limited role in the modern treatment strategies and is associated with significant acute and late toxicity. Irradiation is still used in the treatment of central nervous system (CNS) dissemination of NHL, in case of emergency clinical conditions where a fast reduction of a tumour mass (i.e. mediastinal) is needed or to treat residual lymphoma in selected cases.

Chemotherapy is the treatment of choice in paediatric NHL, which should be considered as a systemic malignancy even in the case of apparently local disease.

In the early 1970s, investigators at St Jude applied chemotherapy regimens used for ALL to treat NHL; more intensive ALL regimens, including the LSA2L2 protocol from Memorial Sloan-Kettering and the APO (adriamycin, prednisone, vincristine) regimen developed at the Dana-Farber Cancer Institute were also introduced. Results of prospective application of these protocols defined some basic concepts used in the following decades. Leukemia regimens were superior in the treatment of LL while short, more intensive chemotherapy protocols achieved better results in BL. Another significant advancement was the introduction of high-dose methotrexate (HD-MTX) which, together with intrathecal administration of MTX, corticosteroids, and cytosine arabynoside (Ara-C), proved effective for CNS prophylaxis without cranial radiation.

Table 17.5 Treatment of disseminated NHL

WHO Classification	Regimen	EFS (%)
Burkitt	FAB/LMB (Group B, C)	70–90
	BFM 90/95	
	No craniospinal irradiation	
Lymphoblastic (T-cell and B-cell precursors)	BFM–NHL 90/95	80–90
	Craniospinal irradiation for CNS (+) only	
DLBCL	FAB/LMB (Group B, C)	85–90
	BFM 90/95	
	No craniospinal irradiation	
ALCL	ALCL99	70–75
	APO, NHL BFM 90	
	No craniospinal irradiation	

FAB, French-American-British; BFM, Berlin-Frankfurt-Munster; CNS, central nervous system; DLBCL, diffuse large B-cell lymphoma; ALCL, anaplastic large cell lymphoma; APO, Adriamycin (doxorubicin), prednisone, and vincristine; EFS, event-free survival; WHO, World Health Organization.

Precursor cell/lymphoblastic lymphoma

The use of ALL regimens has been effective when applied to the treatment of LL. The results of a Children's Cancer Group (CCG) trial that compared a modified LSA2L2 multiagent regimen, initially itroduced at Memorial Sloan-Kettering Cancer Center, with a cyclophosphamide, vincristine, methotrexate and prednisone (COMP) regimen led to the use of ALL regimens for advanced stage LL. Localized disease showed comparable results when treated with either regimen.

Following this study, LSA2L2-based protocols or, more recently, the BFM (Berlin-Frankfurt-Munster) or similar protocols have been used in paediatric LL reaching high cure rates (Table 17.5). Therapeutic components of LL treatment include an initial four- or five-drug induction chemotherapy with intrathecal therapy, followed by a consolidation phase with HD-MTX. A re-induction phase is based on the same drugs as induction therapy, but with lower cumulative doses and the substitution of dexamethasone for prednisone. A maintenance treatment with low dose 6-mercaptupurine and MTX is used to complete a total duration of 24 months treatment. In the most recent trials, prophylactic radiotherapy was omitted without any detrimental effetcs on survival due to the introduction of HD-MTX, but for patients with CNS disease at diagnosis cranial radiotherapy is still used. Presently, survival close to 90 per cent can be achieved in LL by most experienced groups. The oucome of resistant and relapsed LL, particularly of T-cell phenotype, is still dismal (in the range of 20 per cent) and heavily dependent on the possibililty of performing an allogeneic HSCT.

Burkitt lymphoma and other mature B-cell lymphomas

Early experience with African BL showed efficacy of cyclophosphamide as single agent in the treatment of localized disease, whereas advanced stage BL relapsed in the form of disseminated disease often involving also the CNS. Following this pioneering therapy, combination chemotherapy protocols were developed that included MTX and Ara-C in addition to corticosteroids and cyclophosphamide. The French LMB protocols achieved a EFS higher than 95 per cent in completely resected stage I–II BL with a 6-week therapy using the COPAD regimen (cyclophosphamide, vincristine, prednisone, doxorubicin). Similar outcome can be achieved for localized unresected BL treated with four cycles of combination chemotherapy using either the French (LMB) or BFM-based regimens. In the case of more advanced stage BL and B-cell ALL, intensified chemotherapy including a higher dose of cyclophosphamide, HD-MTX and Ara-C, with or without anthracyclines and epipodophyllotoxins, have been used. An important feature of the therapy for BL is the administration of consecutive chemotherapy courses at the shortest interval possibe, i.e. as soon as haematologic recovery is evident, in order to prevent regrowth of lymphoma cells. Because BL tends to disseminate and recur in the CNS; therefore, HD-MTX and HD-Ara-C, drugs that penetrate the CNS, are of critical relevance to obtain systemic antitumour effects, but also to accomplish an efficacious CNS prophylaxis together with intrathecal chemotherapy. By this approach, although with some differences in the structure of chemotherapy cyles, the most recent LMB/FAB and BFM trials achieved EFS of 90 per cent for stage III disease and 80–85 per cent for stage IV BL and B-ALL. Negative prognostic factors identified in these large collaborative studies are high levels of serum lactate dehydrogenase (LDH), little or no response to the cytoreductive chemotherapy (first week of treatment) and CNS involvement. Based on these observations different risk groups were identified that have significantly different prognosis, based on stage, tumour resectability, early response, and LDH values (Table 17.6). Good results of BL therapy rely certainly on the high-dose intensity treatment introduced in the last 15–20 years, but an important element for this success is the availability of adequate supportive care and adequate experience of the treating team. This is of great relevance because the highy effective LMB/FAB and BFM regimens have a high degree of acute toxicity and in the absence of adequate supportive care measures (i.e. prevention of acute cell lysis syndrome, prophylaxix and therapy of infections) the toxicity-related death rate may be significant. Thus, each paediatric oncologist must be aware of the efficacy, but also of the risks of such treatments and should carefully weight potential risks and benefits in relation to local conditions.

Treatment of patients with BL who have refractory or relapsed disease represents a challenge and salvage rates remain below 20 per cent, independently of the treatment used. This underlines

Table 17.6 Risk stratification schema

B-cell NHL (FAB/LMB)	
Stratum	Disease manifestations
A	Completely resected stage I and abdominal stage II
B	Multiple extraabdominal sites. Nonresected stage I and II, III, IV (bone marrow <25% blasts, no CNS disease)
C	mature B-ALL (>25% blasts in bone marrow) and/or CNS disease

B-cell NHL (BFM)	
Stratum	Disease manifestations
R1	Completely resected stage I and abdominal stage II
R2	Nonresected stage I/II and stage III with LDH <500 u/l
R3	Stage III with LDH 500–999 u/l
	Stage IV, B-ALL (>25% blasts), no CNS disease and LDH <1000 u/l
R4	Stage III, IV, B-ALL and LDH ≥1000 u/l
	Any CNS disease

FAB, French-American-British; BFM, Berlin-Frankfurt-Munster; CNS, central nervous system.

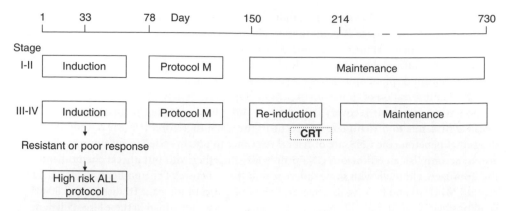

Fig. 17.1 Schema of the BFM-90 protocol for the treatment of pediatric lymphopblastic lymphoma. CRT = cranial radiotherapy

the need of an accurate evaluation of response achieved during first-line therapy, which may include second look-surgery and histological evaluation of residual tumour to assess whether viable lymphoma cells were still present before completion of chemotherapy. In case viable tumour is present at completion of chemotherapy, intensified treatment with autologous haematopietic stem cell rescue should be used. Autologous or allogeneic HSCT as consolidation therapy offers at present the only chance of long-term survival in case of resistant or relapsed disease, but preliminary achievement of a complete remission is essential. Recent analysis of HSCT for refractory or relapsed BL has shown similar long-term EFS for allogeneic or autologous HSCT, differently from LL where autologous HSCT has virtually no chance of cure. Some improvement may be derived from the addition of anti-CD20 monoclonal antibody (rituximab) to second-line chemotherapy, as indicated by studies of small series of relapsed BL/B-ALL patients. However, the role of anti-CD20 antibody in conjunction with first line chemotherapy currently is not clear. This will be one of the main issues to be addressed by future large cooperative trials, taking into consideration its possible detrimental effects on development of the immunological system in young patients.

Paediatric DLBCL are also treated on protocols designed for BL and the largest clinical trials conducted recently showed similar outcome for BL and DLBCL. This is in line with the biological

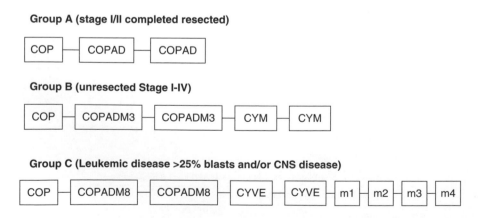

Fig. 17.2 Schema of the FAB-LMB trial for mature B-cell paediatric non-Hodgkin lymphoma.

studies that demonstrated similarities between BL and DLBCL in children, and significant differences between paediatric and adult DLBCL. Whether the addition of anti-CD20 may improve prognosis in paediatric DLBCL, as it was the case for the use of rituximab with CHOP (cyclophosphamide, doxorubicin, vincristine, prednisolone) or CHOP-like regimens in adults, remains to be demonstrated.

Among large B-cell lymphoma, PMBL represents a peculiar entity not only biologically, but also in terms of treatment. The EFS obtained by using BL-based therapies is significantly lower than EFS achieved for BL and DLBCL, although comparable to EFS obtained in adult PMBL treated with MACOP-B or VACOP-B or dose-adjusted EPOCH regimens. It would seem that longer therapy and the addition of rituximab may improve outcome. The use of local radiotherapy in case of mediastinal residue remains controversial.

Anaplastic large cell lymphoma

ALCL responds well to a variety of chemotherapy regimens and, differently from LL and BL, patients with ALCL can be frequently rescued by second line therapy after relapse. Due to its prevalent T-cell phenotype, LSA2L2 derived protocols were applied initially, but shorter treatments have been more recently introduced, such as the BFM and the APO regimens. OS for systemic ALCL is in the range of 90 per cent, although EFS is about 70–75 per cent in most trials. Interestingly, St Jude staging does not appear to correlate with prognosis. A large retrospetive evaluation of numerous prognostic parameters conducted in Europe, identified disease localizations in the mediastinum, liver, spleen, lung, and skin as negative prognostic factors, although more recently minimal disseminated disease has been shown to be perhaps a more significant prognostic feature for lower EFS in children with ALCL. The recent ALCL99 trial was conducted within the European Intergroup for Childhood NHL (EICNHL) by most European national groups and a Japanese collaborative group based on the BFM backbone with six 5-day cycles (similar to B-cell BFM protocol) including, in different combination, dexamethazone, ifosfamide, cyclophosphamide, HD-MTX, etoposide, Ara-C, doxorubicin, and intrathecal chemotherapy. This was the largest randomized study ever conducted in paediatric ALCL and demonstrated that CNS prophylaxis can be omitted when HD-MTX is used, but fail to demonstrate a benefit of addition of vinblastine during the induction phase and weekly during a maintenance treatment to complete 1-year therapy. Overall survival (OS) and EFS of the entire population were 94 per cent and 71 per cent, respectively. The Paediatric Oncology Group (POG) conducted two randomized trials based on the APO (doxorubicin, prednisone, vincristine) which demonstrated no significant benefit of the addition of consolidation cycles with intermediate dose MTX and Ara-C, or the addition of cyclophosphamide to standard APO arm.

Relapsed ALCL can be rescued by various treatments, including single drug therapy. Recently, the French group reported a retrospective analysis of relapsed ALCL treated with vinblastine alone showing efficacy of such an approach even after multiple relapses. Effect of single drug therapy as second-line treatment and increasing evidence of immunological response to ALCL *in vivo*, suggest that treatment intensity may not be a critical issue in this disease. A role for the anti-tumour activity of the immune system is also suggested by the superiority of allogeneic HSCT compared to autologous HSCT in resistant/relapsed ALCL, which suggest a graft-versus-lymphoma effect.

Although systemic ALCL need chemotherapy to be cured, cutaneous ALCL (with no other disease localization) represents a condition that should suggest caution before starting chemotherapy as it may spontaneously regress. In this case, chemotherapy should be initiated only if isolated cutaneous ALCL convert to systemic disease (i.e. involving lymph nodes or other sites).

Future considerations

Refinements in systemic chemotherapy based largely on patterns of spread, risk of relapse, and the immunophenotype of the NHL in children have led to cure rates in approximately 80–85 per cent of all patients. Much of this progress has been by dose intensification of chemotherapy. Dose reductions and the elimination of the routine use of radiotherapy have been demonstrated to be feasible while maintaining excellent outcomes in some patients. With better understanding to the pathogenesis and molecular biology of paediatric NHL, specific molecule/pathway targeting certainly holds much promise. However, the fact remains that almost half the children with BL in Africa can be cured with very minimal therapy. Therefore, improvement of risk classification through more sensitive diagnostic tools and/or identification of patients with disease very sensitive earlier in therapy remains a challenge.

Further reading

Anderson JR, Jenkin RD, Wilson JF, et al. (1993) Long-term follow-up of patients treated with COMP or LSA2L2 therapy for childhood non-Hodgkin's lymphoma: a report of CCG-551 from the Childrens Cancer Group. *J Clin Oncol* **11**, 1024–32.

Burkhardt B (2009) Paediatric lymphoblastic T-cell leukemia and lymphoma: one or two diseases? *Br J Haematol* **149**, 653–8.

Cairo MS, Sposto R, Perkins SL, et al. (2003) Burkitt's and Burkitt-like lymphoma in children and adolescents: a review of the Children's Cancer Group experience. *Br J Haematol* **120**, 660–70.

Damm-Welk C, Busch K, Burkhardt B, et al. (2007) Prognostic significance of circulating tumor cells in bone marrow or peripheral blood as detected by qualitative and quantitative PCR in pediatric NPM-ALK-positive anaplastic large-cell lymphoma. *Blood* **110**, 670–7.

Gross TG, Hale GA, He W, et al. (2010) Hematopoietic stem cell transplantation for refractory or recurrent non-hodgkin lymphoma in children and adolescents. *Biol Blood Marrow Transplant* **16**, 223–30.

Klapper W, Szczepanowski M, Burkhardt B, et al. (2008) Molecular profiling of pediatric mature B-cell lymphoma treated in population-based prospective clinical trials. *Blood* **112**, 1374–81.

Laver JH, Kraveka JM, Hutchinson RE, et al. (2005) Advanced-stage large-cell lymphoma in children and adolescents: results of a randomized trial incorporating intermediate dose methotrexate and high dose ARA-C in the maintenance phase of the APO regimen. A Pediatric Oncology Group phase III trial. *J Clin Oncol* **23**, 541–7.

Le Deley M-C, Reiter A, Williams D, et al. (2008) Prognostic factors in childhood anaplastic large cell lymphoma: results of a large European intergroup study. *Blood* **111**, 1560–6.

Le Deley M-C, Rosolen A, Williams DM, et al. (2010) Vinblastine in children and adolescents with high-risk anaplastic large-cell lymphma: results of the randomized ALCL99-vinblastine. *J Clin Oncol* **28**, 3987–93.

Magrath IT (1991) African Burkitt's lymphoma. History, biology, clinical features, and treatment. *Am J Pediatr Hematol Oncol* **13**, 222–46.

Morris SW, Kirstein MN, Valentine MB, et al. (1994) Fusion of a kinase gene, ALK, to a nucleolar protein gene, NPM, in non-Hodgkin's lymphoma. *Science* **26**, 1281–4.

Murphy SB. (1980) Classification, staging and end results of treatment of childhood non-Hodgkin's lymphomas: dissimilarities from lymphomas in adults. *Semin Oncol* **7**, 332–9.

Mussolin K, Pillon M, d'Amore ES, et al. (2005) Prevalence and clinical implications of bone marrow involvement in pediatric anaplastic large cell lymphoma. *Leukemia* **19**, 1643–7.

Mussolin L, Basso K, Pillon M, et al. (2003) Prospective analysis of minimal bone marrow infiltration in pediatric Burkitt's lymphomas by long-distance polymerase chain reaction for t(8;14)(q24;q32). *Leukemia* **17**, 585–9.

Patte C, Auperin A, Gerrard M, et al. (2007) Results of the randomized international FAB/LMB96 trial for intermediate risk B-cell non-Hodgkin lymphoma in children and adolescents: it is possible to reduce treatment for the early responding patients. *Blood* **109**, 2773–80.

Patte C, Auperin A, Michon J, et al. (2001) The Societe Francaise d'Oncologie Pediatrique LMB89 protocol: highly effective multiagent chemotherapy tailored to the tumor burden and initial response in 561 unselected children with B-cell lymphomas and L3 leukemia. *Blood* **97**, 3370–9.

Percy CL, Smith MA, Linet M, et al. (1999) Lymphomas and reticuloendothelial neoplasms. In: Ries LAG, Smith MA, Gurney JG, et al. (eds) *Cancer incidence and survival among children and adolescents. United States SEER Program 1975–1995.* Bethesda, MD: National Cancer Institute, SEER Program. NIH Pub. No. 99-4649, 35–49.

Perkins, SL (2000) Work-up and diagnosis of pediatric non-Hodgkin's lymphomas. *Pediatr Dev Pathol* **3**, 374–90.

Reiter A, Schrappe M, Ludwig WD, et al. (2000) Intensive ALL-type therapy without local radiotherapy provides a 90% event-free survival for children with T-cell lymphoblastic lymphoma: a BFM group report. *Blood* **95**, 416–21.

Sandlund JT, Santana V, Abromowitch M, et al. (1994) Large cell non-Hodgkin lymphoma of childhood: clinical characteristics and outcome. *Leukemia* **8**, 30–4.

Seidemann K, Tiemann M, Lauterbach I, et al. (2003) Primary mediastinal large B-cell lymphoma with sclerosis in pediatric and adolescent patients: treatment and results from three therapeutic studies of the Berlin-Frankfurt-Munster Group. *J Clin Oncol* **21**, 1782–9.

Seidemann K, Tiemann M, Schrappe M, et al. (2001) Short-pulse B-non-Hodgkin lymphoma-type chemotherapy is efficacious treatment for pediatric anaplastic large cell lymphoma: a report of the Berlin-Frankfurt-Munster Group Trial NHL-BFM 90. *Blood* **97**, 3699–706.

Stein H., Foss HD, Dürkop H, et al. (2000) CD30(+) anaplastic large cell lymphoma: a review of its histopathologic, genetic, and clinical features. *Blood* **96**, 3681–95.

WHO (2008) Classification of Tumours of Haematopoietic and Lymphoid Tissues. Lyon, France: IARC.

Woessmann W, Seidemann K, Mann G, et al. (2005) The impact of the methotrexate administration schedule and dose in the treatment of children and adolescents with B-cell neoplasms: a report of the BFM Group Study NHL-BFM95. *Blood* **105**, 948–58.

Chapter 18

Hodgkin lymphoma: modern management of children and young adults

Robert Johnston, Dieter Korholz
and Hamish Wallace

Introduction

The features of Hodgkin lymphoma (HL) were first documented by Thomas Hodgkin (1798–1866) in 1832 when he described the abnormal appearances of the spleen and lymph nodes in seven patients at post mortem. Wilks further elaborated these findings with 15 additional cases, subsequently naming the disease after Thomas Hodgkin. The classical variant of this malignant condition is characterized histologically by the Hodgkin/Reed Sternberg (HRS) cell, whereas the rare and distinct nodular lymphocyte predominant subtype (NLPHL) has unique clinico-pathological features. This chapter will outline the epidemiological, aetiological, and clinical factors as well as treatment strategies and current issues in the management of this malignancy.

Epidemiology

Lymphoma causes 4 per cent of all malignancy worldwide of which HL contributes 20–30 per cent. In Europe and US, the incidence is approximately 3.6–7 per million children per year and follows a characteristic age-specific bimodal pattern, with two peaks in incidence between 15–30 years and 45–55 years. However, there are complex geographical and ethnical variations in patterns of incidence worldwide. According to Caporaso, there are three epidemiological patterns of disease:

type I where there is a peak in male children and a second peak around the age of 50 years, with mixed cellularity and lymphocyte depleted the predominant histological subtypes

type II in rural areas of developed countries with a childhood peak and a second decade peak among women

type III in urbanized developed countries with a bimodal pattern peaking firstly in young adulthood with nodular sclerosis the predominant histological subtype, rising continuously after the age 40 years.

It is suggested that this pattern is consistent with socioeconomic conditions. For example, in developing countries an earlier onset of HL is seen, possibly associated with poor socio-economic conditions; there the incidence in younger children appears to be higher with the first peak of incidence earlier when compared with those more developed countries. This may reflect the lower standard of environmental hygiene and earlier onset infections. Additionally, in regions such as North Africa and the Middle East, mixed cellularity subgroup occurs in up to 50 per cent of cases, whereas in Western Europe and North America, nodular sclerosing subtype, which is not usually associated with Epstein–Barr virus (EBV), is much more common occurring in two-thirds of all cases. NLPHL is more common in males with a 3:1 preponderance and median age at presentation of 30–40 years.

Aetiology

The aetiology of HL remains unclear although an infectious aetiology is suspected. The characteristic extensive inflammatory component on histology, associated with acute onset disease with fever, night sweats and lymphadenopthy, as well as the increased incidence in immune-deficient individuals lend credence to theories of an infectious aetiology. In contrast to developed countries, the incidence of HL in developing countries is greater in childhood, suggesting that it may be a rare consequence of a common infection, the risk of which is greater at a younger age in less well-developed countries and may be delayed by improving living conditions. Studies from the US and Scandinavia suggest an association with socioeconomic affluence and family structure, with increased risk in young adulthood in first born children and those with greater number of younger siblings, consistent with an infectious aetiology with delayed exposure to a common infectious agent.

Epstein-Barr virus (EBV) has been implicated as an aetiological agent with EBV-positivity seen in up to 90 per cent in developing countries when compared with 30–50 per cent in industrialized countries. Overall, HL is uncommon before the age of 5 years but younger age is also associated with EBV positivity. The clinical syndrome of infectious mononucleosis (IM) related to EBV infection confers a 2.5-fold increased risk to develop HL, increased to 3.5-fold in young adults, possibly because IM typically occurs during adolescence. In addition, elevated anti-EBV antibodies are often seen in patients with, and are associated with increased risk of future HL. EBV has been demonstrated within the HRS cell in 30–40 per cent of cases. EBV readily transforms B lymphocytes *in vitro* and when found in HRS cells the virus is monoclonal, indicating it was present before transformation took place. One hypothesis for the pathogenesis is that, following primary infection, EBV lies latent in the memory B lymphocytes causing chronic stimulation, gene rearrangement, and production of cytokines triggering the development of the HRS cell. In healthy infected individuals, EBV-replication and transformation is prevented by the presence of normal T-cell immunity, not present in some immune-deficient individuals, explaining the increased risk of in these patients.

The HL tumour mass consists largely of inflammatory cells with only around 1 per cent of the mass consisting of neoplastic cells. Thus, the microenvironment and its interaction with the neoplastic cell through cytokines such as IL-13 are important in the development of the disease. Inhibition of IL-13 has been shown to reduce proliferation of HRS cells. The inflammatory component of the tumour mass consists largely of IL-10 secreting T lymphocytes. IL-10 and other cytokines have been shown to be associated with B-symptoms (see below) and high levels correlate with a poorer prognosis.

Classification

Previously a number of different classification systems were used for HL and there was little international consensus. In 1984, with increasing knowledge regarding previously known diagnoses and recognition of new disease entities, the classification was further defined based on current morphologic, immunologic and genetic factors, creating the Revised European-American Lymphoma 'REAL' Classification of HL (see Table 18.1). This classification has subsequently been accepted by the World Health Organization in their most recent classification of lymphomas.

Table 18.1 The revised European-American lymphoma classification

A. Classical Hodgkin Lymphoma	Lymphocyte-rich classical
	Nodular sclerosing
	Mixed cellularity
	Lymphocyte depleted
B. Nodular lymphocyte predominant	

Clinical presentation

Classical HL typically presents with painless cervical lymphadenopathy, the most common present-ing symptom (80 per cent of cases) with mediastinal involvement in 60 per cent, and only 5 per cent affecting the upper cervical nodes. Palpable lymph nodes will typically have a 'rubbery' consistency. Twenty to thirty per cent of children will have systemic features at presentation characterized by unexplained weight loss of 10 per cent body weight over the preceding 6 months, unexplained per-sistent or recurrent fever, or recurrent drenching night sweats. This group of presenting symptoms are termed B-symptoms and have important prognostic significance. Mediastinal lymphadenopa-thy may manifest with cough, dyspnoea or orthopnoea and lead to compression of the airway with resultant respiratory compromise or superior vena cava obstruction. Respiratory symptoms from pulmonary parenchymal involvement are uncommon. Pruritis occurs infrequently, and isolated hepatosplenomegaly is uncommon. Anaemia may be the result of poor utilization of iron or increased red cell destruction and, rarely, Coombs-positive haemolytic anaemia. Bone marrow involvement and resultant cytopenia occurs in approximately 3 per cent of cases at presentation.

Nodular lymphocyte predominant Hodgkin lymphoma (NLPHL) is a rare clinicopathological subtype, distinct from classical HL. It occurs in an older age group, predominantly in males, and presentation is characterized by low stage disease. Prolonged symptom duration prior to diagnosis is characteristic; in 50–60 per cent of cases diagnosis is 6–12 months from initial presentation of lymphadenopathy. There is a propensity for axillae and neck node involvement and mediastinal (15 per cent) and extranodal involvement is uncommon at presentation (spleen 10–15 per cent, liver <10 per cent, bone marrow/lung <5 per cent). When compared with classical HL, NLPHL is characterized by lower stage disease (stage I–II 70–80 per cent) at presentation, with B-symptoms occurring in only 5–10 per cent, and bulky disease in less than 10 per cent.

Investigation and staging

Diagnosis of HL requires detailed histological examination from tissue obtained from excision biopsy of involved tissue. Needle aspiration is not suitable as it will not offer adequate examination of lymph node structure and cellular elements.

Using the WHO criteria, the diagnosis and differentiation of HL requires detailed understanding of the histopathological appearance of the neoplastic cells, the characteristic inflammatory back-ground with surrounding stroma and the immunophenotypic characteristics of the different subtypes. The diagnosis of classical HL requires demonstration of the binucleate Reed/Sternberg cells (HRS cells), characterized by owl-eye-like nucleoli.

The histopathology of nodular sclerosing classical HL is characterized by fewer classical HRS cells and an abundance of lacunar cells, with smaller nuclei and less prominent nucleoli than occurs in the classical HRS cell. The lacunar cells are found in cellular nodules with a back-ground of inflammatory cells. The nodules are surrounded by dense fibrotic layer. In contrast, lymphocyte-depleted classical HL has a variable background with a characteristic predominance of classical HRS cells and, as the name suggests, the inflammatory background contains fewer lymphocytes. Mixed-cellularity classical HL contains much less fibrosis than the nodular sclerosing variant, and the inflammatory background consists of various cells including lymphocytes, neutrophils, and histiocytes. Lymphocyte-rich classical HL is characterized by follicles consisting of lymphocytes and RS cells, with few other inflammatory cells.

NLPHL typically features a nodular growth pattern but this may become more diffuse. HRS cells are not present. Instead, the neoplastic cell (the LP cell) has a broad range of morphological features but lacks the prominent nucleoli of the HRS cell. The immunophenotype differs markedly between the HRS cell and LP cells. Although of B-cell lineage, HRS cells of classical HL do not express the characteristic B-cell markers CD20 and CD79a. In contrast, the LP cell is typically positive for both. Nearly all Classical HL is positive for CD30 with 85 per cent positive for CD15. The LP cell is negative for both.

Blood investigations at presentation may show anaemia as a result of poor iron utilization or rarely haemolytic anaemia. Lymphopenia is suggestive of advanced disease at presentation. Eosinophilia occurs in approximately 15 per cent of cases. Pancytopenia is rare and when present suggests probable bone marrow involvement. Elevated erythrocyte sedimentation rate (ESR), alkaline phosphatase and serum copper are associated with more advanced stage and systemic symptoms but do not offer independent prognostic value.

Accurate staging is essential at diagnosis to define location and extent of disease, to further define clinical manifestations, and outline prognostic factors. Stage at presentation is assigned according to the Ann-Arbor staging system and is utilized to plan treatment. This system was modified in 1988 (see Table 18.2) as, prior to this, staging laparotomy with splenectomy was used

Table 18.2 Ann Arbor staging classification of Hodgkin lymphoma (Cotswold modification)

Stage	
I	Single independent lymph node region (I) or lymphatic structure (e.g. Waldeyer's ring, spleen) or a single extra lymphatic site (I_E)
II	Two or more lymph node regions on the same side of the diaphragm, without (II) or with (II_E) extra lymphatic involvement
III	Lymph node regions on both sides of the diaphragm without (III) or with (III_E) extra lymphatic involvement
IV	Disseminated involvement of extra nodal sites beyond 'E' sites
Systemic symptoms	
A	No symptoms
B	Unexplained weight loss of 10% body weight over preceding 6 months
	Unexplained persistent or recurrent fever (>38°C)
	Recurrent drenching night sweats
Extension	
E	Involvement of a single extra nodal site in close proximity to known nodal site
Bulky disease	Widening of the mediastinum more than one-third of the diameter of the chest at level T5–6 on chest X-ray
X	
	The largest nodal mass measures 10 cm or greater in maximal dimension (in the European childhood trials this definition is not used for upstaging of patients)

to complete staging but this carries no benefit over modern imaging techniques and is no longer utilized, with the added benefit of a reduction in surgical complications and avoidance of risk of overwhelming post-splenectomy sepsis.

A combination of imaging modalities is employed in the initial staging. Chest X-ray is used to document mediastinal mass. Chest computed tomography (CT) is useful to document intrathoracic lymph node enlargement not seen on plain chest radiograph, including the hilar and mediastinal regions. Chest CT is superior to magnetic resonance imaging (MRI) in imaging lung parenchymal disease and is useful to assess pleural, pericardial, and chest wall involvement. MRI, however, has the advantage of improved soft-tissue contrast and does not involve the use of ionizing radiation and is therefore the preferred modality for cross-sectional imaging at sites other than lung parenchyma.

Bone marrow involvement is rare in HL but its presence indicates stage IV disease and documentation of bone marrow status is recommended when staging has already identified disease greater than stage IIA. MRI may be used to image large areas of bone marrow and is highly sensitive in the detection of focal bone marrow involvement.

Overall, however, conventional imaging modalities have limited ability to accurately detect active disease in normally sized lymph nodes or at extranodal sites such as spleen and liver and in the assessment of residual tumour masses after therapy. In the current European study (EuroNet-PHL-C1), FDG-PET (see below) is being used in addition to conventional imaging. The strategy under evaluation is that a lymph node ≥2.0 cm in diameter is considered as involved with HL irrespective of the PET result, whilst lymph nodes <1.0 cm in largest diameter are considered as uninvolved even they are PET positive. Only in case of lymph nodes sized between 1 and 2 cm is the uptake of FDG-PET used to determine tumour involvement.

Treatment of classical Hodgkin lymphoma

Stratification by prognostic factors

In adult trials, increased ESR (erythrocyte sedimentation rate) and alkaline phosphatase levels were associated with a poorer prognosis in advanced stage HL. The International Prognostic Factors Score was established by analysis of > 5000 adult patients with HL and defined risk factors as: albumin level <4.0 g/dl; haemoglobin <10.5 g/dl; male sex and age over 45 years; stage IV disease; leukocytosis >15 x 109/L; lymphopenia <0.6 x 109/l. Patients with five or more risk factors had progression-free survival of 42 per cent compared to 84 per cent in those with no risk factors. However, when treatment intensity was increased, the value of these prognostic factors seemed to disappear. In future, prognostic factors other than stage might re-emerge if new approaches such as that used in the Euronet-PHL-C1 trial indicate that it is possible to maintain a high cure rate while reducing late effects by reducing burden of treatment.

Stratification by response adaption

To limit the late risks of therapy, some studies have tried to avoid the use of radiotherapy after chemoptherapy. Patients in the German GPOH-HD 95 trial received no radiotherapy after end of chemotherapy if they reached a complete remission (defined by volume reduction of >95 per cent and residual tumour volume <2 ml). Using this strategy the 5-year event-free survival (EFS) for patients with early stage disease was no different with (94 per cent) or without (97 per cent) radiotherapy, although patients with intermediate and advanced stage disease fared significantly less well without radiotherapy (5 year EFS 91 per cent vs 79 per cent). The conclusion is that conventional imaging to define adequacy of response to treatment in higher stage disease does not safely inform which patients can avoid radiotherapy.

A similar study by the North American COG studied 501 patients achieving complete remission (CR)—defined either by radiological CR or >70 per cent tumour response with all initially gallium-positive tumour sites becoming negative—who were randomized to receive radiotherapy vs no further treatment. The 3-year EFS was 93 per cent for those receiving radiotherapy and 85 per cent for those who did not but there was no difference in overall outcome.

It is clear that better ways are needed to determine adequacy of response in guiding decisions about the use of radiotherapy. 18-Fluorodeoxyglucose (FDG) is a glucose analogue transported across the cell membrane of highly active cells such as the brain, liver, and most tumours. After intracellular phosphorylation it is not metabolized further and, trapped within the cell, it reflects metabolic activity. Combined with CT, FDG-PET (positron emission tomography) reports a consistently high negative predictive value (81–100 per cent) in identifying patients with an excellent prognosis. In the ongoing EuroNet-PHL-C1 trial, patients with an adequate response to two cycles of OEPA (vincristine, etoposide, prednisone and adriamycin)—defined by a complete metabolic response detected by FDG-PET and at least a partial morphological response detected by CT or MRI—will not receive radiotherapy at the end of chemotherapy.

FDG-PET for response assessment

There are several studies determining the prognostic value of FDG-PET in patients with HL. One study published in children showed that after two cycles and at the end of chemotherapy, PET showed more negative results compared to CT or MRI. The sensitivity and negative predictive value of response by PET was 100 per cent and it now appears that patients with early normalization of PET response have an excellent prognosis. In the European EuroNet-PHL-C1 trial the good prognosis of patients with a negative early response to PET is taken into account to reduce treatment burden. However, until further experience is accrued, it remains the case that PET-guided treatment reduction should still only be performed for patients within the context of a clinical trial.

What is the best treatment for young people with HL?

There is ongoing controversy about the best treatment for adolescent and young adult patients with classical HD. Recent data from the German Hodgkin Study group for advanced stage patients treated with eight cycles of BEACOPP (bleomycin, etoposide, doxorubicin, cyclophosphamide, vincristine, prednisolone and procarbazine) followed by radiotherapy to initial bulky disease and residual tumour after chemotherapy showed 10 year freedom from treatment failure and overall survival rates of 82% and 86% respectively. However, despite these excellent results, the cumulative risk of secondary leukemia was 3 per cent. In contrast, comparable results were achieved for patients with stage IIBE, IIIB and IV disease treated with two cycles of OEPA (vincristine, etoposide, prednisone and adriamycin) followed by four cycles of COPP or COPDAC [vincristine, cyclophosphamide, procarbazine for females (COPP) or dacarbazine for males (COPDAC) and prednisone] and involved field with a risk of secondary leukemia of less than 1 per cent. This highlights the importance of studies to moderate the risk of late sequelae whilst maintaining good survival rates.

Treatment of nodular lymphocyte predominant Hogkin lymphoma (NLPHL)

Previously, NLPHL was treated according to classical HL protocols but it is now recognized that this might be a different entity since it affects mainly boys and characteristically presents at early stages. Preliminary experience from the French study group showed 7/10 patients with complete response after surgery, but 0/4 patients after surgery remained in complete remission without further treatment. Similar results were confirmed by a report from the European study group and the ongoing European trial seeks to confirm these results by using a surgery-alone strategy in patients with completely resectable low stage (Ia) disease. Patients with unresectable stage Ia or IIa disease receive a low-dose chemotherapy combination with cyclophosphamide, vincristine and prednisolone. The few patients with advanced stage NLPHL are treated according to the classical HL protocol.

Management of relapsed and refractory HL

Cure rates following first-line therapy for HL are high. However, 10 per cent of early stage and 20–25 per cent of advanced stage disease classical HL will relapse. Treatment of relapse involves a multimodal approach with radiotherapy in combination with standard dose chemotherapy, high-dose chemotherapy with autologous or allogeneic hemopoietic stem cell transplant (HSCT).

There are no randomized trials in children defining the best treatment of relapse. There is evidence to support a risk-adapted approach to determine which patients may be successfully treated with further standard-dose chemotherapy and involved field radiotherapy, or require high-dose chemotherapy with autologous HSCT. Time to relapse and response to initial salvage chemotherapy are the most important prognostic indicators. Progressive disease on treatment or relapse within 3 moths of completion of first-line therapy carries the worst prognosis (OS rates approximately 50 per cent) and improved outcomes are seen in early relapse (3–12 months from treatment with OS 75–80 per cent) and in late relapse (>12 months off treatment with OS 90 per cent).

Patients who are refractory to salvage chemotherapy have a very poor prognosis (OS < 20 per cent) and additional markers of poor outcome include original stage, stage at relapse, B-symptoms at relapse and high LDH or large residual mediastinal mass at time of autologous HSCT.

A low-risk group comprising late relapse (>12-months after completion of first-line treatment) and limited stage disease may be effectively managed with standard dose chemotherapy with involved-field radiotherapy. Alternating cycles of IEP-ABVD (ifosamide, etoposide, prednisolone and doxorubicin, bleomycin, vinblastine, dacarbazine) are used with radiotherapy to involved sites at relapse and to original sites if radiotherapy was not used in primary therapy. Primary refractory high-risk disease is usually managed with high-dose chemotherapy and autologous HSCT. Options for high-dose chemotherapy include CBV (cyclophosphamide, BCNU and etoposide) which has been most widely used in North America, whereas in Europe the BEAM (BCNU, etoposide, cytarabine, melphalan) regimen is more frequently utilized and is the current strategy in the EuroNet PHL-C1 trial. In this study an intermediate-risk group is also defined for whom the optimal salvage approach remains unclear. In those who achieve a complete response, or a partial morphological response with FDG-PET negativity, after standard dose chemotherapy will proceed with the low-risk strategy of further standard-dose chemotherapy and involved field radiotherapy. Those failing to achieve complete response or who gain a partial response but with residual FDG-PET positivity receive consolidation with high-dose chemotherapy and autologous HSCT. The use of radiotherapy is determined on an individual basis and is dependent on previous radiotherapy exposure, stage at recurrence and toxicity considerations.

Patients with primary progressive and chemo-refractory disease at salvage also have poor outcomes with high-dose chemotherapy. Experience with allogeneic HSCT is limited in paediatric patients but may have a role in primary progressive HL that remains refractory to salvage chemotherapy as this group have a poor outcome with conventional high-dose chemotherapy and autologous HSCT.

As a result of the generally good outcomes achieved with treatment of relapsed HL, there is limited knowledge of the role for novel therapies. Gemcitabine in combination with conventional chemotherapy, and Everolimus have shown promise. CD-30 is expressed on the HRS cell offering a potential target for novel therapies including anti-CD-30 antibodies. There is also interest in rituximab (anti CD-20 monoclonal antibody) and its roles in disrupting the microenvironment of the HRS cell and targeting the putative HRS stem cell as well a direct effect on HRS cells which are CD-20 positive.

Late effects of treatment of HL

Long-term survival following treatment for HL may be compromised by a significant risk of treatment-related late-onset side effects, leading to significant morbidity and mortality. These depend on chemotherapy regimen and dosage as well as radiotherapy dosage and field of treatment but include adverse effects on fertility, thyroid dysfunction, cardiac and pulmonary complications, bone growth and soft tissue effects as well as second malignancy. Risk-adapted treatment protocols have been devised to reduce the frequency and severity of these side-effects but the recognition of the risk, appropriate monitoring for these adverse effects form an important part of ongoing care for survivors of treatment for HL. Although mortality from HL plateaus over time following completion of treatment, death from second malignancy and cardiovascular sequelae continues to increase over time.

Second malignancy is the leading cause of death in survivors of HL and occurs in between 6–8 per cent of survivors of HL during the 15 years following treatment. Wolden reported a relative risk of developing any second malignancy in females 15.4 [95% confidence interval (CI), 10.6–21.5] and 10.6 (95 % CI, 6.6–16.0) in males followed up for a median 13.1years following treatment for HL. Second malignancy can be categorized into three groups—leukaemia, non Hodgkin lymphoma (NHL) and solid tumours. The risk of leukaemia is maximal at 5-years post treatment and associated with the use of alkylating agents in a dose-dependent manner, although the use of large field radiotherapy has been suggested to play a role. There has, however, been a reduction in incidence of leukaemia following the reduction of anthracycline-based chemotherapy in first-line treatment in the 1990s; however the risk of secondary leukaemia remains particularly high following salvage therapy containing alkylating agents.

Although less common than leukaemia, there is an increased risk of NHL following treatment for primary HL. The pathogenesis remains unclear, however it may be related to the mutagenic effects of chemotherapy, altered immune surveillance or, possibly, histologic conversion of HL.

Seventy-five to eighty per cent of all second malignancy is caused by solid tumours, most commonly breast, lung, and gastrointestinal tumours. In contrast to leukaemia, the incidence of solid tumours increases with time after completion of treatment and may persist for many decades. The incidence of breast and lung cancers increases in a dose-dependent manner following radiotherapy. Women who received more than 5 Gy to the breast tissue have a 2.7-fold increased risk compared to those who received less than 5 Gy. This risk increases 8-fold for those who received more than 40 Gy. The risk of breast cancer appears to be reduced in women who have received alkylating agent therapy, probably due to their gonadotoxic effect, however the risk is not further modified in women with a significant family history of breast cancer.

Chemotherapy regimens containing alkylating agents appear to be more gonadotoxic than those without, leading to azoospermia in up to 90 per cent of cases on account of alkylating agent and procarbazine in the former regimens. The BEACOPP regimen developed by the German Hodgkin Study Group is associated with higher risk of sterility. In a recent study, no adult patients had normospermia following BEACOPP although recovery was noted in some patients and longer-term follow-up is required.

The effects of radiation therapy on ovarian function are determined by the site to which the radiotherapy is directed, the fractionation and dose of radiation, and the age of the patient. Additionally, concurrent use of gonadotoxic chemotherapy regimens including alkylating agents will render the patient infertile in almost 100 per cent of cases. Chemotherapy is associated with a 12-fold increased risk of premature menopause. There is a dose–response effect with higher doses of procarbazine and cyclophosphamide leading to an increased incidence of sub-fertility. BEACOPP may result in amenorrhoea in over 50 per cent women, whereas ABVD does not appear to affect fertility. Fertility preservation options including oophorpexy and ovarian cryopreservation should be considered in girls requiring radiation therapy to the pelvis.

Thyroid problems are a common complication of treatment of HL. Radiation therapy to the neck leads to hypothyroidism in almost 50 per cent of patients in the subsequent three decades in a dose-dependent manner. Other thyroid abnormalities are less common; radiation does greater than 35 Gy increase the risk of hyperthyroidism, which is 8-fold greater incidence than controls. Thyroid nodules occur with greater frequency and the incidence of thyroid carcinoma is rare, an estimated 18-fold increase incidence when compared with normal controls.

Further reading

Bhatia S, Yasui Y, Robison LL, et al (2003) Late Effects Study Group. High risk of subsequent neoplasms continues with extended follow-up of childhood Hodgkin's lymphoma: report from the Late Effects Study Group. *J Clin Oncol* **21**, 4386–94.

Caporaso NE, Goldin LR, Anderson WF, Landgren O (2009) Current insight on trends, causes, and mechanisms of Hodgkin's lymphoma. *Cancer J* **15**, 117–23.

Claviez A, Canals C, Dierickx D, et al (2009) Lymphoma and Pediatric Diseases Working Parties. Allogeneic hematopoietic stem cell transplantation in children and adolescents with recurrent and refractory Hodgkin lymphoma: an analysis of the European Group for Blood and Marrow Transplantation. *Blood* **114**, 2060–7.

Daw S, Wynn R, Wallace WH (2011) Management of Relapsed and Refractory Classical Hodgkin's Lymphoma in Children and Adolescents. *Br J Haematol* **152**, 249–60.

Diehl V, Sextro M, Franklin J, et al (1999) Clinical presentation, course, and prognostic factors in lymphocyte-predominant Hodgkin's disease and lymphocyte-rich classical Hodgkin's disease: report from the European Task Force on Lymphoma Project on Lymphocyte-Predominant Hodgkin's Disease. *J Clin Oncol* **17**, 776–83.

Eberle FC, Mani H, Jaffe ES. (2009) Histopathology of Hodgkin's Lmphoma. *Cancer J* **15**, 129–37.

Engert A, Diehl V, Franklin J, et al (2009) Escalated-dose BEACOPP in the treatment of patients with advanced-stage Hodgkin's lymphoma: 10 years of follow-up of the GHSG HD9 study. *J Clin Oncol* **27**, 4548–54.

Furth C, Steffen IG, Amthauer H, et al (2009). Early and late therapy response assessment with [18F] fluorodeoxyglucose positron emission tomography in pediatric Hodgkin's lymphoma: analysis of a prospective multicenter trial. *J Clin Oncol* **27**, 4385–91.

Gutensohn N, Cole P (1981) Childhood social environment and Hodgkin's disease. *N Engl J Med* **304**, 135–40.

Harris NL, Jaffe ES, Stein H, et al. (1994) A revised European-American classification of lymphoid neoplasms: a proposal from the International Lymphoma Study Group *Blood* **84**, 1361–92.

Hasenclever D, Diehl V (1998) A prognostic score for advanced Hodgkin's disease. International Prognostic Factors Project on Advanced Hodgkin's Disease. *N Engl J Med* **339**, 1506–14.

Hudson MM, Poquette CA, Lee J, (1998) Increased mortality after successful treatment for Hodgkin's disease. *J Clin Oncol* **16**, 3592–600.

Jaffe ES, Harris NL, Stein H, Vardiman JW (2001) *World Health Organization Classification of Tumours: Pathology and Genetics of Tumours of Haematopoietic and Lymphoid Tissues.* Lyon: IARC.

Lee AI, LaCasce AS (2009). Nodular lymphocyte predominant Hodgkin lymphoma. *Oncologist* **14**, 739–51.

Loeffler M, Pfreundschuh M, Hasenclever D, et al (1988) Prognostic risk factors in advanced Hodgkin's lymphoma. *Report of the German Hodgkin Study Group. Blut* **56**, 273–81.

Mackie EJ, Radford M, Shalet SM (1996) Gonadal function following chemotherapy for childhood Hodgkin's disease. *Med Pediatr Oncol* **27**, 74–8.

Mani H, Jaffe ES (2009) Hodgkin lymphoma: an update on its biology with new insights into classification. *Clin Lymphoma Myeloma* **9**, 206–16.

Mauz-Körholz C, Gorde-Grosjean S, Hasenclever D, et al (2007) Resection alone in 58 children with limited stage, lymphocyte-predominant Hodgkin lymphoma-experience from the European network group on pediatric Hodgkin lymphoma. *Cancer* **110**, 179–85.

Mauz-Körholz C, Hasenclever D, Dörffel W, et al (2010). Procarbazine-free OEPA-COPDAC chemotherapy in boys and standard OPPA-COPP in girls have comparable effectiveness in pediatric Hodgkin's lymphoma: the GPOH-HD-2002 study. *J Clin Oncol* **28**, 3680–6.

Nachman JB, Sposto R, Herzog P, et al (2002) Children's Cancer Group: Randomized comparison of low-dose involved-field radiotherapy and no radiotherapy for children with Hodgkin's disease who achieve a complete response to chemotherapy. *J Clin Oncol* **20**, 3765–71.

Ng AK, Mauch PM (2009) Late effects of Hodgkin's disease and its treatment. *Cancer J* **15**, 164–8.

Pellegrino B, Terrier-Lacombe MJ, Oberlin O, et al (2003) Study of the French Society of Pediatric Oncology. Lymphocyte-predominant Hodgkin's lymphoma in children: therapeutic abstention after initial lymph node resection—a Study of the French Society of Pediatric Oncology. *J Clin Oncol* **21**, 2948–52.

Rueffer U, Josting A, Franklin J, et al (2001) German Hodgkin's Lymphoma Study Group. Non-Hodgkin's lymphoma after primary Hodgkin's disease in the German Hodgkin's Lymphoma Study Group: incidence, treatment, and prognosis. *J Clin Oncol* **19**, 2026–32.

Sklar C, Whitton J, Mertens A, et al (2000) Abnormalities of the thyroid in survivors of Hodgkin's disease: data from the Childhood Cancer Survivor Study. *J Clin Endocrinol Metab* **85**, 3227–32.

Thorley-Lawson DA, Gross A (2004) Persistence of the Epstein-Barr virus and the origins of associated lymphomas. *N Engl J Med* **350**, 1328–37.

van Leeuwen FE, Chorus AM, van den Belt-Dusebout AW, et al (1994) Leukemia risk following Hodgkin's disease: relation to cumulative dose of alkylating agents, treatment with teniposide combinations, number of episodes of chemotherapy, and bone marrow damage. *J Clin Oncol* **12**, 1063–73.

Wallace WH, Anderson RA, Irvine DI (2005). Fertility preservation for young people with cancer: who is at risk and what can be offered? *Lancet Oncol* **6**, 209–18.

Wilks S (1865) Cases of enlargement of the lymphatic glands and spleen (or Hodgkin's disease), with remarks. *Guy's Hosp Rep* **11**, 56–7.

Wolden SL, Lamborn KR, Cleary SF, et al (1998) Second cancers following pediatric Hodgkin's disease. *J Clin Oncol* **16**, 536–44.

Young H, Baum R, Cremerius U, et al (1999) Measurement of clinical and subclinical tumour response using [18F]-fluorodeoxyglucose and positron emission tomography: review and 1999 EORTC recommendations. European Organization for Research and Treatment of Cancer (EORTC) PET Study Group. *Eur J Cancer* **35**, 1773–82.

Chapter 19

The histiocytoses

Maurizio Aricò and Sheila Weitzman

The term histiocytoses describes a group of disorders characterized by accumulation and/or proliferation of mononuclear phagocytes, comprising dendritic cells and macrophages. They originate from the bone marrow and spread over the body to contribute to immune system function and homeostasis.

The histiocytic disorders are classified into two main groups: dendritic cell-related disorders, the most frequent of which is Langerhans cell histiocytosis (LCH), and macrophage-related disorders represented by haemophagocytic lymphohistiocytosis (HLH).

Langerhans cell histiocytosis

Langerhans cell histiocytosis (LCH) is a rare disease. Its age-adjusted incidence rate has been reported between 5 and 6 cases per million per year. About two thirds of the patients are less than 5 years old at presentation, and the incidence rates decrease with age. The diagnosis is often delayed with only 2 per cent of the LCH cases enrolled in clinical trials being diagnosed within the first month.

The gold standard for diagnosis rests on histology: a lesion that is morphologically appropriate for LCH (cytoplasm-rich pale histiocytes interspersed with inflammatory cells, eosinophils, and lymphocytes), in which lesional cells demonstrate CD1 and Langerin (CD207) positivity. In current practice, electron microscopy for Birbeck granules is now largely obsolete. It is important to note that pathological examination of LCH lesional tissue does not discriminate between lesions that remain localized from those that disseminate.

The pathogenesis of LCH remains elusive. Many attempts to document a specific viral pathogen have been inconclusive. Evidence of clonality of lesional cells was considered by some authors as proof for malignancy of LCH which was, however, not accepted by the majority of investigators in the light of lack of histologic evidence of malignancy, lack of genetic aberrations, and frequent spontaneous regression of the disease. The recent demonstration of mutations in the *BRAF* oncogene in many cases of LCH seems once again to favor a diagnosis of malignancy.

On purely clinical grounds, LCH behaves as a non-familial disorder. Yet, familial clustering has been observed in 1 per cent of cases. Furthermore, concordance for the disease in over 80 per cent of identical twin pairs, versus less than 15 per cent of fraternal twins, suggests a genetic component in the pathogenesis of LCH. Analysis of chromosomes from peripheral blood lymphocytes of patients with LCH, or even of cells from lesional tissue, failed to document specific, recurrent chromosomal aberrations. Evidence of chromosomal instability in patients with active disease might be related to the presence of a viral pathogen.

Recent studies showed that cultures from peripheral blood cells of patients with LCH may provide a model for the lesional granuloma and that IL-17 appears to play a primary role in its pathogenesis. Whether this may provide additional novel insights into the pathogenesis or even disclose novel avenues for non-chemotherapy driven therapeutic approaches, remains to be clarified.

Classification and nosology

The first responsibility of the attending physician upon diagnosis of LCH is to define whether the disease is restricted to one site or tissue (unifocal single system), involves many different sites within one tissue type (multifocal single system usually skin or bone) or whether it involves many different tissues or organs (multisystem). For the purpose of the present review, the different organs will be discussed separately.

Bone LCH

Painful swelling is the most frequent cause for consultation in patients with localized LCH. The skull, long bones, and then the flat bones are most frequently involved, while hands and feet are usually spared. Overall, bone involvement has been observed in 80–100 per cent of cases in large published series. Plain radiography remains the first-line approach for detection of bone lesions and usually shows single or multiple irregularly marginated lytic lesions, sometimes with swelling of adjacent soft tissue. Peripheral sclerosis is considered a sign of initial healing. Periosteal thickening may mimic malignancy in some cases. At the time of diagnosis, combined use of computed tomography (CT) and magnetic resonance imaging (MRI) may better define the lytic lesion and the surrounding soft tissue alteration. Radioisotope scanning has been largely used to screen for subclinical, potentially involved sites and recently FDGP-PET scanning (positron emission tomography using the glucose analogue FDGP) has been suggested to be the most sensitive for diagnosis and follow-up. Clinical features and possible complications of the osteolytic lesions depend on the bone involved. Involvement of the ear and mastoid bone may mimic mastoiditis clinically and radiologically; periorbital involvement may lead to proptosis and mimic orbital sarcomas and vertebral involvement may result in vertebra plana, while an associated soft tissue mass may result in paraplegia.

Skin LCH

Skin involvement is observed in over one third of children with LCH. More frequently affected sites are the scalp and diaper areas, but any area may be affected. The lesions may appear as reddish papules that progress and ulcerate, or depigmentate and heal. Skin is reported as the only affected site in about 10 per cent of cases, especially in male infants, and in such cases spontaneous regression is frequent but early progression to involve 'risk' organs may occur and the patients need to be closely observed. In some cases, isolated skin involvement may be misdiagnosed as seborrhoic dermatitis thus delaying the diagnosis. Interestingly, skin involvement rarely appears in follow up if not present at diagnosis.

Lymph nodes

Nodes may be enlarged in a minority of patients, usually less than 10 per cent at presentation, as part of disseminated disease or as regional nodes associated with local disease affecting skin or bone. The cervical nodes are most frequently involved, and their enlargement may be massive. Occasionally nodal involvement may be the only clinical manifestation, sometime with a recurrent course.

Liver

Although hepatomegaly is very common in patients with disseminated disease, only a minority show altered liver function with evidence of reduced protein synthesis (hypoalbuminemia, ascites) or enzyme function (hyperbilirubinemia). Failure to achieve disease control rapidly may lead to progression, from mild cholestasis to portal infiltration, and sclerosing cholangitis. At this stage, progression of liver damage may be independent of the disease activity, with possible evolution toward end-stage dysfunction requiring liver transplant.

Spleen

Splenomegaly is observed in about 5 per cent of patients at diagnosis. In the course of refractory disease, this may contribute to cytopenia.

Lung

Lung involvement in paediatric LCH is usually part of multisystem disease. The child may have respiratory distress with tachypnea, retractions, and persistent cough. The radiological picture consists of diffuse, interstitial infiltration with nodules, which may evolve into cysts. Rupture of superficial cysts may cause spontaneous pneumothorax, occasionally representing the first manifestation of LCH in adolescents and, far more often, in smoking adults. Similar to the liver, at some point in the disease-course, lung fibrosis and pneumatization may become independent of active LCH and lung transplantation may become necessary.

Endocrine system

Diabetes insipidus (DI) presenting as polyuria and polydipsia, sometime as massive as 6–8 litres of daily water intake, should suggest possible LCH in children. An MRI scan may show loss of the posterior pituitary bright signal, and thickening of the pituitary stalk. Once the central origin of DI has been established, a thorough diagnostic work-up for possibly silent LCH localizations is mandatory. DI may present as the first manifestation of LCH or it may occur later, within months or even many years. DI develops more often in patients with brain or craniofacial lesions. Patients with DI may progress to multiple pituitary hormone deficiencies, the first usually is growth hormone deficiency with a median latency of about one year. Thyroid and gonadal hormone deficiency may follow.

Central nervous system

Cerebral masses, beyond the hypophyseal-pituitary, may be occasionally observed. A minority of patients, most often with preceding DI, develop progressive neurodegeneration with ataxia, coordination disturbances, and cranial nerve and neuropsychological defects during the disease course. A MRI scan shows a characteristic pattern of demyelination starting from the cerebellum, usually bilateral and symmetric. This picture is unfortunately expected to progress both clinically and radiologically, and the prognosis in these cases remains very poor due to lack of effective therapies.

Gastrointenstinal tract

Although unusual, intestinal malabsorption, diarrhoea, or protein-losing enteropathy may occur in patients with multisystem LCH.

Bone marrow

Although anaemia is common in patients with multisystem disease, this usually reflects persistent inflammation, while thrombocytopenia is usually considered a hallmark of aggressive disease. Cytopenia often occurs in the absence of morphologic bone marrow infiltration. Thus, bone marrow examination is not mandatory at the initial staging of patients with documented LCH. Application of a CD1a immunostain may improve detection of LCH cells in the bone marrow.

The diagnosis of LCH is not a difficult one in suspected cases. The clinical picture is suggestive in most cases; radiology usually demonstrates evidence of osteolytic lesions and skin (or bone) lesions may be easily biopsied to document infiltration. In the case of isolated lymphadenopathy, biopsy may provide abundant diagnostic material to rule out possible alternative diagnoses. The diagnosis of isolated central DI should always include a careful screening for undiagnosed LCH. Evidence of haemophagocytosis, seen in severe LCH, is more frequently associated with HLH, which in turn does not feature the peculiar skin rash and bone lesions.

Treatment

The natural course of solitary LCH lesions is usually one of spontaneous healing, supporting observation alone in patients with localized disease outside of vital organs. By contrast, the natural history of patients with multisystem, 'Letterer-Siwe' disease is usually fatal. Thus, the need for specific treatment depends on the number and type of involved sites. To address this issue, as in many other rare disorders, international, cooperative efforts were needed to allow accumulation of sufficient uniformly diagnosed and treated cases. To date, the Histiocyte Society has completed three prospective clinical trials, LCH-I to LCH-III. These trials defined the combination of vinblastine and steroids as the standard of treatment for patients with multifocal bone and multisystem LCH; 6-mercaptopurine was added in continuation phase but the addition of etoposide in LCH-II and methotrexate in LCH-III did not improve outcome. The studies also showed that early response assessment at 6 weeks is important. For poor responders, early move to salvage therapy improves survival and for those in partial remission at 6 weeks, repetition of the 6-week induction therapy appears associated with better disease control. Patients who achieve at least partial disease control within 6 weeks, followed by complete disease resolution, are not at risk for fatal outcome, but rather for possible late sequelae, such as hormone deficiencies or bone deformities. By contrast, multisystem patients, usually young babies, who present with liver dysfunction, splenomegaly or thrombocytopenia and who fail to achieve disease control at 6 weeks, are at significant risk of death, most often due to liver failure or infectious complications. As a consequence, different treatment strategies are needed for the different risk groups. In patients with single osteolytic lesions or skin-only disease, a wait-and-see strategy should be applied following the initial diagnostic procedure, unless there is a risk for deformity of a weight-bearing bone. In patients with multifocal bone disease, treatment should be aimed at prevention of the cascade of bone reactivations over the following months or even years. In children with multisystem, risk organ involvement, aggressive chemotherapy is necessary to prevent a rapidly fatal outcome. For poor responders, treatment intensification with chemotherapy (cytarabine and cladribine) or sometimes even haematopoietic stem cell transplantation (HSCT) is warranted. Radiotherapy, which has been widely employed in the past, has a very limited role today, due to inherent toxicity and risk of cancer.

Late effects

The quality of survival for patients with localized disease or disseminated disease that responds to treatment remains dependent on the morbidity generated by the disease or treatment itself. Bone disease may result in deformities, in the affected bone or associated abnormalities like tooth loss or deafness. Significant bone deformities may be seen in patients previously treated with radiotherapy. The commonest permanent consequence is DI which, with the exception of sporadic reports, is considered as a non-reversible event, only amenable to replacement therapy; other hormonal deficiencies such as growth and thyroid may occur. The neuropsychological conquences of CNS disease may be severe.

Haemophagocytic lymphohistiocytosis (HLH)

Familial haemophagocytic lymphohistiocytosis (FHL) is a genetically heterogeneous disorder characterized by a hyperinflammatory syndrome with fever, hepatosplenomegaly, cytopenia, liver dysfunction, and sometimes CNS involvement. Bone marrow aspiration is usually performed early, enabling the identification of haemophagocytosis by activated macrophages. The absence of haemophagocytosis does not, however, exclude the diagnosis.

Differential diagnosis of HLH may be difficult and diagnostic guidelines for HLH have been established by the Histiocyte Society (Table 19.1). In particular, demonstration of association with common pathogens, together with evidence of impaired natural killer (NK) cytotoxic activity, provided the rationale for considering HLH as a selective immune deficiency.

The pathogenic mechanisms of FHL are based on insufficient control of target antigens by cellular cytotoxicity. As a result, an excessive cytokine production induces lymphocyte overstimulation and limited killing of the dendritic, antigen-presenting cell. In this vicious loop, the patient is unable to get rid of the target, often a common viral pathogen such as Epstein–Barr virus (EBV) or cytomegalovirus (CMV). The disease manifestations are due to excessive inflammatory response caused by hypersecretion of pro-inflammatory cytokines such as interferon-γ, tumor necrosis factor-α, interleukin(IL)-6, IL-10 and macrophage-colony-stimulating factor (M-CSF). These mediators are secreted by activated T lymphocytes and macrophages that infiltrate all tissues, and lead to tissue necrosis and organ failure. In spite of the excessive expansion and activation of cytotoxic cells, patients with FHL have severe impairment of the cytotoxic function of NK cells and CTLs. NK cells and cytotoxic lymphocytes (CTLs) kill their targets through cytolytic granules containing perforin and granzyme. Upon contact between the effector killer cell and the target, an immunological synapse is formed and cytolytic granules traffic to the contact site, dock and fuse with the plasma membrane and release their contents. All known defects in FHL seem to be involved in this process, with the only exception of a small minority of patients with still unassigned defect.

Table 19.1 Diagnostic criteria for haemophagocytic lymphohistiocytosis (HLH)

---

1 Familial disease/known genetic defect

or:

2 Clinical and laboratory criteria (5/8 criteria)

- ◆ Fever
- ◆ Splenomegaly
- ◆ Cytopenia ≥2 cell lines
  - Haemoglobin <90 g/l (below 4 weeks <120 g/l)
  - Neutrophils <1 x 10^9/l
- ◆ Hypertriglyceridemia and/or hypofibrinogenemia
  - fasting triglycerides ≥3 mmol/l
  - fibrinogen <1.5 g/l
- ◆ Ferritin ≥500 µg/l
- ◆ sCD25 ≥2400 U/ml
- ◆ Decreased or absent NK cell activity

Haemophagocytosis in bone marrow, CSF or lymph nodes

In most cases the natural course of FHL is rapidly fatal within a few weeks, unless appropriate treatment, including corticosteroids, cyclosporine, etoposide, or anti-thymocyte globuline, can obtain transient disease control. Yet, due to disease reactivation, rapidly fatal outcome follows, unless HSCT is offered. Prompt identification of such patients is an on-going challenge for the attending physician. The very high transplant–related mortality associated with HSCT for both LCH and HLH has led to the current trials of reduced intensity conditioning for these diseases.

Genetic forms of HLH

The identification of the causative gene(s) for familial haemophagocytic lymphohistiocytosis (FHL) has been a long process. In 1999 the first FHL-related gene was reported, and over 10 years later, we have still not identified all the underlying mutations.

A first mapping approach on consanguineous families of Pakistani origin identified a region on chromosome 9q21.3–22; unfortunately, the underlying defect for this subset of the disease remains unknown (FHL1). Another report documented linkage to a region on chromosome 10q21–22; mutations in the perforin-1 gene (*PRF1*) were soon described at this locus. Perforin is a pore-forming protein with a mechanism of transmembrane channel formation. In patients with FHL2, *PRF1* mutations induce a complete or partial reduction granule-mediated cytotoxicity by NK and T cells. Patients with FHL2 have different ethnic origins, with cases documented from all continents. Age at disease onset is usually very young, median 3 months, but with a wide range reaching the third decade. Mutations of *UNC13D* have been associated with FHL3. It encodes the Munc13–4 protein, a critical effector of the exocytosis of cytotoxic granules including those containing perforin and granzyme. Munc13–4 deficiency, therefore, results in defective cellular cytotoxicity and a clinical picture very similar to that of FHL2. Data on genotype/phenotype correlations showed that ethnic-specific mutations were not identified, that CNS involvement is more frequent than in FHL2 and that age at diagnosis is significantly higher than in FHL2. The combination of the classical clinical picture in association with defective granule release assay suggests FHL3. Most reported patients with FHL4 have been of Turkish/Kurdish descent. FHL4 is due to deficiency of syntaxin 11, a protein contributing to cytotoxic cell degranulation. In 2009, FHL5 was described in patients with mutations in the gene encoding syntaxin-binding protein-2 (*STXBP2* or *Munc18–2*), involved in the regulation of vesicle transport to the plasma membrane. A few additional genetic conditions may have a clinical picture completely overlapping HLH. Chédiak-Higashi syndrome (CHS), Griscelli syndrome type II (GSII), and X-linked lymphoproliferative syndrome (XLP) are immune deficiencies with distinctive clinical features in which the development of HLH is sporadic, though frequent. HLH is often the presenting symptom but may also occur later during the course of disease. Patients with CHS show partial albinism and frequent pyogenic infections. Their white blood cells exhibit decreased chemotaxis and characteristic giant inclusion bodies (lysosomes). Patients with GSII also have hypopigmentation and various degrees of neutrophil dysfunction but lack the giant granules. XLP is mainly characterized by a constitutional defect of a specific effective immune response to EBV. Following exposure to EBV, these subjects are prone to develop HLH; if they survive, they may develop lymphomas or dysgammaglobulinemia.

The clinical approach to the diagnosis of HLH has changed over the years. Initially the diagnosis was based on the identification of a clinical and biochemical constellation of signs and symptoms, supported by very young age and family history. The identification of NK activity defect in FHL became the first milestone in assigning a functional defect to these patients. Yet, NK cell cytotoxicity assay is not easily accessible for most clinicians, thus remaining a confirmative assay, restricted to reference laboratories and normal NK cytotoxicity is seen in some patients.

Identification of the genetic defects allowed investigation of novel tools for rapid screening of FHL. It is now recognized that NK cells and CTLs of patients with *PRF1* mutations lack intracellular perforin detected by flow cytometry, thus providing a reliable and rapid identification of patients with FHL-2. CD-107a (LAMP-1) lines the cytotoxic granule and is expressed on the surface of the NK/T cell after granule exocytosis. Lack of surface CD107a expression represents a rapid tool for identification of patients with FHL3 and degranulation defects, in contrast to healthy control subjects or perforin-deficient NK cells. Thus, this assay rapidly became the standard for identification of patients with FHL-3. Patients with different genetic defects hampering cytotoxic cell degranulation, such as syntaxin 11 (FHL-4) and Munc 18–2 (FHL-5) may also be detected by this granule release assay.

The above diagnostic tools are extremely useful in the diagnostic approach to a child with HLH. The aim is to discriminate those patients who have a genetic defect and thus deserve aggressive therapy followed by HSCT, from those in whom HLH may develop as a temporary complication of an infectious disease, or other underlying conditions such as malignancy, in whom anti-HLH therapy may also be life-saving but who do not usually require HSCT. The term 'macrophage activation syndrome' (MAS) has also been used to describe patients with rheumatologic diseases who develop a clinical syndrome indistinguishable from FHL.

Uncommon histiocytic disorders

The uncommon histiocytic (UCH) disorders are a diverse group of disorders that do not meet the criteria for diagnosis of LCH or HLH. The commonest UCH in childhood are juvenile xanthogranuloma (JXG) and sinus histiocytosis with massive lymphadenopathy (Rosai-Dorfman disease).

The juvenile xanthogranuloma (JXG) family

The JXG family comprises a number of the UCH with identical immunophenotype with lesional cells positive for vimentin, factor XIIIa, CD68, CD163, fascin, CD68, and CD14 and negative for CD1a, S100, and Langerin. Pathologically they show well circumscribed nodules with a dense infiltrates of histiocytes. Touton giant cells, seen in 85 per cent of cases of JXG, but not limited to JXG, are characterized by a wreath of nuclei around a homogenous eosinophilic cytoplasmic centre, while the periphery shows prominent xanthomatization.

The commonest members of the JXG family seen in childhood are benign cephalic histiocytosis (BCH) and JXG. BCH presents with multiple cutaneous lesions confined to the head and neck area in a young child. These lesions either spontaneously disappear or progress to JXG clinically or pathologically, and no therapy is necessary.

JXG is a benign proliferative disorder which usually resolves spontaneously. Median age of onset is 2 years but lesions may be present at birth. Most JXG presents with solitary lesions which vary in size. Children less than 6 months old tend to present with multiple lesions with a predisposition for the head and neck. The male preponderance is much higher (12:1) in young infants with multiple skin lesions. JXG is associated with other diseases including the triad of JXG, neurofibromatosis type 1(NF1), and juvenile myelomonocytic leukemia (JMML). Cutaneous JXG usually follows a benign course with gradual involution over months to several years. Lesions may resolve completely or may leave a residual scar.

Extracutaneous involvement (systemic JXG) occurs in around 4 per cent of children and 30 per cent overall, with half the patients having no skin involvement. Median age at presentation is 0.3 years. The commonest extracutaneous site is a solitary mass in the subcutis and/or deeper soft tissues followed by liver, spleen, CNS and lungs. Most systemic lesions undergo spontaneous involution, but ocular and CNS involvement may cause significant problems. In one series, 2 of 36 children died of progressive CNS disease, while in another two neonates died of hepatic failure.

Ocular JXG occurs in the very young child, (92 per cent are less than 2 years of age), and may occur without skin involvement. When skin lesions co-exist, they are always multiple. Eye involvement is usually unilateral, and commonly presents with an asymptomatic iris tumor, a red eye with signs of uveitis, unilateral glaucoma, spontaneous hyphema, or heterochromia iridis. Other areas of the eye may be involved less commonly. Early diagnosis and treatment determine the final visual outcome.

Therapy of JXG

Patients with JXG isolated to skin should be treated only for pain or ulceration and not for cosmetic appearance. LCH-like therapy with corticosteroids alone or with vinblastine or vincristine appeared to have the highest response rate in systemic JXG, but the response to chemotherapy is less predictable than in LCH. Patients responding to cladribine and cytosine arabinoside, alone and in combination, including two with bone marrow involvement, have been reported. Other published therapies include methotrexate, etoposide, cyclosporine, interferon, and radiation therapy. A trial of different agents may be needed in individual patients.

Rosai-Dorfman Disease

Sinus histiocytosis with massive lymphadenopathy (SHML) or Rosai-Dorfman disease (RDD) is a non-neoplastic, polyclonal, usually self-limited disease due to accumulation of S100+, CD1a–, CD68++, CD163++ histiocytes. Pathologically, lymph nodes show massive sinus infiltration of large histiocytes admixed with lymphocytes and plasma cells. Intact erythrocytes, lymphocytes, and plasma cells may be engulfed by histiocytes, a process known as emperipolesis. Emperipolesis in histiocytes expressing S100 in the appropriate clinicopathologic setting is considered diagnostic of SHML. The mean age of onset is 20.6 years, with a wide age distribution. A familial form of RDD with mutations in *SLC29A3* has recently been described.

The commonest presentation is with bilateral painless cervical adenopathy associated with fever, night sweats, malaise, weight loss and polyclonal hypergammaglobulinemia. Other nodal groups may be involved and involvement of extranodal tissue such as skin, soft tissue, upper respiratory tract, bone, eye, retroorbital tissue and other sites occurs in 43 per cent of cases as the sole initial manifestation or with lymphadenopathy. Involvement of CNS, seen in 4 per cent (8/200) RDD cases in an early series, poses a significant diagnostic and therapeutic challenge, usually occurring without extracranial lymphadenopathy and clinically and radiologically resembling meningioma due to the propensity of all of the intracranial UCH to be dural-based. Pulmonary RDD is uncommon but carries a significantly worse prognosis. While skin involvement occurs commonly, disease limited to skin is uncommon. The clinical course of SHML is unpredictable, with episodes of exacerbation and remission which may extend over many years. The outcome is usually good and disease is often self-limiting, nonetheless about 5 per cent of patients die from disease. A subset of patients with immunologic abnormalities at or prior to presentation, have a less favorable prognosis.

Therapy

Patients with RDD isolated to nodes should be observed without therapy. Surgery may be indicated when nodal obstruction of a vital organ is present. First-line systemic therapy, utilized for patients with vital organ compression or dysfunction, is usually corticosteroids, which are often effective, but off-therapy relapses are common. Chemotherapy—including vinblastine alone or in combination with corticosteroids, cytosine arabinoside, methotrexate, and other agents—produces variable responses. Cladribine alone and in combination has been successful in some patients. Imatinib, targeting platelet-derived growth factor receptor and KIT-positive tumors, has resulted in good responses in some patients but not others. Rituximab therapy induced remission in a child with long-standing refractory disease. Other innovative therapies, including interferon, thalidomide, and retinoids, have been reported and therapies that target cytokines such as TNF-alfa amd IL6 have been used successfully in some patients. Treatment options for CNS and orbital RDD include surgery for diagnosis, relief of compression or excision if possibile, stereotactic fractionated radiotherapy or radiosurgery, or chemotherapy as outlined above. As with JXG, different therapies may have to be tried in individual patient until a response is obtained.

Further reading

Alqanatish JT, Houghton, K, Bond M, et al. (2010) Rituximab treatment in a child with Rosai-Dorfman disease and systemic lupus erythematosus. *J Rheumatol* **37**, 1783–4.

Aricò M, Danesino C, Pende D, Moretta L. (2001) Pathogenesis of haemophagocytic lymphohistiocytosis. *Br J Haematol* **114**, 761–9.

Aricò M, Janka G, Fischer A, et al. (1996) Hemophagocytic lymphohistiocytosis. Report of 122 children from the International Registry. FHL Study Group of the Histiocyte Society. *Leukemia* **10**, 197–203.

Aricò M, Nichols K, Whitlock JA, et al. (1999) Familial clustering of Langerhans cell histiocytosis. *Br J Haematol* **107**, 883–8.

Blouin P, Yvert M, Arbion F, et al. (2010) Juvenile Xanthogranuloma with Hematological dysfunction treated with 2CDA-AraC. *Pediatr Blood Cancer* **55**, 757–60.

Coury F, Annels N, Rivollier A, et al. (2008) Langerhans cell histiocytosis reveals a new IL-17A-dependent pathway of dendritic cell fusion. *Nat Med* **14**, 81–7.

Dehner LP. (2003) Juvenile xanthogranulomas in the first two decades of life: a clinicopathologic study of 174 cases with cutaneous and extracutaneous manifestations. *Am J Surg Pathol* **27**, 579–93.

Favara BE, Feller AC, Pauli M, et al. (1997) Contemporary classification of histiocytic disorders. The WHO Committee On Histiocytic/Reticulum Cell Proliferations. Reclassification Working Group of the Histiocyte Society.[comment]. *Med Pediatr Oncol* **29**, 157–66.

Gadner H, Grois N, Aricò M, et al. (2001) A randomized trial of treatment for multisystem Langerhans' cell histiocytosis. *J Pediatr* **138**, 728–34.

Gadner H, Grois N, Pötschger U, et al. (2008) Improved outcome in multisystem Langerhans cell histiocytosis is associated with therapy intensification. *Blood* **111**, 2556–62.

Grois N, Pötschger U, Prosch H, et al. (2006) Risk factors for diabetes insipidus in langerhans cell histiocytosis. *Pediatr Blood Cancer* **46**, 228–33.

Grois N, Prayer D, Prosch H, et al. (2005) Neuropathology of CNS disease in Langerhans cell histiocytosis. *Brain* **128**, 829–38.

Henter JI, Horne A, Arico M, et al. (2007) HLH-2004: Diagnostic and therapeutic guidelines for Hemophagocytic lymphohistiocytosis. *Pediatr Blood Cancer* **48**, 124–1.

Henter JI, Samuelsson-Horne A, Aricò M, et al. (2002) Treatment of hemophagocytic lymphohistiocytosis with HLH-94 immunochemotherapy and bone marrow transplantation. *Blood* **100**, 2367–73.

Kidd DP, Revesz T, Milller NR. (2006) Rosai-Dorfman diseae presenting with widespread intracranial and spinal cord involvement. *Neurology* **67**, 1551–5.

Kogawa K, Lee SM, Villanueva J, et al (2002) *Blood* **99**, 61–6.

Konca C, Zubeyde N, Ozkurt O, et al. (2009) Extranodal multifocal Rosai-Dorfman disease: response to 2-chlorodeoxyadenosine treatment. *Int J Hematol* **89**, 58–62.

Maghnie M, Cosi G, Genovese E, et al. (2000) Central diabetes insipidus in children and young adults. *N Engl J Med* **343**, 998–1007.

Marcenaro S, Gallo F, Martini S, et al. (2006) Analysis of natural killer-cell function in familial hemophagocytic lymphohistiocytosis (FHL): defective CD107a surface expression heralds Munc13–4 defect and discriminates between genetic subtypes of the disease. *Blood* **108**, 2316–23.

Morgan NV, Morris MR, Cangul H, et al. (2010) Mutations in SLC29A3, encoding an equilibrative nucleoside transporter ENT3, cause a familial histiocytosis syndrome (Faisalabad histiocytosis) and familial Rosai-Dorfman disease. *PLOS genetics*, **6**(2), e1000833.

Sieni E, Cetica V, Santoro A, et al. (2011) Genotype-Phenotype Study Of Familial Hemophagocytic Lymphohistiocytosis Type 3. *J Med Genet* **48,** 343–52.

Stover DG, Alapati S, Regueira O, et al. (2008) Treatment of juvenile xanthogranuloma. *Pediatr Blood Cancer* **51**, 130–3.

Trizzino A, zur Stadt U, Ueda I, et al. (2008) Genotype-phenotype study of familial haemophagocytic lymphohistiocytosis due to perforin mutations. *J Med Genet* **45**, 15–21.

Utikal J, Ugurel, S, Kurzen H, et al. (2007) Imatinib as a treatment option for Systemic Non-Langerhans cell Histiocytoses. *Arch Dermatol* **143**, 736–40.

Chapter 20

Tumours of the central nervous system

Stuart Smith, Franck Bourdeaut, Frank Saran,
Francois Doz and David Walker

Introduction and epidemiology

Brain and spinal cord tumours are the most frequent group of solid tumours, representing up to 25 per cent of all cancers in children under 15 years of age, being second only to leukaemias amongst all childhood malignancies. Central nervous system (CNS) tumour incidence rates vary from the highest in western societies of 25–40 per million to 15 per million in developing countries where they are usually outnumbered by leukaemias and lymphomas. These differences are most likely related to under diagnosis or registration in areas without neurological facilities or pathology departments. Racial or geographical differences are reported within countries which may be related in some, but not all cases, to socio-economic classes.

Aetiology and risk factors

The brain's rate of growth in early childhood is second only to lymphatic tissue proliferation in the same time period, suggesting the contribution of normal growth processes upon tumour development. This is particularly so for the commonest tumour types, low grade astrocytoma and medulloblastoma, where their age incidence is skewed to early age. Overall, childhood tumours predominate within the hind brain including brainstem and cerebellum (50 per cent), approximately 5–7 per cent arise within the spinal cord and the remainder in the midline supratentorial and cerebral cortical regions.

Only a small proportion of CNS tumours in young people arise from recognized tumour predisposition states (see Table 20.1). Their study is of particular importance to developing a biological understanding on how tumours arise in early life within the growing brain and to the identification biological targets for treatment stratification and new drugs, strategies which are currently being explored, holding great promise for the future.

The only established environmental risk factor for CNS tumours in childhood is exposure to ionizing radiation although a viral hypothesis has been proposed and electromagnetic radiation remains a candidate for investigation in epidemiological studies in this early age group. The risk of brain tumour in offspring of individuals with prior astrocytoma and meningioma is increased to the greatest degree in the first 5 years of life (2.5 times and 10.26 times, respectively) and in the first 15 years of life (1.8 and 4.29 times, respectively). Other cancers in parents may predispose to CNS tumours in their offspring during childhood; examples include, ependymoma in offspring of parents with colon cancer and medulloblastoma with parental salivary gland cancer. The presentation of low-grade astrocytomas in childhood has been identified as a marker for family cancer risk.

Table 20.1 Recognized tumour predisposition states linked to CNS tumours

Syndrome	Gene	Chromosome	Nervous system area	Risks	Skin	Other tissues
Neurofibromatosis type 1 (OMIM 162200)	*NF1*	17q11	Neurofibromas, optic nerve gliomas, astrocytomas, MPNST	Optic nerve gliomas, risk 4.4% (15 years) and 5.5% (20 years)	Café au lait spots, axillary freckling	Iris hamartomas, osseous lesions, phaeochromocytoma, leukaemia, soft tissues sarcoma.
Neurofibromatosis type 2 (OMIM 101000)	*NF2*	22q12	Vestibular and peripheral schwannomas, meningioma(s), meningiomatosis, spinal ependymomas, astrocytomas, glial hamartomas, cerebral calcification		-	Schwannosis, meningiomatosis, glial hamartomas, cerebral calcifications, peripheral neuropathy, subcapsular lens opacities, retinal hamartomas
Von Hippel-Lindau (OMIM 193300)	*VHL*	3p25	Hemangioblastoma			Retinal haemangioblastoma, renal cell carcinoma, phaeochromocytoma, visceral cysts
Tuberous sclerosis (OMIM 191100)	*TSC1* *TSC2*	9q34 16p13	Subependymal giant cell astrocytoma, cortical tubers	5–14% associated with subependymal giant cell astrocytomas (SEGA)	Cutaneous angiofibroma, peau chagrin, subungual fibromas	Cardiac rhabdomyomas, adenomatous polyps of small intestine, cysts of lung and kidney, lymphangio-leiomyomatosis, renal angio-myolipoma
Li-Fraumeni Syndrome (OMIM 151623)	*TP53*	17p13	Astrocytomas, PNET			Breast carcinoma, bone and soft tissue sarcoma, adrenocortical carcinoma, leukaemia
Cowden disease (OMIM 158350)	PTEN (MMAC1)	10q23	Dysplastic gangliocytoma of cerebellum (Lhermitte Duclos), megencephaly		Multiple trichilemmomas, fibromas	Hamartomatous polyps of the colon, thyroid neoplasms, breast carcinoma

(continued)

Table 20.1 Continued

Syndrome	Gene	Chromosome	Nervous system area	Risks	Skin	Other tissues
Gardner's syndrome Familial adenomatous polyposis (OMIM 175100)	APC	5q21	Medulloblastoma		Epidermal cysts	Osteomas, supernumerary teeth, desmoid tumours, colorectal and gastroduodenal polyps, congenital hypertrophy of the retinal pigment epithelium (CHRPE), thyroid carcinoma
Turcot syndrome Hereditary non-polyposis colorectal cancer (OMIM 114500)	MSH2 MLH1 PMS2	2p22–21 3p21 7p22	Brain tumour polyposis syndrome (BTP) BTP type 1 predominantly high-grade astrocytoma and familial colorectal adenomas without polyposis BTP type 2 consists of patients with CNS tumour, mainly medulloblastoma and familial adenomatous polyposis (FAP) kindred	Brain tumour risk x 4–6 general population	Café au lait spots	Colorectal polyps
Nevoid basal cell syndrome (Gorlin)	PTCH	9q31	Medulloblastoma		Multiple basal cell carcinomas, palmar and plantar pits	Jaw cysts, ovarian fibromas, skeletal abnormalities
Multiple endocrine neoplasia type 1 (OMIM 131100)	MEN1	11q13	Pituitary tumours Ependymoma			
Down syndrome (OMIM 190685)		Trisomy 21	Negative association with exception of CNS germ cell tumours where there is an enhanced association		Typical facial features Symian crease	Leukaemoid reactions in infancy with enhanced risk of myeloid leukaemia
SMARCB 1 mutation	hSNF5/INI1	22q11	Atypical Teratoid Rhabdoid Tumour, rhaboid tumours at renal and other non-CNS sites, choroid plexus tumours			
Hereditary retinoblastoma	RB1	13q14	Bilateral retinoblastoma, pinealoblastoma, suprasellar PNET	Rare		

Survival

Compared with most other types of childhood cancer, improvements in survival from CNS tumours have been more modest, though some subtypes, notably low-grade astrocytoma, have long had a relatively good prognosis for survival (90 per cent). From the patients' and families' perspective however, survival is only part of the story, as disability rates are high and life-long amongst survivors. In a recent Swedish study, nearly 60 per cent of adult survivors had moderate, and over 25 per cent, severe disability, affecting hearing and sight, communication, mobility, and cognition, which together constrain participation in education, inclusion in work force, forming partnerships leading to marriage, and independent living. The causes and, to some degree, the severity of these disabilities are linked to the speed of diagnosis and the age at which different treatments are initiated in childhood. Focal brain injury is worse with prolonged prediagnostic symptom intervals. Peri-operative brain injury is an unavoidable risk, as is neurotoxicity of radiotherapy and chemotherapy, the severity of which is worse for those receiving radiotherapy, in particular, in the very early ages (<5–8 years).

There have been improvements in overall survival rates in both population registries and clinical trials' reports in almost all tumour types in the past two decades (1990–2010). These improvements have coincided with the establishment of specialist neuro-oncology multidisciplinary teams within children's cancer centres and the increased trials activity of the national and international cooperative groups.

Clinical presentation

Clinical presentations of children and young people with CNS tumours remains a major challenge in most health systems. Figure 20.1 shows results of a meta-analysis of a systematic literature review of symptoms associated with a brain tumour diagnosis, grouped according to tumour site, age and neurofibromatosis (NF) status. This analysis reveals that headache affects only 40 per cent of cases at presentation overall, although it has a higher incidence in sites most strongly associated with hydrocephalus, for example posterior fossa. It is notable that headache is least frequent in supratentorial tumours, followed by brainstem tumours. Focal neurological signs, particularly gait and balance problems, are most common in posterior fossa tumours, brainstem tumours and spinal cord tumours. Finally visual signs or symptoms are particularly common in posterior fossa tumours, midline tumours and supratentorial tumours as well as in patients with neurofibromatosis type 1 (NF1).

Delays in diagnosis are frequent in most health systems although there is considerable variation in reports from country to country, the shortest median symptom intervals are around 5 weeks and the longest greater than 14 weeks with a wide range of times from 1 day to several years, the latter occur in slow growing tumours often with vague symptoms or epilepsy. The experience of prolonged delay in diagnosis causes great concern for the patients and their families and frequently colours the initial contact with clinical teams where confidence can sometimes be very low. There are sadly still reports of children dying from uncontrolled hydrocephalus before a diagnosis can be made.

Communication

Effective communication with children and young people and their families is critical to selecting and managing successful treatment in CNS tumours, as with all malignancies. However the extra challenge is to communicate the risks of treatment-related neurotoxicity and the cognitive consequences of that for education and rehabilitation. The concept of a tumour being inoperable is

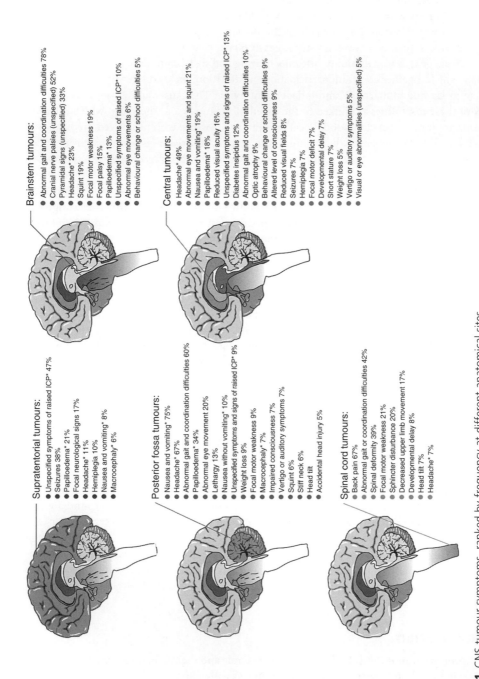

Brainstem tumours:
- Abnormal gait and coordination difficulties 78%
- Cranial nerve palsies (unspecified) 52%
- Pyramidal signs (unspecified) 33%
- Headache* 23%
- Squint 19%
- Focal motor weakness 19%
- Focal palsy 15%
- Papilloedema* 13%
- Unspecified symptoms of raised ICP* 10%
- Abnormal eye movements 6%
- Behavioural change or school difficulties 5%

Central tumours:
- Headache* 49%
- Abnormal eye movements and squint 21%
- Nausea and vomiting* 19%
- Papilloedema* 18%
- Reduced visual acuity 16%
- Unspecified symptoms and signs of raised ICP* 13%
- Diabetes insipidus 12%
- Abnormal gait and coordination difficulties 10%
- Optic atrophy 9%
- Behavioural change or school difficulties 9%
- Altered level of consciousness 9%
- Reduced visual fields 8%
- Seizures 7%
- Hemiplegia 7%
- Focal motor deficit 7%
- Developmental delay 7%
- Short stature 7%
- Weight loss 5%
- Vertigo or auditory symptoms 5%
- Visual or eye abnormalities (unspecified) 5%

Supratentorial tumours:
- Unspecified symptoms of raised ICP* 47%
- Seizures 38%
- Papilloedema* 21%
- Focal neurological signs 17%
- Headache* 11%
- Hemiplegia 10%
- Nausea and vomiting* 8%
- Macrocephaly* 6%

Posterior fossa tumours:
- Nausea and vomiting* 75%
- Headache* 67%
- Abnormal gait and coordination difficulties 60%
- Papilloedema* 34%
- Abnormal eye movement 20%
- Lethargy 13%
- Nausea without vomiting* 10%
- Unspecified symptoms and signs of raised ICP* 9%
- Weight loss 9%
- Focal motor weakness 9%
- Macrocephaly* 7%
- Impaired consciousness 7%
- Vertigo or auditory symptoms 7%
- Squint 6%
- Stiff neck 6%
- Head tilt
- Accidental head injury 5%

Spinal cord tumours:
- Back pain 67%
- Abnormal gait or coordination difficulties 42%
- Spinal deformity 39%
- Focal motor weakness 21%
- Sphincter disturbance 20%
- Decreased upper limb movement 17%
- Developmental delay 8%
- Head tilt 7%
- Headache* 7%

Fig. 20.1 CNS tumour symptoms, ranked by frequency at different anatomical sites.
Reproduced from Wilne S, et al. (2007) Presentation of childhood CNS tumours: a systematic review and meta-analysis, Lancet Oncol 8, 685–95, with permission from Elsevier.

frequently a source of concern, particularly in brainstem tumours and around the hypothalamus and eloquent cortical regions. Clarity of communication regarding the risks of disability or death in these anatomical areas needs to be explained sensitively yet clearly, excessive negative predictions of risks tends to generate disbelief and denial leading to loss of confidence in the clinical team and the need for multiple opinions. Communication needs to be sustained throughout early and late rehabilitation which extends to adulthood as the processes of normal development frequently promote sustained recovery.

Neurosurgery aims, risks and intracranial pressure management

Raised intracranial pressure

Tumour-related raised intracranial pressure may be secondary to the absolute volume of the tumour, to hydrocephalus due to obstruction of CSF drainage pathways (or rarely overproduction of CSF by a choroid plexus tumour) or to tumour-related intracranial haemorrhage. The modified Monroe-Kellie hypothesis proposes that the total volume of all intracranial components (brain, blood, CSF, tumour, etc.) is constant and that a rise in volume of one of these components must be offset by a decrease in another, or intracranial pressure (ICP) will rise. Pressure is distributed roughly evenly throughout the intracranial compartment which is of a fixed volume following fusion of the skull sutures. Symptoms of raised ICP include headache, nausea, vomiting, drowsiness/coma, urinary incontinence, developmental delay/regression, poor appetite, and visual deterioration. Signs include decreased Glasgow Coma Score, papilloedema, gaze sunsetting (failure of upgaze), ptosis, increase in occipito-frontal circumference beyond expected growth, splayed cranial sutures, and pupillary dilation. Critically raised ICP is characterized by Cushing's triad of hypertension, bradycardia, and respiratory irregularity.

Imaging may demonstrate features suggestive of raised ICP such as diminished cerebral sulci but patients with a normal CT scan may still have raised ICP. Raised ICP in one cerebral compartment will cause the contents to attempt to move to an area of lower pressure, resulting in the phenomenon of herniation. Generalized raised pressure will force the cerebellar tonsils down into the foramen magnum ('coning') with subsequent compression of the brainstem respiratory centres and likely death. Locally raised supratentorial pressure may force the medial temporal lobe under the falx–sub-falcine herniation.

The ICP may be directly measured by inserting an intracranial pressure wire allowing the ICP to be monitored via a transduced external ventricular drain. The normal ICP is 1.5–6 mm Hg in infants and rises throughout childhood to the adult value of around 10 mm Hg. The normal ICP trace has a waveform following the cardiac and respiratory cycles, but this may be altered in cases of raised ICP. Pathological ICP changes in response to raised ICP include plateau (Lundberg A) waves of elevations above 50 m mHg for 5–20 minutes. Lundberg B and C (Traube-Hering) waves are lower amplitude rises lasting for shorter periods of time. ICP monitoring may be commenced post-operatively if cerebral swelling is a concern after resection.

Management of raised intracranial pressure

Once the diagnosis of raised ICP has been established on clinical, radiological or monitoring grounds, urgent therapy must be instituted. An ICP elevated above 25 mm Hg for a prolonged period is associated with worsened neurological outcome and critically raised ICP is immediately life threatening. One of the key aims of emergency neurosurgery is to reduce the ICP by removing one of the components of the Monroe-Kellie hypothesis, for examle CSF, blood or tumour, or rarely by increasing the size of the compartment (decompressive craniectomy). Before surgery, medical management can begin this process. Intubation and control of gas exchange can lower the arterial carbon dioxide tension ($paCO_2$), which may be elevated due to poor respiratory effort due to reduced consciousness level. Reducing the CO_2 level to normocapnic levels reduces cerebral vasodilation, thereby reducing the volume of blood inside the cranial compartment and thus ICP. Reducing $paCO_2$ to subnormal levels (< 4 kPa) has been shown to have a counterproductive effect on cerebral perfusion and is no longer advocated. Full sedation, seizure control, normothermia, 30° head up positioning, and maintenance of adequate blood pressure also aid ICP control. Mannitol (an osmotic diuretic) or hypertonic saline can be utilized to produce a temporary reduction in ICP level (possibly with some neuroprotective effects) and facilitate transfer for definitive treatment if the diagnosis is established outside a centre with direct access to paediatric neurosurgical services.

Operative management of raised intracranial pressure

The surgical approach to the patient with critically raised ICP will clearly depend on the exact cause and precise scan findings. Resection of the tumour will aid pressure but this may not be appropriate in an unstable acute patient and is probably usually best done in a planned fashion once full pre-operative investigations have been completed. Haemorrhage associated with tumour may be evacuated via craniotomy. The most common operations performed are to aid CSF drainage to normalize ICP before proceeding to tumour resection.

ICP can be swiftly reduced by an external ventricular drain (EVD) placed into (usually) one of the lateral ventricles via a frontal or lambdoid burrhole. This allows CSF under pressure to drain to a collection bag, with the amount of drainage controlled by the height of the collection bag relative to the ventricular system. An EVD allows CSF drainage to be measured, as well as allowing collection of samples for cytological, biochemical or microbiological analysis. As a connection from the intracranial compartment to the external environment, there is a potential for intracranial infection usually manifesting as ventriculitis. This risk can be reduced by strict aseptic technique when sampling or manipulating the drain, and by the use of antibiotic-impregnated catheters. An EVD is a temporary measure and requires definitive management of the cause of the hydrocephalus or conversion to an indwelling shunt.

A ventricular shunt is an indwelling long-term catheter that drains excess CSF to another body cavity where the fluid is reabsorbed. This can be (most commonly) the abdominal cavity (ventriculo-peritoneal) or. if this is unusable, the pleural cavity or cardiac atrium. CSF flow is controlled by a valve which is set to open at a particular CSF pressure. Shunts can provide good long-term control of CSF pressure, but can block, break or become infected, necessitating shunt revision (with one or more revisions being needed in approximately 25 per cent of children shunted as a result of an intracranial tumour in one series).

Shunt infection can manifest with raised ICP signs/symptoms, sepsis or localized infection or pain. Shunt dysfunction rates are higher in younger children. An alternative to shunting in a selected subset of cases (particularly tumours in the posterior fossa causing aqueduct or fourth ventricle obstruction) is neuroendoscopic third ventriculostomy (NTV). This involves creation of a surgical passage via an endoscope through the floor of the third ventricle into the basal cisterns, allowing drainage of CSF past the obstructed fourth ventricle. If successful, NTV gives good control of hydrocephalus with no foreign material to act as a source of infection and is the preferred option if anatomically feasible. NTV has a good success rate in selected patient groups (e.g. aqueduct blockage or posterior fossa tumours) but may fail (usually soon after surgery) and subsequently require shunt insertion.

General principles of surgical therapy of tumours

Control of CSF pressure/ICP will then be followed by surgical therapy of the underlying tumour. Tumours in the paediatric population are in general less invasive to normal brain parenchyma, and thus more amenable to attempted curative resection. Numerous studies have shown that for all common tumour types, complete or near total resection is associated with a significant survival advantage. Detailed magnetic resonance imaging (MRI) will allow visualization of exact tumour location and the lesion's relationship to surrounding anatomical structures. These relationships will determine the surgeon's estimate of whether complete resection can be achieved. An intimate relationship between the tumour and major blood vessels, cranial nerves or other critical neural structures (e.g. the brainstem) will diminish the chances of achieving a complete resection. Unlike other organs, surgery must be confined to the tumour itself to as great an extent as possible, with little capacity for resection beyond the margin of the tumour in order to avoid the risk of irreversible focal neurological damage.

Anatomic considerations that will influence surgery include the depth of the tumour inside the brain, deep-seated tumours requiring long approaches through normal brain tissue that must be preserved, risking disability. Operating on deep structures also leads to problems of visibility and working space, though the operating microscope can partially compensate for this by improving illumination and magnification. Creating a surgical route to deep structures may also involve retraction of brain tissue which in itself can cause damage if applied for a prolonged period, for example, retraction of the occipital lobe during a supratentorial approach to the pineal region may cause cortical blindness. Some regions of the brain (e.g. the brainstem) are particularly sensitive to disturbance and damage, whereas other lobes (e.g. right frontal) will allow more aggressive surgical strategies.

Decisions on the exact surgical approach are always a balance on an individual case basis between the benefits of more complete resection and the risks of neurological damage leading to potentially permanent disability or even death. More than one approach may have been developed for a particular anatomical site. For example, a pineal region tumour could be accessed by approaches along the superior side or the inferior side of the tentorium, or via the third ventricle, either trans-cortically, trans-callosally or endoscopically. In some cases, the risk of neurological damage precludes radical surgery and in these cases image-guided biopsy only or even no surgery may be the best option. Management of these tumours should be discussed pre and post-operatively in a multidisciplinary meeting and therapeutic plan agreed by all professional groups attending.

Attempted tumour resection will always be preceded by optimization of the patient's medical condition and confirmation that hormonal, haematological, and biochemical status is normal. Blood loss is a key limiting factor in paediatric tumour resection due to both the relatively small patient blood volume and the haemorrhagic nature of some tumours. Blood transfusion or auto-transfusion can be undertaken intra-operatively but this can result in complications of coagulation, calcium levels, hypothermia and immune reactions. If a limiting volume of blood loss is reached then the procedure can be completed in a second stage at a later date if feasible.

Anaesthetic liaison is also key in warning of impending neurological damage in, for example, brainstem surgery. Cardiac decelerations, asystole or blood pressure changes may be a warning of impending brainstem damage. Anaesthesia can also be used to help provide optimal operating conditions, for example by maintaining $paCO_2$ under control and a stable blood pressure. Electrophysiological monitoring (e.g. evoked auditory, sensory or motor potentials) may also be used in selected cases to give warning of impending neurological damage.

Intraoperative adjuncts such as microscopy, image guidance systems, stereotaxy (frame based or frameless), 5-ALA fluorescent dye or intraoperative imaging (MRI or ultrasound) may also increase the chances of achieving a complete resection and minimize the risk to surrounding structures. Post-operative MR imaging is extremely important to assess extent of resection objectively and to provide a post-operative baseline. This imaging should be performed as close to the finish of surgery as possible (under the same anaesthetic or intra-operatively if possible) to minimize the extent of surgical imaging artefacts. Second-look surgery may be indicated if residual tumour remains and is deemed resectable.

Post-operative care on a high dependency or intensive care unit is also appropriate for most cases with close monitoring of haematological, biochemical (especially hyponatraemia), and hormonal status. Frequent neurological observations are required and prompt re-imaging if any significant change occurs. Decreased consciousness level post-operatively can be caused by operative site haemorrhage, hydrocephalus, infection, seizures or biochemical abnormalities.

In selected cases (e.g. leptomeningeal tumour spread) there may be a place for intrathecal chemotherapy after multidisciplinary team (MDT) discussion. In these cases, access to deliver the therapy is required and this can be provided surgically via an Ommaya-type reservoir or Portacath inserted into the ventricular system or the sacral CSF sac. Future developments may include the use of drug infusion systems of intrathecal chemotherapeutic agents.

Radiotherapy planning for CNS tumours

Radiotherapy remains a fundamental component of successful treatment for the majority of malignant primary CNS and spinal cord tumours of childhood. As a treatment modality it has undergone rapid changes in recent years with many more advances in development.

In the paediatric setting, radiotherapy planning and treatment must be deliverable and acceptable to children of all ages, some of which will therefore require treatment under a general anaesthetic (GA).

Recent technological progress has allowed clinicians to come closer to the aim of conforming, maximally, the high doses of radiation to the target (conformal radiotherapy, CRT) using either new more complex techniques (intensity modulated radiotherapy, IMRT) allowing improved critical organ avoidance or dose escalation not previously achievable with conventional techniques. Additionally, the latest imaging techniques visualize normal tissues and tumours with improved anatomical definition as well as providing new functional and biological information, helping to define the target in the first instance (multimodality imaging). In addition, increasing availability of proton therapy facilities can be predicted to further reduce radiation-associated late sequelae, albeit at increased financial cost.

Tumour Classification

The ICD-O classification of nervous system tumours is shown in Table 20.2.

Low-grade astrocytoma (LGA)

LGAs (Grade I and II) constitute 40 per cent of CNS tumours and are therefore the largest group. LGAs are equally common in both sexes. They can occur at any anatomical site within the CNS and are distributed, in descending order of frequency, in hypothalamic-chiasmatic optic nerve regions (36 per cent), cerebellar (31 per cent), cerebral cortical including third and lateral ventricles (16 per cent), brainstem (10 per cent), spinal cord (<5 per cent) and multisite tumours (<2 per cent). LGAs are frequently associated with Neurofibromatosis type 1 (NF1) (15–20 per cent), particularly involving the optic pathway (35 per cent), brainstem, and cerebellum. For patients diagnosed with NF1 there is 5 per cent risk of CNS tumour. Currently. consensus guidelines support visual

Table 20.2 Nervous system tumour classification–ICD-O

Nervous tissue tumours/NS neoplasm/Neuroectodermal tumour (ICD-O 9350–9589) (C70-C72/D32-D33, 191–192/225)			
Endocrine/sellar (9350–9379)	*sellar:* Craniopharyngioma Pituicytoma *other:* Pinealoma		
CNS (9380–9539)	Neuroepithelial (brain tumours, spinal tumours)	Glioma	Astrocyte	Astrocytoma (Pilocytic astrocytoma, Pleomorphic xanthoastrocytoma, Fibrillary (also diffuse or low grade) astrocytomas, Glioblastoma multiforme)
			Oligodendrocyte	Oligodendroglioma
			Ependyma	Ependymoma Subependymoma
			Choroid plexus	Choroid plexus tumour (Choroid plexus papilloma, Choroid plexus carcinoma)
			Multiple/unknown	Oligoastrocytoma Gliomatosis cerebri Gliosarcoma
		Mature neuron		Ganglioneuroma: Ganglioglioma, Retinoblastoma, Neurocytoma, Dysembryoplastic neuroepithelial tumour, Lhermitte-Duclos disease
		PNET		Neuroblastoma (Esthesioneuroblastoma, Ganglioneuroblastoma), Medulloblastoma, Atypical teratoid rhabdoid tumour
		Primitive		Medulloepithelioma
	Meningiomas (meninges)	Meningioma		
	Hematopoietic	Primary central nervous system lymphoma		

screening of NF1 individuals until at least 8 years and subsequent alternate year screening is advocated until adulthood. Imaging screening in early childhood is debated, due to difficult interpretation of visual performances at this age. Where visual signs or symptoms are identified, MRI brain scanning may diagnose an optic pathway glioma but also frequently identifies neurofibromatous bright objects (NBOs) which develop and proliferate during childhood and then regress at the onset of adolescence.

Histologically, LGAs are separated by the WHO classification into grades I and II. Pilocytic astrocytomas (PA; WHO grade I) are most common, accounting for over 60 per cent. Clinically diagnosed tumours, based upon imaging and clinical characteristics, account for about 20 per cent and are presumed to be PA, many being associated with NF1 and involving the hypothalamic-chiasmatic regions (see Fig. 20.2). PAs are not considered premalignant lesions. Pilomixoid astrocytoma is a recently proposed entity that may be associated with younger age at presentation and a more aggressive clinical course.

Diffuse fibrillary astrocytomas (FA, WHO grade II) account for 6 per cent. These are typically more aggressive in their growth pattern, relentlessly progressing unless resected or treated with effective chemo- or radiotherapy. In adulthood they are considered premalignant and malignant

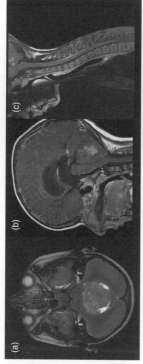

Axial T2 (a) and sagittal T1 (b) showing a primitive tumour of the posterior fossa, with heterogeneous enhancement; (c) leptomeningeal dissemination.

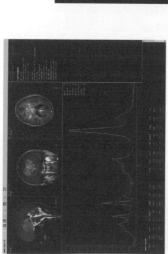

Spectroscopic Imaging of paediatric HGG –Magnetic resonance spectroscopy of a corpus callosum paediatric GBM with a very raised lipid/lactate peak (tallest peak) indicating necrotic tissue, reduced NAA peak (small peak centrally) and increased choline/creatinine ratio

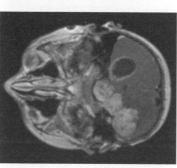

Hypothalamic chiasmatic low grade astrocytoma

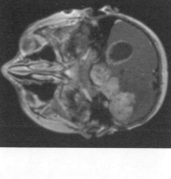

Bilateral ponto-cerebellar tumor in an infant younger than 1 year. Enhancing rim surrounding a cystic necrosis

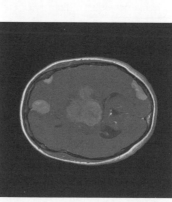

T1 contrast enhanced MRI of multiple meningiomas in a patient with NF2 - Multiple durally based lesions with contrast enhancement in a young adult

Fig. 20.2 Brain tumour imaging.

transformation will occur subsequently although it is not known whether this is similar in children. Recent reports of genetic copy numbers gains at 7q34 in PAs and grade II LGG tumours, tandem duplications involving *BRAF* involving fusion genes *KIAA1549-BRAF* and *SRGAP3-RAF1* as well as their interaction with dysregulated CXCR4 signalling leading to suppression of cAMP have been shown in animal models to promote optic glioma development.

Treatment

Surgical resection, where possible, is the preferred treatment. However, certain anatomical sites such as hypothalamic-chiasmatic or intrinsic brain stem are unsuitable for an attempted complete resection. LGAs may occasionally (<10 per cent) present with leptomeningeal metastases. In unresectable tumours, the selection of patients for non-surgical therapy is a critical decision. Many patients presenting with chiasmatic–hypothalamic-optic nerve tumours present with visual symptoms, reduced acuity and fields, and optic atrophy. The threat of, or evidence of, progressive bilateral vision loss in chiasmatic tumours would seem to identify a sub-group most in need of immediate non-surgical treatment to prevent further vision loss. Non-visual symptoms such as hypothalamic syndrome or progressive focal neurological deficits also justify non-surgical treatment. Endocrine deficits are treated with hormone therapies.

Non-surgical therapy is stratified by age and NF status. Younger children (<8 years) being offered chemotherapy, older children (<8 years) may be offered involved field radiotherapy where the balance of risks and benefits may favour the use of this treatment approach. In NF-positive patients, radiotherapy is contra-indicated as first line treatment because of the increased risks of secondary cerebrovascular events and secondary malignant nerve sheath tumours within the radiation fields. Chemotherapy trials consistently show that further symptomatic/tumour progression can be arrested in about 70 per cent, partial response can be expected in 50 per cent whilst complete response is unusual (<10 per cent). A variety of chemotherapy regimens have been used. Drugs have been selected to offer effective treatment, whilst minimizing the risk of late consequences such as second tumours/leukaemias. Vincristine and carboplatin has been used most extensively, as have cisplatin, actinomycin, vinblastine and the multi-agent regimen including procarbazine, 6-thioguanine, dibromodulcitol, lomustine (CCNU), and vincristine. It should be borne in mind that the biological behaviour of low-grade gliomas can be unpredictable. Incompletely resected or unresected tumours may subsequently progress, remain stable or even occasionally spontaneously involute. The risk of tumour progression seems to reduce beyond their 5th birthday; the biological behaviour of these tumours during adolescence is not completely understood at present.

Other low-grade gliomas account for the remaining 6 per cent and are a heterogeneous collection with particular characteristics.

Subependymal giant cell astrocytoma (SEGA) is a benign tumour arising in 5–15 per cent of patients with tuberous sclerosis, typically within the ventricles, associated with sub-ependymal nodules (SEN) within the sub-ventricular zone. Tumour growth is unpredictable, spontaneous growth arrest being reported. Treatment has been limited to surgical resection which, if impossible, may result in death. Recent reports of SEGAs responding to rapamycin and everolimus, mTOR inhibitors which target the molecular pathway affected by the *TS* gene mutations, is now presenting an opportunity for the use of a medical treatment as a prelude or an alternative to surgical resection where surgical risks are high.

Pleomorphic xanthoastrocytoma (PXA) typically occur within the superficial cortical structures and involving the leptomeninges; typically they present in late childhood or early adulthood. Histologically they are characterized by spindle and giant cell with bizarre multinucleated forms, mitoses and lipid-bearing cells. The majority are grade II lesions with capacity to transform to malignant anaplastic variants. Hypothesized similarities in genetic mutations to diffuse astrocytoma involving the *p53* gene have not been supported by studies. Surgical resection, if complete, can be curative. Radiotherapy in recurrent cases, after re-resection or incomplete resection should be considered.

Ganglioglioma represents the most frequent tumour entity in young patients suffering from chronic focal epilepsies. The majority of which occur within the temporal lobe and reveal a biphasic histological architecture, characterized by a combination of dysplastic neurons and neoplastic glial cell elements. However, gangliogliomas exhibit a considerable variability in their histopathological appearance. The distinction from diffusely infiltrating gliomas is of considerable importance since tumour recurrence or malignant progression are rare events in gangliogliomas. Little is known about the molecular pathogenesis of these glioneuronal tumours. Candidate genes are linked to neurodevelopmental signalling such as reelin and tuberin/insulin-like growth factor receptors rather than cell cycle control or DNA repair mechanisms. Treatment is by surgical resection, where possible, and radiotherapy in progressive tumours.

Dysembryoplastic neuroepithelial tumour (DNET) are benign (WHO grade I), stable or sometimes slow-growing tumours arising from either cortical (vast majority) or deep grey matter, are frequently calcified and not typically associated with vasogenic edema. Imaging typically identifies scalloping of inner table of skull. They are thought to arise from secondary germinal layers and are frequently (up to 80 per cent of cases) associated with co-existent cortical dysplasia and typically the cause of intractable partial seizures. More than 60 per cent occur in temporal lobe and 30 per cent in frontal lobe. They demonstrate essentially no growth over time. The prognosis is excellent so that, if incompletely resected, tumour progression is uncommon yet may be associated with cessation of seizures.

Desmoplastic infantile astrocytoma/ganglioglioma (DIA/DIG) are characterized by their voluminous size, their intense desmoplasia, and the frequent presence of divergent astrocytic and ganglionic differentiation. They predominantly present before 18 months of age, usually within the first 4 months of life, involve the frontal and parietal regions, and are attached to meninges. They are composed predominantly of a dense desmoplastic fibrous tissue admixed with variable numbers of pleomorphic neuroepithelial cells. Divergent astrocytic and neuronal differentiation is observed. Successful total or near-total surgical resection is the favoured treatment.

Cerebral astrocytoma with extensive calcification is rare variant that is recognized but has no specific indications for different approaches to treatment.

Remaining challenges

LGAs, whilst benign and associated with >90 per cent survival rates, represent a significant challenge as they are the commonest cause of potentially treatable blindness in children, they can threaten life in infancy with massive, progressive and symptomatic tumours. Later in childhood they can present with life-threatening raised intracranial pressure. Surgical resection, whilst frequently curative, carries the risk of focal brain injury and life-long disability. Recently described genetic mutations and their interactions with NF1-mediated dysregulation of cAMP has raised the possibility of identifying new targets for therapy, balancing the risk of neurological injury against toxicity of therapy is complex. New genetic mutations in NF1 in particular raise the possibility genetically predicting NF1 rather than relying upon visual surveillance.

High-grade Astrocytoma

Epidemiology

High-grade gliomas (HGG), the most common primary cerebral tumour in adults (including glioblastoma multiforme (GBM) (WHO astrocytoma grade IV), are significantly less common in children. WHO astrocytoma grade III and IV tumours representing around 6.5–10 per cent of intracranial neoplasms. Grade IV astrocytoma is predominantly glioblastoma but also includes small- and large-cell variants, as well as the gliosarcoma, whilst grade III tumours are most commonly anaplastic astrocytoma. High-grade astrocytoma as a group also include the high-grade (WHO grade III) variants of the less aggressive glial tumours such as anaplastic oligodendroglioma, anaplastic oligoastrocytoma or anaplastic pleomorphic xanthoastrocytoma.

Risk factors for the development of astrocytic tumours have not yet been well elucidated. It is clear that previous exposure to therapeutic irradiation (e.g. for CNS directed therapy for acute leukaemias) is associated with an increased risk of CNS tumours including meningiomas and high-grade astrocytomas. It is estimated that this irradiation may give up to a 22-fold increased risk of CNS tumour development. High-grade gliomas are significantly more common in males (up to 1.8 times in adults and 1.6 times in children). Certain familial syndromes have been identified that give an increased risk of astrocytoma development. Turcot syndrome (mismatch repair cancer syndrome) is associated with an increased risk of both colonic polyps and astrocytomas, due to mutations in genes such as mismatch repair endonuclease (PMS2). Changes in the well recognized tumour suppressor p53 are also associated with an increased risk of malignancy generally including brain tumours, as seen in Li-Fraumeni syndrome.

Biology

Molecular features in paediatric HGG have been limited by the rarity of this tumour although in adults global genetic analysis, based on gene expression array technology, has allowed classification into differing groups, with steps being taken towards improved prognostication and targeted therapy. It is apparent that there are important genetically different groups within adult HGG, for example between primary (de-novo) GBM and those that arise from pre-existing lower grade gliomas. Genetic differences are also seen between adult and paediatric HGG, with differences in epidermal growth factor (EGFR), platelet derived growth factor (PDGF), IDH-1 and CDKN2A most significant (Table 20.3).

Imaging

Paediatric HGG can occur anywhere in the CNS with approximately 63 per cent occurring in the cerebral hemispheres, 28 per cent deep supratentorially and 8 per cent in the posterior fossa, with a small number found in the spine. Gliomas can also develop in the brainstem of which approximately 80 per cent are of the diffuse type, generally involving the pons. Their anatomical involvement and imaging characteristics are critical to selection of cases for biopsy, or not. The typical

Table 20.3 Comparison of adult and paediatric glioblastoma, illustrating that different molecular mechanisms are responsible for the two diseases

	Paediatric GBM	**Adult GBM**
IDH-1 mutation	None found	Common in secondary GBM
1q gain	30%	9%
7 gain	13%	74%
Loss of 10q	35%	80%
EGFR amplification	0%	43%
CDKN2A deletion	20%	55%
PDGFR amplification	17%	11%

diffuse intrinsic pontine glioma (DIPG), generally being accepted as a high-grade lesion where the risks of biopsy are not accepted, outside research protocols. Any tumours in the brainstem not meeting these characteristics should be considered for biopsy, as low-grade histology or alternative histological types [e.g. primitive neuro-ectodermal tumours (PNET), ependymoma] is associated with different treatment strategies and improved survival rates, compared to the DIPG after treatment. Imaging features on CT scanning are generally of a ring-enhancing lesion with a hypodense centre and profuse surrounding oedema. They may exert considerable mass effect. On MRI, a similar pattern is seen with ring enhancement, restriction on diffusion imaging, and greatly increased perfusion especially in the enhancing rim on vascular imaging. Differential diagnosis on imaging grounds may include a cerebral abscess and this should be considered if the patient displays any signs of sepsis. Advanced MRI is also now entering routine clinical practice, with techniques such as MR perfusion studies and MR spectroscopy (Fig. 20.2) becoming increasingly important means of assessing tumours. MR perfusion gives a measure of relative blood volume within areas of brain and tumour and higher-grade tumours will have increased vascularity. MR spectroscopic profiles are characteristic for particular tumour types, although interference from bone or CSF remains problematic for some tumour locations. Diffusion-weighted MR gives information regarding level of cellularity within the tumour, discriminating between neoplastic tissue and necrosis, and, with diffusion tensor imaging, may be a better way of assessing the infiltrative growth of a lesion into surrounding brain.

Management

Surgery

Initial management of raised ICP is generally followed by biopsy/attempted resection. The expanding knowledge of the molecular biology of these tumours justifies the emphasis on surgically-collected specimens. Currently in non-brainstem HGG radical (i.e > 90 per cent+) surgical resection is recommended where feasible, with good evidence from both paediatric and adult studies that complete or near complete resection is significantly associated with improved survival. However, due to the highly invasive nature of these tumours, curative surgical resection is rarely achievable. Degree of resection may be aided by adjuncts such as intra-operative MRI or ultrasound imaging, electrocorticography or 5- ALA (fluorescent dye) guided surgery.

Radiotherapy

Treatment for primary HGGs should commence urgently following surgery, ideally no later than 4 weeks from referral, particularly in the presence of progressive symptoms. Gross tumour volume (GTV), clinical target volume (CTV) and planning target volume (PTV) will be determined according to International Commission on Radiation Units guidance (ICRU 50/62). CT planned delineation of all target volumes is mandatory and based on a planning CT with i.v. contrast and/or CT–MR image fusion. The target volumes and organs at risk (according to departmental policies) will be outlined on each slice of the planning scan. Gross Tumour Volume (GTV) is defined by the enhancing tumour on gadolinium contrast-enhanced MR at the time of RT planning together with the cavity following any surgical resection. Thus, the GTV contains any residual enhancing tumour and extends to tissues surrounding the tumour prior to excision. The clinical target volume (CTV) include an additional margin of 2.0–2.5 cm in directions of potential tumour spread and the planning target volume (PTV) will include an addition margin according to department policy. Patients should always be treated using conformal radiation therapy treatment planning and delivery techniques. Generally a conformal 3–4 field arrangement is used with individual shielding, for example by multi-leaf collimators (MLC) or mini multi-leaf collimators (mMLC).

In case of tumours extending in both hemispheres (e.g. bithalamic tumours) a parallel opposed conformal pair may be the best technical solution. Exceptionally, for patients requiring urgent treatment for progressive symptoms, specifically brainstem gliomas, treatment may need to start with a straightforward technique and must not be delayed by the use of complex planning procedures. Such a technique should be modified as soon as possible thereafter, usually within the first week of treatment. IMRT techniques, either delivered via conventional linear accelerators or tomotherapy machines, may allow a more homogeneous dose distribution and better sparing of normal tissues and hence reduce late sequelae. Yet this benefit comes at the cost of a larger amount of normal tissue exposed to lower doses. If this may lead to an increased risk of second malignancies in case of cure, offsetting the benefit from improved conformity remains controversial.

Chemotherapy

Chemotherapeutic regimes were previously based on CCNU/procarbazine and vincristine (PCV) combinations and met with limited success. The new adult standard of care is concomitant and subsequent adjuvant Temozolomide temozolomide with involved field radiotherapy. Similarly, surgically implanted wafers impregnated with chemotherapy (such as Gliadel[R]) can be considered in recurrent tumours able to undergo further aggressive resection and are occasionally used in selected children. Treatments targeting angiogenesis with anti-Vascular Endothelial Growth Factor (VEGF) antibody therapy (Bevacizumab) are increasingly being used in adults and in children, either alone or in combination with cytotoxic drugs (Irinotecan). Other novel agents targeting Platelet Derived Growth Factor Receptor (PDGF-R) or Epidermal Growth Factor Receptor (EGF-R) are under investigation. Similarly, surgically administered genetically modified viral therapy is being investigated. The experience in adult HGG is that the systematic use of combined adjuvant therapies and exploration of additional novel targeted therapies is starting to prolong survival and bring anticipation of improved treatment outcome. There is strong overlap of biology of HGG with adults in older children but less overlap in children with HGG diagnosed at less than 3 years of age. This heterogeneity of biology needs to be included in stratification of trials along biological grounds rather than age- related grounds as this would expand the number of trials suitable for inclusion of children with adults whilst identifying the HGG with unique biological features requiring a separate approach. The remaining areas of serious challenge are diffuse intrinsic pontine gliomas (DIPG). Their critical anatomical location prevents any relevant primary resection and similarly represents a serious threat to life associated with all treatment modalities.

Outcome

Median survival for older children is in the order of 14–18 months, with local recurrence almost inevitable. Grade III tumours in older children do somewhat better with 5-year progression free survival approaching 20–40 per cent. CSF-borne metastasis to distant CNS sites may occur in ~15 per cent of paediatric HGG, whilst metastasis outside the CNS is very rare but has been reported. Diffuse intrinsic pontine gliomas have median survival of 5–12 months, over 90 per cent dying by 2 years. These diffuse intrinsic pontine gliomas are now one of the leading causes of death by brain tumour in children, as survival rates for other paediatric brain tumours improve.

Remaining challenges

The most critical challenge lies in identifying effective non-surgical therapy to complement the existing radiotherapy techniques. The unique biological nature of these high-grade tumours in early life means that research and clinical care must be tailored to tumours arising during growth and development, and stratified by biological factors, whilst remaining aware of the extensive research effort in adult high-grade gliomas and participating selectively in such studies so as to speed up progress in this field.

Medulloblastoma

Epidemiology

Medulloblastoma is the most frequent malignant brain tumour of childhood, with an average incidence of 5 per million children under 15 years of age. By definition, it occurs in posterior fossa, involving mainly vermis and fourth ventricle (80 per cent) and hemispheric tumours being more common in older patients. The mean age at diagnosis is between 5 and 7 years and 85 per cent of all cases occur before the age of 18 years. Sex ratio is males 1.4:1 females. Although most medulloblastomas appear sporadic, they do occur in rare hereditary syndromes such as Turcot (*APC* mutation), Li-Fraumeni (*TP53* mutations) or Rubinstein-Taybi (*CREB/BP* mutation) syndromes, mismatch repair deficiency (*PMS2*, *MLH1*, *MSH2* or *MSH6* mutations), and abnormalities in the *SHH* pathway (Gorlin syndrome with *PTCH1* mutation, *SUFU* mutations). Tumours with PNET features are also encountered in the supratentorial space, they are biologically distinct from medulloblastoma and more resistant to radiotherapy and chemotherapy, currently.

Histological subtypes

Histologically, medulloblastomas are divided in four main WHO subgroups: (i) classical medulloblastoma, (ii) anaplastic/large cell medulloblastoma, (iii) nodular desmoplastic medulloblastoma, and (iv) medulloblastoma with extensive nodularity (MBEN). Classic medulloblastomas are characterized by small round basophilic cells with a high nuclear:cytoplasmic ratio, occasionally organized in Homer-Wright rosettes. Mitoses are abundant, consistent with a frequently high level of Ki67 staining. Large-cell/anaplastic medulloblastoma show an event greater rate of mitosis, together with large round cells showing prominent nucleolus and pleomorphism. Finally, desmoplasia is defined by the presence of dense pericellular collagen deposition, surrounding nodular islets of well-differentiated neurocytic tumour cells. Desmoplastic medulloblastomas are predominant in infants and adults; they are more often located in the hemispheres than other histological subtypes.

Biology: cell of origin

Recent advances in the knowledge of medulloblastoma genetics have identified four distinct patterns:

1) The classic variant show miscellaneous alterations with gain of 17q and loss of 17p, eventually secondary to an iso17q. This is the most frequent type.

2) Those involving the WNT signalling mutations in the beta-catenin gene (*CTNNB1*), *APC* or *AXIN2* associated with loss of chromosome 6. These are associated with a classic histology, an older age at diagnosis, a low rate of metastases, and an overall good prognosis.

3) Those involving alterations in the Sonic Hedgehog pathway, *PTCH1* or *SUFU* mutations (10 per cent of all cases); loss of chromosome 9 is frequent. These are phenotypically desmoplastic or may exhibit extensive nodularity. Within children, this category is mainly observed <3 years of age and has a particularly good outcome.

4) Those involving amplification in any of the three *MYC* genes (*c-MYC*, *MYCN*, *MYCL*, 15 per cent of pediatric cases). These are phenotypically large-cell and anaplastic variants

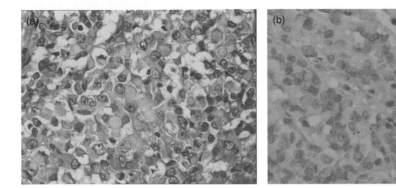

Fig. 20.3 (a) Hematoxylin Eosin Safran, typical rhabdoid features. (b) Anti-BAF47 immunostaining; the arrow shows normal cells with retained nuclear staining. No expression in rhabdoid cells.

An increasingly significant observation is the re-classification of poorly differentiated tumours as atypical teratoid/rhabdoid tumours (ATRT) in view of their extremely resistant phenotyope to current therapies. The observation of rhabdoid cells and/or demonstration of negative SMARCB1 immunostaining facilitates differential diagnosis. The *SMARCB1* gene alterations constantly result in the abolishment of the protein nuclear expression, an immunohistochemical feature that is now widely used for the diagnosis (INI1 staining) (Fig. 21.3). Adult medulloblastomas do not share the same hallmarks of their pediatric counterparts; in particular, iso17q and *MYC* gene amplifications are infrequent, whilst loss of 10q and gain of 17q have a stronger association.

These different histological and biological groups raise the question of the cell of origin. Several lines of evidence suggest that medulloblastoma variants rise from distinct progenitors within the cerebellum. Constitutive activation in the Sonic Hedgehog pathway in mice leads to abnormalities in the normal development of the external granular layer of the cerebellum that result in a tumour formation. *PTCH1*-related desmoplastic medulloblastomas are thought to arise from granule neuron precursor cells. Whilst hyperactivation of the Axin-beta-catenin pathway in granule neuron precursor cell does not give rise to medulloblastoma, CTNNB1-related medulloblastomas may arise from precursors in the primary germinal zone. These clues within the tumour biology are hoped to lead to greater understanding of how the development of these tumours is linked to normal cerebellum development.

Imaging

CT scanning typically demonstrates a hyperdense mass (with calcifications in less than 20 per cent), arising from the vermis, filling the fourth ventricle and leading to obstructive hydrocephalus. MRI is the reference imaging method for diagnosis, staging, and preoperative analysis. Leptomeningeal metastases typically occur in cranial or spinal subarachnoid spaces or along ventricular walls (see Fig. 20.2), more rarely in CNS parenchyma. Systemic metastases can occur, particularly after ventricular peritoneal shunts.

Initial management

Initial management of raised ICP by shunting or neuroendoscopic third ventriculostomy followed by attempted maximal resection is the most common approach. Second resection may occur if there is residuum on post-operative scans. Delayed resections similarly may be undertaken in very ill metastatic patients after biopsy and primary chemotherapy to reduce tumour bulk. One particular complication of surgery that significantly alters management is the presence

Table 20.4 Medulloblastoma risk stratification (Chang)

M0	M1	M2	M3	M4
No dissemination out of the cerebellum	Presence of tumour cells in the cerebrospinal fluid	Metastases in the brain	Metastases in the spine	Metastases out of the central nervous system

of post-operative posterior fossa or cerebellar mutism syndrome. This has been reported in up to 40 per cent of cases and developed within 24–72 hours after surgery, causing progressive cerebellar and long tract signs associated frequently associated with mutism. The signs stabilize and then subsequently recede after a variable period but delays of up 3 or 4 months have been reported. Recovery may not be complete and may be protracted throughout further growth and development until adulthood.

Risk stratification

The existence of distant metastases has for long been linked to a poor outcome. Chang et al. proposed a classification for dissemination that is still currently used (Table 20.4).

Craniospinal MRI is essential to detect distant CNS metastasis and best performed pre-operatively. The presence of tumour cells in the CSF is conventionally evaluated 10–15 days after resection. M1 tumours are considered as metastatic for risk stratification. The degree of tumour resection with an early postoperative (<48 hours) residue >1.5 cm ^{2} should be considered as conferring an adverse outcome. It is important to also take neurosurgical observations into account in risk stratification.

In preschool children (<3/5 years) the risk criteria are affected by the clinical requirement to avoid/minimize radiation doses fields in the early developing brain and the use of more sustained or intensive adjuvant chemotherapy as well as intrathecal chemotherapy as compensation. Currently risk criteria are summarized as:

- Standard risk: Completely resected (T0), non-metastatic (M0) tumours with desmoplastic histology, especially nodular desmoplastic with extensive nodularity
- High risk: Classic/non-desmoplastic histology, any M+.

In contrast, the risk stratification for school age children (>3/5years) children and young people are defined by more extensive data describing clinical tumour and biological factors:

- Standard-risk: localized disease (M0) *and* full resection and no anaplastic/large cells (classic variants), *and* no *MYC* gene amplification. Within standard-risk group, medulloblastomas with beta-catenin nuclear accumulation constitute a low-risk group that being allocated to reduced treatment in the forthcoming clinical trials.
- High-risk: metastatic disease (M1-M2-M3) *or* sub-total resection *or* anaplastic/large cells variant *or* *MYC* gene amplification.

Non-surgical treatment strategies

Preschool age children (<3–5 years)

The risk stratification identifies the new standard risk group with complete resection, no metastases and desmoplastic histology tumours. For this group the use of chemotherapy alone seems sufficient to offer very high cure rates (~80 per cent at 3 years). Treatment regimens have used both systemic and intrathecal chemotherapy. The use of intrathecal chemotherapy is controversial as its added value has not, as yet, been defined within a comparison trial. The high-risk group is predominantly defined by non-desmoplastic or classic histology. This group still has unacceptable outcomes and the use of involved field or neuraxis radiotherapy and chemotherapy is justified. A number of approaches combining different regimens and radiation fields and doses have been proposed and requiring testing. There is therefore no standard of care accepted here.

School age children

The standard of care for standard risk patients is the use of craniospinal radiotherapy and adjuvant chemotherapy. With such approaches ~80 per cent 5-year survival rates can be expected. Recent trials have investigated the use of hyperfractionated radiotherapy as a strategy to minimize neurotoxicity. Adjuvant chemotherapy has been shown to produce imaging response on scanning and be associated with enhanced progression-free survival in randomized trials and enhanced overall survival in a series of single arm studies. The 'Packer Regimen' has been the standard treatment using cisplatin, CCNU, and procarbazine. Careful monitoring of hearing and renal function is essential to avoid the additional problems of high tone hearing loss, substitution of carboplatin or cyclophosphamide being alternatives.

In contrast, the best overall survival rates reported in high-risk medulloblastomas remain around 60 per cent, the worst outcome being observed in M2-M3 diseases (~45 per cent OS). Neo-adjuvant chemotherapies have been evaluated in several trials in order to reduce the tumour burden at the time of radiotherapy and to evaluate the tumour chemosensitivity with limited success despite a wide range of approaches. Currently 'sandwich' high-dose chemotherapy with or without hyperfractionated accelerated craniospinal radiotherapy show promising results (see Gandola et al. in Further reading). Intensification of chemotherapy with myelo-ablative regimens is associated with potentially significant risks of systemic and neurotoxicity. Intrathecal therapy as an alternative strategy (methotrexate, etoposide, topotecan) is under investigation.

Sadly, long-term survival after tumour recurrence when full dose craniospinal radiotherapy has been given previously, is seldom, if ever, successful. Studies testing high-dose chemotherapy salvage surgery and radiotherapy have not been successful in patient rescue strategies. However, tumour recurrence after reduced intensity treatments without radiation therapy were successfully salvaged in a number of cases and experience with patients treated primarily with or without reduced radiation fields and doses are yet to be reported and require further evaluation.

Radiotherapy

There is general agreement that radiotherapy should commence no later than 4–6 weeks postoperatively and last no longer than 50 days, as prolongation of the total radiotherapy treatment time worsens outcome. Given the propensity of medulloblastoma to disseminate via the CSF, current standard practice in the curative setting involves the use of craniospinal irradiation with a boost to the posterior fossa/primary tumour bed. There is evidence suggesting that the quality of radiotherapy is associated with recurrence rate and outcome. Hence strict quality assurance procedures are required to maximize the chance of long-term control and survival.

For radiotherapy planning purposes, the conventional definition of the posterior fossa encompasses: superiorly, the tentorium; inferiorly, the skull at the foramen magnum; anteriorly, the anterior edge of the brain stem; posteriorly, the inner table of the skull; and laterally, the extension of the meninges around the cerebellum. A field arrangement using 3D conformal planning is a mandatory requirement to minimize the radiotherapy dose to the middle ears and temporal lobes. In the past, the dose delivered to the craniospinal axis (i.e. the entire CSF space as identified on MR imaging) was 35 Gy. A number of trials have attempted to reduce the dose and/or volume irradiated in an attempt to reduce the late effects of radiotherapy.

The French SFOP M4 Trial used a volume reduction technique and patients with standard risk medulloblastoma did not receive irradiation to the supratentorial part of the brain. The EFS at

6 years was less than 20 per cent, with 9 out of 13 relapses occurring within the supratentorial compartment, thus demonstrating that irradiation of the entire craniospinal axis is a necessary component. One of the first trials to investigate a reduced dose to the craniospinal axis was the POG 8631/CCG 923 Trial. Patients were randomized to receive craniospinal radiotherapy to a dose of either 36 or 23.4 Gy. This trial closed prematurely due to a statistically significant excess of relapses in the 23.4 Gy arm (67 per cent vs 52 per cent). Between 1990 and 1994 the CCG 9892 pilot study recruited patients to receive reduced dose craniospinal irradiation (23.4 Gy) with concurrent vincristine chemotherapy followed by adjuvant lomustine, vincristine and cisplatin chemotherapy. Due to the promising progression free survival (PFS) rates of 86 per cent at 3 years and 79 per cent at 5 years, this trial formed the basis for a large phase III trial, CCG A9961. This randomized trial included 421 standard risk medulloblastoma patients treated with 23.4 Gy of craniospinal irradiation followed by a posterior fossa boost to 55.8 Gy. All patients included in this trial received concurrent vincristine chemotherapy and were randomized to receive one of two different adjuvant chemotherapy regimens. EFS at 5 years was 81 per cent and OS 86 per cent with no difference between the two chemotherapy arms. This was the first study to demonstrate an excellent clinical outcome with reduced-dose craniospinal irradiation, and this has now become 'standard' treatment across the world.

Attempts to reduce the volume of normal supratentorial brain irradiated to high doses are ongoing. A recently published multi-institution trial used 3D conformal radiotherapy to treat less than the entire posterior fossa with the aim of reducing neurocognitive sequelae; disease control was comparable to that after treatment of the entire posterior fossa, with a 5-year EFS rate of 83 per cent. Importantly, there was a 13 per cent reduction in the volume of posterior fossa receiving 55 Gy and a statistically significant reduction in dose to the temporal lobes, cochleae, and hypothalamus.

Although the use of chemotherapy in standard risk patients is currently perceived as gold standard, attempts have been made to use a 'radiotherapy only' approach by altering the radiotherapy fractionation regime. Some data suggest that the use of hyperfractionated radiotherapy in combination with a reduced boost volume (tumour bed vs whole posterior fossa) can produce an OS rate similar to current combined modality strategies. All patients recruited into this study received 36 Gy craniospinal irradiation twice daily in 1 Gy fractions, with a total dose of 68 Gy boost to the tumour bed. Results are promising, with EFS and OS rates at 6 years of 75 per cent and 78 per cent, respectively. Importantly, they also found a reduction in subsequent decline of full scale IQ.

Consequences of tumour and treatment

This group in particular, present significant challenges for long-term follow up. The combination of risk related to posterior fossa syndrome, craniospinal radiotherapy and its associated risk of cognitive and motor syndromes means that survivors can suffer significant disability affecting their subsequent development and capacity for independent living. The radiotherapy is known to damage white matter tracts and their capacity for myelinization. Endocrine consequences for growth hormone, thyroid hormone, pubertal development, and axial skeletal growth all require careful monitoring and follow up by combined late-effects teams. The risks are all greater for children treated at younger ages and with more disseminated tumours at diagnosis. This experience has promoted the strategies aimed at minimizing the fields and doses of radiation, as well exploring combination of radiotherapy with adjuvant and more recently intrathecal chemotherapy.

Remaining challenges

Comprehensive analyses of medulloblastoma biology will unravel the biological mechanisms of this disease and may offer new targeted treatment strategies for the next decades. *MYC* amplification or *CTNNB1* mutations have already impacted upon the treatment strategies as has the Sonic Hedgehog pathway. The wide variety of biological types, however, means that a single biologically targeted new treatment is unlikely. The current focus upon defining risk stratification and targeting therapies to the brain remain the main focus in standard-risk tumours. The recent introduction of intra-operative MR and proton beam therapy offer the options of enhanced and safer resections, as well as reducing toxicity of radiation therapy. The role of intrathecal chemotherapy requires further explorations as new drugs are identified as candidates for this route (see Further reading).

Ependymomas

Ependymomas are malignant tumours that arise from the ependymal cells lining the ventricles of the brain. They develop preferentially in children rather than in adults; half of them occur before 5 years of age. They are located in supratentorial spaces (25 per cent), posterior fossa (70 per cent) or spinal cord (5 per cent). With an annual incidence of around 2 per million, ependymomas are the third most frequent CNS tumours in children. Ependymomas rarely occur in a context of identified predisposing syndrome except, rarely, in Turcot syndrome and occasionally spinal tumours in NF2.

Four major tumour subtypes of ependymal tumours are defined by the WHO: subependymoma (grade I), myxopapillary ependymoma (grade I), low-grade ependymoma (grade II) and anaplastic ependymoma (grade III), the two latter being the most frequent. Classic low-grade ependymomas harbour some characteristic features: clear cells with eosinophilic cytoplasmic granules, genuine epdendymal rosettes, perivascular pseudorosettes, and canal-like structures. Mitotic figures and pleomorphism may be found, but in lower proportion in low-grade ependymomas than in their anaplastic counterpart. The tumour cells usually express GFAP (glial fibrillary acidic protein). However, the prognostic value of ependymoma grading has not been established between low-grade and anaplastic ependymoma.

Recent studies have demonstrated that the main molecular events driving the oncogenesis, including *CDKN2A* or *NOTCH1*, might differ significantly from one anatomic location to the other, suggesting that the cellular type from which ependymomas arise is not unique and distinguishes supratentorial, infratentorial, and spinal tumours. Several genomic analyses have also led to proposed molecular-based classifications that converge in distinguishing at least three main subtypes of intracranial ependymomas:

i) tumours with numerous aberrations affecting whole chromosomes or chromosomes arms, deletion of chromosome 6 and 22, gains of chromosome 9, 15q and 18

ii) tumours showing a 1q gain, and/or homozygous deletion of 9p (*CDKN2A* locus)

iii) tumours with balanced flat profiles (2).

Strikingly, several studies have observed that balanced profiles are mostly observed in young children (<4 years of age). Among the molecular drivers, *CDKN2A* tumour suppressor gene and *NOTCH1* oncogene may play a major role.

Classic MRI appearance of ependymoma demonstrates a low T1 signal intensity, enhanced with gadolinium, and a heterogeneous T2 hyperintensity. Cystic components may be seen in supratentorial tumours. Posterior fossa ependymomas typically show an extension through the foramina of Luschka into the cerebellopontine angle and/or through the foramen of Magendie. This highly suggestive feature may help to distinguish ependymomas from medulloblastomas. Supratentorial ependymomas, unlike their infratentorial counterparts, frequently arise apart from the ventricles; this suggests that those ependymomas develop from the rest of ependymal cells retained in the parenchyma during development.

Prognostic factors remain in active debate. However, young age at diagnosis, incomplete resection and distant metastasis are usually considered as the main prognostic factors. Merchant et al. reported that age at diagnosis may not be an independent prognostic marker, but rather be linked to the delay to radiotherapy. The prognostic impact of the WHO grading is still debated, even though a large meta-analysis has given evidence in favour of high grade being associated with poorer outcome. In a large array-CGH (comparative genomic hybridization) based analysis, 1q gain and homozygous *CDKN2A* deletion were the strongest factors for overall survival (5-year OS, 30 per cent); this genomic feature was associated with WHO grade 3.

The standard treatment of ependymomas is based on surgery and radiotherapy.

Surgery

The exact approach to surgery depends on the anatomical location of the tumour, but the goal should always be to achieve as complete a resection as possible. Evidence from both, specifically paediatric (e.g. Chakraborty et al., in Further reading) and mixed adult/paediatric series (e.g. Korshunov et al., in Further reading) have consistently shown survival benefit for complete as opposed to subtotal resection. The survival benefit of complete resection applies to supratentorial, posterior fossa and also to spinal lesions. The prognosis for tumours of any grade is improved by complete surgical resection; the introduction of intra-operative MRI and other adjuncts should help surgeons to achieve complete resection in a greater proportion of tumours.

Radiotherapy and chemotherapy

The latest standard for radiotherapy is a focal dose of 59.4 Gy on the clinical target volume with 10 mm margin using a fractionation regime of 1.8 Gy, five times per week. However, since half of the cases occur before 5 years of age, long-term sequelae related to radiotherapy are of serious concern. Hence, several national cooperative groups have aimed at postponing radiotherapy by using post-operative chemotherapy in young children. In the 1990s, the Paediatric Oncology Group first undertook to treat children with 12–24 months of post-operative chemotherapy preceding systematic irradiation. Even though EFS survival was disappointing in these first trials (5-year EFS 27 per cent), other groups have subsequently scheduled radiation-free post-operative chemotherapy for infants, with the following results (Table 20.5).

Ependymoma trials results

These studies combined metastatic and non-metastatic patients, the most promising results came from a UK protocol. This protocol had the highest dose-intensity schedule as the cycles were based on 2-week intervals. Furthermore, high-dose methotrexate was included despite the potential for adverse neurocognitive consequences. This strategy had the attraction that a proportion of patients survive without the need for radiotherapy, reserving the use of radiotherapy for relapse. At relapse, however, there was a consensus upon the use of further surgery and local irradiation: a small number of children are cured after such approaches.

Table 20.5 Ependymoma: comparison of outcomes from international cooperative group protocols

Protocol	No. of patients	3-year PFS	3-year OS	Percentage of patients treated with RT
CCG	74	50%	65%	60
SFOP	73	30%	70%	53
AEIOP	41	28%	48%	66
UKCCSG	89	43%	77%	43

Despite these studies, there is very little evidence for chemosensitivity to any agents in this tumour type. Moreover, long-term sequelae of the combined strategies remain to be investigated and compared with those observed after the more recent trials based upon more intensive use of highly focussed radiation. Experience reported in infants between 18 months and 3 years of age treated with post-operative conformal or intensity-modulated radiotherapy achieved 81 per cent 7-year OS with a local control rate of 87 per cent. These children received 59.4 Gy to the target volume with a 10 mm margin, while infants younger than 18months with total gross resection were given a reduced dose of 54 Gy. The long-term side effects of this strategy remain to be elucidated and other studies have reported reading ability being affected in children receiving conformal radiotherapy with 54–59 Gy. The aim in future studies is to reduce side effects by enhancing tumour-targeting techniques, thereby maximizing sparing of the normal brain tissue.

Future challenges

Since the prognostic impact of histology is largely debated, defining more accurate and widely usable prognostic factors is still needed. In that respect, genomics and transcriptomic large studies should be performed in the coming years, as it has nicely been achieved in medulloblastomas for example.

The genuine benefit of systemic treatment has still to be proven in ependymomas. In particular, enhanced knowledge on the biology of ependymomas might help introducing more efficient adjuvant therapies in incompletely ressected tumours. Alternatively, given their radiosensitivity, ependymomas might also be advantageously further treated by more sparing irradiation techniques, including proton therapy or cyberknife (a robotic radiosurgery technique that delivers highly focussed radiation therapy with great precision, minimizing significant dose to surrounding normal tissues).

Germ cell tumours

Biology

Intracranial germ cell tumours (GCT) usually develop in the midline (pineal gland or suprasellar region) with 10 per cent being bifocal. This midline extragonadal localization may be related to errors in the migration of intra-embryonic mesoderm at the time of primitive streak formation in the beginning of the third week of gestation with resultant localization to the cranial cavity. The molecular mechanisms that account for their migration to these specific sites and latent activation remain unknown. Their relationship to their stem cell origin is under investigation. Prepubertal germ cell tumours demonstrate imbalances at chromosome 1 (loss at 1p, gain at 1q) and 6q, alterations in the sex chromosomes, and, rarely, abnormalities of 12p. A minority of tumours also show evidence for *C-MYC* or *N-MYC* amplification in teratoma in particular. In contrast, pubertal and post-pubertal GCTs are characterized by isochromosome 12p or 12p amplification similar to adult germ cell tumours.

Comparison of genetic mutations in CNS and non-CNS GCTs reveals no difference in patterns of mutations. Intracranial GCTs account for 30 per cent of all GCTs, their histological appearance in the brain is identical to that seen in other anatomical sites. They are classically divided into the 'non-secreting' germinomatous type and the 'secreting' non-germinomatous type. The proteins they secrete are alpha fetoprotein (AFP) and β-human chorionic gonadotropin (β-HCG). Levels of AFP >25 ng/ml and β-HCG levels >50 IU/l define a 'secreting tumour' and act as a diagnostic and staging marker and a marker for monitoring disease response. Placental alkaline phosphatase and the soluble isoform of c-Kit may become clinically relevant in the future.

The 'non-secreting' germinoma is the most common subtype in the teenage and young adult group, although a minority may have syncytiotrophoblastic subtype which secretes low levels of β-HCG. Non-germinomatous germ cell tumours (NGGCT) comprise 18 per cent of CNS germ cell tumours in the 15–29 year age group and, within the WHO classification, include: embryonal carcinoma, yolk sac tumour, choriocarcinoma, immature and mature teratoma, as well as teratoma with malignant transformation and mixed germ cell tumours. The identification of tumour markers in blood or CSF is essential part of tumour assessment as secreting tumours do not need biopsy. Very high levels of AFP and β-HCG were associated with adverse prognosis in the previous generation of studies. 'Non-secreting' tumours require a mandatory biopsy to discriminate between germinoma and other non-germ cell tumour types that can occur in midline structures, for example, pinealoma, pineocytoma, low-grade astrocytoma, PNET, etc. or LCH.

Epidemiology

CNS germ cell tumours are seen exclusively in individuals between the ages of 0–34 years of age with a peak incidence between 15 and 19 years of age. There is a strong male preponderance, particularly in the pineal region, in 'secreting' non-germinomatous tumours, whilst there is equal gender distribution in the pituitary and a lesser preponderance of males in 'non-secreting' germinomatous tumours. There has been a trend for the incidence of CNS germ cell tumours to increase in populations. This is particularly so in Japan, where the incidence is 5–8-fold greater than that seen in the United States. Down Syndrome is the only known predisposing condition. The peak incidence seen during adolescence and early adulthood of both intra- and extra-cranial age-specific germ cell tumours suggests that endocrinological changes occurring during puberty may be involved in the awakening of dormant cells. Melatonin, a hormone secreted by the pineal gland and involved in sleep patterning (which undergoes significant changes in adolescence), interferes with release of the hormone FSH-LH, and may play a role in the activation of those lesions within the pineal region.

Imaging

Radiographic characteristics of CNS GCTs alone are unable to reliably differentiate germinoma from NGGCTs or from other tumours in the typical locations. Leptomeningeal spread as judged by enhanced craniospinal MRI and CSF cell count.

Initial management

Careful ophthalmic and endocrine assessment is essential as urgent treatment may need to be initiated to try to save vision. Endocrinopathies present at diagnosis may compromise early attempts at therapy. In particular, if diabetes insipidus is present, fluid management may be challenging especially where hydration regimes for chemotherapy are required. The endocrinologist will also be needed to deal with the other hypothalamic pituitary axis hormone deficiencies at the time of diagnosis and throughout treatment, and as a consequence of tumour damage and potential late effects of radiation therapy. 'Secreting tumours' do not require biopsy whilst typical midline tumours not associated with raised levels of AFP/β-HCG should be biopsied. Their midline location presents the opportunity of biopsy at the time of neuroendoscopy or stereotaxy. Open approaches are normally reserved for delayed resections after primary chemotherapy.

Non-surgical treatment

'Non-secreting' CNS germinomas

Historically the standard of care was craniospinal radiotherapy to a total dose of 24 Gy followed by a boost to the primary site for a further 16 Gy. Such approaches are highly successful with near 100 per cent cure rates. Current trials are investigating combined chemotherapy and reduced field radiotherapy in order to reduce the volume of brain irradiated, thereby reducing the potential risk of late consequences on cognition, second tumours, endocrinopathies, and vasculopathies. However, the consequences of intense chemotherapy in a predominantly adolescent population cannot be discounted. The results from these studies will take a number of years before the ideal combination of chemotherapy and focal field radiation therapy is determined.

Non-germinomatous CNS germ cell tumours

These are a heterogeneous group which do not require biopsy if the threshold for AFP/β-HCG are exceeded. Primary chemotherapy followed by delayed resection and involved field radiotherapy to known sites of disease is currently being evaluated. For certain patients, such as those with very high level of AFP/β-HCG at diagnosis or those with persistent viable tumour after chemotherapy, the role of additional intensified chemotherapy with stem cell rescue is being explored.

Outcome

The prognosis for pure germinomas, which are exquisitely radio- and chemo-sensitive, remains excellent with 5-year overall and EFS of over 95 per cent. When other more malignant components are present, the prognosis is significantly less optimistic with previous estimated 5-year overall survivals of 40–60 per cent although newer studies have seen an improvement up to 70 per cent. There is a greater reliance on a multidisciplinary approach with platinum-based chemotherapy, reduced field radiotherapy and delayed surgical resection which, in the deep structures of the brain, carries significant surgical risk. Adult oncologists have contributed to the definition of optimal therapy in gonadal germ cell tumours, highlighting the role of cisplatin, while their pediatric counterparts have focused on the need to preserve cognitive function by reducing radiation exposure.

Challenges

GCTs present in older children adolescents and young adults, justifying adult and paediatric neuro-oncology teams to share their respective trial experience and collaborate to investigate new, less toxic treatments. Current combined treatment approaches have been shown to improve survival outcomes in particular for secreting tumours; quality of survival for this group remains a significant challenge given the involvement of anatomical structures critical to normal sexual and cognitive development. Recent population-based studies describing quality of life for adult survivors of childhood CNS tumours identified CNS germ cell tumour group as poorly rehabilitated. In general, endocrine deficits present at the time of diagnosis are not reversed by therapy. Reduction of long-term disability is a major challenge and rests upon achieving an earlier diagnosis to avoid tumour-related irreversible toxicities as well as minimizing the toxic effects of combined treatments.

Craniopharyngioma

Epidemiology

These WHO grade I tumours arise from the anterior superior margin of the pituitary, usually growing superiorly from the sella and impinging on the third ventricle. Overall craniopharyngiomas represent 2.5–4 per cent of brain tumours, with approximately half the cases occurring in childhood. They are the most common non-neuroepithelial tumour of the CNS in childhood (5–10 per cent of paediatric CNS tumours with 0.5–2.5 cases per million population per year). The peak incidence is between the ages of 5 and 10 years. The embryological origin of this tissue is probably from remnants of the Rathke's pouch, the ectodermal pouch that invaginates towards the pituitary region and forms the adenohypophysis region of the pituitary. The pouch normally completely obliterates, but can persist as a Rathke's cleft cyst or as epithelial cell rests, which presumably are the origin of these tumours. They are usually at least partially cystic tumours, with the cysts lined with stratified squamous epithelium. The fluid within craniopharyngioma cysts normally contains cholesterol crystals with their characteristic shimmering oily appearance at operation and the tumour is often partially calcified. Histological subtypes include adamantinomatous and the papillary forms (rare in childhood). Molecular biological studies have revealed frequent mutations of the β-catenin gene.

Imaging

CT scanning demonstrates the cystic/solid nature of these lesions and will demonstrate any calcification clearly. The solid portion of the tumour enhances upon contrast administration. MRI again demonstrates hypointense well-defined cysts surrounded by an irregular mass of solid tumour that grows into the sellar and suprasellar areas, surrounding and enclosing normal structures such as the optic chiasm, anterior cerebral vessels or pituitary stalk. Papillary tumours are usually less cystic on imaging.

Management

Management can be complex and involve several different specialities and is thus best conducted in tertiary referral centres where appropriate multidisciplinary expertise is available. Guidelines such as those developed by the British Society for Paediatric Endocrinology and the UK Children's Cancer and Leukaemia Group (formerly UKCCSG) are available to inform therapy decisions; there is also an active trial programme within SIOP which is refining approaches to management. Treatment of a patient presenting with a craniopharyngioma commences with treatment of acutely raised ICP if present, followed by thorough endocrinological work-up and correction of any significant hormone deficiency (particularly diabetes insipidus and cortisol axis). High-dose dexamethasone is normally commenced (after cortisol investigations) to reduce peri-tumoural oedema. Pre-operative endocrine work-up should also include assessment of serum and urine glucose and electrolytes, gonadotrophin status, thyroid function tests, growth hormone status (e.g. insulin-like growth factor-1 levels), height, weight, pubertal ratings and bone age. Secretory germ cell tumours should also be excluded by measuring β-HCG and AFP levels. Pre- and post-operative involvement of a paediatric endocrinology team is mandatory for all children with craniopharyngioma.

Surgical strategy aims to remove as much tumour as possible whilst avoiding damage to the many critical structures in this area. Radical attempted complete resection may be appropriate for some tumours, but there is increasing recognition that the child may pay an unacceptable price in serious and potentially life threatening complications, particularly hypothalamic damage. The severe disturbances to personality, appetite, thirst, hormonal systems, somnolence, and intellect may have a huge adverse effect on quality of life and also greatly reduce life expectancy. The likelihood of achieving complete resection decreases with tumour size and attempted radical resection is probably only appropriate for tumours less than 2–4 cm high in the midline. Recurrence rates after 'complete' resection range from 5 to 25 per cent. More conservative debulking surgery aiming to remove the bulk of the tumour whilst protecting critical areas is a better option in some cases. The tumour is often relatively slow growing and good survival can be achieved through debulking followed by focussed conformal radiotherapy. Surgical approaches to craniopharyngiomas can include subfrontal, interhemispheric, transfrontal, trans-sphenoidal (microscopic or endoscopic) or a ventriculoscopic approach, depending on the exact growth characteristics of the individual lesion. In cases of incomplete resection or tumour recurrence, problematic larger cysts can be drained by image-guided surgery and placement of catheters to subcutaneous reservoirs.

Once incomplete surgery has been performed, radiotherapy is recommended. This reduces the chance and rate of tumour regrowth, but is not effective in all cases. Side effects can include damage to the local structures such as the optic chiasm or endocrine systems. Radiotherapy may be held back in younger children because of the increased risk of neuronal damage, using repeat surgery for any recurrence to delay the need for radiation. Systemic chemotherapy has had little impact in craniopharyngioma, but some small trials have reported promising results from intra-tumoural agents (e.g. bleomycin or interferon) delivered via an Ommaya-type catheter and reservoir in predominantly cystic tumours.

Survival and recurrence can be very late and their rates vary dramatically between reported series with 5-year survival quoted as between 50 and 90 per cent. Recurrence rates after debulking surgery followed by radiotherapy are around 30 per cent. Thorough endocrinological, ophthalmological and psychological follow up are critical to maintaining quality of life for children with craniopharyngioma in the longer term.

Challenges

This disabling, benign tumour presents great difficulties for neurosurgeons in selecting cases for most effective intervention at each stage. Radiotherapy contributes to controlling recurrence rates with low toxicity, the endocrinologists are faced with assessing hormonal status and managing hormonal fluctuations after surgery and in the long term. The chronic nature of the condition means that these patients need long-term support with good arrangements for transition to adult care.

Meningioma

Epidemiology

Meningiomas are tumours arising from the arachnoid cap cells of the overlying covering membranes of the CNS. They therefore arise outside of the brain or spinal cord, but as they grow can compress the nervous tissue causing disability and, if left unchecked, eventually even death. They are very common, though usually asymptomatic, in adults with up to 3 per cent of post-mortems revealing a meningioma. They are, however, very rare in the paediatric population with, for example, an estimated 5–10 cases per year in the UK. Therefore much of the data, including grading systems and treatment recommendations have only been validated in adults, with their use in childhood cases based on extension of adult protocols. Meningiomas can arise anywhere arachnoid is found, including within the ventricles, and are usually slow growing, well-circumscribed lesions. In childhood up to half of such tumours are secondary to prior ionizing radiation therapy with a lag time of 10–20 years. Other risk factors for the development of meningiomas include inherited genetic syndromes such as neurofibromatosis type 2 (especially tumours of the optic nerve sheath). Molecular abnormalities associated with meningiomas include 1p and 14q deletions, abnormalities of the *NF2* gene and overexpression of progesterone receptors.

Most meningiomas are slow growing WHO grade I lesions with a large number of histological subtypes, but up to 20 per cent of these tumours may be grade II (atypical) tumours. These may have a faster growth rate, are more likely to invade brain and have higher rates of recurrence. Radiation-induced tumours are more likely to be higher grade, as are tumours in males, and a small number of tumours (<1 per cent) are WHO III (anaplastic meningiomas) and these are associated with a very poor prognosis. Meningiomas may de-differentiate to higher grade lesions upon recurrence.

Symptomatology and imaging

Meningiomas usually present with symptoms of compression of surrounding structures and gradually worsening focal neurological signs, though they may present with signs of raised ICP, particularly if there is obstruction of CSF drainage. Imaging features on CT are of a hyperdense durally based lesion with avid contrast enhancement. MRI will more clearly demonstrate the dural attachment, often with a characteristic dural tail and may demonstrate flow voids representing significant vessels within the tumour. Calcification may also be seen as may small cysts and oedema in the adjacent brain parenchyma.

Management

An observational strategy with repeated imaging may be appropriate for small asymptomatic incidentally discovered tumours, with more active therapy only being offered if the tumour shows signs of growth-threatening symptoms. For lesions requiring treatment, complete (including dural origin and any involved bone) or maximal surgical resection is the initial therapy of choice. The completeness of surgical resection (Simpson grade) has a clear relation to recurrence rate, at least in adult tumours, and complete resection can be achieved in the majority of tumours. These tumours can be extremely vascular and pre-operative endovascular embolization by cerebral angiography can be employed to try and minimize blood loss. The tumour usually takes its blood supply from the external carotid circulation and tumours may sometimes compress or occlude major dural venous sinuses.

In grade I tumours, completely resected lesions would not normally require any adjuvant therapy, but radiotherapy may be considered for grade II or III lesions even if resection appears complete to minimize the increased risk of recurrence. Conventional fractionated external beam radiotherapy may improve the progression-free survival rate in incompletely resected grade I tumours from 50 to 80 per cent (adult data). Stereotactic radiosurgery has also been employed for small recurrences or irresectable tumours with apparently good effect, especially in chiasmatic or cavernous sinus tumours. No chemotherapy has been found to be effective for meningiomas, although interest has focused on hormonal therapy and other trials have been undertaken of interferon alpha-2B. These have not been tested in children to our knowledge. Clearly future development of effective chemotherapy and/or molecular targeted therapies would be of significant benefit to those patients with tumours that are progressing despite surgery/radiotherapy.

Challenges

The rarity of meningiomas in early life and the strong association with prior therapeutic radiation provide a clear hypothesis for future research. Their rarity means that research will be limited by access to tissue. The reduction in the use of cranial radiation for acute leukaemia in childhood should already be leading to a reduced incidence of this tumour in early life.

Atypical teratoid rhabdoid tumours (ATRT)

Rhabdoid tumours are classically described as aggressive tumours of infancy. characterized by the presence of tumour cells with the typical rhabdoid phenotype. The so-called rhabdoid phenotype consists of a large nucleus with single prominent nucleolus and uncondensed chromatin, together with intracytoplasmic eosinophilic inclusions. In CNS tumours, rhabdoid cells are frequently observed as a minor component of an otherwise undifferentiated tumours with miscellaneous features, leading to the description of these tumours also as atypical/teratoid rhabdoid tumours (ATRT). The cytogenetic striking feature of ATRT and other rhabdoid tumours is the deletion of chromosome 22q. Further analyses have identified a biallelic inactivation of the tumour suppressor gene *SMARCB1*, located at 22q11.2, in more than 85 per cent of ATRT. The *SMARCB1* gene alterations constantly result in the abolishment of the protein nuclear expression, an immunohistochemical feature that is now widely used for the diagnosis. Hence, and although not fully pathognomonic, loss of SMARCB1 in a CNS tumour is strongly suggestive of ATRT, whatever the morphology of the tumour cells.

The incidence of ATRT, presumably underestimated thus far, is not less than 1 per million children. The median age at diagnosis is approximately 2 years, but ATRT are encountered in older children and even in adults. The younger the age at diagnosis, the highesr the risk of carrying a germline mutation of *SMARCB1*, which is clearly involved in the rhabdoid predisposition syndrome. However, a predisposition syndrome can be found at any age. All studies report a male preponderance. ATRT are equally distributed in the supratentorial and infratentorial space, the latter location being more frequent in younger patients. The diagnosis can be evoked in many tumour locations: pineal gland, cerebral hemispheres, lateral ventricles, pons, cerebellum hemisphere or vermis, pontocereblline angle, cranial nerves, and spine. Wavy band-like enhancing rim surrounding central cystic necrosis is suggestive of ATRT. Leptomeningeal spread is noted in one third of cases. Second tumour locations outside of the CNS (such as kidney tumour) should be systematically searched for.

The prognosis of ATRT is very poor, with 2 years OS being as low as 20 to 30 per cent. The main prognostic factor is the age at diagnosis, at least partly because the intensive therapies required by such aggressive tumours cannot be safely conducted in infants. The total gross resection in localized tumours strongly influences the outcome, as does the use of involved field adjuvant radiotherapy (55 Gy), regardless of the degree of completeness of the resection. Several series suggest that early post-operative irradiation favourably impacts the outcome in comparison with delayed radiotherapy; in particular, the frequent precocious local progression observed during the first cycles of chemotherapy argues in favour of early irradiation. The benefit of craniospinal irradiation is questionable because of the serious consequences of wide field radiation in very young children and the lack of clear evidence of benefit in the literature. Current novel approaches are exploring combined high-intensity systemic and intrathecal chemotherapy; the results are awaited.

Intensive adjuvant chemotherapy is used worldwide, but no specific guidelines for treatment have been established yet. Newly diagnosed and recurrent tumours have shown chemosensitivity to a combination of ifosfamide, carboplatin, and etoposide (ICE). High-dose chemotherapies have not proven to be more effective so far. Because of *in vitro* sensitivity of ATRT cell lines to doxorubicin, anthracyclins are usually part of the treatment despite their poor penetration of the blood–brain barrier. However, retrospective reports of treatment using ICE and anthracycline-based regimens do not clearly show an advanatage. The best survival rates (2 years OS 70 per cent) have been obtained with an intense multimodality treatment including conventional chemotherapy (cisplatinum, carboplatin, vincristin, doxorubicin, cyclophosphamide, and vepeside), intrathecal chemotherapy, maintenance and continuation treatment (with doxorubicin, actino-mycin D and temozolomide). This is, however, a very toxic regimen limiting its applicability in international trials. Further multinational collaborations are needed to improve on current standards.

Chordoma

Biology

These rare tumours arise from the remnants of the primitive developmental notochord which normally forms the nucleus pulposus of the intervertebral discs. They normally arise in either the clivus or the sacrum and are slow growing but osseo-invasive and destructive tumours. On histological examination they show characteristic mucinous physaliphorous (bubble bearing) cells. Differential diagnosis on radiological grounds includes chondrosarcoma or chondroma, and they can often present with lower cranial nerve palsies (clivus lesions) or back pain/root compression (sacral lesions). CT and MRI imaging demonstrate bony destruction and a soft tissue mass.

Management

Treatment is by attempted wide *en bloc* surgical resection, but recurrence rates are high (up to 85 per cent) so radiotherapy is usually considered. Conventional radiotherapy delays but does not prevent recurrence. Recent studies have suggested that highly conformal proton beam therapy may be more effective and this is now the standard treatment, requiring referral to a centre with this facility. Some groups have reported some response to chemotherapy for example imatinib or sirolimus targeting PDGFR and mTOR respectively, targets which have been found to be altered in molecular analysis of chordomas.

Choroid plexus tumours

Choroid plexus tumours (CPT) are intraventricular epithelial neoplasms mainly affecting young children. They account for less than 5 per cent of all brain tumours in childhood, but the propor-tion rises up to 15 per cent within the first year of life. The WHO classification distinguishes three subtypes, namely choroid plexus carcinomas (CPC, WHO grade 3), choroid plexus papillomas (CPP, WHO grade 1) and the most recently identified atypical choroid plexus papillomas (aCPP, WHO grade2). CPT mainly occur in the lateral (80 per cent) or third (15 per cent) ventricles, infratentorial tumours being much rarer (fourth ventricle, cerebellopontine angle). A familial history strongly suggestive of a Li-Fraumeni syndrome might be encountered and should be searched for. Indeed, germline *TP53* mutations are observed in up to 50 per cent of CPC, whereas aCPP and CPP are far less likely to be related to a *TP53* mutation. The presence of a sporadic mutation of *TP53* might be an independent prognostic factor in CPT. Although a malignant transformation of CPP to CPC has been described and despite rare metastases, CPP are usually considered as tumours with low aggressiveness. Therefore, a full resection is frequently achieved and is usually considered sufficient for the definitive treatment of CPP. The 5-year overall survival is approximately 80 per cent without any adjuvant treatment.

In contrast, CPC display a poorer prognosis with an historical 5-year OS of 40–60 per cent. Achieving a complete resection is all the more challenging in that the prominent vascularization of CPC predisposes to severe haemorrhagic complications, and incomplete resection adversely impacts the prognosis. Adjuvant treatments are therefore required, and post-operative chemo-therapy offers at least to delay the start of irradiation. Since few prospective standardized trials have been performed to evaluate adjuvant treatments, the optimal regimen is not established. A meta-analysis encompassing a 20-year period of publication advocates in favour of the craniospinal irradiation which offers a 44 per cent 5-year PFS instead of 15 per cent in case of limited irradiation. A previous UKCCSG-SIOP trial evaluating the efficacy of an irradiation-free strategy using post-operative chemotherapy only for infants with CPC resulted in a dramatically low rate of survival (4/15), the primary tumour bed being the most frequent site of relapse. Conversely, a strategy based on an ICE regimen that allows the avoidance of any radiotherapy in infants with CPC resulted in the survival of eight out of fourteen patients with gross total resection and no irradiation. The CPT-SIOP 2000 trial plans systematic adjuvant chemotherapy (etoposide, vincristine, and carboplatin/or cyclophosphamide) whereas irradiation is stratified according to age at diagnosis; it is withheld in patients younger than 3 years of age provided that the tumour is not metastatic and correctly responses to the first courses of chemotherapy.

Finally, atypical papillomas are deemed to be of intermediate aggressiveness as compared to CPC and CPP, since they show intermediate (Mib-1) proliferation indices. Metastases are encountered in approximately 15 per cent of cases. Complete surgery is achieved in two thirds of patients and might affect the prognosis. Adjuvant chemotherapy and/or radiotherapy are discussed for aCPP in the same ways as for CPC, taking into account that patients are younger at diagnosis than patients with other types of CPT (0.7 years versus 2.5 years for patients with CPC and CPP).

Lymphoma

Primary CNS non-Hodgkin lymphomas (PCNSL) are extremely rare in children. Although immunodeficiency increases the risk of PCNSL, immunocompetent children may also be affected. Clinical symptoms are not specific, including increased ICP, paresis, and cranial nerve palsy. CNS imaging reveal either a solitary tumour or, more suggestive of the disease, a widespread infiltration or multifocal tumour masses. In the only series reported in children, B-cell lymphomas are predominant, but other subtypes are also encountered. With the exception of lymphomas occurring in the context of immunosuppression, it is considered, from a few cases and brief reports, that PCNSL have a better prognosis in children than in adults; a 70 per cent 5-year OS has been reported upon intensive chemotherapy alone, based on high-dose methotrexate and cytarabine regimen. The treatment of PCNSL follows the recommendations used for classical extra-CNS locations. Radiotherapy might be restricted to relapses.

Further reading

Medulloblastoma

Conroy S, Garnett M, Vloeberghs M, et al. (2009) Medulloblastoma in childhood: revisiting intrathecal therapy in infants and children. *Cancer Chemother Pharmacol* **65**, 1173–89.

Ellison DW (2010) Childhood medulloblastoma: novel approaches to the classification of a heterogeneous disease. *Acta Neuropathol* **120**, 305–16.

Gajjar A, Pizer B (2010) Role of high-dose chemotherapy for current medulloblastoma and other CNS primitive neuro-ectodermal tumors. *Pediatr Blood Cancer* **54**, 649–51.

Gandola L, Massimino M, Cefalo G, et al. (2009) Hyperfractionated accelerated radiotherapy in the Milan strategy for metastatic medulloblastoma. *J Clin Oncol* **27**, 566-71.

Rutkowski S, Cohen B, Finlay J, et al. (2010) Medulloblasoma in young children. *Pediatr Blood Cancer* **54**, 635–7.

Ependymoma

Bagley CA, Kothbauer KF, Wilson S, et al. (2007) Resection of myxopapillary ependymomas in children. *J Neurosurg* **106** (4 Suppl), 261–7.

Chakraborty A, Harkness W, Phipps K (2009) Surgical management of supratentorial ependymomas. *Childs Nerv Syst.* **25**, 1215–20.

Korshunov A, Golanov A, Sycheva R, Timirgaz V (2004) The histologic grade is a main prognostic factor for patients with intracranial ependymomas treated in the microneurosurigcal era: an analysis of 258 patients. *Cancer* **100**, 1230–7.

Mack SC, Taylor MD (2009) The genetic and epigenetic basis of ependymoma. *Childs Nerv Syst* **25**, 1195–201.

Zacharoulis S, Moreno L. (2009) Ependymoma: An update. *J Child Neurol* **24**, 1431–8.

ATRT

Biswas A, Goyal S, Puri T, et al. (2009) Atypical teratoid rhabdoid tumor of the brain: case series and review of literature. *Childs Nerv Syst* **25**, 1495–1500.

Roberts CW, Biegel (2009) JA. The role of SMARCB1/INI1 in development of rhabdoid tumor. *Cancer Biol Ther* **8**, 412–6.

Choroid plexus tumours

Gopal P, Parker JR, Debski R, Parker JC Jr. (2008) Choroid plexus carcinoma. *Arch Pathol Lab Med* **132**, 1350–4.

Rickert CH, Paulus W (2001) Tumors of the choroid plexus. *Microsc Res Tech.* **52**, 104–11.

Lymphoma

Abla O, Sandlund JT, Sung L, et al. (2006) A case series of pediatric primary central nervous system lymphoma: favorable outcome without cranial irradiation. *Pediatr Blood Cancer* **47**, 880–5.

Abla O, Weitzman S (2006) Primary central nervous system lymphoma in children. *Neurosurg Focus* **21**, E8.

Makino K, Nakamura H, Yano S, Kuratsu JI. (2007) Pediatric primary CNS lymphoma: long term survival after treatment with radiation monotherapy. *Acta Neurochir* (Wien) **149**, 295–7: discussion 297–8.

Low grade astrocytoma

Evans DGR, Baser ME, McGaughran J, et al. (2002) Malignant peripheral nerve sheath tumours in neurofibromatosis 1. *J Med Genet* **39**, 311–4.

Gneckow A, Packer RJ, Kortman RD. (2004) Astrocytic tumors, low grade. In *Brain & Spinal Tumors of Childhood.* Walker DA, Perilongo G, Punt JAG, Taylor RE. (eds) London: Arnold.

Listernick R, Ferner RE, Liu GT, Gutmann DH (2007) Optic pathway gliomas in neurofibromatosis 1: Controversies and recommendations. *Ann Neurol* **61**, 189–98.

Sharif S, Ferner R, Birch JM, et al. (2006) Secondary primary tumours in Neurofibromatosis 1 (NF1) patients treated for optic glioma: Substantial risks post radiotherapy. *J Clin Oncol* **24**, 2570–5.

Epidemiology

Hemminki K, Li X, Vaittinen P, Dong C (2000) Cancers in the first-degree relatives of children with brain tumours. *Br J Cancer* **83**, 407–11.

Hjern A, Lindblad F, Boman KK (2007) Disability in adult survivors of childhood cancer: A Swedish national cohort study. *J Clin Oncol* **25**, 5262–6.

Surgery

Reddy GK, Bollam P, Caldito G, et al. (2011) Ventriculoperitoneal shunt complications in hydrocephalus patients with intracranial tumors: an analysis of relevant risk factors. *J Neurooncol* **103**, 333–42.

Craniopharyngioma

Helen Spoudeas, H (ed) (2005) *Paediatric Endocrine Tumors–A Multi-Disciplinary Consensus Statement of Best Practice from a Working Group Convened Under the Auspices of the BSPED and UKCCSG (rare tumor working groups)* Crawley, UK: Novo Nordisk Ltd.

Meningioma

Traunecker H, Mallucci C, Grundy R, et al. (2008) Children's Cancer and Leukaemia Group (CCLG): guidelines for the management of intracranial meningioma in children and young people. *Br J Neurosurg* **22**. 13–25; discussion 24–5.

Chapter 21

Soft tissue sarcomas

Gianni Bisogno and Andrea Ferrari

Introduction

Soft tissue sarcomas (STS) are a heterogeneous group of tumours derived from mesenchymal cells. As these cells normally mature into muscle, fibrous structures, fat, etc., the different histotypes of STS are designated according to the line of differentiation that may be recognized in the tumour.

STS comprise approximately 8 per cent of all paediatric malignancies. They are conventionally divided in rhabdomyosarcoma (RMS), which accounts for 50-60 per cent of the whole group, and the non-rhabdomyosarcoma soft tissue sarcomas (NRSTS) (Fig. 21.1).

Rhabdomyosarcoma

Rhabdomyosarcoma (RMS) is an aggressive tumour that typically affects young children and can develop in almost any part of the body where mesenchymal tissue is present. Historically, until the 1960s, less than one third of children survived. In the 1970s, large co-operative national and international study groups started to adopt a systematic multidisciplinary approach including multidrug chemotherapy coordinated with surgery and radiotherapy. This led to a progressive increase of survival (now above 70 per cent) and to the identification of a number of prognostic factors that can be utilized to tailor the treatment. More recently, clinical protocols have been linked to pathology and biological studies that have added important insight in the nature of RMS and may provide new therapeutic opportunities in the near future.

Epidemiology and aetiology

RMS is a rare tumour with an annual incidence of 4.5 per million children under the age of 20. A male predominance is generally reported. In two thirds of cases, RMS arises before 6 years of age, but a second, smaller peak is evident in adolescence and the number of adults with RMS should not be neglected. The aetiology is not known. Genetic factors may play an important role, as demonstrated by an association between RMS and a familial cancer syndrome (Li-Fraumeni), congenital anomalies (involving the genitourinary and central nervous system), and other genetic conditions.

Pathology and biology

RMS is characterized by a variable degree of myogenic differentiation, a feature that results from the biological impact of aberrant transcription signals and the resultant production of myogenic proteins. Classically, RMS is histologically distinguished in two main subtypes: embryonal RMS (E-RMS), which accounts for approximately 70 per cent of all RMS, and alveolar RMS (A-RMS) (20 per cent). A third subtype, pleomorphic RMS, is described in adults but very rarely encountered in children; this entity is probably more closely related to adult pleomorphic STS than to other RMS subtypes.

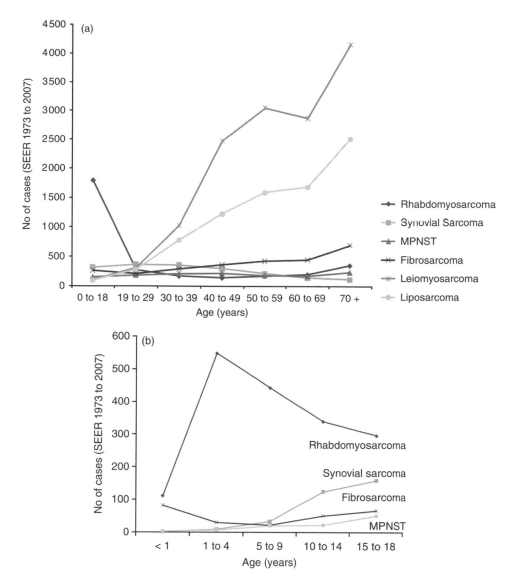

Fig. 21.1 Frequency of soft tissue sarcoma subtypes (a) at all ages and (b) for patients aged 0–18 years.
Data from the Survival Epidemiology and End result (SEER) public-access database (1973–2007) (www.seer.cancer.gov).

E-RMS is characterized by a spindle and/or round cell tumour in a loose myxoid or dense collagenous stroma. Two variants have been described:

The **botryoid subtype**, found typically at vaginal or nasopharyngeal sites, where tumour grows into organ cavities. Histologically, it shows a characteristic condensed layer of tumour cells (cambium layer) under the overlying mucosa

The **spindle cell variant**, with either collagen-poor or rich leiomyomatous forms, with a storiform pattern, arising in paratesticular locations. Its distinction from other forms of STS relies on the presence of well-differentiated rhabdomyoblasts in the spindle cell population.

Classical A-RMS displays well defined alveolar-like spaces separated by thick collagenous bands and lined with round tumour cells showing variable myogenic features. A solid alveolar variant has been described and tumours exist with a mixed embryonal-alveolar appearance. Previously it was generally accepted that the percentage of cells showing an alveolar pattern was unimportant and that even a focal presence was sufficient to justify the diagnosis of A-RMS. More recently, this concept has been challenged and it is likely that the definition of A-RMS will be further revised taking into account its molecular characteristics.

Other variants have been proposed such as pseudovascular sclerosing, rhabdoid or anaplastic RMS, but the clinical significance of these entities is yet to be confirmed.

Desmin and muscle-specific actin are relatively sensitive immunohistochemical markers of RMS but the most sensitive markers are the muscle transcription factors MyoD and myogenin. A high degree of nuclear staining of myogenin seems correlated with the alveolar subtype. Recently, gene expression data have identified AP2Beta and P-cadherin as specific markers for A-RMS, and epidermal growth factor (EGF) receptor and fibrillin-2 as markers for E-RMS. The search for specific genetic alterations has identified two chromosomal translocations specifically associated with A-RMS, and the t(2;13)(q35;q14), and t(1;13)(p36;q14) translocations are found in more than 80 per cent of cases. These abnormalities fuse the *FKHR* locus on chromosome 13 to either the *PAX3* gene on chromosome 2 or the *PAX7* gene on chromosome 1, producing the PAX3–FKHR and PAX7–FKHR chimeric proteins that are powerful transcription factors influencing cell growth, differentiation, and apoptosis. A minority of A-RMS do not show known translocations: this may be explained by the presence of rare alternative translocations [e.g. t(2;2) and t(2;8)]. It seems however that most translocation-negative A-RMS are clinically and molecularly indistinguishable from embryonal cases and significantly different from fusion-positive A-RMS. As a consequence, it has been suggested that fusion gene status should be used in risk stratification of RMS irrespective of histology. No specific genetic alterations have been found in E-RMS but many of them exhibit a loss of heterozygosity at chromosome 11p15.5 although the biological implications of this are not yet understood.

The International Classification of Rhabdomyosarcoma identified three risk groups:

(a) superior prognosis: botryoid and spindle cell RMS

(b) intermediate prognosis: E-RMS

(c) poor prognosis: A-RMS.

This was shown to be strongly predictive of survival but it does not take into account the recent advances of molecular biology.

Clinical presentation and diagnosis

RMS is encountered at almost all anatomic sites although the head and neck (40 per cent), genitourinary (20 per cent) and extremities (20 per cent) are the most common locations. It tends to invade nearby organs and regional lymph nodes. Metastases at diagnosis are present in approximately 20 per cent of cases, more frequently in the lungs, bone marrow, bones, and distant lymph nodes. Clinical presentation is strongly influenced by site: for example, tumours within the orbit tend to present early with obvious displacement of the globe and are rarely associated with regional lymph node or distant metastatic spread (Fig. 21.2), whilst tumours in the nasopharynx may result in a history of nasal discharge and obstruction and frequently involve local extension to the skull base, with the potential for associated cranial nerve palsies or visual loss. The definition of certain head-neck sites as 'parameningeal' relates to the risk of direct tumour extension into the meninges and beyond intracranially. Tumours within the genitourinary tract may present with urinary obstruction (in bladder and prostate sites), as a scrotal mass (paratesticular) or as a vaginal polyp or discharge (vaginal and uterine tumours).

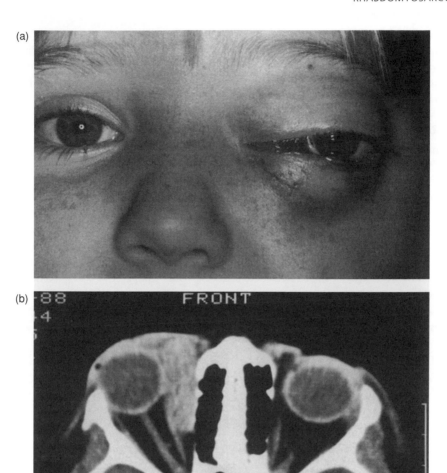

Fig. 21.2 Orbital tumour. (a) Clinical presentation with proptosis and deviation of globe. (b) CT scan shows large antero-medial soft-tissue mass without bone erosion.

Diagnostic and staging investigations

These must include adequate imaging of the primary site and regional lymph nodes by computed tomography (CT) or magnetic resonance imaging (MRI) scans, and accurate assessment of sites of potential metastatic spread (lung CT scan, radionuclide bone scan, bone marrow biopsy and aspirates). Cerebrospinal fluid should be sampled in the case of parameningeal tumours. The risk of involvement of regional lymph nodes depends on the primary site and there is a general consensus to biopsy nodes when the RMS arises in the extremities (the use of sentinel lymph node mapping technique may be of help). Different strategies are adopted when RMS occurs in other sites; for example, systematic retroperitoneal lymph node sampling is recommended in older children with paratesticular RMS in North American protocols, while radiological evaluation and selective biopsy is considered sufficient in Europe.

Diagnosis must be confirmed histologically and, although needle biopsy may be the simplest approach favoured by some clinicians, it has the disadvantage of limiting the tissue available for conventional histological examination, including immunohistochemistry, and may limit the fresh and frozen tissue for cytogenetic and molecular genetic investigation. Open biopsy is therefore frequently preferred and should, when possible, be undertaken at the oncology centre where the initial surgical approach can determined by the multi disciplinary team responsible for the child's subsequent treatment, with the optimal use of diagnostic material.

Treatment

The multi disciplinary risk-adapted management of RMS promotes chemotherapy as systemic treatment for both local and metastatic lesions, coordinated with local treatment that includes surgery and/or radiotherapy. Since the early 1970s, patients have been enrolled in large multi-institutional trials sequentially addressing crucial questions. In particular, the studies coordinated by the Intergroup Rhabdomyosarcoma Study (IRS) Group [now the Soft Tissue Sarcoma Committee of the Children's Oncology Group (COG)] are examples of successful models of clinical coordination to research rare diseases. In Europe, three independent cooperative groups have coordinated paediatric STS studies: the International Society of Paediatric Oncology—Malignant Mesenchymal Tumour Committee (SIOP-MMT); the German Soft Tissue Sarcoma Cooperative Group (CWS); and the Italian Cooperative Group (ICG) [now the Associazione Italiana Ematologia Oncologia Pediatrica Soft Tissue Sarcoma Committee (AIEOP-STSC)] Recently the SIOP-MMT and the AIEOP-STSC Groups merged to form the European Paediatric Soft tissue sarcoma Group (EpSSG).

Prognostic factors and staging

The presence of metastasis at diagnosis is the most powerful factor in determining an adverse outcome and groups of patients with localized or metastatic disease have often been investigated separately for the search of prognostic factors.

Table 21.1 Prognostic factors in localized rhabdomyosarcoma

	Favourable	Unfavourable
Histology	Embryonal Spindle cell Botryoid RMS Alveolar fusion negative (?)	Alveolar, including the solid-alveolar variant Anaplastic features (?)
Tumour site	Orbit Genito-urinary non bladder prostate (i.e. paratesticular and vagina/uterus) Head and neck non parameningeal	Parameningeal Extremities Genito-urinary bladder-prostate 'Other' (i.e. trunk, pelvis)
Tumour size	Maximum diameter <5 cm	>5 cm
Tumour invasiveness*	T1: tumour confined to the organ or tissue of origin	T2: tumour involving one or more contiguous organs or tissues
Lymph node involvement*	N0 = no clinical or pathological node involvement	N1 = clinical or pathological nodal involvement
Initial surgery	Complete (IRS Group I)	Incomplete (IRS Group II or III)
Patient age	1–9 years	<1 year and ≥10 years

*TNM system.
(?) Factors that need to be confirmed

Localized disease

For non-metastatic RMS patients, several prognostic factors have emerged with the evolution of treatment. Table 21.1 describes the tumour and patient characteristics currently used to assign risk group and treatment strategy.

Histology—The IRS IV Study showed 88 per cent relapse-free survival in E-RMS versus 66 per cent in A-RMS. This prognostic distinction has been confirmed in most other studies and may become more striking if only fusion-positive A-RMS are compared with E-RMS.

Tumour site and size—Site is a major determinant of treatment strategy and outcome: orbit, non-bladder prostate genitourinary (i.e. paratesticular and vagina/uterus), and non-parameningeal head-neck sites are associated to a better prognosis. Tumour dimension >5 cm in maximum diameter is the usually adopted point for identifying tumour size as an adverse factor within treatment stratification systems although recent evidence suggests that tumour dimension should be correlated with patient size and the use of a fixed size cut-off may be questioned in the future.

Post-surgical status—The IRS grouping system is used:

group I: completely-excised tumours with negative microscopic margins

group II: grossly-resected tumours with microscopic residual disease and/or regional lymph node spread

group III: macroscopic residual disease after incomplete resection or initial biopsy;

group IV: metastatic disease.

Age—Prognosis is worse in patients over 10 years of age. Young children (below 1 year) generally have worse prognosis, maybe associated with constraints on the use of radiotherapy due to the higher risk of sequelae.

It is important to note that factors predictive of prognosis are often interdependent: limb tumours are generally of the alveolar type and tend to spread more frequently both to regional nodes and to distant metastatic sites. The surgical status is also strongly determined by the site; for example, complete tumour resection is usually impossible for parameningeal RMS but easily performed for paratesticular tumour.

Metastatic disease

A pooled analysis of 788 patients treated in nine studies performed by European and American cooperative groups identified factors with an independent and significant negative impact on survival: age, alveolar histology, unfavourable primary site (extremity and 'other' sites), presence of three or more sites of metastatic disease, and the specific presence of bone or bone marrow involvement. Patients without any of these unfavourable characteristics showed a 50 per cent event-free survival (EFS) in comparison with 42, 12, and 5 per cent in patients with one, two or more than two adverse factors.

Treatment stratification

To take into account all the known prognostic factors, risk-adapted treatment strategies are currently based on complex staging systems. As an example, the EpSSG stratification takes into consideration six different prognostic factors leading to the identification of eight subgroups that receive different treatments according to the four derived risk groups.

Low-risk group: includes 6–8 per cent of the whole population of localized RMS. These children present with a small (<5cm) tumour, completely resected at diagnosis (IRS group I) with favourable histology and site. Most of these patients are represented by children with paratesticular RMS. The 5-year EFS is approximately 90 per cent, so the goal for this selected group of patients is to avoid aggressive treatment. In the current EpSSG protocol these children are treated with a relatively short course of non-intensive chemotherapy (vincristine and actinomycin-D).

Intermediate-risk group: includes patients with favourable histology and site, with a survival around 70–80 per cent. The goal for this group includes is to reduce treatment cautiously without compromising survival. Intensive alkylating agent-based chemotherapy is utilized but there is an attempt to reduce cumulative dose exposure and to limit the use of radiotherapy.

High-risk group: this group includes patients with large E-RMS localized in unfavourable sites or with nodal involvement, and most A-RMS. These patients have an unsatisfactory prognosis (survival below 60 per cent) and are therefore the major focus of randomized trials to identify more effective strategies.

Very high-risk group: this includes mainly metastatic RMS. In this group survival is between 20 and 30 per cent and has not improved in the past 40 years. Experimental approaches are therefore needed for these patients.

Therapeutic strategy

Surgery, radiotherapy and chemotherapy have been combined differently over the years by international cooperative groups, in an attempt to improve outcome whilst finding the correct balance between the intensity of treatment and its possible cost in terms of late effects. In general there is concordance on the use of intensive chemotherapy and aggressive non-mutilating surgery. Controversies relate more to the method and timing of local treatment, and, more specifically, to the place of radiotherapy in guaranteeing local control for patients who appear to achieve complete remission with chemotherapy with or without surgery. This represented an important philosophical difference between the SIOP MMT studies and those of the IRS Group and, to some extent, those of the German and Italian Co-operative groups. Local relapse rates are higher when radiotherapy is not systematically used, although the SIOP experience has also made it clear that a significant number of patients who relapse may be cured with salvage treatment. In the context of such differences in approach to local treatment, overall survival rather than disease-free or progression-free survival may become the most important criteria for measuring outcome.

Surgery

Tumour resection at diagnosis should be attempted only if the tumour can be realistically excised with clear margins without danger, functional impairment or mutilation. If this is not possible, a diagnostic biopsy is required. An attempt at surgical resection which leaves microscopic residual disease makes treatment decisions more complicated because the patient is unassessable for the efficacy of chemotherapy and may still require further local treatment. Primary re-excision (i.e. a second surgical resection before chemotherapy) may be worthwhile in cases when there is confidence that clear margins of excision can be achieved without functional or cosmetic disadvantage: this may be particularly useful in limb and paratesticular tumours.

RMS usually shrinks significantly with initial chemotherapy and secondary conservative surgery to achieve local control may become more feasible and remains an important aspect of treatment. Its implementation depends, however, on the site of disease: for example, surgery has little or no role in the primary management of orbital or parameningeal RMS. At other sites, surgery should aim to completely resect the residual tumour, although marginal resections may be acceptable provided that they are followed by radiotherapy. The efficacy and the potential morbidity of surgery and radiotherapy must be carefully assessed: in some cases, the morbidity of radiotherapy may be more acceptable than radical operations which result in important functional (e.g. total cystectomy) and/or cosmetic (e.g. amputation) consequences; in other circumstances, the morbidity of radical surgery to achieve local control may be preferred, for example to avoid pelvic or extremity irradiation in very young children.

Radiotherapy

The role of radiotherapy in the local control of RMS is unquestionable but the awareness of the possible late effects, especially in young children, has led to attempts to identify groups of patients where irradiation can be withheld or modulated in its dose and target volume.

Strategies determining the use of radiotherapy require consideration of diverse factors including histological subtype, patient age, tumour size and site, response to initial chemotherapy, and presence of residual tumour after surgery. The only patients where radiotherapy can be safely withheld are those with E-RMS completely resected at diagnosis. It is also known that a certain proportion of patients with E-RMS can be cured without radiotherapy when the tumour is completely resected at secondary surgery but, as most studies suggest a survival advantage for radiotherapy, this strategy is often limited to very young children.

Studies from the European groups have attempted to relate the use of radiotherapy to the response to initial chemotherapy. The most radical approach has been used in the SIOP protocols, where radiotherapy was avoided if complete remission was achieved after initial chemotherapy, with or without second surgery (except for parameningeal RMS). This approach has proved feasible, especially in the subsets of patients with orbital embryonal RMS where up to 40 per cent of patients were cured without irradiation. However, the higher rate of relapse observed in this population requires consideration of the burden of second-line therapy, and the psychological impact of relapse, in the total cost of cure. There is good evidence from all groups that survival is improved when radiotherapy is given to all patients with A-RMS and to those with E-RMS with microscopic or macroscopic residual disease. The timing of radiotherapy in treatment may be important and, at least in some subgroups such as those with parameningeal RMS, there is evidence that early irradiation may improve local control.

Current guidelines for therapy within the COG and EpSSG Groups recommend doses from 40 to 55 Gy, given by conventional fractionation (single daily doses of 1.8 Gy) depending on the various clinical variables. A reduction of dose to 32–36 Gy is under exploration in children with favourable characteristics. Hyperfractionated schedules have been explored but did not show any advantage in terms of local control or survival.

The reduction of side effects can be pursued not only by avoiding or reducing the doses of radiotherapy but also through better treatment planning and the use of the most modern techniques. Radiotherapy should be performed only in a limited number of experienced centres and 3D-conformal planning is recommended to reduce irradiation of critical structures near the target volume. The target volume should be selected as the initial tumour volume plus adequate margins (1–2 cm), but after good response to chemotherapy the use of residual tumour volume can be considered (plus margins). In large tumours, a boost can be delivered to a more limited field. Interstitial radiotherapy (brachytherapy) using intracavitary moulds or implanted wires may be of particular relevance for small tumours at selected sites, notably in the vagina and perineum. Occasionally this technique is utilized at other genitourinary sites, including tumours of the bladder base and prostate, and there is emerging experience of its application to head and neck sites. The use of intensity modulated radiotherapy (IMRT) and proton therapy awaits clinical studies to understand their indications and potential advantages although both are already increasingly utilized.

Chemotherapy

Chemotherapy is an essential component of treatment for all children with RMS. Chemotherapy is effective in the adjuvant setting to control occult metastasis after the primary tumour has been completely resected; it is given to patients with large infiltrating tumours to reduce the extent of subsequent surgery or radiation therapy; finally, it is the only available tool against metastatic lesions not otherwise amenable to local therapy, for example bone marrow involvement.

Experience since the 1970s has defined the efficacy of a variety of individually active chemotherapeutic agents, subsequently combined in different multidrug regimens to increase their effect. Vincristine, actinomycin D, cyclophosphamide and doxorubicin have been the most frequently utilized agents in the treatment of RMS. Early experience from the IRS group failed to show a convincing difference in survival when patients were treated with VAC (vincristine, actinomycin and cyclophosphamide) with or without doxorubicin and concern about potential cardiotoxicity justifies caution over its incorporation into primary treatment. Nevertheless, doxorubicin has convincing single agent activity and its role is being re evaluated in a more dose-intense combination (IVADo: ifosfamide, vincristine, actinomycin D, doxorubicin) as part of the current EpSSG RMS 2005 study.

The substitution of cyclophosphamide by ifosfamide in combination with vincristine and actinomycin D (with or without doxorubicin) has been the hallmark of all recent European studies. There is no evidence that an ifosfamide-based combination with vincristine and actinomycin D (IVA) is superior to VAC although ifosfamide appears to convey some advantages over its analogue, showing a lack of cross resistance, a lower myelotoxicity profile and (probably) a lower risk of gonadal toxicity, but it carries a risk of renal toxicity. Currently, VAC remains the combination of choice for North American studies, while the IVA regimen is the gold standard for European groups.

The addition of newer drugs (originally cisplatin and etoposide, later epirubicin and carboplatin and, more recently, topotecan) has failed to demonstrate any convincing evidence for superiority over VAC or IVA although some or all may have value in second line therapies. The role of irinotecan is currently under investigation.

Approaches to high-dose and dose-intensified chemotherapy

The very poor prognosis presented by subgroups of patients, particularly those with metastases detectable at diagnosis, has justified the search for novel strategies. The place of high-dose chemotherapy (HDCT) followed by haematopoietic stem cell rescue (HSCR) has been explored in different trials although there has been no direct randomized comparison with conventional does chemotherapy. The closest study was a non randomized European protocol that compared 12 cycles of a six-drug regimen (CEVAIE: carboplatin, epirubicin, vincristine, actinomycin D, ifosfamide, and etoposide) to six courses of CEVAIE followed by high-dose melphalan as consolidation therapy for patients who achieved complete remission. No obvious difference in survival was identified. Similarly unsatisfactory results were achieved with other high-dose regimens (including combinations of melphalan, etoposide, carboplatin, thiotepa, and cyclophosphamide) and with attempts to use rapid sequential HDCT with HSRC earlier in the treatment pathway. In contrast, recent data from the German group suggested a survival advantage for metastatic patients who received low-dose 'maintenance' chemotherapy with oral trofosfamide and idarubicin when compared (albeit in a non-random manner) with patients undergoing HDCT. Nevertheless, the strategy to add a 'metronomic' (regular and frequent low doses) maintenance treatment after completing conventional chemotherapy is a promising alternative approach which aims to control presumed minimal residual disease resistant to standard chemotherapy. The current EpSSG RMS 2005 protocol is investigating the role of a six-month schedule of maintenance treatment using vinorelbine and low-dose oral cyclophosphamide in high-risk patients. An alternative way to increase dose intensity is by compressing the interval between cycles of chemotherapy with granulocyte colony-stimulating growth factor (G-CSF) support: this strategy is now part of a current COG trial for high-risk metastatic patients.

Experimental approaches

A number of potentially new approaches are being investigated in preclinical and clinical studies, including the use of novel antineoplastic agents, immunotherapy, and molecules directed against specific biological targets. Various new antineoplastic agents are in current phase I-II trials (as single agents or in combination). Preclinical studies have shown that RMS expresses high levels of a number of cellular growth factors including insulin-like growth factors IGF-I and -II, EGF and ErbB-2. This provides the rationale for testing agents such as IGF-receptor inhibitor molecules or gefitinib, a small molecule that competes with ATP for the intracellular catalytic site of EGF receptor.

The observation that RMS cell lines express vascular endothelial growth factor (VEGF) and that VEGF-receptor-1 antibody inhibits VEGF signalling and delays RMS proliferation, has made anti-angiogenic treatment an attractive option. A study on the use of bevacizumab, a humanized monoclonal antibody which blocks the binding of human VEGF to its receptors, in association with IVADo chemotherapy is ongoing in Europe under the auspices of the EpSSG.

The demonstration of a graft effect against some solid tumour cells has prompted the consideration of allogeneic bone marrow transplantation in paediatric STS. Data from bone marrow transplant (BMT) registries and other small series are inconclusive but have provided the basis for ongoing prospective trials in very high-risk patients (mainly with recurrent disease) using related or unrelated donors as the source of stem cells, with or without post-transplant immunomodulation. A more specific approach to immunotherapy in RMS includes attempts to generate cytotoxic T lymphocytes against A-RMS cells expressing the PAX3-FKHR fusion protein.

Outcome

The advent of multidisciplinary protocols dramatically increased the overall survival of patients with RMS from around 20 per cent in the 1970s to over 70 per cent in the early 1990s since which time further improvement has been less noticeable. Treatment failures usually occur within 3 years from diagnosis, and are represented mostly by local or regional relapse (accounting for approximately 60 per cent of all relapses). Survival after relapse is generally poor (below 30 per cent at 5 years), but patients with favourable tumour characteristics (embryonal histology, favourable primary site) who did not receive radiotherapy during first line treatment have a realistic chance of cure with further therapy.

Late effects of treatment

The cost of the cure is the difficult, yet essential, issue to be addressed when reviewing the outcome of survivors of all forms of cancer in childhood, particularly when survival is achieved using different philosophies and treatment modalities. The importance of accurate prognostic assessment at diagnosis is as much to ensure that patients with good prognosis are not over treated as to identify those with a poorer prognosis who require a more aggressive approach. Much concern has been focused on the late sequelae of local treatment for RMS, particularly in patients with head-neck and genitourinary primaries. Chemotherapy is also associated with significant sequelae in some patients, and the concept that more intensive chemotherapy may help to reduce the use of local treatment must be balanced against the additional toxicity that the chemotherapy may bring. The more recent use of ifosfamide has raised concern about long-term renal damage although risks seem acceptably low with cumulative doses below 60 g/m^2 as in all current European protocols. The continuing use of high doses of alkylating agents (and etoposide) has been linked to an increased risk of second malignancy and the long-term follow up and prospective evaluation of survivors of current protocols is required in order to document the frequency and functional significance of all possible late effects of therapy.

Non-rhabdomyosarcoma soft tissue sarcomas

The term non-rhabdomyosarcoma soft tissue sarcoma (NRSTS) describes a very heterogeneous group of mesenchymal extra skeletal malignant tumours, with different biology and clinical history, classified on the basis of their differentiation according to the adult tissue they resemble. The term NRSTS is in widespread use, reflecting the fact that these tumours have often been treated in the past according to the principles adopted for RMS despite the fact that this is a clearly different entity.

Most of the NRSTS histotypes are more common in adults than in children but the frequency of the different subtypes differs significantly according to age: infantile fibrosarcoma is a peculiar entity of young children, synovial sarcoma and malignant peripheral nerve sheath tumour (MPNST) are typical of adolescents and young adults, liposarcoma and leiomyosarcoma occur typically in adults and are very rare in children (Fig. 21.1).

The pathogenesis of NRSTS is still unknown and there are no well-established risk factors. Ionizing radiation (angiosarcoma) and oncogenic viruses (leiomyosarcoma in immunocompromised patients) have been variously associated to the development of some type of sarcomas, but the aetiological relation is yet unclear. A well-known association is that between MPNST and neurofibromatosis type 1 (NF1). The life-time risk of developing MPNST in NF1 patients has been estimated at 8–13 per cent compared to 0.001 per cent in the general population and the incidence of NF1 in patients with MPNST has been variously reported from 15 per cent to 70 per cent. Both NF1-associated and sporadic MPNST show loss or mutation of the *NF-1* gene (chromosome 17q11.2).

Local behaviour and the propensity to local relapse, as well as the risk of distant metastases, are features that correlate with different diagnoses and, importantly, with tumour grade. In general, it is possible to say that low-grade tumours are often locally aggressive but unlikely to metastasize, whilst high-grade tumours are more aggressive and have a high risk of metastasis (Table 21.2).

Diagnosis

As with RMS, NRSTS can arise anywhere in the soft tissues of the body although the most common clinical presentation is that of a painless, growing mass localized in lower extremities; less frequent sites are the trunk or the head and neck region.

In general, the paediatric oncology community adopts the same diagnostic work-up (MRI is the recommended investigation) and staging systems (tumour-node-metastasis (TNM) classification and IRS post-surgical grouping system) as used for RMS. After the radiologic assessment to assess local tumour extent, biopsy should be done to define the histological diagnosis before any definitive surgery or other therapy, since the surgical and therapeutic approach may vary depending on histotype and grading; in case of large and deep soft tissue mass, biopsy should be always the initial surgical procedure, as there is no benefit from initial surgical debulking.

The precise definition of histotype and grading is of paramount importance in the planning of therapy. The WHO Classification of STS, last updated in 2002, classifies tumours on the basis of

Table 21.2 Peak age of incidence, details of characteristic chromosomal translocation and fusion transcripts, and major clinical characteristics of some NRSTS subtypes

Histotype	Peak age of incidence	Molecular findings	Clinical characteristics
Synovial sarcoma	Second to third decade	t(X;18)(p11;q11) SYT-SSX1, SYT-SSX2, SYT-SSX4	Extremity site (but it is the most frequent subtype in lung, pleura and mediastinum) 60% response rate to chemotherapy (halfway between adult soft tissue sarcomas and pediatric small round cell sarcomas)
Malignant peripheral nerve sheath tumour (MPNST)	Third to fourth decade	Loss or rearrangement of 10p, 11q, 17q and 22q	30% associated with neurofibromatosis type 1 (NF-1) Frequently located in the trunk Poor response to chemotherapy Poor prognosis
Infantile fibrosarcoma	First year of life	t(12;15;)(p13;q25) ETVG(TEL)-NTRK3 (as in mesoblastic nephroma)	Rapid growth Relatively high chemosensitivity to alkylating and anthracycline-free regimens Overall good prognosis
Adult-type fibrosarcoma	Fourth to fifth decade	t(2,5) and t(7,22)	Tendency to metastatic spread according to tumour grade
Epithelioid sarcoma	Third decade	-	Superficial, distant sites (fingers) Indolent course Lymph nodal spread
Liposarcoma	Sixth to seventh decade but earlier (before fourth decade) for myxoid-type	myxoid liposarcoma: t(12;16)(q13;p11) t(12;22)(q13;q12) FUS-CHOP	Different biology and clinical behaviour according to the subtype, i.e. well-differentiated, dedifferentiated or myxoid/round cell subtype Retroperitoneal location
Leiomyosarcoma	Sixth decade	-	Retroperitoneum Immunocompromised patients
Alveolar soft part sarcoma	Third decade	t(X;17)(p11.2;q25) TFE3-ASPL	Head and neck and other unusual locations Poor response to chemotherapy Poor prognosis
Clear cell sarcoma	Third to fourth decade	t(12;22)(q13;q12) t(9;22)(q22;q12) ATF1-EWS	Extremity site, deep-seated Poor response to chemotherapy Poor prognosis

(continued)

Table 21.2 (continued)

Histotype	Peak age of incidence	Molecular findings	Clinical characteristics
Angiosarcoma	Fourth to sixth decade	-	Associated with lymphoedema, after radiotherapy
			Superficial or deep
			Breast
			Poor prognosis
Dermatofibrosarcoma protuberans	Third to fifth decade	t(17;22)	Subcutaneous
		t(2;17)(p23;q23)	Indolent growth
		ALK-CLTC	
		PDGFβ-COL1A1	
Extraskeletal myxoid chondrosarcoma	Fifth to sixth decade	t(9;22)(q22;q12)	Slow-growing tumour of extremity
		t(9;17)(q22;q11.2)	
		EWS-CHN	
Extraskeletal mesenchymal chondrosarcoma	Second to third decade	Complex cytogenetic alteration	Head-neck region (orbit)
			Highly aggressive tumour
		t(11;22) (q24;q12) (as Ewing family tumours)	
Desmoplastic small round cell tumour	Second to third decade	t(11;22) (p13;q12)	Abdominal mass widely disseminated at onset
		EWS-WT1	Peritoneal seeding
			Metastases
			Poor outcome
Extracranial extrarenal rhabdoid tumour	Infants and young children	hSNF5/INI 1 gene mutations	Poor prognosis

their differentiation as adipocytic, fibroblastic/myofibroblastic, fibrohistiocytic, smooth muscle, pericytic/perivascular, skeletal muscle, and vascular, and tumours of uncertain differentiation. In most cases the diagnosis of histotype requires the use of immunohistochemistry and cytogenetic/molecular evaluation and a number of specific translocations have been identified in NRSTS (Table 21.2). Once the histotype is defined, the grade of malignancy should be estimated. Although this usually indicates how aggressively a tumour will behave, some diagnoses (e.g. synovial sarcoma, alveolar sarcoma, angiosarcoma) should be considered high grade regardless of their morphological parameters, whereas in others (e.g. clear cell sarcoma, extraskeletal myxoid chondrosarcoma) biological behaviour is less predictable. Tumour grade is usually established from a combined assessment of histological features including degree of cellularity, cellular pleomorphism or anaplasia, mitotic activity, and degree of necrosis. Over the years, two different grading systems have emerged: the Pediatric Oncology Group (POG) system and the French system (FNCLCC) developed for adult STS but also used in Europe for pediatric NRSTS.

Treatment strategy

The rarity and heterogeneity of these tumours suggest that children and adolescents with NRSTS should be referred to selected institutions with adequate experience in the diagnosis and treatment of paediatric STS, and with a commitment to enrolling patients in clinical trials. A critical step is the assessment of patients according to histotype and grading in order to modulate the indication and intensity of multimodal therapy (surgery, radiotherapy, and chemotherapy).

Synovial sarcoma is an adult-type sarcoma but it should be treated and analysed separately from the other histotypes, not only because it is the most common NRSTS in childhood and adolescents, but also because its chemosensitivity probably stands midway between that of most typical adult STS (in which less than 40 per cent of patients respond to chemotherapy) and that of RMS (up to 80 per cent respond to chemotherapy).

For many of the other specific diagnoses seen amongst NRSTS, allocation of a treatment strategy within a group loosely described as 'adult-type' NRSTS seems most appropriate. Histotypes that are typical of adulthood, definitely malignant, with morphological features resembling differentiated/mature tissues, include adult-type fibrosarcoma, MPNST, epithelioid sarcoma, leiomyosarcoma, clear cell sarcoma of soft part, liposarcoma, alveolar soft part sarcoma, undifferentiated polymorphous sarcomas, malignant solitary fibrous tumour/hemangiopericytoma, angiosarcoma, dermatofibrosarcoma. This definition excludes infantile fibrosarcoma, other small round cell tumours (extra-osseous Ewing sarcoma) and a group of 'other histotypes' which includes various entities that are characterized by unique biology and clinical course, and require separate consideration.

Although the overall cure rate for NRSTS patients is around 70 per cent, this correlated to risk group based on prognostic variables which include:

(1) extent of disease at diagnosis—survival is very poor in children with disseminated disease (<20 per cent can be cured)

(2) completeness of initial surgery:—5-year OS is around 90 per cent in patients who achieve complete resection at diagnosis (group I according to the post-surgical IRS classification), 80 per cent in those who had marginal resection (group II) and 50 per cent in initially unresected cases (group III)

(3) tumour grade—5-year OS: 90 per cent for G1, 80 per cent for G2 and 65 per cent for G3

(4) tumour site—5-year OS: 80 per cent for extremity tumours and 60 per cent for axial location

(5) tumour size—5-year OS: 95 per cent for tumour ≤5 cm, 55 per cent for size >5 cm.

Tumour invasiveness (T-stage) and superficial/deep location are often linked to tumour size and site and are not commonly used in risk-stratification of NRSTS in children. Many of these prognostic variables are inter-related, for example, MPNST are often large, axial tumours and unresectable at diagnosis.

Synovial sarcoma

Synovial sarcoma is the most frequent NRSTS in childhood and adolescence and since relatively high rates of response to chemotherapy were recorded in previous pediatric experience, synovial sarcoma was traditionally considered as an 'RMS-like' tumour by many pediatric oncologists, particularly in Europe. In the adult setting, chemotherapy is less frequently used but outcomes have generally been better in pediatric experience with 5-year OS rates of around 80 per cent. Comparative studies have highlighted that cancer-specific mortality from synovial sarcoma is higher in adults than in children and that the adverse outcome for adults remains even after correction for the presence of unfavourable risk factors. This might reflect differences in the biology of the tumour at different ages although there is, as yet, no data to support this and there is a

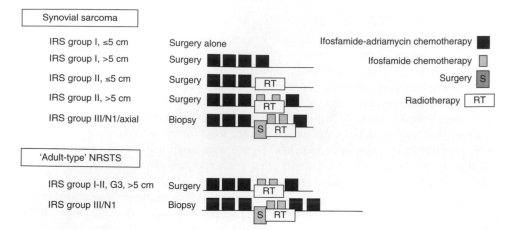

Fig. 21.3 Risk-adapted treatment strategy for synovial sarcoma and 'adult-type' soft tissue sarcoma in the European Paediatric Soft Tissue Sarcoma Study Group (EpSSG) NRSTS 2005 protocol. IRS, Intergroup Rhabdomyosarcoma Study; G, tumour grade.

suggestion that the difference might relate to the different use made of chemotherapy. A retrospective single-institutional analysis undertaken at the Istituto Nazionale Tumori in Milan on patients of all ages, showed that adjuvant chemotherapy (administered to most of the children and to a minority of the older patients) improved patient outcome. However, a formal demonstration of the efficacy of adjuvant chemotherapy in synovial sarcoma is still not available and it is possible that its use for all synovial sarcoma patients (as in RMS) is unnecessary: recent data suggest that chemotherapy can be omitted from a subset of low-risk patients (completely resected tumours <5 cm) without jeopardizing the results. The choice of chemotherapy for synovial sarcoma has shifted away from classic RMS regimens to the use of the standard adult STS chemotherapy combination of ifosfamide and doxorubicin (Fig. 21.3). Radiotherapy is reserved for synovial sarcoma that is incompletely resected (IRS group II and III).

Adult-type NRSTS

These tumour types are not usually considered very sensitive to chemotherapy and surgery remains the key element of therapy with the aim of obtaining adequate margins with limited or no long-term sequelae. The definition of 'adequate margins' depends on the quality and the quantity of healthy tissues surrounding the tumour. There is no consensus on the definition of a safe distance between tumour and resection margin: 'adequate' might be considered those >1 cm of healthy tissue around the tumour, in all directions, when the tumour arises in muscle or adipose tissue, but when the tumour is resected adjacent to periostium, vessel sheath, epineurium, or muscular fascia, a rim of healthy tissue >1 mm may be considered sufficient.

Radiotherapy plays a well-defined role in local control for adult STS but its indications are more strictly controlled in children, given the higher risk of late effects. In general, the indication for post-operative irradiation seems clear after initial marginal resection (IRS group II) but it is still debated after wide resection (IRS group I). In patients whose tumours are judged unresectable at diagnosis (group III), initial chemotherapy is usually given to try to shrink the tumour after which the best approach (with surgery and/or radiotherapy) to local treatment is planned, taking into account the anatomical site, tumour size, patient's age, response to initial chemotherapy, and the need to minimize sequelae and preserve function.

Table 21.3 Histology-directed therapeutic options in adult-type NRSTS

Histotype	Agent
Synovial sarcoma	Ifosfamide
Angiosarcoma	Taxanes
	Gemcitabine
	Vascular endothelial growth factor (VEGF) inhibitors
Leiomyosarcoma	Gemcitabine
	Gemcitabine and docetaxel
	Trabectedine
	Vascular endothelial growth factor (VEGF) inhibitors
	Mammalian targets of rapamycin (mTOR) inhibitors
Liposarcoma (myxoid/round cell)	Trabectedine
Dermatofibrosarcoma protuberans	Imatinib
Alveolar soft part sarcoma	Sunitinib, cedarinibid
Clear cell sarcoma	Sunitinib

The place of chemotherapy is still debated, particularly whether or not to provide adjuvant chemotherapy to minimize distant recurrence after initial surgery. Overall, however, the outcome after initial tumour resection alone is good in patients with small, low-grade tumours (5 year OS 90 per cent), whilst the prognosis for patients with high-grade, large and invasive tumours is unsatisfactory, even after initial microscopically complete resection, as there is a high risk of developing lung metastases if the treatment is limited to local therapy alone. This would suggest, in principle, the use of systemic chemotherapy to try to improve survival despite the fact that most randomized trials in adult STS have shown no statistically significant benefit for patients given adjuvant chemotherapy and the only randomized trial of adjuvant chemotherapy in pediatric NRSTS also failed to achieve an informative result. In the current EpSSG NRSTS 2005 protocol, ifosfamide-doxorubicin adjuvant chemotherapy is recommended for patients with large, high grade tumours (Fig. 21.3).

The role of front-line (neo-adjuvant) chemotherapy in patients with advanced unresectable disease at diagnosis is more established. Neo-adjuvant chemotherapy may improve the chance of subsequent complete resection and may play an important role in treating presumed micrometastases. Experience suggests that approximately 40 per cent of these patients may achieve a worthwhile response that may translate into a survival advantage.

In recent years, various drugs other than the ifosfamide-doxorubicin combination have shown some activity against particular STS histotypes (Table 21.3) and the next step in the treatment of NRSTS should be in the direction of histology-determined therapies. Furthermore, better understanding of the characteristic chromosomal translocations occurring in some NRSTS may reveal targets for new small molecular drugs.

Other histotypes

Other rare and very specific tumour types are included in this heterogeneous group. A brief description of some of them is given below.

Infantile fibrosarcoma

This is a tumour typical of very early childhood and is the most common STS under 1 year of age. In the past, this entity was defined according to age (occurring at less than 2 years), but it is currently recognized that it should be identified biologically by the presence of a characteristic (12;15) translocation. The tumour usually arises in the distal extremities, and presents as a painless, rapidly enlarging mass. Despite rapid growth, evolution may be indolent but metastatic spread is not uncommon, yet spontaneous regressions have been described. The overall prognosis is very good (survival rates are between 80–100 per cent). Surgery is the mainstay of treatment and a conservative approach should be taken to decisions about the use of chemotherapy, utilizing low toxicity alkylating/anthracycline free regimens, typically, VA (vincristine and actinomycin D): more intensive chemotherapy should be reserved in the event of non-response. The use of radiotherapy is very restricted in view of patient age.

Extra-osseous peripheral primitive neuroectodermal tumour (pPNET)/Ewing sarcoma

Extra-osseous Ewing family tumours are less frequent than the skeletal Ewing sarcoma but share the same chromosomal translocation and it is unlikely there are any biological differences between Ewing sarcomas arising at different sites. Although previously treated like RMS in many studies, in many groups they are now enrolled into the same protocols used for bony Ewing sarcoma (see Chapter 22).

Desmoplastic small round cell tumour (DSRCT)

DSRCT is a very aggressive neoplasm, identified by the specific translocation t(11;22)(p13;q12), with the chimeric transcript EWS-WT1. It usually arises in the abdominal cavity, often disseminated at onset, and is characterized by a poor outcome despite the various intensive multimodality treatment approaches (including aggressive surgery, intensive chemotherapy, and radiotherapy) attempted over the years. New tailored therapeutic approaches are urgently needed for this tumour.

Malignant rhabdoid tumour (MRT)

Soft tissue MRT represents the soft tissue counterpart of the intracranial and renal entities of the same name. These are very rare and aggressive tumours characterized by *hSNF5/INI1* gene deletions and mutations. They are currently treated with intensive chemotherapeutic strategies (multidrug therapy with vincristine, ifosfamide, carboplatin, etoposide, doxorubicin, and cyclophosphamide), but prognosis is poor and new approaches to treatment are required.

Epithelioid hemangioendothelioma

This particular entity has distinctive clinical features and is regarded as borderline tumour. Two distinct subtypes are described: (1) epithelioid hemangioendothelioma of soft tissues, usually characterized by a single lesion located in the extremities or cervical region, with little propensity to metastasize or become fatal; (2) epithelioid hemangioendothelioma of bone, lung or liver, which is often multifocal or metastatic, and although it may take an indolent course, death from disease progression is not negligible (around 35–65 per cent). While surgery is the only treatment for the former, optimal treatment is not so clear for the latter diagnosis. Some reports suggest that whilst conventional chemotherapy is ineffectual, the use of alpha-interferon (α-IFN) may have a significant role, probably due to an anti-angiogenic effect. Liver transplantation is a treatment option for cases with inoperable disease in the liver.

Aggressive fibromatosis

Aggressive fibromatosis (AF), also known as desmoid tumour, is a rare, deep-seated, fibroblastic tumour of borderline malignancy. It arises in musculo-aponeurotic structures, mainly in extremities and deep structures in abdomen and pelvis. Tumours usually grow fairly slowly but diffusely along muscle bundles and fascial planes, lacking a pseudocapsule, which contributes to the difficulty in defining the border of the tumour at resection. AF has a strong tendency for local recurrence (from 24 to 77 per cent), but does not metastasize to other organs as truly malignant tumours may do. Overall survival rates at 10 years are favourable at about 90 per cent but many patients experience long-term morbidity from repeated attempts at surgical resection.

The pathogenesis of AF is most likely multifactorial: genetic predisposition, endocrine factors, and trauma all seem to play an important part. The incidence is higher in families with familial adenomatous polyposis (FAP) within which there is a particular association with intra-abdominal fibromatosis (Gardner's syndrome).

Surgery retains a principal place in the treatment of these tumours, but treatment strategies are currently changing to some degree, from a strategy of aggressive surgery to a multidisciplinary approach that takes the functional and cosmetic sequelae of treatments into account too. Various pharmacological treatments have proved to be relatively effective; options include non-cytotoxic agents [including hormonal treatment (tamoxifen), non-steroidal anti-inflammatory drugs and interferon-α] or cytotoxic agents, including the regimens usually adopted for RMS and NRSTS. There is interest in the value of prolonged low-dose chemotherapy using combinations such weekly low-dose methotrexate plus a vinca alkaloid (vinblastine or vinorelbine). Interesting responses have been seen using target therapy (imatinib). The observation that desmoid tumours can remain stable for a long time, with or without primary treatment, has prompted the suggestion that a 'wait-and-see' strategy (i.e. clinical-radiological monitoring alone) may be suitable in cases where tumour growth is slow or static.

Further reading

Arndt CA, Stoner JA, Hawkins DS, et al. (2009) Vincristine, actinomycin, and cyclophosphamide compared with vincristine, actinomycin, and cyclophosphamide alternating with vincristine, topotecan, and cyclophosphamide for intermediate-risk rhabdomyosarcoma: Children's Oncology Group study D9803. *J Clin Oncol* **27**, 5182–8.

Bisogno G, Ferrari A, Bergeron C, et al. (2005) The IVADo regimen—a pilot study with ifosfamide, vincristine, actinomycin D, and doxorubicin in children with metastatic soft tissue sarcoma: a pilot study of behalf of the European pediatric Soft tissue sarcoma Study Group. *Cancer* **103**, 1719–24.

Bisogno G, Ferrari A, Prete A, et al. (2009) Sequential high-dose chemotherapy for children with metastatic rhabdomyosarcoma. *Eur J Cancer* **45**, 3035–41.

Breitfeld PP, Meyer WH (2005) Rhabdomyosarcoma: new windows of opportunity. *Oncologist* **10**, 518–27.

Carli M, Ferrari A, Mattke A, et al. (2005) Malignant peripheral nerve sheath tumours in pediatric age: a report from the Italian and German Soft Tissue Sarcoma Cooperative Group. *J Clin Oncol* **23**, 8422–30.

Casanova M, Ferrari A, Bisogno G, et al. (2004) Vinorelbine and low-dose cyclophosphamide in the treatment of pediatric sarcomas: pilot study for the upcoming European Rhabdomyosarcoma Protocol. *Cancer* **101**, 1664–71.

Crist WM, Anderson JR, Meza JL, et al. (2001) Intergroup rhabdomyosarcoma study-IV: results for patients with nonmetastatic disease. *J Clin Oncol* **19**, 3091–102.

Davicioni E, Anderson JR, Buckley JD, et al. (2010) Gene expression profiling for survival prediction in pediatric rhabdomyosarcomas: a report from the Children's Oncology Group. *J Clin Oncol* **28**, 1240–6.

Ferrari A, Bisogno G, Casanova M, et al. (2002) Paratesticular rhabdomyosarcoma: report from the Italian and German Cooperative Group. *J Clin Oncol* **20**, 449–55.

Ferrari A, Casanova M, Meazza C, et al. (2005) Adult-type soft tissue sarcomas in pediatric age: experience at the Istituto Nazionale Tumori in Milan. *J Clin Oncol* **23**, 4021–30.

Ferrari A, Casanova M. (2005) New concepts for the treatment of pediatric non-rhabdomyosarcoma soft tissue sarcomas. *Expert Rev Anticancer Ther* **5**, 307–318.

Ferrari A, Gronchi A, Casanova M, et al. (2004) Synovial sarcoma: a retrospective analysis of 271 patients of all ages treated at a single institution. *Cancer* **101**, 627–34.

Klingebiel T, Boos J, Beske F, et al. (2008) Treatment of children withmetastatic soft tissue sarcoma with oral maintenance compared to high dose chemotherapy: report of the HD CWS-96 trial. *Pediatr Blood Cancer* **50**, 739–45.

Martelli H, Oberlin O, Rey A, et al. (1999) Conservative treatment for girls with nonmetastatic rhabdomyosarcoma of the genital tract: A report from the Study Committee of the International Society of Pediatric Oncology. *J Clin Oncol* **17**, 2117–22.

Meazza C, Bisogno G, Gronchi A, et al. (2010) Aggressive fibromatosis in children and adolescents: the Italian experience. *Cancer* **116**, 233–40.

Meza JL, Anderson J, Pappo AS, et al. (2006) Analysis of prognostic factors in patients with nonmetastatic rhabdomyosarcoma treated on intergroup rhabdomyosarcoma studies III and IV: the Children's Oncology Group. *J Clin Oncol* **24**, 3844–51.

Oberlin O, Rey A, Lyden E, et al. (2008) Prognostic factors in metastatic rhabdomyosarcomas: results of a pooled analysis from United States and European cooperative groups. *J Clin Oncol* **26**, 2384–9.

Okcu MF, Munsell M, Treuner J, et al. (2003) Synovial sarcoma of childhood and adolescence: a multicenter, multivariate analysis of outcome. *J Clin Oncol* **21**, 1602–11.

Orbach D, Rey A, Cecchetto G, et al. (2010) Infantile fibrosarcoma: place of chemotherapy and treatment proposals based on the European experience. *J Clin Oncol* **28**, 318–23.

Pappo AS, Devidas M, Jenkins J, et al. (2005) Phase II trial of neoadjuvant vincristine, ifosfamide, and doxorubicin with granulocyte colony-stimulating factor support in children and adolescents with advanced-stage nonrhabdomyosarcomatous soft tissue sarcomas: a Pediatric Oncology Group Study. *J Clin Oncol* **23**, 4031–38.

Stevens MC, Rey A, Bouvet N, et al. (2005) Treatment of nonmetastatic rhabdomyosarcoma in childhood and adolescence: third study of the International Society of Paediatric Oncology—SIOP Malignant Mesenchymal Tumor 89. *J Clin Oncol* **23**, 2618–28.

Stevens MC (2005) Treatment for childhood rhabdomyosarcoma: the cost of cure. *Lancet Oncol* **6**, 77–84.

Sultan I, Ferrari A (2010) Selecting Multimodal Therapy for Rhabdomyosarcoma. *Expert Rev Anticancer Ther* **10**, 1285–301.

Wachtel M, Schäfer BW (2010) Targets for cancer therapy in childhood sarcomas *Cancer Treat Rev* **36**, 318–27.

Williamson D, Missiaglia E, de Reyniès A, et al. (2010) Fusion gene-negative alveolar rhabdomyosarcoma is clinically and molecularly indistinguishable from embryonal rhabdomyosarcoma. *J Clin Oncol* **28**, 2151–8.

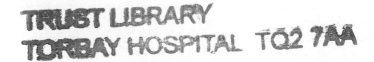

Chapter 22

Bone tumours

Michael Paulussen, Stefan Bielack, Heinrich Kovar, Herbert Jürgens and Mark Bernstein

Epidemiology

Osteosarcoma and Ewing sarcoma (ES), including peripheral neuroectodermal tumour (PNET) and Askin tumours of the chest wall, account for the majority of malignant bone tumours in children and adolescents. In both, males are affected approximately 1.5 times as often as females. The median age at presentation is around age 15 years and at least half of all diagnoses are made in the second decade of life.

Incidence

Osteosarcoma is the most frequent primary bone cancer. Its approximate annual incidence is 2–3 per million in the general population, peaking at 8–11 per million at age 15–19. A second, smaller peak in older patients is due to osteosarcoma arising in abnormal bones, such as those affected by Paget disease or prior irradiation. In paediatric and adolescent populations of Caucasian descent, Ewing sarcoma is the second most common primary malignancy of bone. Annual incidence rates are approximately 2–3 per million in children, adolescents and young adults below age 25. It is almost unheard of in African and Chinese populations.

Predisposition and genetic links

In most paediatric and adolescent patients, the aetiology remains obscure. Trauma has been implicated but little evidence exists to support this relationship. There are no known predisposing factors for ES. The predilection of osteosarcoma for the age of the pubertal growth spurt and sites of maximum growth suggest a correlation with bone growth. The incidence of osteosarcoma is increased in several disorders associated with germline alterations of tumour suppressor genes but these account for only a few per cent of all osteosarcoma. Survivors of hereditary retinoblastoma with germline mutations of the retinoblastoma gene RB1 carry a risk that is 500–1000 times greater than in the general population. The Li-Fraumeni cancer family syndrome, caused by mutations in the *p53* gene, is associated with a 15-fold increase. Radiation is another risk factor for osteosarcoma, the risk being related to the dose administered. Exposure to alkylating agents may also contribute. The use of radiation and alkylating agent chemotherapy, together with genetic tumour predisposition, make osteosarcoma one of the most frequent secondary solid malignancies following therapy for childhood cancer.

Clinical presentation

Primary osteosarcoma is usually located in the metaphysis of long extremity bones, particularly the distal femur or the proximal tibia, followed by the proximal humerus. In total, two thirds of

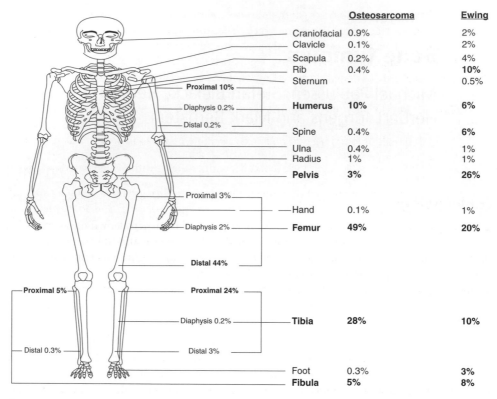

	Osteosarcoma	Ewing
Craniofacial	0.9%	2%
Clavicle	0.1%	2%
Scapula	0.2%	4%
Rib	0.4%	**10%**
Sternum	-	0.5%
Humerus	**10%**	6%
Spine	0.4%	**6%**
Ulna	0.4%	1%
Radius	1%	1%
Pelvis	**3%**	**26%**
Hand	0.1%	1%
Femur	**49%**	**20%**
Tibia	**28%**	**10%**
Foot	0.3%	3%
Fibula	**5%**	**8%**

Fig. 22.1 Skeletal distribution of osteosarcoma and Ewing sarcoma, based on 1791 primary high-grade central osteosarcomas and 1426 ES from Cooperative Osteosarcoma Study Group (COSS) and European Intergroup Cooperative Ewing's Sarcoma Study [(EI)CESS], respectively. The percentages shown for proximal, diaphyseal, and distal extremity locations are for osteosarcoma.

all paediatric osteosarcomas arise around the knee (Fig. 22.1). Osteosarcomas of the axial skeleton or craniofacial bones generally occur in older patients. Sites most frequently affected by ES of bone are the pelvis, long bones of the extremities, ribs, scapulae, and vertebrae. Compared to osteosarcoma, involvement of flat bones of the trunk is much more common (Fig. 22.1). If ES arises in long extremity bones, it usually does so in the diaphysis, in distinction to the typical metaphyseal presentation of osteosarcoma.

At diagnosis, accurate staging will reveal metastases in only 10–30 per cent. Without systemic therapy, however, most patients with seemingly localized bone sarcomas will develop metachronous metastases within 1–2 years. In osteosarcoma, primary and secondary metastases are limited to the lungs in 80 per cent of affected individuals. The remainder has bone metastases with or without additional pulmonary involvement. Skip metastases, defined as isolated tumour foci within the same bone as the primary tumour, occur in a minority of patients. In ES, lungs and bones contain metastatic deposits at diagnosis in approximately equal proportions (~10 per cent of patients each), and there may be bone marrow involvement (~5 per cent). In both diseases, lymph node metastases are rare and other sites of metastatic disease are almost never involved at initial diagnosis.

Patients with bone tumours usually do not feel ill until late in the course of their disease. They typically seek medical attention because of, at first, intermittent and then continuous pain, often erroneously attributed to recent trauma. Tumour-related swelling and loss of function of adjacent joints usually develop later. In approximately 10 per cent, the first sign of disease is a pathological fracture. Pain at bony sites other than the primary may represent metastatic involvement. Metastases in the lungs produce respiratory symptoms only with extensive involvement. Systemic symptoms, particularly fever, may be present in ES.

Diagnosis

Most patients present with a history of pain of the involved region and physical examination is typically remarkable only for a mass at the primary site. Loss of motion of neighbouring joints, infiltration of the skin, and neurological deficits may occur, depending on the location and extent of the tumour. There are no laboratory tests that can identify patients with malignant bone tumours. Blood tests may show moderately elevated erythrocyte sedimentation rates and may reveal some degree of anaemia and leucocytosis. Elevated serum levels of lactate dehydrogenase or alkaline phosphatase may correlate with tumour burden or bone destruction, or, in osteosarcoma, with tumour phenotype, and can thus be of prognostic significance.

Imaging of the primary tumour

Plain radiographs and cross-sectional imaging, preferably by magnetic resonance imaging (MRI), are required to assess tumour size and its loco-regional extension.

Plain radiographs are used to describe the bony compartment. Osteosarcoma can present with lytic or sclerotic changes, or both. Ossification in the soft tissues in a radial or 'sunburst' pattern is typical, but neither sensitive nor specific. Periosteal bone formation with lifting of the cortex may lead to the appearance of Codman's triangle (Fig. 22.2). The typical radiograph of ES shows a destructive osteolytic lesion of the diaphysis with destruction of the osseous cortex, elevation of the periosteum and infiltration of surrounding soft tissue. The layered periosteal reaction may give rise to a classic 'onion-skin' appearance. MRI is the most useful tool to define the intramedullary tumour extent, its soft tissue component, and the relation to vessels and nerves (Fig. 22.2). Serial MRIs can also be used to monitor response to induction chemotherapy. In ES, a marked shrinkage of the soft tissue component can be used as a surrogate marker for response. In osteosarcoma, where the osteoid matrix often prevents tumour shrinkage, response can be predicted based upon the results of serial dynamic contrast enhanced MRIs. Other methods used to predict response pre-operatively include serial evaluation by angiography, quantitative bone scans, or positron emission tomography (PET).

Systemic staging

The search for metastases focuses on those sites where the majority occur: lungs and bones. The bone marrow is evaluated in ES. Plain radiographs and a CT scan of the thorax must be performed to rule out pulmonary metastases. Bone metastases are searched for by a ^{99m}Tc-MDP bone scan. Skip metastases may also be visualized on the bone scan, but MRI of the whole bone is more sensitive. Whole body MRI may lead to a higher detection rate of bone metastases, but its exact role remains to be defined. There is currently no established role for PET in osteosarcoma staging as it is inferior to CT for the detection of lung metastases and may also be inferior to bone scintigraphy for bone metastases. Prospective evaluation of PET is ongoing in ES.

Ewing sarcoma cells may be inhomogeneously distributed within the bone marrow. It is therefore recommended that marrow samples be obtained from several sites distant from the primary. In addition to standard pathology assessment, marrow micro-metastases can be detected by reverse transcriptase polymerase chain reaction (RT-PCR) for tumour-specific ES gene (*EWS*)

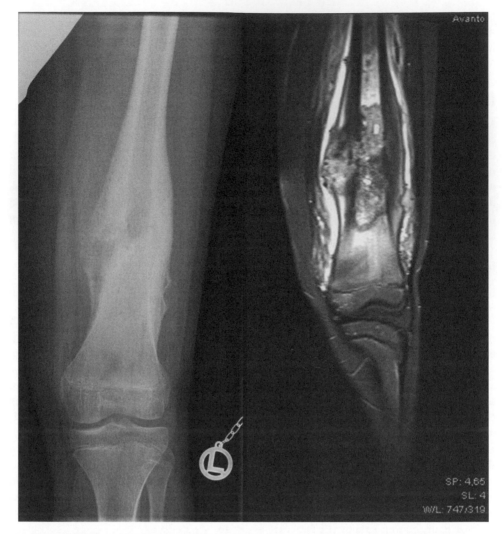

Fig. 22.2 Conventional radiograph (left) and MRI (right) of an osteosarcoma of the left distal femur. X-ray shows cortical destruction and Codman's triangles on the medial aspect, and 'onion skin' appearance of the periosteum on the lateral aspect of the tumour.
(Images courtesy of Prof. P. Winkler, Stuttgart).

fusion transcripts. While involvement detectable by light microscopy carries adverse prognostic implications, assessment of micro-metastatic dissemination by RT-PCR is still investigational.

Biopsy

Imaging will often result in a high index of suspicion, but diagnosis must always be verified histologically. In order to ensure appropriate biopsy techniques and optimal evaluation of the obtained material, it is strongly recommended that biopsies should be performed in specialized centres. Open biopsy is most suitable to obtain sufficient material for histological evaluation and ancillary studies. The biopsy specimen should be forwarded to the pathologist without prior fixation. Tissue is required for standard histology, immunohistochemistry, and fresh/frozen samples are required for molecular biology studies. The biopsy track and adjacent tissues must be regarded as tumour-contaminated and the approach should be planned so that these can subsequently be included into definitive local treatment. If metastases are suspected, but there is no unequivocal evidence from imaging, histological confirmation should be attempted.

Differential diagnosis

The differential diagnosis of osteosarcoma includes traumatic lesions, osteomyelitis, benign tumours such as exostosis, fibroma, osteoid osteoma, chondroma, giant-cell tumour of bone, bone cysts, and others, as well as other primary malignant lesions of bone such as ES or lymphoma, and metastases from malignancies such as neuroblastoma or soft tissue sarcoma. The most important clinical differential diagnosis of ES is osteomyelitis. The radiological appearance may be very similar and, on occasion, ES may be secondarily infected. On histological examination, ES must be differentiated from other small round-cell tumours, in particular embryonal rhabdomyosarcoma, neuroblastoma, small-cell osteosarcoma, and non-Hodgkin lymphoma.

Histopathology

By definition, osteosarcoma is a mesenchymal malignancy in which the malignant cell population produces osteoid, but production can vary considerably. Both abundant production, leading to hard sclerotic tumours, and very scanty production of osteoid are consistent with the diagnosis. Conventional osteosarcoma, a high-grade central malignancy of bone, accounts for 80–90 per cent of all osteosarcomas. Its most frequent subtypes are osteoblastic, chondroblastic, and fibroblastic, but various less frequent subtypes are also considered conventional osteosarcomas. Conventional, telangiectatic, high-grade surface and small-cell osteosarcomas all have a similar clinical course and are treated by multimodal regimens that include chemotherapy. Low-grade central and parosteal osteosarcomas are treated by surgery only. Craniofacial osteosarcomas, apart from those of the skull, metastasize less frequently than conventional osteosarcomas, as do periosteal osteosarcomas, and there is no general consensus whether these should be treated by surgery alone or by surgery plus chemotherapy. Extraskeletal osteosarcomas, usually high-grade malignancies, are exceedingly rare in young people.

Ewing sarcomas of bone are composed of firm, grey-white soft tissue with a glistening, moist appearance on sectioning. Macroscopically, the intraosseous component of the tumour is usually firm, while the extraosseous component tends to be less firm with areas of haemorrhage and cystic degeneration secondary to tumour necrosis. All ES are high-grade malignancies. When stained with haematoxylin and eosin, they appear as a monomorphic small blue round primitive cell population, with round nuclei and scanty cytoplasm. Variable amounts of glycogen deposition stain periodic-acid-Schiff (PAS) positive. Peripheral primitive neuroectodermal tumour (pPNET) cells differ from other ES and show features of neural differentiation with prominent neurite-like cell processes containing neurosecretory granules and neurofilaments on electron microscopy; infrequently, rosettes and Homer-Wright pseudorosettes are also identified. S-100 protein, neuron-specific enolase (NSE) and synaptophysin may also be expressed. Ewing sarcoma cannot be differentiated from other PAS-positive small blue round-cell tumours on morphological features alone and the diagnosis must be assisted by immunocytochemistry. CD99 (Mic-2 antigen) expression is positive in > 95 per cent of cases but is not unique for ES. Other useful markers include vimentin, desmin, smooth muscle actin, and CD45 (leukocyte common antigen). These help to differentiate between small round-cell tumours of myogenic, fibrogenic, and haematopoetic origin.

Biology

Biology of osteosarcoma

Although germline mutations of *p53* and *RB* are rare, these genes are altered in many osteosarcoma tumour samples. Consequently, loss of function of the *p53* and *RB* tumour suppressor genes, which regulate cell cycle progression, are believed to have important roles in osteosarcoma tumorigenesis. Rothmund-Thomson syndrome and Bloom syndrome, rare conditions caused by mutations in tumour suppressor genes coding for helicases, are also associated with an increase in osteosarcoma, as is Werner syndrome (adult progeria).

Numerous oncogenes are also altered in osteosarcoma tumour cells. These include amplifications of the product of the murine double minute 2 gene, amplification of cyclin-dependent kinase 4 and over-expression of human epidermal growth factor receptor 2. Although it is clear that alterations in tumour suppressor genes and oncogenes are necessary to produce osteosarcomas, it is not clear which of these events occurs first and why or how it occurs. Moreover, it is not clear which, if any, of the alterations are essential to tumour development and might therefore represent therapeutic targets.

Biology of Ewing sarcoma

The molecular key to ES is the rearrangement of the ES gene *EWS* on chromosome 22q12 with the *FLI-1* gene on 11q24. *EWS* encodes a ubiquitously expressed RNA binding protein which appears to be involved in transcription and processing of messenger RNA. *FLI-1* codes for a protein with a carboxy-terminal DNA binding domain that is characteristic for members of the ETS transcription factor family. As a consequence of gene fusion, the EWS RNA binding domain is replaced by the FLI-1-derived ETS DNA binding domain, resulting in a novel transcription factor with strong *in vitro* transactivation potential (Fig. 22.3). The most frequent gene fusions in ES result in the type 1 (EWS exon 7 to FLI1 exon 6: 50 per cent of cases) or type 2 (EWS 7/FLI1 5: 27 per cent) fusions. In 10–15 per cent, alternative *EWS* gene fusions to other *ETS* gene family members (predominantly *ERG*) can be observed (Table 22.1). While *EWS*, as well as its close relatives *TLS* (*FUS*) and *RPB56* (*hTAF$_{II}$68*)], and *ERG* genes are involved in several chromosomal translocations in other solid tumours and in acute leukaemia, the specific combination of *EWS* with an *ETS* gene is restricted to, and therefore diagnostic of, ES. *EWS–ETS* fusion is essential for ES pathogenesis.

The classical cytogenetic demonstration of t(11;22)(q24;q12) has been largely replaced by fluorescence *in situ* hybridization (FISH) using probes flanking the *EWS* breakpoint region on chromosome 22. Using this method, even complex chromosomal rearrangements and rare *EWS* translocations with other *ETS* partner genes can be revealed. However, the most frequently used method to detect the fusion gene is RT-PCR. This requires immediate snap freezing of the biopsy since it relies on extraction of good-quality RNA. The strength of the method lies in its high sensitivity, enabling identification of single tumour cells among 10^5–10^6 normal cells.

Risk classification

Staging

Many clinicians, especially tumour surgeons, prefer a staging system developed by the Musculoskeletal Tumor Society (MSTS) to the TNM classification. The MSTS (Enneking) system categorizes localized malignant bone tumours by grade (low grade—stage I or high grade—stage II) and anatomic extent (intracompartmental—A or extracompartmental—B). The compartmental status

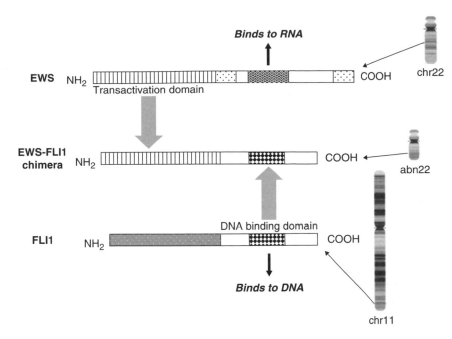

Fig. 22.3 Chromosomal translocation t(11;22)(q24;q12) in Ewing sarcoma. This leads to the generation of a DNA binding fusion protein. The gene for the RNA binding protein EWS is located on chromosome 22 (chr22) in the region q12, the gene for the DNA binding transcription factor FLI1 on chromosome 11 (chr11) at q24. The EWS–FLI1 chimeric protein is expressed from the abnormal chromosome 22 (abn22), while the reciprocal translocation product on chromosome 11 has no gene product.

is determined by whether or not the tumour extends through the cortex of the bone. The current (6th) edition of the TNM classification is an expansion of the MSTS system (Table 22.2).

Prognostic factors

Several prognostic factors have been identified in osteosarcoma. Primary metastases, axial or proximal extremity location, and large tumour size are of independent negative prognostic value. Factors associated with an adverse outcome in some series also include very young or older age, high levels of alkaline phosphatase or lactic dehydrogenase, and the immunohistochemical detection of p-glycoprotein or HER2/erbB2. The relative risk associated with any presenting factor, however, is lower than that of two treatment-related variables: incomplete surgery is the most important

Table 22.1 Gene fusions in Ewing sarcoma

Gene fusion	Cytogenetic equivalent	Observed frequency
EWS–FLI1	t(11;22)(q24;q12)	85%
EWS–ERG	t(21;22)(q22;q12)	10%
EWS–ETV1	t(7;22)(p22;q12)	<1%
EWS–ETV4	t(17 ;22)(q12;q12)	<1%
EWS–FEV	t(2 ;21 ;22)	1%

Table 22.2 TNM classification (7th ed.) for malignant bone tumours and suggested staging system

Tx	Primary tumour cannot be assessed			
T0	No evidence of primary tumour			
T1	Tumour ≤ 8 cm in greatest dimension			
T2	Tumour > 8 cm in greatest dimension			
T3	Discontinuous tumours in the primary bone site			
NX	Regional lymph nodes cannot be assessed			
N0	No regional lymph node metastasis			
N1	Regional lymph node metastasis			
MX	Distant metastases cannot be assessed			
M0	No distant metastases			
M1	Distant metastases			
M1a - lung				
M1b -other distant sites				
Stage IA	T1	N0, NX	M0;	(low grade)
Stage IB	T2	N0, NX	M0;	(low grade)
Stage IIA	T1	N0, NX	M0	(high grade)
Stage IIB	T2	N0, NX	M0	(high grade)
Stage III	T3	N0, NX	M0	(any grade)
Stage IVA	any T	N0, NX	M1a	(any grade)
Stage IVB	any T	N1	any M	(any grade)
	any T	any N	M1b	(any grade)

negative prognostic indicator, and response to induction chemotherapy is the most important prognostic factor for resectable osteosarcoma. Response, however, is not all or nothing, even a very moderate response is associated with better outcomes than none at all.

The classical factors related to poor prognosis in ES include presence of metastases, older age, large tumours, and primary site in the trunk and pelvis. Specific prognostic factors that currently influence the choice of treatment regimens include initial tumour size, the presence of pulmonary and/or extrapulmonary metastases, the presence of tumour cells at the surgical margins, and poor histological response to induction chemotherapy. The previously suggested prognostic importance of the specific *EWS–FLI1* gene fusion type has recently been refuted. As in osteosarcoma, the most clear-cut treatment-related prognostic indicator is tumour response to induction chemotherapy. Several large analyses have shown that early relapse (within 2 years from the time of initial diagnosis) is another predictor of death.

Treatment

Treatment principles and strategy

Many children and adolescents can be cured with appropriate therapy (Fig. 22.4). Inappropriate use of diagnostic tools and suboptimal initial therapy can irrevocably compromise a patient's chances and patients should be treated in specialized, experienced centres able to provide access

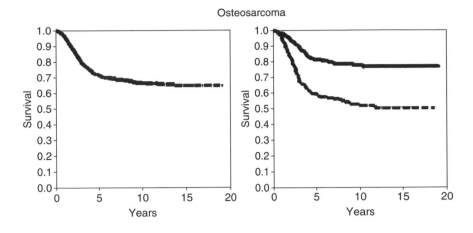

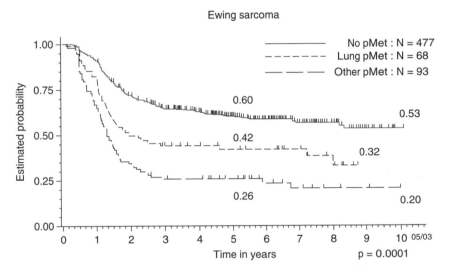

Fig. 22.4 Osteosarcoma (top): left—overall survival with multimodal therapy; right—comparison of good responders (solid line) and poor responders (dashed line), good response = <10 per cent viable tumour. Results are from 1152 COSS patients under 20 years with localized extremity osteosarcoma. Ewing sarcoma (bottom): event-free survival by disease stage at initial presentation. Without primary metastases (no pMet), with lung or pleural metastases only (lung pMet), and with metastases to bones and/or bone marrow (other pMet).
(CESS/EICESS data).

to the full diagnostic and therapeutic spectrum. Treatment within prospective clinical trials is considered standard clinical practice in many countries. Multinational trials such as the European and American Osteosarcoma Study EURAMOS-1 or the studies of the COG and EURO-E.W.I.N.G. groups are current examples.

Local treatment (surgery in osteosarcoma, surgery and/or radiotherapy in ES) is an essential part of curative therapy. Most patients, however, will already have micro-metastatic disease by the time their sarcoma is detected. Prior to the 1970s, when treatment was exclusively targeted towards the primary, the outcome was extremely poor. This dismal outlook was dramatically improved when multi-agent chemotherapy was added to local treatment. Many trials have since reported disease-free survival rates in the range of 50–70 per cent. A multimodal approach has therefore emerged as the undisputed standard of care.

Currently, most institutions use an approach consisting of pre-operative chemotherapy (also called neoadjuvant or induction chemotherapy), followed by definitive local therapy, and post-operative, adjuvant chemotherapy both for osteosarcoma and ES. Theoretical advantages of this approach include early treatment of micro-metastatic disease and facilitation of subsequent local therapy because of shrinkage and decreased vascularity of the tumour. Furthermore, pre-operative treatment permits tumour response to induction chemotherapy to be evaluated. A theoretical concern is that delayed removal of the bulk tumour could lead to the emergence of chemotherapy resistance. Only one relatively small, randomized osteosarcoma trial has prospectively compared patients treated by both pre- and post-operative chemotherapy with patients treated by primary surgery followed by the same chemotherapy. Treatment results did not differ between the two arms. Similarly, the Cooperative Osteosarcoma Study Group could not detect a survival difference between both approaches in a retrospective comparison of 157 patients undergoing primary surgery and 1451 who received initial chemotherapy. As the delivery of initial chemotherapy also facilitates preparation for limb salvage surgery, as well as offering the value of measuring early response, induction chemotherapy has become standard.

Local therapy

Choice of modality

In osteosarcoma, complete surgical removal of the primary tumour and, if present, all metastases is the local treatment of choice. Indications for radiotherapy are limited and basically restricted to inoperable tumours.

The radiosensitivity of ES was first recognized by James Ewing in 1921 and has long played a major role. Currently, however, radiotherapy is no longer the local treatment of first choice for most ES. Increasing awareness of the risk of local recurrence has encouraged the use of surgery, and its use was associated with a survival advantage in several series. Situations in which surgery is preferable to irradiation include lesions in expendable bones, pathologic fractures, distal extremity sites, bulky primary tumours, and in patients with poor response to initial chemotherapy. Pre-operative radiotherapy may be indicated when there is tumour progression during chemotherapy, in emergencies such as spinal cord compression, or when incomplete surgery is anticipated. Post-operative radiotherapy is indicated after incomplete resection or, in the opinion of some, in patients with poor histologic response to induction chemotherapy.

Principles of bone sarcoma surgery

Bone sarcoma surgery has three aims. First and foremost, the tumour must be removed. Second, the patient should be left with good function. Third, it should, if possible, result in a cosmetically acceptable appearance. Complete tumour removal is of paramount importance, functional and cosmetic aspects are secondary goals. The aim should be that the tumour, including the biopsy scar and biopsy track, should be removed together with an intact cuff of the surrounding normal tissue, corresponding to the definition of 'wide' margins within the MSTS definition (Table 22.3). Wide and radical margins are considered adequate, whilst marginal or intralesional margins are associated with an increased risk of local recurrence, which in turn carry a grave prognosis.

The location, size, and regional anatomy of the tumour, its relation to nerves and vessels as well as neighbouring joints, the bones, soft tissues, and skin which will remain after wide resection, and the patient's growth expectancy must all be evaluated before deciding upon the type of surgery.

Table 22.3 Surgical margins in musculoskeletal oncology

Type	Resection
Intralesional	Within the lesion
Marginal	Through the pseudocapsule or reactive tissue
Wide	Lesion (including biopsy scar), pseudocapsule and/or reactive zone, and an intact cuff of normal tissue completely surrounding the mass removed as a single block
Radical	Entire anatomic compartment containing the tumour removed as one block

En bloc resection with limb salvage is possible in many cases. Amputation, however, may still be the most appropriate type of surgery for selected patients with unfavourable tumour characteristics. Advantages of amputation include oncologic safety, low complication rates, and a low rate of revision surgery. Disadvantages include mutilation and phantom sensations. The functional outcome is often rather poor after proximal amputations, but better with below the knee amputations.

Rotation-plasty, used for sarcomas of the distal femur and occasionally the proximal tibia, is the classic example of a resection-reimplantation procedure. The knee is removed *en bloc* together with the tumour, the only structure left *in situ* being the popliteal nerve bundle. The distal part of the tibia together with the foot is then rotated by 180°, the tibia is fused with the femoral stump, and anastomoses between the femoral and tibial vessels are created. The result of this reimplantation is a shortened extremity, in which the rotated foot substitutes for the knee and carries the prosthesis. Advantages of rotation-plasty include oncologic safety even in very large tumours, lack of phantom sensations, and an infrequent need for revision surgery, as well as an extremity function rivalling that of limb-salvage. The highly unusual cosmetic appearance is its main disadvantage.

Retaining the extremity requires reconstruction of bony and soft tissue defects. Only a minority of tumours are situated in expendable bones, such as the proximal fibula. Far more often, limb salvage implies replacement of a major joint. Allografts are used by some surgeons, but modular endoprosthetic systems, assembled to fit in the operating room, are employed more commonly. Autologous bones, such as vascularized fibulae bridging diaphyseal defects, can be used in selected situations. Special expandable endoprostheses are available for growing extremities. Innovative models can be lengthened noninvasively, markedly reducing the number of revision procedures. Disadvantages of limb salvage include a significant complication risk, to which infections, fractures, and prosthetic wear contribute. Several publications report local recurrence rates approximately three times higher than after ablative procedures, suggesting that resection margins may sometimes not be as wide as expected.

Principles of radiotherapy

In osteosarcoma, radiotherapy is limited to few indications. Post-operative irradiation is indicated when definitive surgery did not result in safe margins and in which revision surgery, even when mutilating, could not do so. Radio-sensitization with drugs such as the histone deacetylase inhibitors is being investigated pre-clinally.

In ES, whole bone irradiation had traditionally been advised because the tumour was thought to arise in the bone marrow, putting the whole marrow cavity at risk. The advent of MRI, which accurately demonstrated the extent of marrow involvement, and of effective chemotherapy, questioned this approach. A randomized study undertaken by the North American Pediatric Oncology Group (POG) group has demonstrated that radiotherapy to the initial tumour volume plus a 2 cm safety margin produced results that were equivalent to that achieved by whole bone irradiation. Scars after biopsy or tumour resection should be included in the radiation field. To avoid constrictive fibrosis, an adequate strip of skin and subcutaneous tissue should be left when irradiating limb sites and epiphyseal plates should be spared if possible, particularly in children.

In inoperable ES, a compartment dose of 44.8 Gy is recommended, with a tumour boost to at least 54.4 Gy: whether this can be achieved depends on the site of tumour and the age of the patient. For pre-operative radiotherapy, the standard target volume dose is 54.4 Gy. For post-operative radiotherapy, dosage recommendations depend on histological assessment of the resection margins and the tumour response to induction chemotherapy, and vary between 44.8 and 54.4 Gy.

Systemic therapy for osteosarcoma

The majority of current treatment protocols are based upon combinations of only four active agents: doxorubicin, cisplatin, high-dose methotrexate, and ifosfamide. Even after several decades and numerous clinical trials, the exact role of each of these, and the optimal way in which they are to be combined and delivered, are still being debated, as is the potential benefit of additional drugs.

Doxorubicin was introduced into osteosarcoma treatment in the 1970s and has remained an integral part ever since. Some protocols include measures aimed towards reducing doxorubicin cardiotoxicity, cardioprotectants such as dexrazoxane and the reduction of anthracycline peak levels by continuous doxorubicin infusions featuring most prominently. Sequential studies by American and European groups suggest that there is no major loss of efficacy with these approaches, but no controlled studies have been reported.

Methotrexate, a folate antagonist, blocks the action of dihydrofolate reductase, the enzyme responsible for reducing folate to its active form, tetrahydrofolic acid. In osteosarcoma, methotrexate is given at very high doses in the range of $8–12$ g/m^2. Toxicity must be antagonized by the use of leucovorin, activated folate. The treatment concept of high-dose methotrexate is based on the assumption that normal cells can be rescued more effectively than tumour cells, which may lack active folate transporters. High-dose methotrexate therapy requires meticulous attention to detail and extensive supportive measures, including hydration, alkalinization of the urine, and leucovorin administration adapted to methotrexate serum levels. Inadequate supportive care will result in severely delayed methotrexate clearance and excessive toxicity, including myelosuppression, renal toxicity, and mucositis. Some patients will experience such toxicity despite adequate supportive care, the risk apparently increasing with increasing patient age. The enzyme glucarpidase, which cleaves methotrexate, may be of benefit in selected patients with renal failure and severely delayed methotrexate clearance, but most cases of delayed methotrexate clearance can be handled by maintaining hydration and increasing leucovorin dose and frequency.

Given that, under most circumstances, patients do not experience significant myelotoxicity and the resulting ability to schedule methotrexate at times when other agents cannot be administered, most groups incorporate high-dose methotrexate into their treatment protocols.

The efficacy of cisplatin against osteosarcoma was proven in early phase II trials. Cisplatin therapy requires supportive hyperhydration. Oto- and nephrotoxicity are dose limiting but both can be reduced by administering the drug as a continuous infusion. Intra-arterial administration of cisplatin into the vessel supplying the tumour was previously tried but has largely been abandoned since comparative trials failed to demonstrate enhanced antitumour effects compared to intravenous administration.

Following positive phase II trials, ifosfamide has been part of many osteosarcoma protocols since the mid-1980s. Its efficacy may be related to the dose administered. Supportive measures necessary to prevent haemorrhagic uropathy include hyperhydration and Mesna (Uromitexan). Ifosfamide may also lead to chronic renal tubular toxicity and to sterility.

Data from two European trials (by the Istituto Rizzoli and the COSS group) supported the use of ifosfamide but a randomized trial by the North American groups (POG and CCG) could not demonstrate that adding standard dose ifosfamide to high-dose methotrexate, doxorubicin, and cisplatin improved outcomes. The results of the North American trial, (INT0133) should, however, be interpreted with caution as a second randomization of liposomal muramyl tripeptide (MTP-PE) may have interfered with the ifosfamide question. Furthermore, the ifosfamide arm contained no pre-operative cisplatin. Results of a French trial, SFOP-91, which did not add, but rather substituted ifosfamide, suggest that favourable results may be obtained by regimens that rely on ifosfamide rather than on doxorubicin.

No other cytostatic agents have come close to replacing the four standard substances described above. A combination of bleomycin, cyclophosphamide, and actinomycin D (BCD) was used in the early days of chemotherapy but was largely abandoned due to questionable efficacy. Carboplatin has some activity against osteosarcoma, but less than cisplatin. Etoposide is almost inactive when given as a single agent, but may enhance the effect of carboplatin or ifosfamide. Negative phase II studies have been reported for paclitaxel, docetaxel, and topotecan. Gemcitabine seems to be marginally active, with stable disease achieved in some patients.

Overall, progress in the treatment of osteosarcoma has been slow and survival rates have improved little over more than two decades. Attempts to improve prognosis through treatment intensification by interval compression achieved with G-CSF support or by combining maximally tolerated doses of high-dose ifosfamide, high-dose methotrexate, cisplatin, and doxorubicin have failed to show benefit. High-dose chemotherapy with autologous peripheral blood stem cell transplantation was also unsuccessful in the few reported series. Improving the prognosis for patients with poor response to induction chemotherapy remains a particular challenge. Early reports from the Memorial Sloan-Kettering Cancer Center had suggested that it could be improved by altering post-operative chemotherapy. However, a prospective trial by the Cooperative Osteosarcoma Study Group and a later reanalysis of the Sloan-Kettering results failed to confirm this salvage effect. Several other attempts to improve outcomes for poor responders by altering post-operative chemotherapy have been explored, but none as a randomized trial in which a salvage approach was compared to unaltered post-operative chemotherapy. The only trial suggesting positive benefit from salvage chemotherapy comes from the Rizzoli Institute, Bologna, where, within an uncontrolled setting, ifosfamide/etoposide was added post-operatively for poor responders to an ifosfamide-free pre-operative regimen. Such an approach is currently subject of a prospective, randomized, European-American Intergroup trial, EURAMOS-1. The same trial will also evaluate whether outcomes for good responders to induction chemotherapy can be improved by maintenance therapy with pegylated interferon α.

Whether the addition of the immunomodulator L-MTP-PE (liposomal muramyl tripeptide phenol ethanolamine) to chemotherapy improves prognosis, as evaluated in the randomized North American POG/CCG, INT0133 trial, is currently a matter of intense debate. A first analysis of INT0133 concluded that there was an interaction between L-MTP-PE and ifosfamide, which, within a rather complex factorial trial design, was evaluated in the same study. A later publication reported a survival advantage for L-MTP-PE, but could still not prove that adding L-MTP-PE improved event-free survival. It has been argued that further trials are needed before the agent might be considered for routine use.

Systemic therapy for Ewing sarcoma

Ewing sarcoma is responsive to alkylating agents such as ifosfamide and cyclophosphamide, to doxorubicin, and to other agents such as vincristine, actinomycin D, or the topoisomerase II inhibitor etoposide. Combinations of these agents with complementary mechanisms of action have improved disease-free survival rates. The Intergroup Ewing Sarcoma (IESS) studies demonstrated the superiority of a four-drug regimen using vincristine (V), actinomycin D (A), cyclophosphamide (C) and doxorubicin (D) over three-drug VAC in terms of both disease-free survival (60 per cent vs. 24 per cent) and local control (96 per cent vs. 86 per cent). Rosen, from the Memorial Sloan-Kettering Cancer Center (MSKCC), reported an advantage of using these drugs in combination rather than sequentially as early as 1978 but it is important to realize that a considerable number of patients in earlier series received cumulative doxorubicin doses of over $700 \, mg/m^2$ before its use was restricted to a maximum of $400–500 \, mg/m^2$ because of the risk of doxorubicin-related cardiomyopathy.

The IESS and MSKCC experience led to the widespread use of similar four-drug regimens and treatment was later extended to incorporate ifosfamide (I) and etoposide (E). In the European EICESS-92 study, patients with localized high-risk disease (tumour volume >200 ml) receiving VIDA benefited from the addition of etoposide, and in the randomized POG-CCG Ewing trial (VACD versus EVADI), patients treated with EVADI appeared to have a more favourable outcome.

The incorporation of granulocyte colony-stimulating growth factor (G-CSF) into treatment regimens allows dose intensification by increasing the dose per cycle or by shortening the interval between treatments. The IESS-II study compared high-dose intermittent chemotherapy with moderate-dose continuous chemotherapy, resulting in a significant benefit from the more intensive regimen (68 per cent vs. 48 per cent disease-free survival at 5 years). Another POG-CCG randomized study explored dose intensification (maintaining a dosing interval of 21 days) by condensing treatment duration to 30 weeks by increasing the individual doses of chemotherapy in comparison to the delivery of the same cumulative doses over 48 weeks: so far, results between the standard and the dose intensified arms do not differ. More recently, COG has explored dose intensification with the use of G-CSF by decreasing the intervals between cycles (interval compression) while maintaining the same dose-per-cycle. Results seem to confirm that relapse rates are lower and toxicity was manageable, but final publication is pending.

The treatment of metastatic and recurrent disease

Primary metastases

In osteosarcoma, all detectable metastases must be removed by surgery if therapy is to be curative. As most metastases develop in the lung, this usually implies thoracotomy. There is evidence that a significant proportion of patients with apparently unilateral lung metastases may indeed have bilateral disease. Complete resection of osteosarcoma pulmonary metastases requires palpation of the lung. Acceptable surgical approaches include bilateral thoracotomy or median sternotomy. Approximately one quarter of all osteosarcoma patients with proven metastatic disease at diagnosis and 40 per cent of those who achieve a complete surgical remission of both the primary and all metastases in the context of an intensive polychemotherapy regimen will go on to become long-term survivors. Solitary primary metastases may have a prognosis similar to that of localized disease.

Metastatic disease at diagnosis is also a major adverse prognostic factor in ES. A recently published analysis of the Euro-EWING consortium described survival rates of 10–40 per cent at 3 years, with patient age, tumour size, and site and number of metastases defining distinct prognostic groups. Patients with isolated lung metastases have a better prognosis than those with extrapulmonary metastases (Fig. 22.4). If pulmonary disease is present, patients also receive bilateral pulmonary irradiation at doses of 14–20 Gy. Patients with solitary or circumscribed bony lesions can receive irradiation to those sites at doses of 40–50 Gy. However, survival rates for patients with multiple bony and/or bone marrow metastases are below 10 per cent at 2 years. These discouraging results have led to more aggressive approaches utilizing high-dose chemotherapy with autologous stem cell reinfusion. A variety of agents such as busulfan, treosulfan, melphalan, cyclophosphamide, thiotepa, etoposide and carboplatin have been employed but without definitive evidence of improved outcome. Total body irradiation does not seem to offer benefit, but significantly contributes to toxicity. Local therapy aimed at identified metastases may improve survival.

Recurrent disease

Osteosarcoma recurrences usually involve the lung. Bone metastases and local recurrences are much less common, and other sites are rarely affected. Unfortunately, survival rates are below 20 per cent. A short latency period and the presence of more than one or two metastases are associated with particularly poor outcomes. Complete surgery of all sites of recurrence is the only therapy with unequivocally proven impact on survival. Selected patients may be cured after multiple recurrences, provided that surgery results in a renewed complete remission. It may be prudent to irradiate suitable inoperable lesions in order to slow the progression of disease, but this is unlikely to lead to cure. Patients with inoperable recurrent osteosarcoma who receive chemotherapy may survive longer than those who do not. The exact role of adjuvant chemotherapy in recurrent operable osteosarcoma is under debate. Success has been limited, and there is no universally accepted standard regimen although many would consider the use of a combination of ifosfamide and etoposide in patients who had not previously received those drugs.

The survival of ES patients who develop local or metastatic recurrence is poor and second remissions are usually short-lived. Patients with a longer disease-free interval represent the subset of patients most likely to survive. The role of local therapy is less clear than in osteosarcoma. Chemotherapy and radiotherapy are commonly applied in an attempt to prolong survival. Chemotherapy regimens currently used include combinations of previously used drugs, or of platinum compounds with ifosfamide and etoposide, topotecan and cyclophosphamide, or irinotecan and temozolomide.

Follow up

Suggestions for follow-up are given in Table 22.4. Intervals between visits mirror the declining risk of relapse with time. As there have been no prospective trials, suggestions must necessarily remain somewhat arbitrary. Follow up should, however, include regular assessments of remission as well as tests for possible late effects of treatment.

Remission status

Tumour directed follow up focuses on the few organ systems where relapses are likely to occur. Pulmonary metastases contribute to over 80 per cent of recurrences of osteosarcoma and approximately half of all recurrences of ES. They will not usually cause symptoms until they have reached a very large size or penetrated the pleura. In order to detect them at an earlier stage, they must be searched for by appropriate imaging, which includes serial X-rays and/or C -scans of the thorax. In ES, where bone metastases occur more frequently, technetium bone scans may be included. Local recurrences are often first detected because of symptoms, most noticeably pain. Most centres still include sequential imaging of the primary site into their follow-up program.

Late effects

Fortunately, many former bone sarcoma patients can lead relatively normal and productive lives. Nevertheless, they are more likely to suffer from chronic health conditions than survivors of most other paediatric cancers. Late complications may be caused by the tumour itself or by surgery,

Table 22.4 Suggestions for follow-up after multimodal therapy for bone sarcoma

Time	Tumour directed investigations	Late effects monitoring
Baseline	Chest X-ray & CT X-ray & MRI of primary site	Echocardiogram, audiogram*, liver & kidney function
Years 1 & 2	Chest X-ray q 6–12 wk X-ray of primary site q 4 mo	Echocardiogram q 1–2 yr, audiogram*, liver** & kidney** function
Years 3 & 4	Chest X-ray q 2–4 mo X-ray of primary site q 4 mo	Echocardiogram q 1–2 yr
Years 5–10	Chest X-ray q 6 mo***	Echocardiogram q (1-)2–4 yr****
Thereafter	A few relapses reported as late as 2 decades after treatment: discuss with patient whether to continue chest X-ray monitoring	Echocardiogram q (1-)2–4 yr

Every clinic visit should include detailed history & physical examination. Many institutions will add complete blood counts. Evaluate any site with unexplained pain or swelling. Chest CT scan is optional, but should always be performed if chest X-ray shows metastasis or is inconclusive. Add consultation with orthopedic surgery and physical therapy as indicated. Offer fertility testing for males. Additional investigations may be indicated.
* If treatment included cisplatin.
** Need not be repeated if normal at one year.
*** Some groups recommend annual radiographs of the primary site until year 10.
**** Longer interval if normal function and post pubertal at diagnosis.

radiotherapy, or chemotherapy. Functional and cosmetic consequences for the musculoskeletal system depend on the location and extent of the tumour as well as the type of local treatment employed. Amputations and rotation-plasties carry the stigma of mutilation, but may lead to functional results that are similar to those after limb-salvage procedures. Revision surgery is more frequently needed after limb-salvage procedures, where periprosthetic infection, loosening, fractures, and prosthetic wear can occur. The use of expandable prostheses in skeletally immature patients is predictably associated with the need for multiple revision procedures. Radiotherapy may lead to growth reduction, functional limitations, and secondary cancers. The late consequences of chemotherapy are more completely described in Chapter 12.

Future and remaining challenges

Osteosarcoma remains a challenging disease. It is sensitive to a small number of medications, all having significant short- and long-term toxicities. Radiation is of limited value and even sensitive tumours are incompletely eliminated by chemotherapy, mandating surgical resection and reconstruction, with their attendant morbidity. Patients with recurrent disease are difficult to cure, with a somewhat better outlook for those with resectable metastases. The role of MTP-PE (mifurmatide) therapy in osteosarcoma requires better definition. A study using a standard chemotherapy backbone with the randomized addition of mifurmatide is being discussed to more definitively answer its efficacy in patients with newly diagnosed osteosarcoma.

New initiatives are required. Bisphosphonates target the bone microenvironment and reduce the risk of skeletal events as well as recurrence in some adult cancers. Zoledronic acid is the most potent of the available bisphosphonates, affecting both osteolytic and osteoblastic metastatic lesions. Bisphosphonates inhibit osteosarcoma growth *in vitro*, and have shown activity in preclinal xenograft models. A COG study to demonstrate the tolerability of standard dose zoledronic acid in combination with multi-agent chemotherapy in patients with newly diagnosed metastatic osteosarcoma is nearing completion, and a randomized study of the addition of zoledronic acid to a somewhat different multi-agent chemotherapy regimen is underway in the French Society of Pediatric Oncology.

Another way to affect the osteoclastic activity important for the progression of bone lesions is to interfere with the receptor activator for nuclear factor kappa-B (RANK) pathway. RANK, RANK-Ligand, and osteoprotegrin maintain normal bone metabolism. Osteosarcoma cells express RANK-Ligand. Those resistant to chemotherapy show increased expression of genes involved in osteoclast activation. Denosumab, a humanized antibody that binds RANK-Ligand, inhibiting osteoclasts and therefore bone resorption, has been successfully used in patients with giant cell tumour of bone, and has decreased skeletal-related events in patients with some adult cancers. A study is under development in COG.

Metformin is a drug widely used in the therapy of type 2 diabetes. Recently, metformin has been shown to have several antineoplastic actions: a reduction in insulin resistance, decreasing signalling through the insulin growth factor pathway, and, most prominently, activation of AMP-activated protein kinase (AMPK), reducing signalling through the mammalian target of rapamycin (mTOR) pathway. Preclinical activity has been seen in a variety of adult cancers. Trials either alone or in combination with chemotherapy are ongoing in adult malignancies. Preclinal activity has been seen with concomitant doxorubicin, albeit in breast cancer cell lines, not osteosarcoma. More direct interference with the mTOR pathway is possible, using rapamycin or one of its analogues. The tolerability of their addition to cytotoxic chemotherapy remains to be demonstrated and the optimal dose and schedule require definition. Similarly, the insulin growth factor receptor pathway can be interrupted, but the tolerability of the addition of a receptor inhibitor is the first step, prior to studying the efficacy of such a combination.

In patients with ES, the addition of multi-agent chemotherapy to local control with radiation and/or surgery has improved disease-free survival from 10 per cent to 50–70 per cent. High throughput microarray-based gene expression profiling studies comparing different types of small blue round-cell tumours have identified a unique gene expression pattern in ES and gene expression studies on large cohorts may lead to the discrimination of prognostically distinct groups, allowing better treatment stratification.

The combinations of topotecan-cyclophosphamide and irinotecan-temozolomide have shown activity in patients with recurrent ES. Topotecan and cyclophosphamide combined with vincristine (VTC) has been added to the compressed vincristine, doxorubicin, cyclophosphamide, ifosfamide, etoposide (VDC-IE) schedule to study the feasibility of interval compression with that additional combination. Once the tolerable interval has been established, it is likely that a randomized study of compressed VDC-IE compared with VDC-IE-VTC will follow.

A target of particular interest in ES is the vascular endothelial growth factor (VEGF) pathway. Bevacizumab is a humanized anti-VEGF antibody that may sensitize endothelial cells to cytotoxic cell death. By encouraging pruning of the abnormal vasculature, decreasing vasogenic oedema by decreasing vascular permeability and decreasing interstitial pressure within the tumour, anti-angiogenic drugs may improve the delivery of cytotoxic chemotherapy to tumour cells. Tumour tissue oxygenation may also be increased. The characteristic *ews/fli1* oncogene downregulates thrombospondins (angiogenic inhibitors) and upregulates VEGF. Preclinal combination therapy with cytotoxic chemotherapy shows added efficacy and a European study randomizing the addition of bevacizumab to chemotherapy for patients with newly diagnosed metastatic soft tissue sarcomas is underway, as is a study in patients with newly diagnosed ES at St Jude's Children's Research Hospital. On a cautionary note, 6 of 17 adult patients with metastatic sarcoma treated with the combination of bevacizumab and doxorubicin developed at least grade 2 cardiotoxicity, despite cardioprotection with dexrazoxane. Many other anti-angiogenic compounds are being developed, including pazopanib, sunitinib, sorafenib, and cilengitide. The exact role of each of these will be challenging to define.

Initial studies targeting the insulin-like growth factor 1 receptor (IGF-1R) and the mTOR pathway, or engaging other apoptotic mechanisms like TRAIL are promising, but only preclinical and very early clinical data are currently available.

Conclusions

The prognosis for bone sarcoma patients is determined primarily by local treatment options, tumour dissemination and tumour burden, as well as by response to treatment. Tumour burden can only be limited by early diagnosis but response is subject to the impact of better therapies: These include: the design of more effective chemotherapy combinations, increased drug intensity with improved supportive care, and surgical removal of all tumour. In addition, more precise determination of prognostic factors should result in opportunities to better stratify treatment intensity, offering the opportunity to limit the risk of late effects from treatment in patients with favourable disease. Because of the rarity of these tumours, treatment should always be performed in centres experienced in bone sarcoma treatment, and within the framework of controlled clinical trials. The evaluation of experimental approaches to treatment should be restricted to clinical trial settings.

Further reading

Abed R, Grimer R (2010) Surgical modalities in the treatment of bone sarcoma in children. *Cancer Treat Rev* **36**, 342–47.

Bernstein M, Kovar H, Paulussen M, et al. (2006) Ewing's sarcoma family of tumors: Current management. *The Oncologist* **11**, 503–519.

Bielack S (2010) Editorial comment—Osteosarcoma: Time to move on? *Eur J Cancer* **46**, 1942–5.

Bielack S, Kempf-Bielack B, Delling G, et al. (2002) Prognostic factors in high-grade osteosarcoma of the extremities or trunk. An analysis of 1,702 patients treated on neoadjuvant Cooperative Osteosarcoma Study Group protocols. *J Clin Oncol* **20**, 776–90.

DuBois SG, Marina N, Glade-Bender J (2010) Angiogenesis and vascular targeting in Ewing sarcoma: a review of preclinical and clinical data. *Cancer* **116**, 749–57.

Ferrari S, Briccoli A, Mercuri M, et al. (2003) Postrelapse survival in osteosarcoma of the extremities: prognostic factors for long-term survival. *J Clin Oncol* **21**, 710–5.

Fletcher CDM, Unni K, Mertens K (Eds) (2002) *WHO Classification of tumours. Pathology and genetics of tumours of soft tissue and bone.* Lyon: IARC.

Grier HE, Krailo MD, Tarbell NJ, et al. (2003) Addition of ifosfamide and etoposide to standard chemotherapy for Ewing's sarcoma and primitive neuroectodermal tumor of bone. *N Engl J Med* **34**, 694–701.

Hattinger AM, Pasello M, Ferrari S, et al. (2010): Emerging drugs for high-grade osteosarcoma. *Expert Opin Emerg Drugs* **15**, 615–34.

Heymann D, Ory B, Blanchard F, et al. (2005) Enhanced tumor regression and tissue repair when zoledronic acid is combined with ifosfamide in rat osteosarcoma. *Bone* **37**, 74–86.

Jaffe N, Bruland Ø, Bielack S (Eds) (2010) *Pediatric and adolescent osteosarcoma. Series: Cancer Treatment and Research, Vol. 152* , New York: Springer.

Jalving M, Gietema JA, Lefrandt JD, et al. (2010) Metformin: Taking away the candy for cancer? *Eur J Cancer* 2010 **46**, 2369–80.

Khanna C (2008) Novel targets with potential therapeutic applications in osteosarcoma. *Curr Oncol Rep* **10**, 350–8.

Kempf-Bielack B, Bielack S, Jürgens H, et al. (2005) Osteosarcoma relapse after combined modality therapy: an analysis of unselected patients in the Cooperative Osteosarcoma Study Group (COSS). *J Clin Oncol* **23**, 559–68.

Ladenstein R, Pötschger U, Le Deley MC, et al. (2010) Primary disseminated multifocal Ewing sarcoma: results of the Euro-EWING 99 trial. *J Clin Oncol* **28**, 3284–91.

Meyers PA, Schwartz C, Krailo M, et al. (2008) Osteosarcoma: The addition of muramyl tripeptide to chemotherapy improves overall survival. A report from the Children's Oncology Group. *J Clin Oncol* **26**, 633–8.

Oeffinger KC, Mertens AC, Sklar CA, et al. (2006) Chronic health conditions in adult survivors of childhood cancer. *N Engl J Med* **355**, 1572–82.

Paulussen M, Craft AW, Lewis I, et al. (2008) Results of the EICESS-92 Study: two randomized trials of Ewing's sarcoma treatment—cyclophosphamide compared with ifosfamide in standard-risk patients and assessment of benefit of etoposide added to standard treatment in high-risk patients. *J Clin Oncol* **26**, 4385–93.

Picci P, Sangiorgi L, Rongraff BT, et al. (1994) The relationship of chemotherapy- induced necrosis and surgical margins to local recurrence in osteosarcoma. *J Clin Oncol* **12**, 2699–705.

Schuck A, Ahrens S, Paulussen M, et al. (2003) Local therapy in localized Ewing tumors: results of 1058 patients treated in the CESS 81, CESS 86, and EICESS 92 trials. *Int J Radiat Oncol Biol Phys* **55**, 168–77.

Scotlandi K, Picci P, Kovar H (2009) Targeted therapies in bone sarcomas. *Curr Cancer Drug Targets* **9**, 843–53.

Sobin LH, Gospodarowicz MK, Wittekind C (2009) *UICC TNM classification of malignant tumors*. 7th. edn. New York: Wiley.

Subbiah V, Anderson P, Lazar AJ, et al. (2009) Ewing's Sarcoma: *Standard and experimental treatment options* **10**, 126–40.

Vallet S, Smith MR, Raje N (2010) Novel bone-targeted strategies in oncology. *Clin Cancer Res* **16**, 4084–93.

Womer RB, West DC, Krailo MD (2008) Randomized comparison of every-two-week v. every-three-week chemotherapy in Ewing sarcoma family tumors (ESFT) *Journal of Clinical Oncology, 2008 ASCO Annual Meeting Proceedings (Post-Meeting Edition). Vol 26, No 15S (May 20 Supplement), 2008: 10504).*

Chapter 23

Wilms and other renal tumours

Norbert Graf and Christophe Bergeron

Wilms tumour (nephroblastoma)

Introduction

In 1814, Rance classified Wilms Tumour (WT) or nephroblastoma for the first time as a renal neoplasia. In 1899, the surgeon Max Wilms described this tumour entity in a 90-page monograph *Die Mischgeschwülste der Niere* in much more detail. Today, this tumour is regarded as a prime example of a curable malignant disease. The improvements in the treatment of nephroblastoma are particularly based on the progress in surgery, radiotherapy, and in the development of effective chemotherapies. Interdisciplinary cooperation and prospective randomized trials have made considerable contributions to this success.

Epidemiology

The incidence of the WT is 7 per million children less than 15 years of age. With 6–7 per cent of all childhood malignancies, nephroblastoma represents the most frequent malignant renal tumour. Worldwide WT are more common in girls than boys. The age distribution shows a peak between the second and third year of life. Children with a bilateral tumour are younger.

Aetiology and risk factors

In 1964, Miller and colleagues reported for the first time an association between WT and aniridia. Today, different malformations linked to WT are known, in particular, hemihypertrophy and urogenital malformations (cryptorchidism, hypospadias, pseudohermaphroditism, and gonadal dysgenesis). Aniridia and hemihypertrophy are very rare syndromes justifying regular check-ups in children with such anomalies for an early diagnosis. A high incidence of WT is seen in children with hemihypertrophy, the WAGR syndrome (WT, aniridia, genital deformity, retardation), the Beckwith–Wiedemann syndrome (BWS; hemihypertrophy, omphalocele, and macrosomy, macroglossia, hypoglycaemia, deep-rooted ears), the Denys–Drash syndrome (DDS; pseudohermaphroditism, glomerulopathy, and WT), the Perlman syndrome (macrocephaly, deep-rooted eyes and ears, macrosomia and organomegalia) and neurofibromatosis type 1. Environmental factors do not play a major role in the genesis of nephroblastoma.

Pathogenesis

Molecular biology and genetics

Nephroblastoma is a genetically heterogeneous tumour. As well as gene mutations, loss of heterozygosity (LOH) and imprinting (LOI) are know to contribute to tumour development. Nephroblastomas mainly show an euploid set of chromosomes and the frequency of LOH is less than 5 per cent.

Several genes are known which play a decisive role in the emergence of nephroblastoma. Only the WT suppressor gene *wtl* on chromosome 11p13 has been cloned so far. Deletions of this gene are found in 10–30 per cent of the WT. Other WT candidate genes are on chromosomes 11p15.5 (*wt2*), 16q (*wt3*), 17q12-q21 (*wt4; fwt1*), and 7p15-p11.2 (*wt5*). Numeric and structural changes concern particularly chromosomes 1, 6, 7, 8, 11, 12, 16, 17, and 18. LOH are mainly found on 11p (40 per cent), and in a lower frequency in 1p, 7p, and 16q. Epigenetic alterations primarily affect 11p15.5 and 11 p13.

The genetics of the overgrowth syndromes are complex. As with the Beckwith–Wiedemann syndrome (BWS) they arise from abnormalities of imprinting in 11p15.5, with differences between BWS and hemi-hypertrophy. The WAGR syndrome is caused by a complete deletion of one copy of the Wilms tumour gene, *WT1*, and the adjacent aniridia gene, *PAX6* on chromosome 11p13. In patients with aniridia this information helps to identify those patients, who are at risk for developing Wilms tumour, by screening them for the combined deletion of *WT1* and *PAX6*. *WT1* is also involved in the Denys–Drash syndrome caused by a germline point mutation. In familial Wilms tumours, accounting for approximately 1 per cent of patients, there is usually no associated congenital abnormality or predisposition to other tumour types. They show an autosomal dominant inheritance with a variable penetrance. Genetic linkage studies in different families have shown no association to 11p13 or 11p15.5. One gene for familial Wilms tumour, *FWT1*, could be localized on chromosome 17q and another, *FWT2*, on 19q.

Nephrogenic rest and nephroblastomatosis

Nephrogenic rests can appear as preliminary stages of a nephroblastoma. Nephroblastomatosis is defined as the diffuse or multifocal occurrence of nephrogenic rests. Different forms of nephrogenic rests are distinguished according to their localization in the renal lobe:

- perilobar nephroblastomatosis
- intralobar nephroblastomatosis
- mixed peri-/intralobar nephroblastomatosis
- panlobar nephroblastomatosis.

Despite the histological similarity to WT, nephroblastomatosis behaves like residua of primitive embryonic tissue and does not seem to have any invasive or metastatic behaviour. The malignant potential of nephrogenic rests is justified in their high mitotic activity and the narrow association with WT. They occur in approximately 40 per cent of all children with WT. A progression of nephroblastomatosis to a true nephroblastoma is possible.

Histopathology

Despite enormous progress in the molecular genetic characterization of nephroblastoma, the diagnosis of this tumour is still based on histopathological classification. Multicentric growth of the tumour in one or both kidneys is possible and approximately 5 per cent are bilateral. In accordance with Wilms' concept, nephroblastoma is a tumour of mesodermal origin and develops in the embryonic kidney. Classic nephroblastomas (mixed type) are renal tumours with a blastemic, epithelial (tubules) and mesenchymal component (stroma). The distribution of these three components can vary, explaining epithelial, stromal, and blastemal types of nephroblastoma.

The pathohistological classification of childhood renal tumours depends on the initial treatment. Patients receiving pre-operative chemotherapy are classified according to the Stockholm-Working classification (1995, revised 2002) and patients undergoing primary surgery are classified according to the classification of the Children's Oncology Group (COG). formerly the National

Wilms Tumor Study Group. According to the Stockholm classification, three risk groups can be distinguished [low, intermediate and high] whereas in COG only favourable and unfavourable risk groups are defined. The tumours with a low and intermediate risk in the International Society of Paediatric Oncology (SIOP) classification of childhood renal tumours correspond largely to tumours of the group with a favourable histology of COG (Table 23.1).

Prognostic factors

As a result of a pre-operative chemotherapy, the distribution of the different histological sub-types changes. In particular, the percentage of the blastemal type goes down from 40 to 10 per cent. As the remaining blastema after pre-operative chemotherapy is chemo-resistant, these tumours are treated as high risk in SIOP.

Table 23.1 The SIOP classification of childhood renal tumours for patients with a preoperative chemotherapy

---

A. For pre-treated cases

I. Low risk tumours

Mesoblastic nephroma

Cystic partially differentiated nephroblastoma

Completely necrotic nephroblastoma

II. Intermediate risk tumours

Nephroblastoma - epithelial type

Nephroblastoma - stromal type

Nephroblastoma - mixed type

Nephroblastoma - regressive type

Nephroblastoma - focal anaplasia

III. High risk tumours

Nephroblastoma - blastemal type

Nephroblastoma - diffuse anaplasia

Clear cell sarcoma of the kidney

Rhabdoid tumour of the kidney

B. For primary nephrectomy cases

I. Low risk tumours

Mesoblastic nephroma

Cystic partially differentiated nephroblastoma

II. Intermediate risk tumours

Non-anaplastic nephroblastoma and its variants

Nephroblastoma - focal anaplasia

III. High risk tumours

Nephroblastoma - diffuse anaplasia

Clear cell sarcoma of the kidney

Rhabdoid tumour of the kidney

Tumours in Italic are non Wilms tumours.

After pre-operative chemotherapy, some tumours become completely necrotic or regressive in the form of necroses, fibrosis, and a collection of xanthomatous cells. The detection of anaplasia is of prognostic importance.

The extension of the tumour (staging) must be described exactly and is essential for correct treatment stratification after surgery. Growth of the tumour beyond the tumour capsule represents the decisive feature between stage I and II. Tumour in vessels is indicative of stage II. Incomplete operative removal, tumour rupture or open tumour biopsy and a lymph node infiltration are all assigned to stage III. In stage IV, distant metastases are diagnosed. Bilateral tumours indicate a stage V (Table 23.2).

Table 23.2 SIOP staging criteria for renal tumours of childhood

Stage I

a. The tumour limited to kidney or surrounded with fibrous pseudocapsule if outside of the normal contours of the kidney, the renal capsule or pseudocapsule may be infiltrated with the tumour but it does not reach the outer surface, and it is completely resected (resection margins 'clear')

b. The tumour may be protruding ('bulging') into the pelvic system and 'dipping' into the ureter (but it is not infiltrating their walls)

c. The vessels of the renal sinus are not involved

d. Intrarenal vessel involvement may be present.

Fine needle aspiration or percutaneous core needle biopsy ('tru-cut') do not upstage the tumour. The presence of necrotic tumour or chemotherapy induced changes in the renal sinus/hilus fat and/or outside of the kidney should not be regarded as a reason for upstaging a tumour.

Stage II

a. The tumour extends beyond kidney or penetrates through the renal capsule and/or fibrous pseudocapsule into perirenal fat but is completely resected (resection margins 'clear')

b. The tumour infiltrates the renal sinus and/or invades blood and lymphatic vessels outside the renal parenchyma but it is completely resected

c. The tumour infiltrates adjacent organs or vena cava but is completely resected.

Stage III

a. Incomplete excision of the tumour which extends beyond resection margins (gross or microscopical tumour remains postoperatively)

b. Any abdominal lymph nodes are involved

c. Tumour rupture before or intra-operatively (irrespective of other criteria for staging)

d. The tumour has penetrated through the peritoneal surface

e. Tumour implants are found on the peritoneal surface

f. The tumour thrombi present at resection margins of vessels or ureter, transsected or removed piecemeal by surgeon

g. The tumour has been surgically biopsied (wedge biopsy) prior to preoperative chemotherapy or surgery

The presence of necrotic tumour or chemotherapy-induced changes in a lymph node or at the resection margins should be regarded as stage III.

Stage IV

Haematogenous metastases (lung, liver, bone, brain, etc.) or lymph node metastases outside the abdomino-pelvic region.

Stage V

Bilateral renal tumours at diagnosis. Each side should be sub-staged according to the above criteria.

The prognosis of nephroblastoma depends primarily on tumour stage, histological type, and response to preoperative chemotherapy. In addition, some molecular markers correlate with a poor prognosis (LOH 1p, 11q, 16q, 22q; and *p53* mutations).

Ninety per cent of all children with a nephroblastoma can be cured today, that is, those with a low- and intermediate-risk tumour without metastasis. Patients with a tumour of diffuse anaplasia have a considerably poorer outcome. In stage IV, the prognosis of patients depends on treatment response. Patients with a complete remission after pre-operative chemotherapy and tumour nephrectomy have an overall survival of 80 per cent. The prognosis of clear cell sarcoma has improved considerably with overall survival rates of 80 per cent, whereas the prognosis of patients with a rhabdoid tumour remains dismal and below 20 per cent.

Prevention and early diagnosis

Most WTs appear sporadically. A general screening is not possible because there are no tumour markers. On the other hand, in those children with syndromes associated with nephroblastoma, the individual risk of developing a nephroblastoma can be defined by molecular genetic examinations. Ultrasound scans are recommended at 3-month intervals in such children. In Germany, 10 per cent of children with nephroblastoma are diagnosed in the context of preventive medical check-ups by paediatricians.

Clinical symptoms

The typical first sign of a WT is an asymptomatic palpable or visible abdominal mass. Pain or haematuria are rare (Table 23.3). In addition, WT is known to present with

- Hypertension that is caused by an increase in renin activity and is sometimes difficult to control
- Coagulopathy caused by an acquired von Willebrand syndrome

In most cases, an acquired coagulation disorder and the hypertension will resolve after tumour nephrectomy. Intratumoural haemorrhage may occur, resulting in an emergency situation with a rapid abdominal enlargement that requires urgent surgery. Prenatal diagnoses by ultrasound are described.

Diagnostic procedures

Besides clinical examination, the diagnosis of nephroblastoma is primarily based on imaging studies [abdominal ultrasound, computed tomography (CT) and/or magnetic resonance imaging (MRI);

Table 23.3 First symptoms at diagnosis in children with a nephroblastoma

Symptom	Frequency [%]
Asymptomatic tumour swelling	61.6
Haematuria	15.1
Preventive medical check-up	9.2
Constipation	4.3
Weight loss	3.8
Urinary tract infection	3.2
Diarrhoea	3.2
Diagnosis at trauma	2.7
Nausea, vomiting, pain, hernia, pleural effusion, high blood pressure	Rare

Fig. 23.1]. As patients in the SIOP trials and studies are treated without histological diagnosis, all imaging studies need to be of high quality to reduce the risk of a false diagnosis and unnecessary chemotherapy. By using abdominal ultrasound, this risk was assessed below 2 per cent for SIOP 6 and SIOP 9. The most important criteria allowing a safe diagnosis are listed in Table 23.4.

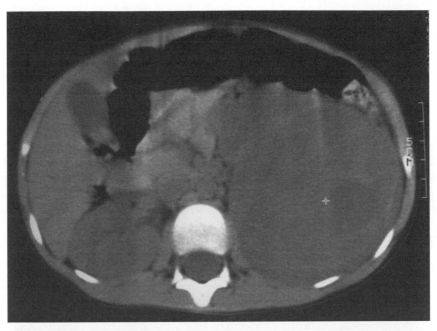

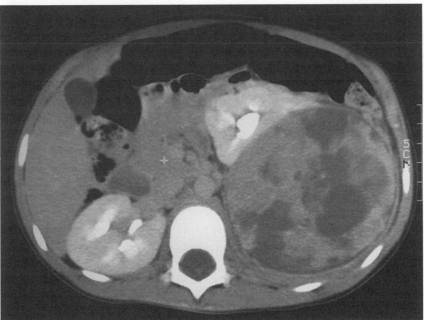

Fig. 23.1 CT scan with and without contrast enhancement in a patient with unilateral nephroblastoma.

Table 23.4 Criteria for a safe diagnosis of nephroblastoma using imaging studies

The intra-renal tumour is solid and heterogeneous with partly cystic areas
The tumour has a sharp border
The surrounding tissue is replaced rather than infiltrated
The destruction, inclination and replacement of calices and the renal pelvis is characteristic
The heterogeneity of the tumour increases after contrast enhancement
Intratumoral bleedings are relatively frequent (27%)
Calcifications in the tumour are rare (8%)

Differential diagnoses

The following diseases need to be ruled out: neuroblastoma, lymphoma of the kidney, renal cell carcinoma, nephroblastomatosis, rhabdoid tumour, teratoma, ganglioneuroma, cystic nephroma, hamartoma, renal cysts, hematoma, renal abscess, xanthogranulomatosis pyelonephritis, angiomyolipoma, and adenoma.

The diagnosis of the nephroblastomatosis can only be proven by histology. It is of utmost importance that the pathologist is aware of the history of the patient and the imaging studies.

Treatment

The treatment of this tumour should always be carried out in prospective trials in which surgery, chemotherapy, and radiotherapy are combined according to the individual risk of a patient. There are currently two major study groups. The fundamental difference between the groups is their initial treatment approach: primary surgery (COG: Children's Oncology Group, North America) and pre-operative chemotherapy (SIOP: International Society of Paediatric Oncology). Arguments for pre-operative chemotherapy are the reduction of the tumour volume (down staging) with the possibility to measure the *in vivo* response. The number of intra-operative tumour ruptures is decreased and the number of patients with a post-operative local stage I is raised (Table 23.5 and Fig. 23.2). Moreover, the chemotherapy response gives some additional prognostic factors. For more than 40 years both study groups have gained a lot of success in treating these patients. The most important results of their trials form the basis of today's treatment and are listed in Table 23.6.

Surgery

Surgery of a WT is almost always an elective intervention and rarely due to emergency situations after traumatic or spontaneous tumour rupture. Even if the tumour nephrectomy seems technically simple, the most experienced team of surgeons and anaesthesiologists should carry out the intervention. The tumour has to be removed radically and the tumour spread has to be

Table 23.5 Number of tumour ruptures at primary surgery and after preoperative treatment in SIOP 1 and SIOP 2

SIOP 1	Rupture		SIOP 2	Rupture	
	[%]			[%]	
Preoperative irradiation	4	$p = 0.001$	Preoperative chemotherapy	5	$p = 0.0025$
Primary surgery	32		Primary surgery including small tumours	20	

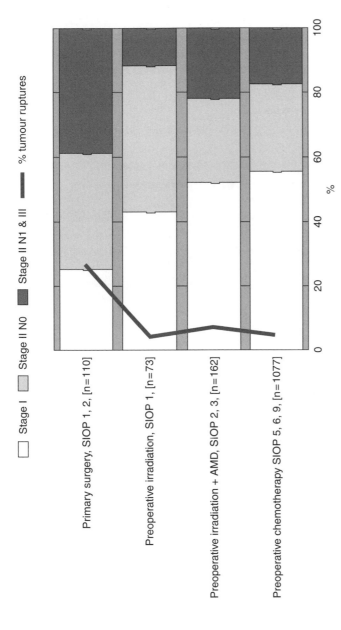

□ Stage I   ▨ Stage II N0   ▨ Stage II N1 & III   —— % tumour ruptures

Primary surgery, SIOP 1, 2, [n=110]

Preoperative irradiation, SIOP 1, [n=73]

Preoperative irradiation + AMD, SIOP 2, 3, [n=162]

Preoperative chemotherapy SIOP 5, 6, 9, [n=1077]

Fig. 23.2 Postoperative stage distribution and rupture rate in different SIOP studies.

Table 23.6 Major findings of NWTSG (COG), SIOP and UK trials

Treatment needs to be stratified according to stage and histology
The combination of vincristine and actinomycin D is more effective than the use of a single drug with the exception of single VCR in stage I after primary surgery
In stage I no irradiation is needed
In stage II and intermediate risk or favourable histology no irradiation is needed
With the addition of doxorubicine in stage III the dose of radiation can be reduced
Cyclophosphamid does not increase prognosis in stage IV, however, in case of anaplasia
Anthracyclines are decisive for the prognosis of clear cell sarcoma
A single bolus of actinomycin D is as effective as a split dose
The duration of treatment is 8 weeks in stage I and up to 6 months in stage II and III in intermediate risk or favourable histology
A tumour volume of more than 500 ml after preoperative chemotherapy is of prognostic significance
The number of tumour ruptures decreases as the number of stage I increases significantly after preoperative treatment
A preoperative chemotherapy with vincristine and actinomycin D is as effective as a preoperative irradiation with 20 Gy
After 4 and 8 weeks of preoperative chemotherapy with vincristine and actinomycin D the same stage distribution is achieved
Patients with pulmonary metastases and complete remission after preoperative chemotherapy do not need lung irradiation
Some patients with very low risk can be cured by surgery alone
LOH of 1 p and 16q are of prognostic significance
Remaining blastema after preoperative chemotherapy is a bad prognostic feature

documented simultaneously. The quality of the imaging studies has improved fundamentally and can rule out a bilateral disease with a great safety. If the contralateral kidney looks normal in good-quality imaging studies, the normal kidney need not be exposed during surgery. If there are doubts about the diagnosis of a nephroblastoma before or during surgery, a biopsy or puncture of the tumour may only be considered in case of a clearly inoperable tumour since there is a high risk of a peritoneal tumour cell seed. On the other hand, a primary complete tumour removal should always be preferred where malignancy is supected. Renal sparing surgeries in unilateral tumours should only be done in special cases and by experienced surgeons. Surgery of thromboses of the vena cava often requires the use of the heart-lung machine. Prognosis of these patients remains good after adequate surgery. Experienced surgeons should remove primary liver metastases after pre-operative chemotherapy.

Congenital mesoblastic nephromas (CMN) show an unusual growth pattern with fine finger-shaped extensions into the adjacent kidney fat capsule. Because of these extensions, the fat capsule needs to be removed with wide excision margins.

Irradiation

Nephroblastoma is a radiosensitive tumour. With the development of effective chemotherapeutic combinations, its place can be restricted to local risk situations and, in a few cases, for the treatment of pulmonary metastases.

Radiotherapy is given in SIOP and COG studies in local stage III in non high-risk or unfavourable histology. The total dose is 15 Gy in intermediate- and 30 Gy in high-risk histology in the SIOP studies. A local boost of 10–15 Gy is given for macroscopic remains. In COG, the irradiation dose is 10.2 Gy. Whole abdominal irradiation is needed in case of diffuse peritoneal seeding due to a tumour rupture. A dose reduction is required to the liver and particularly to the unaffected kidney (12 Gy). According to the data of the SIOP studies, irradiation of the lungs can be avoided if a complete remission of the metastases is achieved after chemotherapy. It has to be taken into account that treatment planning should take into account the whole spinal column particularly at doses of more than 15 Gy, to avoid disturbances of growth with a later scoliosis. The dose to the genital organs has to be taken into account and should be below 2 Gy for at least at one ovary and under 1 Gy for both testicles if possible.

Chemotherapy

SIOP studies Pre-operative chemotherapy **is** carried out in all patients aged over 6 months and less than 18 years after diagnosis of WT by imaging studies. Vincristine and actinomycin D are given for 4 weeks in localized stages. Anthracyclines are added in the case of metastatic disease and treatment is prolonged for 6 weeks. Patients with a bilateral disease are treated individually with vincristine and actinomycin D as long as there is tumour regression but not longer than 12 weeks. Babies less than 6 months of age and teenagers over 18 years are primarily treated surgically in the context of the SIOP studies, as other renal tumours (CMN, renal cell carcinoma) are more common in these patients.

Post-operative treatment is always carried out on the basis of the local stage and the histological type. The following guidelines apply to the individual sub-types:

Low-risk tumours: In stage I, no further treatment is given. In stage II and III, vincristine and actinomycin D are given for 26 weeks.

Intermediate-risk tumours: The relapse-free survival (RFS) of patients with stage 1 is 90 per cent with only 4 weeks of postoperative treatment. In stage II and III patients receive only 2 drugs for 26 weeks as the results of SIOP 2001 showed that doxorubicin can be avoided.

High-risk tumours: Having a RFS below 50 per cent treatment is intensified with carboplatin and etoposide. In the high-risk schema both drugs are alternatively given with a combination of cyclophosphamide and doxorubicine. Patients with stage II and III need local irradiation.

Stage IV disease: Post-operative treatment depends on the response to pre-operative chemotherapy. In case of complete remission (CR) after preoperative treatment (good responder), postoperative treatment is given according to local stage and histology as in non-metastatic tumours but at least according to stage II including doxorubicin. Patients with incomplete remission do need a more intensified treatment (VP16, cyclophosphamide, doxorubicine, carboplatin). Radiotherapy to the lung is necessary in patients with incomplete remission or with high-risk tumours.

COG studies Pre-operative chemotherapy is not done as immediate nephrectomy is attempted under almost all circumstances. Post-operative treatment is always carried out on the basis of age, local stage, histological type, LOH 1p and 16q, and response to chemotherapy in case of stage IV. The most important drugs in the treatment are vincristine, actinomycin D, and doxorubicine. The NWTS 4 study evaluated an early intensification of the treatment. It turned out that this so-called 'pulse intensive treatment' is equal to the standard treatment and more cost effective by minimizing hospital visits. The duration of the treatment is shortened to 6 months at the longest. In the NWTS 5 study the necessity of a post-operative therapy was evaluated in children below

2 years of age with a unilateral nephroblastoma, favourable histology, stage I and a tumour weight of less than 550 g. This observation arm of the study had to be closed early because of a too high number of relapses. As nearly all of these patients could be rescued by an effective relapse regimen a very low risk group will be continued to receive no chemotherapy after surgery if they fulfil the same criteria. In the ongoing COG trial LOH of 1p and 16q are used for stratification. Patients with LOH 1p and LOH 16q do receive a more intensified treatment to improve their survival rates.

Treatment of nephroblastomatosis

The treatment of nephroblastomatosis is still controversial. Initial nephrectomy should be avoided, and treatment orientates on WT. In case of a simultaneous WT, treatment is done according to the histological results and the stage of the tumour. For a diffuse perilobar nephroblastomatosis (without WT), a prolonged chemotherapy with vincristine and actinomycin D is recommended. Impressive regressions are described. The indication for radiation treatment has to be very restrictive. During the course of the treatment regular abdominal ultrasounds are needed throughout treatment at short intervals so that the development of a possible anaplastic WT can be detected as soon as possible.

Treatment of bilateral nephroblastomas

The therapeutic goal is to preserve as much healthy kidney as possible. Pre-operative chemotherapy is always indicated. This should be individualized and be carried out as long as renal sparing surgeries are possible but should not exceed 12 weeks. Renal sparing surgeries on both sides are possible in more than 50 per cent of patients. The post-operative therapy is determined by the histology and the local stage in which the highest risk group and the highest local stage of the two sides are decisive for the treatment. The choice of chemotherapy will be as given for unilateral cases. Essential drugs in the treatment are vincristine and actinomycin D, sometimes supplemented with doxorubicine. Surgery is of utmost importance when preoperative chemotherapy fails to shrink the tumour. The treatment of high-risk tumours is the same as for unilateral cases. The prognosis of bilateral tumours is good, with survival rates of about 70 per cent after 10 years. Late effects on kidney function are observed that can lead to renal failure making dialysis and renal transplantation necessary. In every case, the treatment of such a patient should be carried out in a paediatric oncology centre.

Treatment of adults with a nephroblastoma

A nephroblastoma is rarely diagnosed in adults. The treatment can be carried out following paediatric protocols. In adults, the tumour is operated on first. The tumour is frequently more advanced than in children with a high rate of patients with initial metastases. The reason for a poorer outcome can be attributed to non-standardized treatments in adulthood. Adult patients who are treated according to the guidelines of children have a better outcome. The increased neurotoxicity of vincristine needs to be considered in this age group.

Treatment of relapses

Approximately 15 per cent of patients with favourable histology WT and 50 per cent of patients with anaplastic WT experience recurrence. Most recurrences occur within 2 years of diagnosis. The general profile of relapse site shows that the lungs and pleura alone account for 50–60 per cent; abdominal recurrences make up to 30 per cent (isolated abdomen or combined to other sites), while other sites (brain or bone) are involved in less than 10 per cent of cases.

Treatment regimens for recurrent WT include drugs that are not used during primary chemotherapy. Therapy of recurrent disease depends on the nature of initial treatment, and of recognized prognostic factors of the primary tumour. Only children with a first and late relapse (>6 months after nephrectomy) in a non-irradiated field without lymph node involvement and no high-risk histology have a high chance of survival with conventional therapy. The chance of survival is less than 40 per cent in all other cases.

Several highly effective chemotherapy regimens, including ifosfamide, carboplatin and etoposide (ICE) are considered first-choice treatment for recurrent high-risk disease. How far the prognosis can be improved in such patients by giving high-dose chemotherapy with following stem cell rescue is unclear. International cooperation is needed to achieve a better outcome for these patients.

Follow up

The most important acute toxicity is VOD (veno occlusive disease) of the liver, which is associated with the use of actinomycin D. Further risk factors are right-sided tumours with post-operative radiotherapy including liver. Other acute side effects are rare and concern mainly infections, neuropathies (vincristine) and gastrointestinal side effects after abdominal radiation. Operative complications are lower after pre-operative treatment and lie within a range of 5 per cent. In the longer term, one needs to pay attention to skeletal and soft tissue growth as a result of radiotherapy. The extent of the impairment is dependent on the radiation dose, the treatment volume and the age of the child at the time of irradiation. Manifestations include kyphoscoliosis and bone and soft tissue hypoplasia in the area of the spinal column, pelvis, ribs and soft tissue of the flank, as well as the development of osteochondromas. Impairments are minimized with low doses (15 Gy). Delayed cardiotoxicity (anthracycline related) and renal impairment are possible. Second malignant neoplasms occur in around 1 per cent of cases. A follow-up schema for patients with nephroblastoma is given in Table 23.7.

Clear cell sarcoma of the kidney (CCSK)

Clear cell sarcoma of the kidney (CCSK) represents 3 per cent of malignant tumours of the kidney. It occurs with a peak incidence at 1–4 years of age, predominantly affecting boys (2:1). Four per cent of CCSK have metastasis at the time of diagnosis. In addition to pulmonary and bone metastases, CCSK may also spread to brain and soft tissue. The prognosis for CCSK improved after the introduction of anthracyclines to modern treatment regimens, with survival rates approaching 90 per cent for non-metastatic tumours.

Imaging studies do not distinguish this tumour from WT. Bone scintigraphy and cranial MRI have to be done in the work-up of this tumour.

A large series of cases from the NWTSG Pathology Center has provided detailed insight into the pathology of CCSK and its microscopic and immunohistochemical features. According to the NWTS-5 study, 25 per cent of patients had stage I disease; 37 per cent stage II; 34 per cent stage III; and 4 per cent stage IV disease. These tumours are characteristically composed of a mixture of cord cells and very clear septal cells with an extensive capillary network. However, many variant patterns explain the difficulties in making a correct diagnosis at the first attempt. CCSK is considered as a high-risk renal tumour. Immunohistochemical staining has shown positivity for vimentin but without any characteristic pattern of immune markers. Gene expression profiling studies have reported apparent expression of neural markers (e.g. nerve growth factor receptor) and a 100 per cent expression of epidermal growth factor receptor (EGFR).

Cytogenetic studies of CCSK have reported balanced translocations t(10;17)(q22;p13) and t(10;17)(q11;p12) and del(14)(q24.1q31.1).

Table 23.7 Follow up schema for children with nephroblastoma

	End of therapy	1st year	2nd year	3rd–5th year	6th year
Psychosocial history	+	Every 12 m	Every 12 m	Every 12 Mo	Every 12 m
Clinical examination, RR	+	Every 3 m	Every 3 m	Every 6 m	Every 12 m
Imaging studies					
X-ray of the lung	+	Every 3 m	Every 3 m	Every 6 m	Every 12 m
Sonography, abdomen	+	Every 3 m	Every 3 m	Every 3 m	Every 12 m
Laboratory					
Blood picture	+	Every 4 w	Every 3 m	Every 6 m	Every 12 m
Urinalysis	+	Every 4 w	Every 3 m	Every 6 m	Every 12 m
Kidney values	+	Every 2 m	Every 3 m	Every 6 m	Every 12 m
Fanconi syndrome*	+	Every 3 m	Every 3 m	Every 6 m	Every 12 m
Vaccination status, HBV, HCV, HIV	+	At end of 1st year	After vaccination		At end of 5th year
T3, T4, TSH**	+	Every 6 m	Every 12 m	Every 12 m	
Audiogram***	+	once	once, if path.	once, if path.	once, if path.
ECG/Echocardiography****	+	Every 6 m	Every 12 m	Every 12 m	Every 24 m
Bone scintigraphy*****	+	Every 6 m	Only at relapse	Only at relapse	Only at relapse

* after ifosfamide, ** after lung irradiation, ***after carboplatin, ****after anthracyclines, ***** in case of clear cell sarcoma.

The experience of NWTS1–2-3 in patients with CCSK showed that the combination of doxorubicine with vincristine and actinomycin D improved the 6-year RFS. The 6-year OS for stages I, II, III, and IV is 97, 75, 77, and 50 per cent. Similar results are reported by UK and SIOP. Today NWTS/COG as well as SIOP use four drugs to treat this tumour (cyclophosphamide, VP16, vincristine and doxorubicin). Prognosis of patients with CCSK is excellent, if they receive adequate therapy.

Rhabdoid tumour of the kidney

Rhabdoid tumours of the kidney (RTKs) are rare (2 per cent of all renal malignancies) and extremely aggressive. Eighty per cent of the patients are younger than 2 years of age and 60 per cent are under the age of 1 year. There is an overall male predominance (ratio 1·5:1). The kidney is the most common location, but brain and soft tissue could be involved. Fever and haematuria in a young patient with a renal malignancy with lung metastasis and hypercalcemia should suggest the diagnosis of RTK. As reported by van den Heuvel-Eibrink et al, 2008, among 639 cases of kidney tumours in the first 7 months of life with specified histology and stage, 9/11 stage IV tumours were RTK. Up to 15 per cent of patients with RTK have brain lesions. Because of the coincidence with brain metastasis, a cerebral MRI is always indicated.

Rhabdoid tumours commonly have deletions of the tumour suppressor gene *SMARCB1* (hSNF5/INI1) on chromosome 22. Today mutations can be detected at least in 80 per cent of cases on chromosome 22q11.2. Germline mutations of *SMARCB1* should be searched for especially in very young children and in those with synchronous rhabdoid tumours of the CNS and the kidney.

The diagnosis of RTK can only be done by histology, and now can be confirmed by immuno-histochemical and/or molecular genetic techniques showing the loss of INI1 protein expression resulting from *SMARCB1* mutations.

The prognosis of patients with RTK remains dismal despite aggressive treatments. RTK is a very chemo-resistant tumour. Common therapeutic regimens use intensive anthracycline-based regimens and aggressive local therapy. In all NWTS studies, 142 children showed an OS of 23.2 per cent after 4 years. Additionally the outcome of infants under 6 months of age at diagnosis was only 8 per cent compared to 41 per cent in patients 2 years of age or older ($p<0.0001$). In most reports, treatment is based on regimens with vincristine, dactinomycin, and doxorubicin with or without cyclophosphamide. In today's strategies, radical nephrectomy is followed by carboplatin and etoposide alternating with cyclophosphamide and doxorubicine for 6 months, as well as radiotherapy. The use of high-dose chemotherapy followed by autologous stem cell transplantation is controversial. Treatment of these patients should be centralized and done according to prospective trials. A registry for all rhabdoid tumours independent of their primary site is open in Europe to see if there is a difference between intra- and extracranial rhabdoid tumours.

Renal cell carcinoma

Renal cell carcinoma (RCC) is a rare malignancy in the kidney of children and accounts for only 1.9–5 per cent of paediatric renal tumours. The average age of children diagnosed with a RCC is about 10 (range 9– 5) years with a male predominance. Metastases to the lungs, bone, liver, or brain are identified in about 20 per cent of cases. Imaging is uncharacteristic and shows a non-specific solid intrarenal lesion with little enhancement and is often smaller than WT. Calcifications are more frequent in RCC than in Wilms tumour (25 per cent and 9 per cent, respectively).

The signs and symptoms of RCC in children are most frequently abdominal pain and haema-turia, sometimes accompanied by fever. Recent data suggest that paediatric RCC may be different from adult RCC with distinct morphologic characteristics and unique genetic abnormalities. Some studies have shown that most RCCs can be classified according to genetic translocations that involve chromosome Xp11.2, resulting in *TFE3* fusions. Childhood RCCs are more fre-quently of the papillary subtype and the Xp11 translocation type or the related t(6;11) transloca-tion type. An association of RCC to neuroblastoma is found in children as well as to other syndromes (tuberous sclerosis, urogenital malformations, Saethre-Chotzen, XYY syndrome). The clear-cell RCC with 3p25 abnormalities is rare in children.

Survival of children with RCC depends on the stage of disease at presentation and the possibility of complete resection, with an overall survival rate of 60–90 per cent. The 5-year survival rate is between 90 and 100 per cent for stage I, 50– 80 per cent for stage II-III and 10 per cent for stage IV. The surgical resection of tumour and metastases remains the crucial mainstay of successful treat-ment in paediatric RCC even in stage IV. RCC in children, as in adult, is not chemo-sensitive. In patients with distant metastasis, a combination of surgery, radiotherapy and immunotherapy (IL-2 or IFN-α) needs to be discussed in every single case. Most of the localized RCCs can be cured by surgery alone. The prognosis of disseminated RCC is still dismal and an efficient treatment needs to be defined. Because of the small number of patients, an international multicentre approach including adult oncologists is needed. Novel targeted therapies such as sunitinib, sorafenib and/or others need to be evaluated.

Congenital mesoblastic nephroma

Congenital mesoblastic nephroma (CMN) is a rare paediatric tumour with a favourable clinical outcome. Although the most common renal tumour under the age of 7 months is a WT, a relatively high percentage of children suffer from congenital mesoblastic nephroma (CMN), especially in the first 2 months of life. Metastatic disease at diagnosis is very unlikely. In a series of 750 patients with kidney tumours below the age of 7 months the proportion of CMN decreased markedly with increasing age, being 54 per cent of those diagnosed in the first month, 33 per cent in the second month, 16 per cent in the third and <10 per cent of all tumours diagnosed in the fourth and subsequent months of life. CMNs were stage I or II in 74 per cent of the cases and III in 13 per cent.

CMN is a spindle cell neoplasm with a low malignant potential that may exhibit several subtypes including classical, cellular and mixed, identified on the basis of molecular characterizations and morphological features. The cellular variant, which represents 40–60 per cent of CMN, shows a t(12;15)(p13;q25) translocation with resultant *ETV6–NTRK3* fusion. An identical gene-fusion transcript has also been reported in congenital or infantile fibrosarcoma (IFS), which also affects the same age group and shows similar morphology, suggesting that cellular CMN represents intrarenal IFS. The use of RT-PCR may be helpful for diagnosis, even though transcript expression levels are variable.

The clinical presentation of CMN is similar to other paediatric renal neoplasms. CMN usually presents as an asymptomatic abdominal mass in an infant. As CMN patients usually have a good outcome, immediate nephrectomy is advocated and no further treatment needed. Overall event-free survival is >95 per cent but occasional Stage III cellular CMN in older patients has a worse prognosis. The main risk factors for local recurrence are cellular subtype and incomplete local excision at primary surgery. Relapse usually occurs within 12 months of diagnosis, so close follow-up is recommended.

Further reading

Nephroblastoma

Coppes MJ, Pritchard-Jones K (2000) Principles of Wilms' tumor biology. *Urol Clin North Am* **27**, 423–33.

de Kraker J, Graf N, van Tinteren H, et al. (2004) Reduction of postoperative chemotherapy in children with stage I intermediate risk and anaplasia Wilms'Tumour. The SIOP 93–01 randomised trial. *Lancet* **364**, 229–1235.

Graf N, Tournade MF, de Kraker J (2000) The role of preoperative chemotherapy in the management of Wilms Tumor–The SIOP Studies. *Urol Clin North Am* **27**, 443–54.

Green DM, Breslow NE, Beckwith JB et al. (2001) Treatment with nephrectomy only for small, stage I/favorable histology Wilms'tumor: a report from the National Wilms' Tumor Study Group. *J Clin Oncol* **19**, 3719–24.

Grundy PE, Breslow NE, Li S, et al. (2005) Loss of heterozygosity for chromosomes 1p and 16q is an adverse prognostic factor in favorable-histology Wilms tumor: a report from the National Wilms Tumor Study Group. *J Clin Oncol* **23**, 7312–21.

Mitchell C, Jones PM, Kelsey A et al. (2000) The treatment of Wilms' tumour: results of the United Kingdom Children's cancer study group (UKCCSG) second Wilms' tumour study. *Br J Cancer* **83**, 602–8.

Neville HL, Ritchey ML (2000) Wilms' tumor. Overview of National Wilms' Tumor Study Group results. *Urol Clin North Am* **27**, 435–42.

Pastore G, Znaor A, Spreafico F, et al. (2006) Malignant renal tumours incidence and survival in European children (1978–1997): report from the Automated Childhood Cancer Information System project. *Eur J Cancer* **42**, 2103–14.

Pein F, Michon J, Valteau-Couanet D et al. (1998) High-dose melphalan, etoposide, and carboplatin followed by autologous stem-cell rescue pediatric high-risk recurrent Wilms' tumor: a French Society of Pediatric Oncology study. *J Clin Oncol* **16**, 3295–3301.

Perlman EJ, Faria P, Soares A, et al. (2006). Hyperplastic perilobar nephroblastomatosis: long-term survival of 52 patients. *Pediatr Blood Cancer* **46**, 203–21.

Pritchard-Jones K (2002) Controversies and advances in the management of Wilms' tumour. *Arch Dis Child* **87**, 241–4.

Reinhard H, Aliani S, Rübe C, et al. (2004) Wilms Tumor in Adults–Results of the SIOP 93–01/GPOH study. *J Clin Oncol* **22**, 4500–6.

Ritchey M, Panayotis PK, Breslow N, et al. (1992) Surgical complications after nephrectomy for Wilms' tumor. *Surg Gynecol Obstetr* **175**, 507–14.

Spreafico F, Pritchard Jones K, Malogolowkin MH, et al. (2009) Treatment of relapsed Wilms tumors: lessons learned. *Expert Rev Anticancer Ther* **12**, 1807–15.

Vujanic GM, Sandstedt (2010) The pathology of Wilms' tumour (nephroblastoma: the International Society of paediatric Oncology approach. *J Clin Pathol* **63**, 102–9.

Weirich A, Leuschner I, Harms D, et al. (2001) Clinical impact of histologic subtypes in localized non-anaplastic nephroblastoma treated according to the trial and study SIOP-9/GPOH. *Annals of Oncology* **12**, 311–9.

CCSK

Argani P, Perlman EJ, Breslow NE, et al. (2000). Clear cell sarcoma of the kidney: a review of 351 cases from the National Wilms Tumour Study Pathology Center. *Am J Surg* **24**, 4–18.

Seibel NL, Li S, Breslow NE, Beckwith JB et al. (2004) Effect of duration of treatment on treatment outcome for patients with clear-cell sarcoma of the kidney: a report from the National Wilms' Tumor Study Group. *J Clin Oncol* **22**, 468–73.

Rhabdoid tumour

Biegel JA, Zhou JY, Rorke LB, et al. (1999) Germ-line and acquired mutations of INI1 in atypical teratoid and rhabdoid tumors. *Cancer Res* **59**, 74–9.

Chi, S.N., Zimmerman, M.A., Yao, X., et al. (2008). Intensive Multimodality Treatment for Children With Newly Diagnosed CNS Atypical Teratoid Rhabdoid Tumor. *J Clin Oncol* **8**, 8–14.

Weeks DA, Beckwith JB, Mierau GW, et al. (1989) Rhabdoid tumour of kidney: a report of 111 cases from the NWTS pathology center. *Am J Surg Pathol* **13**, 439–58.

RCC

Selle B, Furtwängler R, Graf N, et al. (2006) Population-based study of Renal cell carcinoma in children in Germany, 1980–2005. More frequently localized tumors and underlying disorders compared with adult counterparts. *Cancer* **107**, 2906–14.

Argani P, Ldanyi M (2006) The evolving story of renal translocation carcinomas. *Am. J. Clin Pathol* **126**, 332–4.

CMN

Sebire NJ, Vujanic GM (2009) Paediatric renal tumours: recent developments, new entities and pathological features. *Histopathology* **54**, 516–28.

van den Heuvel-Eibrink MM, Grundy P, Graf N, et al., (2008). Characteristics and survival of 750 children diagnosed with a renal tumor in the first seven months of life: A collaborative study by the SIOP/GPOH/SFOP, NWTSG, and UKCCSG Wilms tumor study groups. *Pediatr Blood Cancer* **50**, 1130–4.

Chapter 24

Neuroblastoma

Angelika Eggert and Alberto Garaventa

Introduction

Neuroblastoma represents the most frequent extracranial tumour of children. A century ago, in 1910, Wright introduced the term neuroblastoma after demonstrating its origin from embryonal neuroblasts of the sympathetic peripheral nervous system. He also described the diagnostic aspect of metastatic disease in the bone marrow, which he called the 'pseudorosette'. The tumour was first described by Virchow in 1864 in a child with an abdominal mass. In 1901, Pepper described six cases of newborns with an adrenal tumour, and six cases of infants with massive hepatic metastases that regressed spontaneously.

Despite the presence of more than 30 000 publications in PubMed and a great deal of progress in understanding the biology, diagnosis and treatment of neuroblastoma, the biological reasons for its clinical aspects remain unclear and the prognosis of patients with advanced disease remains dismal, with a long-term event-free survival (EFS) less than 50 per cent.

Epidemiology

Neuroblastoma represents 6–10 per cent of all pediatric cancers. Its age distribution is character-ized by a peak of incidence in the first year of life, followed by a rapid decline in the following years. After the age of 6, it becomes rare and exceptional among adolescents and adults. Neuroblastoma occurs at slightly higher rates in males than in females (M/F ratio 1.1–1.2). Its mean annual inci-dence is 7–12 cases per million children in western countries, and it occurs in 1 of 7000 live births. However, incidence rates are rather heterogeneous, except for the extremely low rates observed in some African regions. Screening programs were implemented in regions of several countries including Japan, Germany, and Canada, and an increase in the incidence of neuroblastoma has been reported in these regions. It will be of interest to determine whether this increase is partly due to increased surveillance and screening, or rather to an increase in potential risk factor distribution.

The overall influence of known environmental agents on the etiology of neuroblastic tumours is very low. The predisposing effect of alcohol and recreational drug use as well as codeine intake during pregnancy warrants further investigation, as do the potentially protective effect of folic acid and of vitamin supplementations. Congenital anomalies may be associated with neuroblas-toma, especially in infants. However, the consistent incidence rates of neuroblastoma in children support the hypothesis of a major role of genetic factors.

Tumour predisposition and genetics

Familial neuroblastoma

A familial history of neuroblastoma is observed in ~ 1 per cent of patients with an estimated pen-etrance of 11 per cent in hereditary cases. Neuroblastoma pedigrees usually show an autosomal dominant pattern of inheritance with incomplete penetrance. Two main neural crest-derived developmental disorders are associated with an increased risk to develop neuroblastoma: (1) Hirschsprung's disease, characterized by an absence of ganglion cells in the distal colon resulting in functional obstruction and (2) Ondine's curse, a disorder characterized by a failure of the autonomic control of ventilation during sleep. Both diseases are frequently associated with each other, and most cases are linked to mutation of the *PHOX2B* gene. Interestingly, associations between neuroblastic tumours and various 'neuro-cardio-facial-cutaneous' syndromes, including Noonan and Costello syndromes and neurofibromatosis type 1, defined by the constitutive activation of the RAS–MAPK pathway have been also reported. Although the involvement of *PHOX2B* in familial cases of neuroblastoma is compelling, its contribution to the development of sporadic neuroblastoma is much less obvious since somatic mutations are extremely rare. The molecular mechanisms underlying the role of these mutations in neuroblastoma predisposition remain unclear.

More recently, the anaplastic lymphoma kinase (*ALK*) gene was identified as a second neuroblastoma predisposition gene, when several groups demonstrated germline *ALK* mutations in neuroblastoma pedigrees. The *ALK* gene encodes a transmembrane receptor tyrosine kinase (RTK) preferentially expressed in the central and peripheral nervous systems. The function of the full-length ALK receptor is poorly understood. Three types of *ALK* germline mutations have been described to date in neuroblastoma families, the R1275Q mutation being the most frequent. Although detailed clinical information is still lacking for several families, it is apparent that the penetrance of these mutations may be incomplete, and that neuroblastic tumours of variable aggressiveness can be observed in *ALK* mutation carriers.

Germline mutations of *NF1*, *ALK* and *PHOX2B* do not account for all familial neuroblastoma cases. Interestingly, various types of abnormal constitutional karyotypes have been observed in patients with neuroblastoma, including constitutional copy number anomalies, balanced and unbalanced translocations as well as specific chromosome deletions.

Sporadic neuroblastoma

Although neuroblastomas may occur in familial contexts, most cases occur sporadically. Decades ago, chromosome banding techniques revealed that neuroblastoma cells frequently harbour gross cytogenetic aberrations such as double-minute chromosomes (DM), homogeneously staining regions of chromosomes (HSR) or deletions of the short arm of chromosome 1. In 1983, Schwab, et al. demonstrated that HSR and DM in neuroblastoma contained ectopic amplifications of a gene designated *MYCN* and located at the chromosomal site 2p24. The presence of such amplicons was highly associated with advanced stage of disease and poor outcome. *MYCN* amplification (NMA) with copy numbers from 5- to more than 100-fold is observed in around 25 per cent of neuroblastomas, and is associated with advanced-stage disease and rapid tumour progression. The adverse prognostic effect of NMA on neuroblastoma patients has been confirmed in many studies. The *MYCN* status is routinely used in clinical practice to assign therapeutic intensity. Several lines of evidence indicate that overexpression of MYC proteins has a major role in oncogenesis through the deregulation of proliferation. In particular, transgenic mice overexpressing MYCN in neuroectodermal cells develop tumours in peripheral neural crest-derived structures, and show typical histopathological features of human neuroblastoma, therefore, demonstrating that MYCN can contribute to the transformation of neuroblasts *in vivo*.

In addition to NMA, numerous non-random cytogenetic alterations have been described in primary neuroblastomas, the majority of which represent allelic losses of chromosomal material. The development of high-resolution, microarray-based comparative genomic hybridization (array-CGH) has allowed the comprehensive examination of whole genome aberration patterns of neuroblastoma tumours and cell lines.

Segmental copy number alterations, mainly including deletions of chromosome 1p, 3p, 11q and gain of 1q, 2p, and 17q, occur frequently in neuroblastoma, and are usually associated with a poor outcome. Although strongly associated with NMA, 1p deletion is also observed in cases without NMA. Deletions at 1p have been analysed thoroughly, resulting in the definition of a deleted consensus region at 1p36. Loss of 1p36 has been observed in 23–35 per cent of cases, and was demonstrated to be significantly associated with prognostic markers of aggressive neuroblastoma. In addition, loss of chromosome 1p has been shown to predict survival in multivariate analyses. Therefore, the genomic region at 1p36 might contain one or more neuroblastoma tumour suppressor genes.

More recently, the effect of chromosome 11q loss on neuroblastoma outcome has been investigated. Deletions of 11q in a consensus region at 11q23 have been detected in 26–44 per cent of cases in large patient cohorts. Interestingly, although loss of 11q is related to features of unfavourable neuroblastoma, it is inversely correlated with NMA. Thus, the presence of 11q deletions and NMA appears to delineate two molecularly distinct subgroups of unfavourable neuroblastoma. In multivariate analyses of relevant prognostic variables, allelic loss of 11q turned out to be an independent marker of decreased EFS in the entire cohorts as well as in subgroups of low and intermediate risk. Thus, 11q alterations represent a promising prognostic marker that could improve risk estimation of neuroblastoma in future risk-stratification systems.

Partial 17q gain is often observed in primary neuroblastomas exhibiting segmental alterations, independent of their *MYCN* status. Recurrent segmental alterations are thought to lead to the loss of putative tumour suppressor genes and/or to the gain of oncogenes.

The recent identification of somatic and activating mutations of the *ALK* gene in approximately 8 per cent of neuroblastomas represents a breakthrough in the understanding of neuroblastoma pathogenesis. Interestingly, the spectra of somatic and germline *ALK* mutations are different. The existence of a potential link between *ALK* mutations and tumour biology remains to be fully determined, since *ALK* mutations have not consistently correlated with aggressive neuroblastoma subtypes in the studies published to date. The analysis of larger neuroblastoma series will provide further information about the precise relationship between *ALK* mutations, ALK expression, other genomic alterations, and tumour phenotype.

Pathology

The peripheral neuroblastic tumours (pNTs) including neuroblastoma belong to the 'small blue round cell' neoplasms of childhood. They are derived from progenitor cells of the sympathetic nervous system: the sympathogonia of the sympathoadrenal lineage. After migrating from the neural crest, these pluripotent sympathogonia form the sympathetic ganglia, the chromaffin cells of the adrenal medulla, and the paraganglia, reflecting the typical localizations of neuroblastic tumours.

The International Neuroblastoma Pathology Classification (INPC) assigns pNTs to one of four basic morphological categories.

Neuroblastoma (Schwannian stroma-poor) A tumour composed of neuroblastic cells forming groups or nests separated by stromal septa with Schwannian proliferation ranging from none to limited. This category consists of the three subtypes: (1) undifferentiated, (2) poorly differentiated, and (3) differentiating.

Ganglioneuroblastoma, intermixed (Schwannian stroma-rich) A tumour containing well-defined microscopic nests of neuroblastic cells intermixed or randomly distributed in the ganglioneuromatous stroma. The nests are composed of a mixture of neuroblastic cells in various stages of differentiation.

Ganglioneuroblastoma, nodular (composite Schwannian stroma-rich/stroma-dominant and stroma-poor) This lesion is characterized by the presence of grossly visible, usually haemorrhagic neuroblastic nodules (stroma-poor component, representing an aggressive clone) co-existing with intermixed ganglioneuroblastoma (stroma-rich component) or with ganglioneuroma (stroma-dominant component), both representing a non-aggressive clone. The term 'composite' implies that the tumour is composed of biologically different clones.

Ganglioneuroma (Schwannian stroma-dominant) This variant has two subtypes: maturing and mature. The maturing subtype is predominantly composed of ganglioneuromatous stroma with scattered collections of differentiating neuroblasts and/or maturing ganglion cells in addition to fully mature ganglion cells. The mature subtype is composed of mature Schwannian stroma and ganglion cells.

There is a significant correlation between morphological features of the INPC and biological properties of the pNTS, such as *MYCN* amplification or TrkA expression.

Biological aspects

A number of biological pathways regulating major hallmarks of cancer appear to be disrupted or at least affected in neuroblastoma. Important biological characteristics include abnormal patterns of gene or protein expression in the areas of tumour differentiation, apoptosis, drug resistance, angiogenesis, invasion, and metastasis. Insight into the molecular regulation of these biological features will ultimately lead to the identification of novel drug targets.

As neurotrophin signalling has a central role in normal neuronal development and may be involved in both differentiation and regression of neuroblastoma, there has been a particular interest in alterations of these pathways. The clinical and biological roles of Trk receptors and their corresponding ligands have been extensively investigated, and Trk receptors were identified as important prognostic factors influencing the clinical and biological behaviour of neuroblastoma.

Delayed activation or disruption of normal apoptotic pathways may also be an important phenomenon involved in spontaneous regression as well as therapy resistance of neuroblastoma. Major elements of the apoptotic signalling cascade with abnormal expression or activation patterns include the BCL2 family, survivin, and caspase-8. The latter is mainly affected by inactivation due to epigenetic silencing. Alterations in DNA methylation represent one of the most common molecular events in neoplasia, and CpG-island hypermethylation of gene promoters is a frequent mechanism for functional inactivation of relevant tumour-associated genes. Hypermethylation of these genes might be a major event leading to therapy resistance of neuroblastoma cells. Therefore, the anti-tumour effects of demethylating agents including decitabine are currently being investigated.

Acquired resistance to chemotherapeutic agents may also be conferred by enhanced drug efflux via overexpression of classical multidrug resistance proteins, including the multidrug resistance gene 1 (*MDR1*) and the gene for the multidrug resistance-related protein (*MRP*). Their potential clinical significance in neuroblastoma has been addressed in several studies.

Enhanced tumour angiogenesis and elevated expression of pro-angiogenic factors, such as vascular endothelial growth factor (VEGF) are both correlated with an aggressive phenotype in neuroblastoma, making angiogenesis inhibitors an attractive treatment option that is currently being evaluated in preclinical studies. Further advances in our understanding of the molecular biology of neuroblastoma are currently supported by the use of high-throughput, array-based methods, not only with the goal of patient-tailored precise prognostication, but also to identify key targets for therapeutic exploitation.

Clinical presentation, diagnosis and staging

Neuroblastoma can arise at any site along the sympathetic nervous system chain, but the distribution of the primary tumours at diagnosis varies across the sites with age. Most primary tumours occur within the abdomen (~70 per cent), and over half of these arise in the adrenal gland. Infants more frequently have adrenal, thoracic, and cervical primary tumours. The clinical presentation of neuroblastoma reflects the site of tumour origin, the extent of regional and metastatic disease, as well as the presence of paraneoplastic syndrome (Table 24.1).

Cervical neuroblastomas (4 per cent of cases) mimic aspecific adenopathies, and often include Horner syndrome (ptosis, miosis, enophthalmos) and heterochromia. Thoracic neuroblastomas represent 15 per cent of all cases. Tumours in the upper mediastinum cause respiratory distress, as well as Horner syndrome and heterochromia, while tumours arising in the middle and lower mediastinum are usually asymptomatic and discovered by routine chest X-ray. The typical neuroblastoma patient is a toddler failing to grow, with abdominal distension and a palpable lateral or central hard, fixed mass. Pelvic tumours are uncommon and present as suprapubic masses, causing constipation and urinary disturbances. Approximately half of all patients have disseminated disease at the time of diagnosis. The most commonly involved organs are the bone marrow, skeleton, liver, and lymph nodes, with less common involvement of the lung and central nervous system. Disseminated disease is usually associated with aspecific symptoms, including fever, pallor, anorexia, and bone pain with consequent refusal to walk and mood changes. Retro-orbital and orbital metastases are rather frequent, and produce a typical appearance of proptosis and periorbital ecchymoses (Fig. 24.1). In infants, stage 4S is characterized by massive liver involvement, with or without the presence of bluish nodules in the subcutaneous tissue, and infiltration of the bone marrow. Infants with stage 4S can present with significant respiratory distress due to a massively enlarged liver. By definition, stage 4S patients do not have bone lesions. Neuroblastoma in adolescents and adults has a slow, indolent clinical course compared to that of children, although the distribution of primary tumours and sites and patterns of metastases are similar.

The anatomical connection between the sympathetic nervous system and the spinal cord accounts for the propensity of neuroblastoma to infiltrate the intervertebral foramina. Paraspinal tumours tend to grow through the neural foramina of the vertebral bodies, causing compression of the spinal cord as a presenting sign of the tumour. Motor deficits are the most frequent symptoms experienced by patients with paraspinal tumours, followed by radicular or back pain, bladder or bowel dysfunction, and rarely, sensorial manifestations. Only 4–5 per cent of patients have clinical evidence of epidural compression. Early detection of this phenomenon is crucial because symptoms may rapidly worsen, leading to irreversible paraplegia.

Ganglioneuroblastoma (GNB) are well-differentiated locoregional tumours, and may occasionally cause symptoms not directly related to the effects of the tumour mass, but related to the paracrine secretion of various substances. Vasoactive intestinal peptide (VIP) causes watery diarrhea, and antineuronal antibodies can trigger an autoimmune reaction that may occur as a

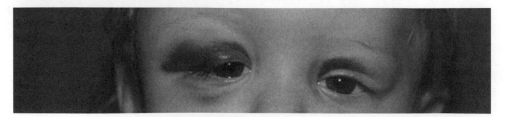

Fig. 24.1 Retro-orbital and orbital metastases with a typical appearance of proptosis and periorbital ecchymoses in a child with stage 4 neuroblastoma.

Table 24.1 Tumour site and clinical characteristics

Tumour site	Main symptoms and signs	Incidence (%)	Metastases (%)	Outcome
Neck	Mass mimicking lymphadenopathy, Horner Syndrome	4	2	Good
Thorax: *Upper*	Respiratory symptoms	6	5	Good
Lower	Incidental X-ray detection	6	2	Good
Abdomen	Central or lateral mass, symptoms related to metastatic disease (fever, pallor, anorexia, bone pain, irritability)	70	75	Poor
Pelvis	Lower abdominal mass, dysuria, constipation	5	5	Good
Not identified	Fever, pallor, anorexia, bone pain, irritability	1	100	Very Poor

cerebellar or an opsoclonus-myoclonus syndrome (OMS). OMS occurs in 2–3 per cent of neuroblastoma patients, and is characterized by multidirectional rapid eye movement (opsoclonus), myoclonus, and brainstem ataxia. These symptoms may precede the detection of a tumoural mass by several months, and improve if the primary tumour is removed, but in many cases patients require specific immunosuppressive treatment. Symptoms may reappear during infectious episodes and the majority of these children appear to have neurological deficits.

Increased catecholamine levels may cause high blood pressure, although hypertensive crises are very rare in patients with neuroblastoma. Hypertension may also be caused by the stimulation of the renin-angiotensin system due to pressure on the renal artery by the retroperitoneal mass.

Tumour markers

Urinary metabolites produced by catecholamine degradation, namely vanillylmandelic acid (VMA) and homovanillic acid (HVA), are the most sensitive (90 per cent positive cases in large series) and specific disease markers. Overall levels and the ratio of VMA to HVA in the urine have prognostic value, and are related to age, histology, stage, and *MYCN* amplification. Screening for neuroblastoma using a urinary assay for catecholamines at 6 months of age was pioneered in Japan in the early 1970s. Two large population-based studies in Quebec and Germany showed that screening detected many neuroblastomas that would never have been diagnosed clinically, and observed no reduction in the incidence of advanced stage neuroblastoma. Cumulative mortality was no different from concurrent or retrospective mortality. As a result, routine screening was ceased because of the low clinical impact in treating neuroblastoma. However, a great deal of biological information on neuroblastoma with favourable outcome has been derived from these studies. Lactate dehydrogenase (LDH), ferritin and neuron specific enolase (NSE) have been identified as markers for neuroblastoma in patient serum, and correlate with tumour stage, extension, and prognosis. Other serum tumour markers such as chromogranin, and neuropeptide Y have been reported, but their clinical use is less well established.

Diagnostic criteria

The following examinations are required for accurate diagnosis and staging, as indicated by the International Neuroblastoma Staging System (INSS):

- CT or MR of the primary tumour site
- Histological evaluation of a biopsy from the primary tumour or metastatic site
- Bone marrow aspirate and trephine biopsy at two different sites

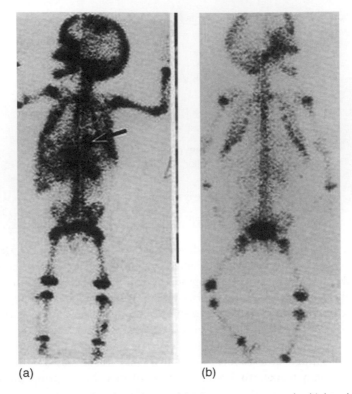

(a)   (b)

Fig. 24.2 Metaiodobenzylguanidine (MIBG) scan. (a) Primary tumour uptake (right adrenal gland) as well as bone and bone marrow metastases are visualized. (b) Normal radioelement uptake after chemotherapy.

- Meta-iodo-benzylguanidine (MIBG) scintigraphy before tumour excision to evaluate the primary tumour site and detect metastatic sites (Fig. 24.2). Detection of a single equivocal lesion requires confirmation by another imaging modality
- Technetium-99 bone scintigraphy is required only in exceptional cases when I-MIBG cannot confirm a primary tumour. An isolated bone uptake should be confirmed by another imaging modality and/or a biopsy
- Assay of the urinary catecholamine levels (HVA and VMA). Additional assays should include levels of serum ferritin, LDH and NSE.

Staging

Disease staging is necessary in order to define prognosis and to design the treatment program. The INSS definitions are based on the local and distant extension and the resectability of the tumour (Table 24.2).

Since the INSS stage of locoregional tumours is based on the degree of surgical resection, the International Neuroblastoma Risk Group (INRG) classification system was developed to facilitate the comparison of risk-based clinical trials conducted in different regions of the world by defining homogeneous pretreatment patient cohorts. The premise is that a staging system based on preoperative, diagnostic images will be more robust and reproducible than one based on operative findings and approaches. Since the surgical risk factors are based on radiographic

Table 24.2 The International Neuroblastoma Staging System (INSS)

Stage 1	Localized tumour with complete gross excision, with or without microscopic residual disease. Representative ipsilateral lymph node microscopically negative for tumour
Stage 2A	Localized tumour with incomplete gross excision. Representative ipsilateral non-adherent lymph nodes microscopically negative for tumour
Stage 2B	Localized tumour with or without complete gross excision, with ipsilateral non-adherent lymph nodes positive for tumour. Enlarged contralateral lymph nodes must be microscopically negative for tumour
Stage 3	Unresectable unilateral tumour, infiltrating across the midline*, with or without regional lymph node involvement; or localized unilateral tumour with contralateral lymph node involvement; or midline tumour with bilateral extension by infiltration or lymph node involvement
Stage 4	Any primary tumour with dissemination to distant lymph nodes, bone, bone marrow, liver and/or other organs (except as defined for Stage 4S)
Stage 4S	Localized primary tumour (as defined for Stage 1, 2A or 2B), with dissemination limited to liver, skin and/or bone marrow**. Limited to infants <1 year of age

Multifocal primary tumours should be staged according to the greatest extent of disease and be followed by a subscript 'M' (i.e. Stage 3_M).
* The midline is defined as the vertebral column. Tumours originating on one side and crossing the midline must infiltrate to or beyond the opposite side of the vertebral column.
** Marrow involvement in Stage 4S should be minimal (i.e. <10% nucleated cells in bone marrow biopsy). More extensive marrow involvement should be considered Stage 4. The MIBG scan should be negative in the marrow for Stage 4S.

images, the term, image-defined risk factors (IDRFs), was chosen and a consensus was reached for the IDRFs listed in Table 24.3.

These criteria, based on the relation of the tumour with the adjacent structures and vasculature, (Fig. 24.3) predict severe surgical complications and are the basis for the new International Neuroblastoma Risk Group Staging System (INRGSS; Table 24.4).

Several international groups have developed a model of risk stratification to facilitate the delivery of risk-adapted treatments. Various biological features were added to the different clinical characteristics, and currently the most important prognostic factors include age, stage, and *MYCN* amplification. These parameters define at least two different patterns of disease. The first is neuroblastoma that arises in the first months of life, with some patients showing spontaneous regression of the disease and most having excellent survival with minimal treatment, provided the tumour is not *MYCN* amplified. The second pattern contrasts greatly, with an unfavourable outcome expected for children with *MYCN*-amplified tumours or children older than 18 months at diagnosis with metastatic tumours. Between these two extremes there is at least one less well-defined group with intermediate characteristics. Additional prognostic markers, including histopathological classification, tumour ploidy, chromosomal anomalies, as well as gene- or expression-level anomalies identified in molecular profiling, could help to better define prognosis and consequently enable physicians to tailor different treatment strategies to individuals in this patient subgroup. The INRG Task force has developed the INRG Consensus Pretreatment Classification Schema to establish a consensus approach for current pretreatment risk stratification. The prognostic effect of 13 variables in an 8800-patient cohort was analyzed, and a schema with four main prognostic groups (Table 24.5) and 16 pretreatment designations was developed (Table 24.6). This approach will greatly facilitate the comparison of risk-based clinical trials conducted in different regions of the world.

Table 24.3 Image-defined risk factors (IDRFs) in neuroblastic tumours

Ipsilateral tumour extension within two body compartments
Neck
Tumour encasing carotid and/or vertebral artery and/or internal jugular vein
Tumour extending to base of the skull
Tumour compressing the trachea
Cervico-thoracic junction
Tumour encasing brachial plexus roots
Tumour encasing subclavian vessels and/or vertebral and/or carotid artery
Tumour compressing the trachea
Thorax
Tumour encasing the aorta and/or major branches
Tumour compressing the trachea and/or principal bronchi
Lower mediastinal tumour, infiltrating the costo-vertebral junction between T9 and T12
Thoraco-abdominal
Tumour encasing the aorta and/or the vena cava
Abdomen/pelvis
Tumour infiltrating the porta hepatis and/or the hepatoduodenal ligament
Tumour encasing branches of the superior mesenteric artery and the mesentery root
Tumour encasing the origin of celiac axis and/or of the superior mesenteric artery
Tumour invading one or both renal pedicles
Tumour encasing the aorta and/or the vena cava
Tumour encasing the iliac vessels
Pelvic tumour across the sciatic notch
Intraspinal tumour
Extension, regardless of location, provided that more than one-third of the spinal canal in the axial plane is invaded and/or the perimedullary leptomeningeal spaces are not visible and/or the spinal cord signal is abnormal
Infiltration of adjacent organs/structures
Pericardium, diaphragm, kidney, liver, duodeno-pancreatic block and mesentery
Conditions to be recorded, but not considered as IDRFs
Multifocal primary tumours
Pleural effusion, with or without malignant cells
Ascites, with or without malignant cells

Treatment

The treatment of children with neuroblastoma primarily depends on patient age, disease extension, and histological and biological features. The currently employed treatment modalities include surgery, chemotherapy, and radiotherapy.

Surgery

Surgery plays a key role for both diagnosis and treatment. The goals of primary surgery are to confirm the diagnosis, acquire tissue samples for classification, histological and biological studies,

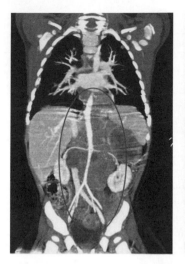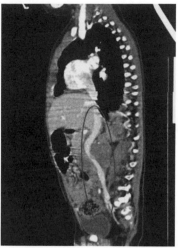

Fig. 24.3 Angio-CT, coronal view, showing a large abdominal neuroblastoma encasing the major retroperitoneal vessels.

and to resect the tumour with minimal morbidity. When the anatomical characteristics (site, size, relationship with the surrounding structures and presence of a pseudo-capsule) indicate that surgical resection is feasible, surgery is the treatment of choice for patients presenting with localized disease. An international panel of surgeons and radiologists, who identified surgical risk factors detectable by computer tomography (CT) or magnetic resonance imaging (MRI), has established radiological criteria for a safe resection. Surgery is the only treatment necessary to cure the majority of patients with localized disease, even if macroscopic remnants of the tumour are left behind. If surgical risk factors are detected, pre-surgical chemotherapy is necessary to shrink the tumour prior to resection. Since neuroblastoma has an elevated tropism towards lymphatic vessels and lymph node infiltration, it is important to perform a surgical exploration of the locoregional lymph nodes, especially in abdominal and pelvic sites. With regard to paravertebral sites with infiltration through the intervertebral foramina, laminectomy is indicated only in selected cases with severe neurological symptoms. In fact, chemotherapy can rapidly reduce both tumour size and the magnitude of spinal cord compression in these cases.

In contrast to its pivotal role in treating localized disease, the function of surgery is somewhat controversial for metastatic disease. Considering the high incidence of local relapse, the current indication in most treatment protocols is resection of the primary tumour after inducing remission of the metastases. In delayed primary or second-look surgery, the surgeon evaluates the response to therapy, and removes the residual tumour whenever possible.

Table 24.4 International Neuroblastoma Risk Group Staging System (INRGSS)

Stage L1	Radiological risk factors absent. Localized tumour not involving vital structures as defined by the list of image-defined risk factors and confined to one body compartment
Stage L2	Locoregional tumour with presence of one or more image-defined risk factors
Stage M	Distant metastatic disease (in contrast to stage MS)
Stage MS	Metastatic disease in children <18 months with metastases confined to the skin, liver and/or bone marrow (bone marrow involvement should be limited to <10% of total nucleated cells on smears or biopsy)

Table 24.5 The four main prognostic groups

Pretreatment Risk Group	5-year EFS (%)	Proportion of patients (%)[*]
Very Low	>85	28.2
Low	>75 to ≤85	26.8
Intermediate	≥50 to ≤75	9.0
High	<50	36.1

Radiotherapy

Neuroblastoma is a radiosensitive tumour, and tumouricidal doses range from 15 to 32 Gy (with fractional radiation doses ranging from 150 to 400cGy) depending on tumour site, volume, and age of the patient. The definition of the role of external beam radiotherapy (EBRT) is under continuous refinement due to the identification of risk factors that can limit its use in low-risk patients. The lack of randomized trials addressing the contribution of radiotherapy hampers proper evaluation of the impact of this treatment modality on clinical outcome. However, the more recent trend is towards the use of radiotherapy in possible combination with surgery at the primary tumour site in patients with *MYCN*-amplified tumours in stage 4 and stage 3

Table 24.6 International Neuroblastoma Treatment Risk Groups

INRG Stage	Age (months)	Histological classification	Grade of tumour differentiation	MYCN	11q Aberration	Ploidy	Pretreatment risk group
L1/L2	Any	GN maturing GNB intermixed					A Very Low
L1	Any	Any except GN maturing or GNB intermixed		NA Amp			B Very Low K High
L2	<18	Any except GN maturing or GNB intermixed		NA	No Yes		D Low G Intermediate
	≥18	GNB nodular; neuroblastoma	Differentiating	NA	No		E Low
			Poorly differentiating or undifferentiating	NA	Yes H Intermediate		
M	<18			NA		Hyperdiploid	F Low
	<12			NA		Diploid	I Intermediate
	12 to <18			NA		Diploid	J Intermediate
	<18			Amp			O High
	≥18						P High
MS	<18			NA	No Yes		C Very Low Q High
				Amp			R High

Amp = amplified; GN = ganglioneuroma; GNB = ganglioneuroblastoma; NA = not amplified disease with unfavourable prognostic factors. EBRT is also successfully used as palliative care on painful sites.

A radio-metabolic therapy is used for stages 3 and 4 neuroblastomas and utilizes I^{131} carried by I-MIBG, a noradrenalin analogue that is incorporated in the neurosecretory granules of neuroblastoma cells. Dosimetry problems, together with the non-homogeneous uptake of I-MIBG throughout the tumour, and toxicity have limited the use of this therapeutic approach to selected treatment centres. Some groups have used radio-metabolic therapy as first-line treatment, but the results from long-term patient follow up were not favourable in these cases. Other approaches have included radio-metabolic therapy using I-MIBG in the conditioning phase prior to haematopoietic stem cell transplantation, and current use as consolidation treatment is under investigation.

Chemotherapy

Chemotherapy has an important role in treating neuroblastoma, since the majority of patients present with metastatic or locally advanced disease at diagnosis and require systemic treatment. Alkylating agents (cyclophosphamide, ifosfamide, busulfan, melphalan), platinum analogues (cis-platinum and carboplatinum), vinca alkaloids (vincristine), epipodophyllotoxins (VP16, VM26), and anthracyclines (doxorubicin) have well-established activities and efficacies against neuroblastoma, and are considered standard options. Over the last few years other agents, such as topotecan, irinotecan or temozolomide, have also proven to be effective, and combinations including these drugs are being tested in ongoing phase II studies. High-dose chemotherapy with various combinations of busulfan, melphalan, carboplatin, and etoposide, followed by autologous peripheral blood stem cell (PBSC) rescue, is currently used as consolidation treatment in high-risk patients.

Risk-adapted treatment

Low- and very low-risk group

This group includes children with INSS stage 1 and 2, infants with stage 3(L2) and 4S neuroblastomas without unfavourable biological markers. As all these patients have an excellent prognosis, the goal is to reduce the risk of short-term side effects, while maintaining high survival rates. The predicted survival is near to 100 per cent, both for patients who are treated with a moderate dose of chemotherapy [Children Oncology Group (COG) and International Society of Paediatric Oncology European Neuroblastoma Network (SIOPEN) groups] and patients who are treated without cytotoxic agents [Memorial Sloan-Kettering Cancer Center (MSKCC) and German groups]. German studies have shown that infants with neuroblastomas detected in screening programs may safely be observed over time without obtaining a definitive intraoperative histologic diagnosis, thus avoiding the potential complications of surgery. SIOPEN has recently started a randomized study of these two approaches. Chemotherapy is mandatory if severe symptoms are present or if tumour progression occurs. Stage 4S group: neuroblastoma without *MYCN* amplification undergoes spontaneous regression in the majority of cases. Chemotherapy or low-dose radiotherapy should be reserved for patients with large tumours or massive hepatomegaly causing mechanical obstructions, respiratory insufficiency or liver dysfunction.

Intermediate-risk group

The intermediate-risk group encompasses a wide spectrum of conditions, including patients with *MYCN* nonamplified tumours >12 months of age, stage 3 (L2) and stage 4 (M) patients <18 months. Stage 1(L1) *MYCN*-amplified tumours have also recently been included by SIOPEN in this group. Survival of this group is nearly 90 per cent, and the challenge is to identify patients for whom therapy may be further reduced. Surgical resection and moderate-dose, multiagent chemotherapy are the backbone of therapy. High-dose chemotherapy with PBSC rescue is not necessary, while the role of radiotherapy is less well defined.

High-risk group

This group includes all stage 4 (M) patients > 12 months of age and stage 2, 3 and 4S patients with *MYCN*-amplified tumours. These patients are generally treated with dose-intensive multiagent chemotherapy consisting of high-dose cisplatin with etoposide, vincristine, doxorubicin, and cyclophosphamide and, more recently, topotecan. Chemotherapy is followed by resection of the primary tumour, where possible, then myeloablative chemotherapy with PBSC rescue. Irradiation of the tumour bed or residual primary tumour is performed after myeloablative therapy. The indication for irradiation of metastatic lesions is less clear, but current protocols usually employ a dose of 21 Gy to the primary site as consolidation therapy, though randomized trials have not been performed. Most high-risk neuroblastomas initially respond to therapy, but subsequently relapse.

The European Neuroblastoma Group Fifth Study (ENSG5) study has shown a considerable beneficial effect on event-free and overall survival of the rapid COJEC schedule (cisplatin, vincristine, carboplatin, etoposide and cyclophosphamide), which achieved a 1.8-fold increase in dose intensity over conventional OPEC/OJEC induction employing the same drugs. In the standard regimen, chemotherapy was administered every 21 days if patients achieved haematological recovery, whereas the rapid regimen was administered every 10 days irrespective of haematological recovery. The idea of eliminating resistant tumour clones with supralethal chemotherapy has been studied in neuroblastoma since the early 1980s, and the results of a randomized phase III cooperative study (COG 4) has shown improved EFS. Since most patients still relapsed despite such an intensive strategy, much attention has been given to biological therapies including differentiation-inducing agents such as retinoid derivatives or immunotherapy with GD2 monoclonal antibodies. Retinoids are a class of compounds inducing terminal differentiation of neuroblastoma cells *in vitro*. The cohort of patients assigned to receive post-transplantation 13-cis-retinoic acid therapy in a randomized phase III trial by the COG had better EFS, and toxicity was acceptable.

Although the profound immunosuppression produced by high-dose chemotherapy regimens provides unfavourable conditions for the application of active immunotherapy, the use of passive immunotherapy is feasible. Disialoganglioside (GD2) is a surface glycolipid antigen present on neuroblastoma cells. Its expression in normal tissues is restricted to neurons protected from the effects of intravenous monoclonal antibodies (MoAbs) by the blood–brain barrier. Therapies using various MoAbs have been assessed in phase I and II settings, and their safety profile has been established. GD2 therapies are currently being studied, together with or without cytokines, in phase III trials for neuroblastoma patients in first response. Recent early data from the COG randomized phase III trial of anti-GD2 MoAb ch14.18 plus cytokines after PBSC rescue demonstrated a clear survival advantage in patients receiving immunotherapy compared to untreated controls.

Treatment of spinal cord compression

The use of MRI has increased the number of cases with documented infiltration of the foramina. In the majority of cases, no neurological symptoms arise and no specific treatment is required. There is very little evidence that an asymptomatic intraspinal tumour will continue to grow after resection of the extraspinal component. Some cases suggest that intraspinal neuroblastoma in patients with no neurological symptoms tends to remain stable or even regress without specific treatment. If >50 per cent of the spinal canal is taken up by the tumour, dexamethasone in addition to chemotherapy (carboplatin plus VP 16 is currently the best option) should be administered.

Patients with localized neuroblastoma who present with signs of spinal cord compression require urgent specific treatment. Rapid therapeutic decisions must be made within a few hours if neurological deficits and clinical progression are detected. The decision regarding whether to administer emergency chemotherapy should be made immediately after detailed conference between the oncologist and neurosurgeon and treatment start should never be delayed. Laminectomy or laminotomy is preferable only in infants showing very rapid neurological deterioration. The tumour should be biopsied when the patient is stable a few days after chemotherapy.

Treatment of relapse

The survival rate of children with relapsing or resistant neuroblastoma is very poor. A small cohort of patients, mainly represented by children with stages 1 and 2 who underwent local recurrence or developed late relapse, may still benefit from further conventional treatment including aggressive surgery, external or metabolic radiotherapy, and chemotherapy. However, experimental therapies are proposed for the majority of patients. In these cases, the patient's quality of life has to be carefully discussed with the parents.

New drugs

The molecular characterization of tumours from high-risk neuroblastoma patients with poor outcome is likely to disclose potential targets for the development of novel therapies for the most aggressive forms of this malignancy.

Targetting MYC

In light of the frequency and importance of *MYCN* amplification in the pathogenesis of high-risk neuroblastoma, blockade of MYCN signalling represents an important approach for the development of new therapeutics. Transcription factors have long been considered as targets for cancer therapy. However, clinical approaches to block this class of molecules remain elusive. The most direct means of silencing these molecules would be to disrupt MYC synthesis directly using RNA interference (RNAi) methods. These approaches are extremely useful tools in the laboratory, but they have yet to achieve regular use in the clinic, largely because of difficulties with delivery *in vivo*.

Targeting Aurora kinases

Aurora kinase A represents a suitable therapeutic target, since it has critical functions in cell cycle regulation and spindle assembly, and contributes to the stabilization of phosphorylated and ubiquitinated MYCN. Expression of Aurora kinase A is a negative prognostic factor in neuroblastoma. Emerging data regarding the functions of inhibitors of Aurora kinase A in cancer therapy suggests that they may have unique functions when utilized in therapy for neuroblastoma.

Targeting RTKs and PI3K

MYCN degradation is a critical downstream factor for the efficacy of the PI3K/mTOR pathway, and suggests that clinical inhibitors of phosphatidylinositol-3-kinase (PI3K) should show activity against MYCN-driven neuroblastomas. Inhibitors for signalling effectors downstream of RTKs, including PI3K, mTOR, AKT, and dual inhibitors for PI3K/mTOR, are all currently in clinical trials. Allosteric inhibitors of mTORC1, which block mTOR independently of ATP binding, are currently being tested for neuroblastoma, and have shown mixed results preclinically. Specific ALK and TRK inhibitors are in development, and have shown promising results preclinically and in phase I trials. The availability of clinical inhibitors presents an important translational opportunity to test these agents in children with high-risk neuroblastoma. Because of the complex interrelation of pathway members, inhibition at one point often induces feedback activation in other signalling pathways, justifying the need to test these agents in combination.

Targetting ALK

Pharmacological inhibition of activated ALK may represent a promising novel therapeutic approach for neuroblastoma treatment. The knockdown of ALK expression in *ALK*-mutated cells, but also in several neuroblastoma cell lines overexpressing an apparently normal ALK protein, led to a dramatic decrease in cell proliferation. In agreement with these observations, neuroblastoma cell lines harbouring activating *ALK* mutations responded to the ALK inhibitors, NVP-TAE684, and PF-02341066. These data provide a strong molecular rationale for ALK-targeted therapy for neuroblastoma.

Targeting Histone deacetylases

Histone deacetylases (HDAC) inhibitors are an emerging class of promising novel anticancer drugs. Initial phase I/II trials have shown that unselective inhibition of HDACs causes a variety of side effects. Therefore, identification and selective targeting of the most critical tumour entity-relevant HDAC family member may reduce unspecific effects and increase antitumour efficacy in the future. Neuroblastoma is the first tumour entity in which expression of all classical HDAC family members has been investigated systematically. Expression of all 11 classical HDAC family members was detected, but HDAC8 was the only isozyme that significantly correlated with advanced disease stage, age, unfavourable tumour histology, 11q aberration and poor survival. As HDAC8-selective inhibitors are available, HDAC8 may be a promising drug target for neuroblastoma differentiation therapy.

Conclusion

For many decades, neuroblastoma has remained a challenging disease for both clinicians and researchers. Novel high-throughput techniques have provided molecular markers that indicate tumour behaviour and patient outcome with very high accuracy. Once the anticipated value of these markers has been confirmed in ongoing studies, patients may profit from more accurate risk assessment by integrating these markers into the clinical routine. Moreover, discovery of further tumour-initiating events, such as the recently revealed oncogenic mutations of *ALK*, will further promote the elucidation of the genetic etiology of the disease. Together with recent information on altered signalling pathways in aggressively growing tumours, this knowledge will help to establish therapeutic strategies specifically targeting molecular key factors of neuroblastoma tumour progression.

Further reading

Bourdeaut F, Trochet D, Janoueix-Lerosey I, et al. (2005) Germline mutations of the paired-like homeobox 2B (PHOX2B) gene in neuroblastoma. *Cancer Lett* **228**, 51–8.

Brodeur GM (2003) Neuroblastoma: Biological insights into a clinical enigma. *Nat. Rev Cancer* **3**, 203–216.

Brodeur GM, Pritchard J, Berthold F, et al. (1993) Revisions of the international criteria diagnosis, staging, and response to treatment. *J Clin Oncol* **11**, 1466–77.

Capasso M, Diskin SJ (2010) Genetics and genomics of neuroblastoma. *Cancer Treat Res* **155**, 65–84.

Cecchetto G, Mosseri V, De Bernardi B, et al. (2005) Surgical risk factors in primary surgery for localized neuroblastoma: The LNESG1 study of the European International Society of Pediatric Oncology Neuroblastoma Group. *J Clin Oncol* **23**, 8483–89.

Cohn SL, Pearson AD, London WB, et al. (2004) The International Neuroblastoma Risk Group (INRG) Classiication System: AN INRG Task Force *J Clin Oncol* **27**, 289–97.

De Bernardi B, Pistoia V, Gambini C, et al. (2008) Peripheral Neuroblastic Tumors. In: Hay ID and Wass JAH (eds) *Clinical Endocrine Oncology* pp 360–69 Oxford: Wiley–Blackwell.

De Bernardi B, Balwierzb W, Bejentc J, et al. (2005) Epidural compression in neuroblastoma: Diagnostic and therapeutic aspects. *Cancer Letters* **228**, 283–99.

De Grandis E, Parodi S, Conte M et al. (2009) Long-term follow-up neuroblastoma-associated opsoclonus-myoclonus-ataxia syndrome. *Neuropediatrics* **40**, 103–11.

DuBois SG, Matthay KK (2008) Radiolabeled metaiodobenzylguanidine for the treatment of neuroblastoma *Nucl Med Biol* **35**(S1), S35–48.

Fulda S (2009) The PI3K/Akt/mTOR pathway as therapeutic target in neuroblastoma. *Curr Cancer Drug Targets* **9**, 729–37.

Garaventa A, Parodi S, De Bernardi B, et al. (2009) Outcome of children with neuroblastoa after progression or relapse. A retrospective study of the Italian neuroblastoma registry. *Eur J Cancer* **16**, 2835–42.

Haas-Kogan DA, Swift PS, Selch M, et al. (2003) Impact of radiotherapy for high-risk neuroblastoma: a Children's Cancer Group study. *Int J Radiat Oncol Biol Phys* **56**, 28–39.

Houghton PJ, Morton CL, Kolb EA, et al. (2008) Initial testing (stage 1) of the mTOR inhibitor rapamycin by the pediatric preclinical testing program. *Pediatr Blood Cancer* **50**, 799–805.

Janoueix-Lerosey I, Lequin D, Brugières L, et al. (2008) Somatic and germline activating mutations of the ALK kinase receptor in neuroblastoma. *Nature* **455**, 967–70.

Janoueix-Lerosey I, Schleiermacher G, Delattre O (2010) Molecular pathogenesis of peripheral neuroblastic tumors. *Oncogene* **29**, 1566–79.

Maris JM (2010) Recent advances in neuroblastoma. *N Engl J Med* **362**, 2202–11.

Maris JM, Hogarty MD, Bagatell R, Cohn SL. (2007) Neuroblastoma. *Lancet* **369**, 2106–20.

Matthay K, Reynolds P, Seiger RC et al. (2009) Long-Term Results for Children With High-Risk Neuroblastoma Treated on a Randomized Trial of Myeloablative Therapy Followed by 13-cis-Retinoic Acid: A Children's Oncology Group Study *J Clin Oncol* **7**, 1007–13.

Modak S, Cheung NK (2010) Neuroblastoma: Therapeutic strategies for a clinical enigma. *Cancer Treat Rev* **36**, 307–17.

Monclair T, Brodeur, GM, Ambros PF, et al. (2009) The International Neuroblastoma Risk group Staging System: an INRG Task Force Report. *J Clin Oncol* **27**, 298–303.

Ohira M, Nakagawara A (2010) Global genomic and RNA profiles for novel risk stratification of neuroblastoma. *Cancer Sci* **101**, 2295–301.

Otto T, Horn S, Brockmann M, et al. (2009) Stabilization of N-Myc is a critical function of Aurora A in human neuroblastoma. *Cancer Cell* **15**, 67–78.

Parodi S, Papio F, Haupt R, et al. (2007) The prognostic role of urinary catecholamines in infants with disseminated neuroblastoma may be mediated by MYCN amplification. *Ped Blood Cancer* **48**, 593.

Schramm A, Schulte JH, Astrahantseff K, et al. (2005) Biological effects of TrkA and TrkB receptor signaling in neuroblastoma. *Cancer Lett* **228**, 143–53.

Schwab M, Alitalo K, Klempnauer KH, et al. (1983) Amplified DNA with limited homology to myc cellular oncogene is shared by human neuroblastoma cell lines and a neuroblastoma tumour. *Nature* **305**, 245–8.

Shimada H, Ambros IM, Dehner LP, et al. (1999) Terminology and morphologic criteria of neuroblastic tumors: recommendations by the International Neuroblastoma Pathology Committee. *Cancer* **86**, 349–63.

Weiss WA, Aldape K, Mohapatra G, et al. (1997) Targeted expression of MYCN causes neuroblastoma in transgenic mice. *EMBO J* **16**, 2985–95.

Witt O, Deubzer HE, Lodrini M, et al. (2009) Targeting histone deacetylases in neuroblastoma. *Curr Pharm Des* **15**, 436–47.

Yalçin B, Kremer LC, Caron HN, van Dalen EC (2010) High-dose chemotherapy and autologous haematopoietic stem cell rescue for children with high-risk neuroblastoma.*Cochrane Database Syst Rev* **5**, cd 006301.

Yu AL, Gilman AL, Ozkaynak MF, et al. (2010) Anti-GD2 antibody with GM-CSF, interleukin-2, and isotretinoin for neuroblastoma. *N Engl J Med* **363**, 1324–34.

Chapter 25

Germ cell tumours

Gabriele Calaminus and James Nicholson

Introduction

Germ cell tumours (GCT) constitute a highly heterogeneous group of tumours characterized by a wide range of histologies, benign and malignant, and clinical presentation at many different anatomical sites. In adolescents and adults, over 90 per cent of cases develop within the gonads, mostly in males, whilst around half of childhood GCT occur at extra-gonadal midline sites such as the sacrococcygeal region, CNS, and mediastinum. The diverse nature of GCT necessitates cooperation between paediatric oncologists and surgeons (according to tumour site) and radiotherapists, as well as related disciplines of endocrinology and neurology. Coordination of this multidisciplinary care is critical in the success of treatment.

During the past three decades, a dramatic improvement in prognosis of malignant GCT has been achieved. This progress can mainly be attributed to national and international cooperative therapeutic protocols using platinum-based combination chemotherapy as part of a multimodal therapeutic approach. Identification of risk groups relating to age, histology, primary site, and stage have led to stratification of chemotherapy.

Epidemiology and biology

Germ cell tumours can occur in all age groups, ranging from the foetal period to adulthood. The annual incidence is approximately 0.5 per 100 000 in children under 15. However, the overall incidence of teratomas is likely to be underestimated because of under reporting to registries.

Registry and trial data show a distinct distribution pattern with regard to site and tumour histology of GCT (Fig. 25.1). The histological subtypes of GCT in neonates are almost exclusively mature and immature teratomas (0.9 per 100 000 in girls; 2.6 per 100 000 in boys), sometimes admixed with subtle foci of yolk sac tumour (YST). YST predominate later in infancy and during early childhood. Whilst the incidence of GCT drops steadily during childhood to below 0.1 per 100 000, a significant increase is observed after the onset of puberty.

In children, the most frequent primary sites of GCT are the testes (25 per cent), ovaries (25 per cent), sacrococcygeal region (20 per cent), and the CNS (20 per cent); they may also arise in the head-neck region, anterior mediastinum, retroperitoneum, and urogenital system (10 per cent).

Sacrococcygeal, vaginal, and head and neck GCT develop during the neonatal period and during infancy and early childhood. Histologically, they present as teratomas and YSTs (Fig. 25.2). Testicular GCT may also develop during infancy and childhood; however, they show a bimodal age distribution with a second incidence peak during adolescence and adulthood. In this age group, GCT present as seminomas and malignant non-seminomatous GCT, which may include embryonal carcinoma, YST, and choriocarcinoma, often with mixed histology. In contrast, ovarian and CNS GCT predominantly develop after the onset of puberty and during the second (and third) decade of life.

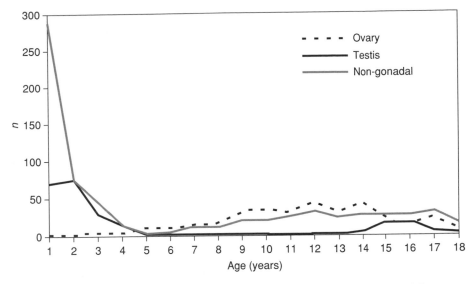

Fig. 25.1 Age distribution with respect to primary tumour site in 1307 children and adolescents with germ cell tumours registered to the MAKEI protocols. Reproduced from Schneider *et al.* (2004) with permission.

Conditions predisposing to GCT

In adolescents, there is an association between testicular GCT and testicular dysgenesis, resulting from inadequately treated undescended testes. GCT are also associated with constitutional disturbances of sex chromosomes such as Klinefelter syndrome. The risk of developing GCT is increased in phenotypic females with testicular feminization and streak gonads (frequently associated with ambiguous sexual differentiation, Swyer syndrome), and in Turner syndrome; in these patents, Y-chromosome fragments are often detected and dysgerminoma can occur in association

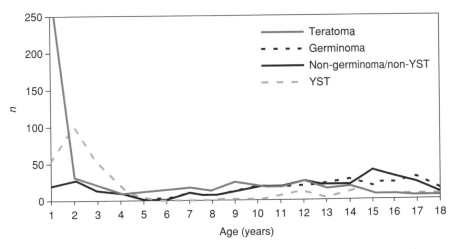

Fig. 25.2 Age distribution with respect to histology in 1307 children and adolescents with germ cell tumours registered to the MAKEI protocols. Reproduced from Schneider *et al.* (2004) with permission.

with gonadoblastoma. Maternal exposure to oestrogen may influence the appearance of testicular GCT in young men, an association not seen for GCT in infants and childhood.

Embryology and histological classification

GCT are believed to arise from primordial germ cells (PGCs), which are totipotent and capable of differentiating into all GCT subtypes. During normal development, PGCs migrate from the extra-embryonic yolk sac to the gonads; the occurrence of GCT at midline extra-gonadal sites is thought to result from aberrant migration. Despite their common origin, GCT are characterized by marked heterogeneity, impacting on their behaviour and management. Their complex classification reflects their degree of differentiation, and is based on the WHO classification of testicular cancer (2004) with modifications from Dehner (Fig. 25.3).

Germinomatous tumours [synonyms: seminoma (testis), dysgerminoma (ovary), germinoma (extra-gonadal)] arise from cells that remain in the pluripotent undifferentiated state with morphological features of undifferentiated germ cell epithelium. Yolk sac tumours (YST) and choriocarcinoma (CHC) follow an extra-embryonic differentiation pattern and are characterized by secretion of alpha-1-fetoprotein (AFP) or human choriogonadotropin (HCG or β-HCG) respectively. Embryonal carcinoma (EC) consists of immature totipotent cells resulting from embryonic differentiation. Somatic differentiation results in the formation of teratomas, mature or immature, and mimicking structures of all germ layers. The histological grade of immaturity is defined by the extent of immature (predominantly neuroepithelial) elements (Table 25.1). This correlates with the risk of loco-regional relapse, particularly after incomplete resection, and is therefore essential in risk assessment of pure teratomas. Gonadoblastoma is a benign but pre-malignant condition, with stromal components associated with dysgenetic gonads, occurring only in the presence of the Y chromosome. Left untreated it may become malignant, typically as a germinoma.

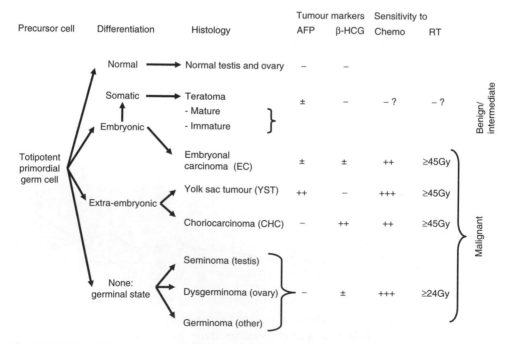

Fig. 25.3 Biological characteristics of GCT.

Table 25.1 Histological classification of paediatric germ cell tumours

I Germinoma*

  a. Intratubular

  b. Invasive

II Teratoma:

  A Mature

  B Immature**

    Grade 1 Immature tissue <1 Low Power(x 4) Field (LPF)/slide

    Grade 2 Immature tissue 1–3 LPF/slide

    Grade 3 Immature tissue >4 LPF/slide

Common to each of these: +/– microfoci of probable yolk sac tumour (Heifetz lesion [Am J Surg Pathol. (1998) 9,1115–24.])

  C Malignant teratoma (Teratoma with non germ cell malignant component)

III Embryonal carcinoma

IV Yolk sac tumour***

V Choriocarcinoma

VI Gonadoblastoma

VII Mixed malignant germ cell tumour (each component to be listed)

---

* Synonyms: dysgerminoma (ovary), seminoma (testis), germinoma (extra-gonadal)
** Degree of immaturity is sometimes expressed according to Gonzalez-Crussi in terms of % of sampled surface
  (grade 1, <10%; grade 2, 10–50%; grade 3, >50%)
*** Yolk sac tumour is also known as endodermal sinus tumour

In contrast to testicular GCT of adult patients, there is no evidence to suggest that paediatric GCT develop from carcinoma *in situ*.

In most patients, response to different treatment modalities can be predicted from histology and tumour marker profile. Paediatric GCT often present with more than one histological subtype; in this situation selection of therapy is based on the strategy employed for the most aggressive malignant component.

Tumour markers

The secretion of AFP and HCG by some subtypes of GCT is well recognized, and can be exploited in diagnosis and monitoring, on and off treatment. AFP, an α-globulin, has very high levels at birth as it is the main foetal serum binding protein but falls to adult levels of <12ng/ml (<10kU/l; 1 ng/ml $\equiv$ 0.84 KU/l) between 1 and 2 years of age, so isolated AFP levels should be interpreted cautiously in children under 2 years. AFP is produced by YST, and at low levels, by some embryonal carcinomas and immature teratomas.

HCG is a glycoprotein produced by the placenta and made up of α and β subunits. The α subunit is structurally similar to other hormones including LH, FSH, so the more specific β subunit is used in assays to avoid cross-reactivity with other hormones. β-HCG secretion by tumour is seen typically in the presence of choriocarcinoma, with lower levels produced by some germinomas, indicating the presence of syncytiotrophoblastic giant cells. Since relative levels of 'free β' and intact dimer (α+β) vary between different tumour subtypes, measurement of total HCG (both free β and dimer) is recommended.

Lactate dehydrogenase (LDH) and placental alkaline phosphatase (PLAP) are sometimes measured in GCT. LDH is a non-specific marker of malignancy of limited value in the assessment of paediatric tumours and PLAP is raised in only around 20 per cent of germinoma, and may therefore be used as an additional diagnostic tool if elevated.

Molecular biology

The rarity of GCT and their subtypes has hampered progress in understanding their biology although patterns are now emerging in terms of genomic changes and gene expression.

Gain of the short arm of chromosome 12 (12p) is a well recognized abnormality found almost universally in adult testicular GCT, usually arising by isochromosome formation. It has also been observed in ovarian and mediastinal GCT but is relatively rare in children. The incidence of 12p gain increases through childhood and the pattern of imbalances seen on chromosomes 1, 6, 13 and 20 differs between pre- and post-pubertal patients with mediastinal GCT. No consistent correlation between cytogenetic imbalance and primary site has been observed, and teratomas are associated with complete absence of chromosome imbalance.

Molecular studies of the imprinting status of GCT support the hypothesis that GCT at all sites share a common cellular origin in the primordial germ cell, and that extra-gonadal GCT develop from germ cells that have migrated aberrantly during embryonic development. More recent work has suggested an association between global methylation patterns and resistance to treatment.

In addition, paediatric and adult malignant germ cell tumours (MGCT) differ significantly in their protein-coding gene expression profiles (messenger RNA, mRNA) supporting the suggestion that they differ biologically, segregating by both histology and age. In contrast, and in keeping with their presumed primordial germ cell origin, it has also been shown that MGCT all over-express two microRNA clusters, regardless of patient age, histological subtype, and anatomical site of the tumour.

Diagnosis

Clinical presentation

GCT tend to occur as relatively indolent masses, with clinical symptoms determined by their site of origin. Gonadal GCT comprise around half of childhood GCT. Ovarian tumours typically occur in girls over the age of 5 years; they are usually teratoma or dysgerminoma, more complex mixed tumours being seen during adolescence. They present as palpable abdominal masses, often with visible distension, and there may be pain associated with torsion or rupture. Symptoms associated with hormonal disturbances such as virilization and menstrual disturbance may be seen in post-pubertal patients with ovarian primaries. Testicular GCT present as painless scrotal swellings, either in the first years of life when yolk sac tumours and teratomas predominate, or in adolescence, when seminomas and mixed MGCT are seen.

The most common sites for extra-gonadal GCT are the CNS (these are discussed in Chapter 20), sacrococcygeal region, mediastinum, retroperitoneum and head and neck, typically in the midline. Most sacrococcygeal tumours are teratomas (mature or immature) and occur more commonly in girls than boys. They may be diagnosed antenatally, by routine scanning, or as a visible mass on neonatal examination. Cases that present later, with partly or exclusively internal tumours, are more likely to have malignant components, typically YST, and to present with functional disturbances resulting from the effects of tumour bulk or nerve damage. Mediastinal GCT are more common in boys than girls and the majority occur from adolescence onwards, almost exclusively in the anterior mediastinum. Symptoms may result from airway compression, superior vena cava obstruction, and occasionally aberrant hormone production.

Approximately 20 per cent of malignant GCT have metastases at the time of diagnosis, although they are rarely associated with presenting symptoms, and mostly identified as a result of staging investigations. GCT most commonly spread to the lungs, but occasionally to liver, bone or bone marrow. Metastasis to the CNS is associated with CHC, and may be seen in approximately 4 per cent of young males with malignant testicular GCT, but in less than 1 per cent of cases in younger children; this possibility should therefore be borne in mind in patients with very high levels of HCG.

Investigations

Radiology and staging

In many patients with extra-cranial GCT, initial assessment will be made with ultrasound of the abdomen and pelvis, and should include assessment of tumour position and size, as well as the presence of lymphatic spread or peritoneal seeding. This is followed by detailed three-dimensional imaging with computed tomography (CT) or magnetic resonance imaging (MRI) scan; a CT scan is required for assessment of lung metastases and extent of abdominal disease. MRI is the investigation of choice for sacrococcygeal GCT, in order to define extension into the sacral and spinal canal. Plain X-rays have limited value in initial assessment, except for mediastinal tumours, but are valuable in follow up, particularly chest X-ray. Skeletal metastases and bone marrow involvement are seen in less than 10 per cent of patients overall, and are rare in the absence of pulmonary metastases, but are particularly associated with malignant sacrococcygeal GCT. Technetium bone scan should therefore be considered in the presence of organ metastases. CNS imaging only needs to be considered in patients (mainly adolescent males) in which CHC is identified histologically or by markers.

Laboratory investigations

AFP and total HCG should be measured in all cases of suspected GCT, as raised tumour markers may be of value in diagnosis and monitoring of GCT, both on and off treatment: caution should be exercised in interpretation of AFP levels in infants. GCT may be treated without tissue diagnosis on the basis of radiological findings and raised tumour markers, although histological confirmation is usually available at diagnosis in gonadal tumours, for which primary excision is part of treatment. Neo-adjuvant chemotherapy with delayed surgery may be the treatment of choice for some extra-gonadal GCT, in which case raised markers may obviate the need for potentially hazardous biopsy. However, in equivocal cases (non-diagnostic markers, hepatic or upper retroperitoneal tumours), a diagnostic biopsy should be performed, and should include storage of fresh tumour tissue for genetic and biological studies. Where a biopsy is performed in a mixed tumour, the GCT components in the tissue diagnosis may differ from the subtype suggested by marker estimation, or may under report the range of histologies present as result of sampling error. This is unlikely to influence treatment, provided that the tumour is fully staged. Thresholds above which marker levels can be considered diagnostic are controversial. For AFP, moderately elevated levels may be consistent with the presence of microfoci of YST in immature teratoma. HCG may be moderately elevated in germinoma, and levels up to 50 IU/l are usually considered consistent with this diagnosis, although caution should be exercised in labelling levels any higher than this as CHC, given that CHC are rare in young people and typically associated with HCG levels over 1000 IU/l.

In female patients with ovarian GCT and in male patients with mediastinal GCT, constitutional karyotyping is also recommended.

In addition to routine blood tests before chemotherapy, special consideration should be given to assessment of renal function as most regimens used for treatment of GCT incorporate nephrotoxic agents including platinum compounds and ifosfamide.

Treatment

Surgery

Most extra-cranial GCT are amenable to primary resection, and this is the treatment of first choice for localized tumours. If the diagnosis of a malignant GCT has been made histologically or with raised markers, and the initial radiological assessment shows infiltration or metastatic spread, preoperative chemotherapy will increase the likelihood of microscopically complete resection. In general, there is no role for debulking surgery in pediatric GCT. In patients with tumour residual after initial resection, second-look surgery is essential. Surgical removal of metastases is not indicated unless they show insufficient response to chemotherapy. Close attention to surgical recommendations for GCT is essential to optimize outcomes whilst minimizing morbidity.

Testis

The resection of testicular tumours is performed as unilateral orchidectomy after high inguinal incision, to avoid scrotal contamination; trans-scrotal surgery will lead to upstaging of tumours that might otherwise be stage 1, with the result that patients may receive chemotherapy that could have been avoided. There is no evidence that retroperitoneal lymph node dissection improves prognosis in children, and it leads to increased morbidity including risk to future sexual function.

Ovary

Primary surgical resection (salpingo-oopherectomy) is standard management in ovarian GCT. Ascitic fluid or peritoneal washings should be collected for cytological examination, and biopsies of any suspicious area on peritoneal surfaces, lymph nodes, omentum or contralateral ovary performed. Unresectable or bilateral tumours should be biopsied with a view to fertility-preserving surgery where possible following neo-adjuvant chemotherapy, except in the presence of gonadoblastoma or XY gonadal dysgenesis, when bilateral gonadectomy is recommended.

Coccyx

A dorsal approach to sacrococcygeal tumours is appropriate for most cases in view of their predominantly external components. Some have substantial internal components deep in the pelvis for which an additional anterior approach via laparotomy is required. The coccyx should be resected *en bloc* to avoid tumour rupture and infiltrated skin areas should also be removed *en bloc* with the tumour. Separation of tumour and rectum is mostly possible with digital control, and bowel and bladder function recover postoperatively in the majority of patients.

Other sites

Malignant GCT at other extra-gonadal sites such as mediastinum, retroperitoneum, and genitourinary tract are less likely to be amenable to complete resection and the surgical approach should be individualized.

Evolution of chemotherapeutic strategies

Until 1980, the prognosis of children with malignant GCT was poor. The modern era of GCT chemotherapy began in the mid 1970s with the identification of the efficacy of cisplatin in testicular GCT, given in combination with vinblastine and bleomycin (PVB) following tumour resection. With this regimen, the overall good response rate was also translated into durable remissions. Nevertheless, the challenge of relapsed or refractory tumours established the need for second-line therapies. Etoposide soon emerged as an active drug with a single agent efficacy superior to vinblastine.

The resulting combination of cisplatin, etoposide and bleomycin (BEP) is now standard chemotherapy for GCT in adult patients. The efficacy of ifosfamide in cisplatin-refractory GCT has since been demonstrated and combinations of cisplatin with ifosfamide and either etoposide or vinblastine for recurrent testicular GCT are considered standard relapse treatment. These observations led to studies incorporating ifosfamide into the first-line treatment of GCT and although the inclusion of ifosfamide with cisplatin and etoposide (PEI) did not result in significantly improved outcome, this demonstrated that malignant GCT could be treated successfully with combination chemotherapy from which bleomycin is excluded.

Side effects of chemotherapy

Selection of suitable chemotherapeutic regimes is based on a balance between efficacy and adverse effects. Cisplatin has been retained in the majority of first-line treatment approaches for GCT but it is associated with a risk of toxicity to kidneys and hearing. For this reason, strategies employing carboplatin instead of cisplatin have been explored. However, although the auditory and renal toxicity of carboplatin-based regimens are less than for cisplatin, carboplatin is more myelotoxic at therapeutically equivalent doses. Whilst this has not been found to be a dose-limiting effect in children, adult patients may tolerate this less well and there has been some reluctance to pursue a carboplatin-based approach in adult protocols. Pulmonary toxicity is the main concern associated with the use of bleomycin, particularly in older patients and the very young, and in the presence of renal impairment. These concerns have led to the development of regimens omitting bleomycin or using it at a reduced dose. The PEI combination is associated with a higher degree of myelosuppression and also carries a risk of tubular nephropathy, particularly in small children. Etoposide, used in the majority of GCT strategies in both adults and children, carries the risk of secondary leukaemia, estimated to be in the region of 1 per cent over 10 years of follow up.

Development of cooperative protocols

Prospective trials for gonadal and nongonadal GCT in children and adolescents were initiated by national groups in the 1980s. Early experience from North American (CCG) studies showed that patients with ovarian GCT had a better prognosis than children with nongonadal GCT due to the higher rate of incomplete tumour resections in nongonadal tumours. A subsequent US Intergroup protocol adopted the watch-and-wait policy for stage I testicular GCT and achieved good results for intermediate-risk patients (testicular stage II, ovarian and nongonadal stage I–II) with four cycles of cisplatin, etoposide, and bleomycin. In high-risk patients (stage III-IV), the therapeutic impact of cisplatin dose intensification (200 mg/m^2/cycle) was evaluated, indicating that higher doses of cisplatin may result in higher response and complete remission rates, but without improvement in overall survival. Furthermore, high-dose cisplatin was also associated with higher rates of renal and auditory toxicity. A subsequent report from this study group failed to demonstrate a protective benefit of amifostine against hearing loss during cisplatin therapy at escalated doses.

UK experience with the UKCCSG GC I and GC II protocols also demonstrated the high therapeutic efficacy of platinum-based regimens and promoted the use of carboplatin-based chemotherapy (JEB utilizing carboplatin at 600 mg/m^2/cycle with etoposide and bleomycin) in preference to cisplatin (BEP). Results of 184 patients treated between 1989 and 1997 confirmed the high efficacy of the JEB regimen with 5-year event-free survival (EFS) of 88 per cent and overall survival (OS) of 93 per cent, comparable to outcomes with cisplatin-based strategies from other national groups and with a favorable toxicity profile.

The French cooperative protocol TGM 85 used a similar chemotherapeutic approach, and in the consecutive TGM 90 protocol, cisplatin was replaced by carboplatin (400 mg/m^2/cycle).

The results were less favorable than with the UKCCSG JEB regimen, the difference attributed mainly to the lower dose of carboplatin. In both the French TGM 90 and the UK GC II studies, the analysis of prognostic factors revealed the prognostic impact of high serum AFP levels at diagnosis, a finding that was not reproduced by other studies that used a cisplatin-based regimen.

From 1982, the German protocols for testicular (MAHO) and non-testicular (MAKEI) GCT included cisplatin and etoposide-based chemotherapy regimens with recommendations for delayed tumour resection after neo-adjuvant chemotherapy. These protocols also focused on minimizing the risk of bleomycin-associated pulmonary toxicity. From 1989, the bleomycin dose was reduced in children younger than 2 years of age, and withheld in children less than 1 year. Event-free survival rates above 80 per cent were achieved with the first MAKEI and MAHO protocols, resulting in a step-wise reduction in duration of chemotherapy from a maximum of eight cycles to six and, currently, four to five cycles, with no adverse impact on outcomes. The omission of bleomycin in infants was also achieved without detriment to outcome. As with strategies used by other national groups, an expectant 'watch-and-wait' strategy was introduced in the MAKEI 96 protocol for patients with completely resected low-stage tumours. This resulted in sparing of chemotherapy for almost 75 per cent of patients with stage Ia malignant GCT, although more intensive chemotherapy was required for those patients who subsequently relapsed. A neo-adjuvant approach to locally invasive and/or metastatic tumours was shown to facilitate complete tumour resection and thereby reduce the need for second-look surgery. In malignant sacrococcygeal tumours, it was demonstrated that bone involvement had no impact on prognosis and did not necessitate treatment intensification.

In a further attempt to reduce the toxicity of treatment, the Brazilian group reported the results of a two drug regimen in standard risk patients, comprising five cycles of cisplatin and etoposide delivered over 14 weeks. This strategy seems to be sufficient to achieve complete remission rates of over 80 per cent.

Current therapeutic approaches

In general, current paediatric GCT strategies stratify therapy according to initial diagnostic parameters, and only in cases of insufficient response to treatment is therapy further intensified. Although there is some variation between protocols in the application of risk factors, there are common themes, summarized Table 25.2.

Gonadal tumours are considered lower risk than extra-gonadal, but this is largely because they are more likely to be completely resected. Increasing age is generally associated with increased risk, and often associated in older teenagers with higher risk, adult-type histology. The impact of metastases on risk and the need for treatment intensity varies according to type of tumour, and the risk associated with high levels of AFP is of uncertain significance. Complete control of disease at primary and metastatic sites is essential in all cases and residual disease following treatment confers a relatively adverse prognosis.

A summary of the approach to treatment of malignant GCT is as follows:

◆ Surgical resection at diagnosis where possible with inguinal approach for testicular tumours, and sampling of ascites and nodules for ovarian tumours

◆ Biopsy or marker diagnosis in unresectable tumours

◆ Watch-and-wait for completely resected stage 1 gonadal primaries avoids chemotherapy in over 70 per cent of cases, and effective salvage is available for the remainder

◆ Platinum based chemotherapy for all stage II–IV patients; ranging from two cycles of a two drug regimen for completely resected stage II (MAKEI) to four to six cycles of three drug regimen for highest risk (stage IV extra-gonadal)

Table 25.2 Standard chemotherapy regimens in pediatric extra-cranial GCT

PEI		**(MAKEI 96, MAHO 98)**	
Cisplatin*	20 mg/m²	over 1 h	day 1,2,3,4,5
Etoposide	100 mg/m²	over 3 h	day 1,2,3
Ifosfamide**	1500 mg/m²	over 3 or 20 h	day 1,2,3,4,5
2 to 4 cycles			
PVB		**(MAHO 98)**	
Cisplatin*	20 mg/m²	over 1 h	day 4,5,6,7,8
Vinblastin	3 mg/m² or 0.15 mg/kg	i.v. bolus	day 1,2
Bleomycin***	15 mg/m²	over 24 h	day 1,2,3
3 cycles			
BEP		**(MAHO 98)**	
Bleomycin***	15 mg/m²	over 24 h	day 1,2,3
Etoposide	80 mg/m²	over 3 h	day 1,2,3
Cisplatin*	20 mg/m²	over 1 h	day 4,5,6,7,8
3 cycles			
BEP		**(US-Childrens Oncology Group)**	
Bleomycin	15 mg/m²	over 24 h	day 1
Etoposide	100 mg/m²	over 3 h	day 1,2,3,4,5
Cisplatin*	20 mg/m²	over 1 h	day 1,2,3,4,5
4 cycles			
High-dose BEP		**(US-Childrens Oncology Group)**	
Bleomycin	15 mg/m²	over 24 h	day 1
Etoposide	100 mg/m²	over 3 h	day 1,2,3,4,5
Cisplatin*	40 mg/m²	over 1 h	day 1,2,3,4,5
4 cycles			
JEB		**(UKCCSG/CCLG GC3)**	
Carboplatin	600 mg/m²	over 1 h	day 2
Etoposide	120 mg/m²	over 1 h	day 1,2,3
Bleomycin***	15 mg/m²	over 15 min	day 3
4 or 6 cycles			
PE		**(Brazilian GCT group)**	
Cisplatin	20/30 mg/m²	over 1 h	day 1,2,3,
Etoposide	100/120 mg/m²	over 1 h	day 1,2,3,4,5
5 cycles			

*Given with mannitol forced diuresis; **given with Mesna uroprotection; ***omitted in children <1 year, and at reduced dose (7.5 mg/m²) in children <2 years.

- Surgery following chemotherapy for residual tumour
- There is no place for radiotherapy in the first line treatment of extra-cranial GCT.

Treatment of teratoma

Mature teratoma are considered benign and are cured by surgical excision which should be complete in order to avoid recurrence. Sacroccoccygeal teratomas may recur as malignant tumours in around 10 per cent of cases, underlining the need to aim for complete excision and also to monitor AFP closely for recurrence. Surgical excision is also the mainstay of treatment for immature teratoma and although they may show clinical features of malignancy, a role for chemotherapy has not been established. The risk of recurrence can be estimated from the primary site of the tumour, histologic grade of immaturity, and completeness of the tumour resection. Pure immature teratoma of the ovary may be associated with secondary peritoneal deposits for which surgery remains the treatment of choice. The significance of small foci of YST and/or mildly raised AFP in immature teratoma is uncertain and management subject to controversy, particularly with respect to the role of chemotherapy.

Follow up

Most relapses occur within the first 2 years after diagnosis, although much later recurrences have been observed. Most groups would therefore recommend close monitoring of markers for secreting GCT and imaging, at least for marker negative GCT, for 3–5 years from the end of treatment. AFP and β-HCG are usually monitored weekly until they reach the normal range, then at reduced frequency (1–3 monthly) for the remaining period of follow up. In watch-and-wait patients, the decline of AFP level should be evaluated with respect to its serum half-life of approximately 6–7 days. The interpretation of AFP may be difficult in infants but a slowing of the rate of decline or a secondary rise in AFP level strongly suggests the presence of residual or recurrent YST.

Imaging of the primary site of tumour should be undertaken at the end of treatment. In case of residual abnormalities after chemotherapy, further surgery is indicated even in a secreting tumour with normalized markers, since mature teratoma may remain after successful treatment of the malignant component of a mixed tumour, imposing a risk of tumour progression. Positron emission tomography (PET) scans have not been proven useful in this situation, as they cannot readily distinguish between mature teratoma and residual necrosis or fibrosis.

Monitoring for late effects of treatment needs to be tailored to the treatment received. Audiometry should be performed during and at the end of treatment in patients who have received cisplatin therapy. Patients who have received bleomycin require lung function testing. Although routine monitoring of blood counts is not indicated, the risk of treatment related secondary leukemia should be considered as part of routine follow-up, in patients who have received etoposide.

Relapse treatment

There is no international consensus on strategies for treatment of recurrent GCT. In patients previously treated with a carboplatin-based or non-platinum based therapy, cisplatin-based regimens such as PEI or VIP (vinblastine, ifosfamide, cisplatin) have been used successfully. Failure following primary treatment with cisplatin may be treated with carboplatin and etoposide. Other relapse strategies have included 'Adria VAC' (vincristine, actinomycin D, cyclophosphamide and doxorubicin) and, more recently, combinations of gemcitabine, oxaliplatin and taxol.

A standardized strategy is used for patients with recurrent extra-cranial malignant GCT in Germany which includes high dose carboplatin and etoposide. Aggressive local therapy is central to the strategy because most relapse occurs at the primary site. Local radiotherapy, at doses above 45 Gy, has shown some benefit after incomplete resection of the recurrent tumour.

The therapeutic value of high dose chemotherapy with autologous stem cell transplantation has been investigated in a small number of patients with relapsed or refractory disease. Long term survival is likely to be achieved only in those patients in whom a clinical complete remission can be achieved by other treatment prior to high dose chemotherapy.

Future perspectives

In view of the high cure rates achieved by current protocols for standard risk GCT, research should now focus on the better identification of patients more likely to fail first-line treatment, the intensification of treatment in high-risk patients and reduction of therapy with its attendant toxicities in low-risk cases.

As insufficient local tumour control at the primary site represents the main problem in most relapsing patients, further advances in outcomes for relapsed GCT may depend on improvements in local therapy. Novel approaches need to be explored for high risk GCT. Loco-regional hyperthermia combined with platinum-based chemotherapy may offer a therapeutic concept in locally recurrent extra-cranial tumours and augmentation of standard treatment with the development of targeted therapies to oncogenes, growth factors, and receptors should be a goal for the future.

Timely progress in these areas for such a rare tumour group requires multinational cooperation in both biological studies and clinical trials. A strong focus is also needed on the rehabilitation and quality of life of the survivors of GCT and such outcomes should be taken into consideration when planning treatment.

Further reading

Baranzelli MC, Kramar A, Bouffet E, et al. (1999) Prognostic factors in children with localized malignant nonseminomatous germ cell tumours. *J Clin Oncol* **17**, 1212–19.

Billmire D, Vinocur C, Rescorla F, et al. (2004) Outcome and staging evaluation in malignant germ cell tumors of the ovary in children and adolescents: an intergroup study. *J Pediatr Surg* **39**, 424–9; discussion 424–9.

Blohm ME, Vesterling-Horner D, Calaminus G, et al. (1998) Alpha 1-fetoprotein (AFP) reference values in infants up to 2 years of age. *Pediatr Hematol Oncol* **15**, 135–42.

Calaminus G, Schneider DT, Bökkerink JP, et al. (2003) Prognostic value of tumour size, metastases, extension into bone, and increased tumour marker in children with malignant sacrococcygeal germ cell tumours: a prospective evaluation of 71 patients treated in the German cooperative protocols Maligne Keimzelltumouren (MAKEI) 83/86 and MAKEI 89. *J Clin Oncol* **21**, 781–6.

Cushing B, Giller R, Cullen JW, et al. (2004) Randomized comparison of combination chemotherapy with etoposide, bleomycin, and either high-dose or standard-dose cisplatin in children and adolescents with high-risk malignant germ cell tumors: a pediatric intergroup study—Pediatric Oncology Group 9049 and Children's Cancer Group 8882. *J Clin Oncol* **22**, 2691–700.

De Giorgi U, Rosti G, Slavin S, et al. (2005) European Group for Blood and Marrow Transplantation Solid Tumours and Paediatric Disease Working Parties. Salvage high-dose chemotherapy for children with extragonadal germ-cell tumours. *Br J Cancer* **93**, 412–7.

Eble JN, Sauter G, Epstein JI, Sesterhenn IA (eds) (2004) Pathology and Genetics of Tumours of the Urinary System and Male Genital Organs. World Health Organization Classification of Tumours.

Einhorn LH, Donohue JP (1977) Chemotherapy for disseminated testicular cancer. *Urol Clin North Am* **4**, 407–26.

Göbel U, Schneider DT, Calaminus G, et al. (2001) Multimodal treatment of malignant sacrococcygeal germ cell tumours: a prospective analysis of 66 patients of the german cooperative protocols MAKEI 83/86 and 89. *J Clin Oncol* **19**, 1943–50.

Göbel U, Schneider DT, Teske C, et al. (2010) Brain metastases in children and adolescents with extracranial germ cell tumor - data of the MAHO/MAKEI-registry. *Klin Padiatr* **222**, 140–4.

Lopes LF, Macedo CR, Pontes EM, et al. (2009) Cisplatin and etoposide in childhood germ cell tumor: brazilian pediatric oncology society protocol GCT-91. *J Clin Oncol* **27**, 1297–303.

Mann JR, Raafat F, Robinson K, et al. (1998) UKCCSG's germ cell tumour (GCT) studies: improving outcome for children with malignant extracranial non-gonadal tumours—carboplatin, etoposide, and bleomycin are effective and less toxic than previous regimens. United Kingdom Children's Cancer Study Group. *Med Pediatr Oncol* **30**, 217–27.

Mann JR, Raafat F, Robinson K, et al. (2000) The United Kingdom Children's Cancer Study Group's Second Germ Cell Tumour Study: Carboplatin, Etoposide, and Bleomycin Are Effective Treatment for Children With Malignant Extracranial Germ Cell Tumours, With Acceptable Toxicity. *J Clin Oncol* **18**, 3809–18.

Marina M, Chang KW, Malogolowkin M, et al. (2005) Children's Oncology Group. Amifostine does not protect against the ototoxicity of high-dose cisplatin combined with etoposide and bleomycin in pediatric germ-cell tumors: a Children's Oncology Group study. *Cancer* **104**, 841–7.

Palmer RD, Foster NA, Vowler SL, et al. (2007) Malignant germ cell tumours of childhood: new associations of genomic imbalance. *Br J Cancer* **96**(4), 667–76.

Palmer RD, Murray MJ, Saini HK, et al. (2010) Malignant Germ Cell Tumours Display Common MicroRNA Profiles Resulting in Global Changes in Expression of Messenger RNA Targets. *Cancer Research* **70**, 2911–23.

Perlman EJ, Hu J, Ho D, et al. (2000) Genetic analysis of childhood endodermal sinus tumours by comparative genomic hybridization. *J Pediatr Hematol Oncol* **22**, 100–5.

Schmoll HJ, Kollmannsberger C, Metzner B, et al. (2003) German Testicular Cancer Study Group, Long-term results of first-line sequential high-dose etoposide, ifosfamide, and cisplatin chemotherapy plus autologous stem cell support for patients with advanced metastatic germ cell cancer: an extended phase I/II study of the German Testicular Cancer Study Group. *J Clin Oncol* **21**, 4083–91.

Schneider DT, Calaminus G, Koch S, et al. (2004) Epidemiological Analysis of 1442 Children and Adolescents Registered in the German Germ Cell Tumor Protocols. *Pediatr Blood Cancer* **42**, 169–75.

Schneider DT, Schuster AE, Fritsch MK, et al. (2001) Multipoint Imprinting Analysis Indicates a Common Precursor Cell for Gonadal and Nongonadal Pediatric Germ Cell Tumours. *Cancer Res* **61**, 7268–76.

Schneider DT, Schuster AE, Fritsch MK, et al. (2002) Genetic analysis of mediastinal nonseminomatous germ cell tumours in children and adolescents. *Genes Chromosomes Cancer* **34**, 115–25.

Veltman I, Veltman J, Janssen I, et al. (2005) Identification of recurrent chromosomal aberrations in germ cell tumours of neonates and infants using genomewide array-based comparative genomic hybridization. *Genes Chromosomes Cancer* **43**, 367–76.

Wermann H, Stoop H, Gillis AJ, et al. (2010) Global DNA methylation in fetal human germ cells and germ cell tumours: association with differentiation and cisplatin resistance. *J Pathol* **221**, 433–42.

Wessalowski R, Kruck H, Pape H, et al. (1998) Hyperthermia for the treatment of patients with malignant germ cell tumours: a phase I/II study in ten children and adolescents with recurrent or refractory tumours. *Cancer* **82**, 793–800.

Chapter 26

Childhood liver tumours

Giorgio Perilongo and Jozsef Zsiros

Introduction

Childhood liver tumours are a heterogeneous group of neoplasms encompassing individually rare histological varieties. Hepatoblastoma and hepatocellular carcinoma are the two most frequent subtypes; undifferentiated sarcoma of the liver, atypical teratoid/rhabdoid tumour, primary hepatic germ cell tumour, lymphoma, angiosarcoma are examples of other, very rare primary liver tumours in childhood. This chapter will focus only on hepatoblastoma and hepatocellular carcinoma.

Hepatoblastoma

Biology

Hepatoblastoma is an embryonal tumour of the liver. The term 'embryonal' implies that its origin is related to a derangement in the mechanisms regulating normal hepatic organogenesis. Various hypotheses have already linked the different histologic subtypes of hepatoblastoma to specific stages of the arrest of normal hepatic organogenesis. Further investigation is required to clarify which developmental, signaling, and transcriptional pathways are affected, at what level, and for what reason such changes occur. Nevertheless, different genetic abnormalities have been described in association with hepatoblastoma.

Abnormalities of the Wnt/β-catenin transcription pathway have been consistently reported. Due to mutations in the β-catenin (*CTNNB1*) gene, β-catenin bypasses the proteasomal degradation pathway and is translocated to the nucleus where it can be detected by immunohistochemistry. A potential prognostic relevance of this finding has been proposed.

Microarray analysis shows that the glypican 3 (*GPC3*) gene, mutated in the Simpson-Golabi-Behmel tissue overgrowth syndrome, in which an association with an increased risk of hepatoblastoma development has been hypothesized, is one of the most over-expressed genes in hepatoblastoma.

Growth regulation of hepatoblastoma involves the insulin-like growth factor II (IGF2) signalling pathway. IGF2 is a maternally imprinted gene and encodes a fetal peptide hormone that regulates cell proliferation, differentiation, and cell migration. IGF2 is expressed in hepatoblastoma, inversely correlated with the degree of differentiation: it is lacking in fetal-type cells and high in embryonal-type cells. High expression of IGF2 is the hallmark of the Beckwith–Wiedemann syndrome and this finding could explain the higher incidence of hepatoblastoma in children affected by this condition.

Epidemiology

The estimated incidence of hepatoblastoma is 1.2 per million, with a male prevalence, but no geographic variations have been reported. Little is know about the risk factors for hepatoblastoma development. A consistent association appears to exist between risk of hepatoblastoma and very low birth weight; duration of oxygen therapy has been identified as a significant factor associated with that risk. The International Agency for Research on Cancer has recently classified tobacco smoke (via parental smoking) as a human carcinogen for childhood hepatoblastoma.

Most cases of hepatoblastoma are sporadic but at least three congenital conditions have been linked to an excess risk: trisomy 18, Beckwith–Wiedemann syndrome and familial adenomatous polyposis. The suggestion that hepatoblastoma is a developmental aberration is supported by the fact that a wide spectrum of congenital malformation syndromes and isolated anomalies have been reported in cases of hepatoblastoma. The overall frequency of anomalies among children with hepatoblastoma appears to be higher than for any pediatric tumour other than Wilms.

Clinical presentation

Hepatoblastoma is a tumour of early childhood, with more than 80% of the patients being diagnosed under the age of 2 years. An asymptomatic abdominal mass in an otherwise healthy young child is the classical presenting feature of hepatoblastoma and systemic symptoms are rarely present. The presence of clinical signs of associated syndromes, such as Beckwith–Wiedemann syndrome, should always be sought and may dominate the clinical picture. The hallmark of hepatoblastoma is an elevated serum level of alpha fetoprotein (AFP) although tumours associated with normal or low (<100 ng/ml) levels of AFP do occur, but are very rare (less than 2 per cent). Levels may be more difficult to interpret in very young infants because of high physiological production of AFP and should always be interpreted in relation to the normal range for age. Extremely high levels of AFP in some patients can generate erroneously low results on standard laboratory testing and require appropriate serum dilution for a reliable assessment. Paraneoplastic abnormalities of calcium metabolism can occur with a picture of pseudo-osteoporosis and spontaneous fractures. Rarely hepatoblastoma can also secrete β-human chorionic gonadotropin (β-HCG) which may result in pseudo-precocious puberty in males. Thrombocytosis, related to the hyperproduction of thrombopoietin by tumour cells, is frequently documented at presentation. Rarely a child with hepatoblastoma will present with an acute abdomen due to tumour rupture or intra-tumoural haemorrhage

Diagnosis

Whilst the presence of a hepatic mass in a young child, associated with an elevated alpha fetoprotein, is extremely suggestive of the diagnosis of hepatoblastoma, surgical biopsy is required to establish histological diagnosis.

Radiological investigation is required to define the extent of the primary disease and confirm or exclude the possibility of metastases. Abdominal ultrasound and computed tomography (CT) and/or magnetic resonance imaging (MRI) scans are the conventional tools to document the presence, extension, and characteristics of a hepatic mass. As slightly more than 20 per cent of patients present with lung metastases, a contrast enhanced CT of the lung is part of the diagnostic work-up for any child presenting with hepatoblastoma.

Laboratory investigations should include a full blood count and serum AFP and β-HCG. In most children with hepatoblastoma, liver function tests are with the normal limits.

Histologic classification

A variety of histologic classifications for hepatoblastoma have been used in the past but criteria for modern classifications of hepatoblastoma have recently been reviewed. Table 26.1 shows the classification currently employed by International Childhood Liver Tumour Strategy Group (SIOPEL).

About 55 per cent of hepatoblastomas are epithelial (30 per cent fetal, 20 per cent fetal-embryonal, 3 per cent macrotrabecular, 2 per cent small-cell undifferentiated), and 45 per cent are mixed epithelial and mesenchymal, but when all types are considered, around 85 per cent contain both fetal and embryonal components in variable proportions. Evidence is accumulating that small-cell undifferentiated hepatoblastoma is associated with unfavourable outcome whilst pure fetal hepatoblastoma with a mitotic index [<2 mitoses/10 HPF (high power fields)], if completely resected, has an excellent outcome even without adjuvant treatment.

Transitional liver cell tumour (TLCT) is a recently described malignant liver cell neoplasm that chiefly occurs in older children and young adolescents. The term 'transitional' has been proposed based on the hypothesis that the relevant tumour cell might be located between a hepatoblastoma cell and a hepatocyte, but this requires further evaluation. These tumours are highly aggressive and usually present as large masses associated with high or very high serum AFP levels.

Staging and prognosis

Two different systems to describe tumour extension or stage are presently in use: one used by the North American Cooperative Group on Childhood Hepatic Tumors and another one by the International Childhood Liver Tumor Strategy Group—SIOPEL group—consisting mainly of European investigators. The American system is based on the results of the initial surgical procedure (post-surgical system). It encompasses four stages:

stage I—complete tumour resection without microscopical residual

stage II— tumour grossly resected with evidence of microscopical residual

stage III— tumour unresectable or resected with gross residual tumour or positive lymph nodes

stage IV— tumours presenting with metastases.

A progressive decline in the survival rate with evolution of stage in this system has been firmly documented.

The SIOPEL group developed an alternative system that describes tumour extension before any surgery (pre-surgical system); this is known as the PRETEXT system (*Pre*treatment *Ex*tension of the disease). It has been developed in accordance with the surgical anatomy of the liver, based on the vascular structures, This indentifies four sectors, two in each lobe. The PRETEXT category is defined by the number of sectors involved by the tumour (see Table 26.4). The presence of distant metastases is identified by the addition of the letter 'M'; extension of tumour into portal vein is indicated by the letter 'P'; extension into the vena cava and/or hepatic veins by the letter 'V'; and

Table 26.1. SIOPEL Classification of hepatoblastomas

Hepatoblastoma, wholly epithelial type
Fetal subtype
Mixed embryonal/fetal subtype
Macrotrabecular subtype
Small-cell undifferentiated subtype
Hepatoblastoma, mixed epithelial and mesenchymal type
Without teratoid features
With teratoid features
Hepatoblastoma, not otherwise specified (NOS)

the presence of intra-abdominal extra-hepatic disease by the letter 'E'. The prognostic relevance of the PRETEXT system has also been well documented.

The completeness of surgical resection still remains the most important single prognostic factor for hepatoblastoma and only those children in whom complete tumour resection is achieved can hope for cure. The second most important, negative, prognostic factor is the presence of metastases at diagnosis. It is now generally accepted that a normal (for age) or low level (<100 ng/ml) of AFP is a hallmark of a poorer prognosis: in the SIOPEL group experience, 3-year overall survival of children presenting with low or normal AFP was around 15 per cent. An association between small-cell undifferentiated hepatoblastoma and low or normal for age AFP has been proposed.

Different study groups have developed different risk stratifications systems for determining treatment but, although these are based on known prognostic factors, there is not full agreement between the study groups in defining risk categories. The SIOPEL group uses a risk stratification that is mainly based on pretreatment tumour extent according to the PRETEXT system and the initial AFP level, while the American system is based mainly on postsurgical stage and histology.

Treatment strategies

The goal of any therapeutic strategy directed at the cure of children with hepatoblastoma is to achieve complete tumour resection, although surgery alone is not sufficient and the best chance of cure can only be achieved with a multidisciplinary treatment strategy also using systemic chemotherapy. The two major cooperative groups offer different approaches to primary treatment. The North American Children's Oncology Group (COG) utilizes a strategy based on an initial attempt at surgical resection (primary surgery) regardless of the tumour extension within and/or outside the liver. In contrast, the SIOPEL group takes an approach based on the use of primary chemotherapy before definitive surgery (neo-adjuvant chemotherapy) regardless of the initial tumour extension. The rationale for using primary chemotherapy is to reduce the tumour volume, to make tumour more solid, less prone to bleed, and better demarcated from the surrounding healthy liver parenchyma and, ultimately, more easily resected. The results of these two strategies have been comparable, both achieving 5-year overall and event-free survival rates of over 70 per cent.

Historically, the most significant step in improving the prognosis of hepatoblastoma was introduction of cisplatin-based chemotherapy after which resection rate and 3-year overall survival improved from historical rates of 44 per cent and 30 per cent to more than 80 per cent and 70 per cent, respectively.

COG conducted a trial that compared cisplatin (90 mg/m^2 as an infusion over 6 hours) followed by doxorubicin (80mg/m^2 as a continuous infusion over 96 hours) with the combination of cisplatin (delivered as per above) on day 1, and vincristine (1.5 mg/m^2) and 5-fluorouracil (600 mg/m^2) on day 2 (C5V). They subsequently chose C5V as their standard chemotherapy, not because there was a significant difference between the two regimens but because of a difference in toxicity profiles. It should be noted, however, that while tumour progression accounted for 86 per cent of all reported events for patients treated with C5V, it represented only 56 per cent of all events observed in those patients treated with cisplatin/doxorubicin. The SIOPEL group has adopted the combination cisplatin (90 mg/m^2 as an infusion over 24 hours) followed by doxorubicin (60 mg/m^2 infusion over 48 hours) as its therapeutic gold standard.

Risk-adapted treatment

In the course of the subsequent clinical trials, these two principal regimens have been further refined. The COG group achieved 100 per cent 3-year survival in children with pure fetal hepatoblastoma after gross complete resection (Stage I and II, favourable histology) with adjuvant chemotherapy using four cycles of C5V. These excellent results have prompted the further reduction of chemotherapy to only two cycles for most of these patients and, for children with completely resected (Stage I) pure fetal hepatoblastoma and low mitotic index (<2 mitoses/10 HPF), omission of all adjuvant chemotherapy. On the other hand, children with unresectable and metastatic tumour, still do not enjoy satisfactory long-term outcome and have an overall survival of approximately 50 and 30 per cent respectively. The current COG strategy is to explore whether the addition of doxorubicin will benefit patients with unresectable localized disease, whilst the very poor results achieved in patients with metastases at diagnosis has promoted a search for new agents using a therapeutic 'window approach'.

The SIOPEL group have been able to show that cisplatin alone is as effective as the combination cisplatin/doxorubicin in children with standard risk hepatoblastoma (data from SIOPEL 3 SR study—see Table 26.3). For children with high-risk hepatoblastoma, the SIOPEL group undertook a trial (SIOPEL 4) exploring the use of alternating courses of cisplatin and the combination of carboplatin/doxorubicin. The results were encouraging with improved EFS and OS estimates at 3 years of 65 per cent (95% CI 57–73%) and 69 per cent (95% CI 62–77%) for the whole group; 75 per cent and 77 per cent for patients with PRETEXT-IV tumours: and 57 per cent and 63 per cent for those with lung metastases.

In the most recent generation of clinical trials directed to children with advanced hepatoblastoma, the SIOPEL group is looking into a further intensification in the use of cisplatin, based on the weekly administration of the drug and in a recently closed phase II trial the SIOPEL group has shown some efficacy of irinotecan in relapsing hepatoblastoma, confirming preliminary data reported by the COG group The incorporation of irinotecan into the treatment regimen for (very) high-risk hepatoblastoma is presently under consideration by both groups.

Concerns about the oto- and nephrotoxicity of cisplatin have stimulated both the COG and the SIOPEL groups to investigate the possibility of integrating the use of toxicity protective agents within their standard regimens.

The results of the series of trials so far run by the North American Study Group and by the SIOPEL are reported in Tables 26.2 and 26.3 while their present therapeutic recommendations are summarized in Table 26.4.

Orthotopic liver transplantation

In the past two decades, the role of orthotopic liver transplantation for children with hepatoblastoma has been quite clearly delineated. In summary, children with hepatoblastoma eligible for transplant should meet the following criteria: (a) have had a response to chemotherapy, a criterion which implies that any child with hepatoblastoma should be treated with chemotherapy regardless of the type of resection which is envisaged; (b) have a tumour completely confined to the liver but deemed unresectable (usually these are those clearly involving all four sectors of the liver as judged by MRI scan and/or angiography; or which lie so close to the main vessels at the hilum of the liver and/or to the hepatic veins to make a tumour-free excision margin highly unlikely. The presence of metastases at diagnosis is not an absolute contraindication to transplant but requires complete clearing of the lungs with chemotherapy. In managing a child who may be a potential candidate for transplantation, it is important to ensure early assessment by a transplant team, so that the treatment strategy can be carefully timed.

Hepatocellular carcinoma

Hepatocellular carcinoma is an even rarer tumour than hepatoblastoma. Among the 213 liver tumour cases diagnosed in the UK National Registry of Childhood Tumours between 1995 and

Table 26.2 Results of the North American trials for childhood hepatoblastoma

Trial	Type of trial/ inclusion criteria	Regimen	Outcome
CCG 862	Single arm All patients	Vincristine+ cyclophosphamide/ doxorubicin alternating with vincristine, cyclophosphamide, 5-fluorouracil	3-year OS Stage I = 94 Stage II = 57% Stage III = 20% Stage IV = 14%
CCG 823F	Single arm	Cisplatin/doxorubicin	2-year OS Stage II = 86% Stage III = 58% Stage IV = 32%
POG 8697	Single arm	Cisplatin/vincristine/ 5-fluorouracil	4-year OS Stage I/PFH = 100%* Stage I/II = 90% Stage III = 67% Stage IV = 12%
INT 0089	Prospective randomized trial	Cisplatin/vincristine/ 5-fluorouracil vs cisplatin/doxorubicn	4-year OS Stage I/II 100% vs 96% Stage III 66% vs 71% Stage IV 33% vs 42%
POG 9345	Single arm Stage III/IV	Carboplatin followed by carboplatin/vincristine/ 5-fluorouracil	4-year OS Stage III =73% Stage IV = 27%
COG P9645	Prospective randomized Stage III/IV	Cisplatin/vincristine/ 5-fluorouracil vs cisplatin/carboplatin	3-year OS All patients = 75% vs 56%

*Stage I = microscopic complete resection; Stage II = microscopical residuals; Stage III macroscopical residual; Stage IV = presence of metastases; OS = Overall survival.

2006, there were 154 (72.3 per cent) cases of hepatoblastoma and 22 hepatocellular carcinoma, including five fibrolamellar tumours (10.3 per cent). All other diagnoses represented a heterogeneous group of even rarer primary liver tumours. Hepatoblastoma dominated the under 1 and 1–4 year age groups with low rates for other tumours. In 5–9 and 10–14 year olds there was a more even distribution of rates between the tumour groups, but hepatocellular carcinoma had a higher incidence than other tumours in 10–14 year olds, albeit still very low in absolute terms.

The majority of hepatocellular carcinoma cases across all ages seen in developing countries are due to hepatitis B virus infection (HBV) and to aflatoxin exposure, while in developed countries, the more common aetiological links are to alcohol abuse and smoking. Hepatitis C virus (HCV) is also a factor, especially in Japan. The incidence of hepatocellular carcinoma in HBV hyper-endemic areas in China and Thailand appears to have fallen. Hepatocellular carcinoma may also arise in children with various inherited metabolic disorders.

Table 26.3 Results of the International Childhood Liver Tumor Strategy Group (SIOPEL) trials for childhood hepatoblastoma

Trial	Type of trial/inclusion criteria*	Regimen	Outcomes*
SIOPEL 1	Single arm/all patients	Cisplatin/doxorubicin	5-year OS 66%
			3-year EFS 75%
SIOPEL 2 SR	Single arm	Cisplatin alone	3-year OS 91(±7)%
	SR-HB		3-year PFS 89(±7)%
SIOPEL 2 HR	Single arm	Cisplatin and carboplatin/doxorubicin	3-year OS 53(±13)%
	HR-HB*		3-year PFS 48(±13)%
SIOPEL 3 SR	Prospective randomized trial	Cisplatin/doxorubicin vs cisplatin alone	Cisplatin/doxorubicin
	SR-HB		3-year OS 93(±5)%
			3-year EFS 85(±7)%
			Cisplatin alone
			3-year OS 95(±4)%
			3-year EFS 83(±7)%
SIOPEL 3 HR	Single arm	Cisplatin and carboplatin/doxorubicn	3-year OS 69(±7)%
[Zsiros, 2010]	HR-HB		3-year EFS 65(±8)%

*SR-HB = Standard risk hepatoblastoma: tumour confined to the liver, involving at the most thee hepatic sectors associated with alpha-fetoprotein >100 ng/ml; HR-HB = high risk hepatoblastoma: tumour involving the entire liver, and/or presenting with metastases; and/or with vascular invasion and/or with extra-hepatic abdominal disease and/or with alpha-fetoprotein <100 ng/ml; EFS = event-free survival; OS= overall survival; PFS = progression free survival.

Similar to hepatoblastoma, a hard abdominal mass is the classical presenting symptom of hepatocellular carcinoma, but more commonly associated with systemic symptoms such as fatigue, anorexia, and abdominal pain. Jaundice is rare but has been reported. In cases that arise in the context of pre-existing liver conditions, the clinical features of the underlying disease may dominate the clinical picture. Seventy per cent of patients with hepatocellular carcinoma presented with an elevated AFP. In patients with a fibrolamellar carcinoma, AFP level is normal but high serum vitamin B12 binding capacity (transcobalamin) has been shown to be elevated and may be used as a tumour marker. Finally, the serological evidence of pre-existing infection, or of metabolic conditions may be present in the affected patients.

The diagnostic strategy is similar to that described for hepatoblastoma. Abdominal ultrasound and contrast enhanced CT or MRI scans serve to delineate tumour extension within the liver and abdomen, chest CT is recommended to rule out lung metastases and the definitive diagnosis relies on the histological assessment of a biopsy.

The prognosis of children with hepatocellular carcinoma is unsatisfactory. Results from the use of cisplatin and doxorubicin, with surgery, in the first SIOPEL study gave 5-year EFS and OS of 17 per cent and 28 per cent, respectively. No improvement in the prognosis was observed in the subsequent study, where an alternating regimen with cisplatin, carboplatin, and doxorubicin was used and long-term survival is reported only among the group of patients who achieve complete resection. The experience of the North American group is comparable: 46 patients were enrolled in the INT-0098 trial which compared treatment with cisplatin/doxorubicin with the C5V regimen. EFS at 5 years was 19 per cent for the whole cohort but ranged from 88 per cent for children with completely resected (stage I) tumour, to 0 per cent for those with metastatic disease.

Table 26.4 Hepatoblastoma: summary of the therapeutic recommendations of the Children's Oncology Group and of the SIOPEL group according to the PRETEXT system

Figurative tumour extension	PRETEXT	Children's Oncology Group*	SIOPEL Group*
	I/M-	Surgery at diagnosis (primary surgery)	Primary chemotherapy with cisplatin monotherapy
		Completely resected UH–minimal adjuvant therapy with C5V	Treatment schema: 4 doses—S—2 doses ± cisplatin toxicity protective agents
		If complete resection and pure fetal histology, no further therapy	
	II/M-	As per above	As per above
	III/M-	Surgery at diagnosis if feasible (primary surgery) and if complete resection as per above	As per above
		If complete resection not feasible—C5V + doxorubicin and recommendations for transplant	
	IV/M-	Primary chemotherapy: C5V + doxorubicin; treatment chemotherapy 4 cycles+S+2 cycles	Primary chemotherapy
			Intensified cisplatin therapy associated with doxorubicin and carboplatin
		Recommendations for transplant	Recommendations for transplant
	M+	Experimental 'window approach' (with irinotecan/vincristine)	Primary chemotherapy
		followed by C5V + doxorubicin	Intensified cisplatin therapy associated with doxorubicin and carboplatin
			? + irinotecan

*C5V = cisplatin, vincristine 5-fluorouracil (600mg/m^2 on day 2), M- or M+= absence or presence of metastases; S= Surgery, UH = Unfavourable histology, meaning no- pure fetal hepatoblastoma with low mitotic index.

There is still some uncertainty about the role of chemotherapy in hepatocellular carcinoma and the place of liver transplantation is less well established than for hepatoblastoma. However, the introduction of biological agents, specifically sorafenib, a small-molecule multikinase inhibitor, is opening new approaches to the treatment of this challenging tumour.

Further reading

Alkhouri N, Franciosi JP, Mamula P (2010) Familial Adenomatous Polyposis in Children and Adolescents. *J Pediatr Gastroenterol Nutr* 2010 **51**, 727–32.

Aronson DC, Schnater JM, Staalman CR, et al. (2005) Predictive value of the pretreatment extent of disease system in hepatoblastoma: results from the International Society of Paediatric Oncology Liver Tumour Study Group SIOPEL-1 study. *J Clin Oncol* **23**, 1245–52.

Brown J, Perilongo G, Shafford E, et al. (2000) Pretreatment prognostic factors for children with hepatoblastoma—results from the International Society of Paediatric Oncology (SIOP) study SIOPEL 1. *European Journal of Cancer* **36**, 1418–25.

Bulterys M, Goodman MT, Smith MA et al. (1999) Cancer Incidence, Survival among Children, Adolescents: United States SEER Program 1975–1995. SEER program, NIH Pub No 99–4649: 91–7.

Czauderna P, Mackinlay G, Perilongo G, et al. (2002) Hepatocellular carcinoma in children; results of the first prospective study of the International Society of Pediatric Oncology *J Clin Oncol* **20**, 2798–804.

De Ioris M, Brugieres L, Zimmermann A, et al. (2008). Hepatoblastoma with a low serum alpha-fetoprotein level at diagnosis: the SIOPEL group experience. *Eur J Cancer* **44**, 545–50.

Katzenstein HM, London WB, Douglass EC, et al. (2002). Treatment of Unresectable and Metastatic Hepatobalstoma: A Pediatric Oncology Group Phase II Study. *J Clin Oncol* **20**, 3438–44.

Katzenstein HM Krailo MD, Malogolowkin MH, et al. (2002) Hepatocellular carcinoma in children and adolescents: results from the Pediatric Oncology Group and the Children's Cancer Group Intergroup Study. *J Clin Oncol* **20**, 2789–97.

Kitanovski L, Ovcak Z, Jazbec J (2009) Multifocal hepatoblastoma in a 6-month-old girl with trisomy 18: a case report. *J Med Case Reports* **3**, 8319.

Li J, Thompson TD, Miller W, et al (2008) Cancer Incidence Among Children and Adolescents in the United States, 2001–2003. *Pediatrics* **121**, e1470–77.

Ortega JA, Douglass EC, Feusner JH, et al. (2000) Randomized comparison of cisplatin/vincristine/fluorouracil and cisplatin/continuous infusion doxorubicin for treatment of pediatric hepatoblastoma: A report from the Children's Cancer Group and the Pediatric Oncology Group. *J Clin Oncol* **18**, 2665–75.

Malogolowkin MH, Katzenstein H, Krailo MD, et al. (2006) Intensified platinum therapy is an ineffective strategy for improving outcome in pediatric patients with advanced hepatoblastoma. *J Clin Oncol* **24**, 2879–84.

Malogolowkin MH, Katzenstein HM, Krailo M, et al. (2008) Redefining the Role of doxorubicin for the Treatment of Children with Hepatoblastoma. *J Clin Oncol* **26**, 2379–83.

Ortega JA, Krailo MD, Haas JE, al. E (1991). Effective treatment of unresectable or metastatic hepatoblastoma with cisplatin and continuous infusion doxorubicin chemotherapy: A report from the Children's Cancer Study Group. *J Clin Oncol* **9**, 2167–76.

Ortega JA, Douglass EC, Feusner JH, et al. (2000) Randomized comparison of cisplatin/vincristine/fluorouracil and cisplatin/continuous infusion doxorubicin for treatment of pediatric hepatoblastoma: A report from the Children's Cancer Group and the Pediatric Oncology Group. *J Clin Oncol* **18**, 2665–75.

Otte JB, Pritchard J, Aronson DC, et al. (2004) Liver Transplantation for Hepatoblastoma: Results From the International Society of Pediatric Oncology (SIOP) Study SIOPEL-1 and Review of the World Experience. *Pediatr Blood Cancer* **42**, 74–83.

Perilongo G, Brown J, Shafford E, et al. (2000) Hepatoblastoma presenting with lung metastases: treatment results of the first cooperative, prospective study of the International Society of Paediatric Oncology on childhood liver tumors. *Cancer* **89**, 1845–53.

Perilongo G, Shafford E, Maibach R, et al: (2004) Risk-adapted treatment for childhood hepatoblastoma. Final report of the second study of the International Society of Paediatric Oncology—SIOPEL 2. *Eur J Cancer* **40**, 411–21.

Perilongo G, Maibach R, Shafford F, et al. (2009) Cisplatin versus cisplatin plus doxorubicin for standard risk hepatoblastoma. *N Engl J Med* **361**, 1662–70.

Pritchard J, Brown J, Shafford E, et al. (2000) Cisplatin, doxorubicin, and delayed surgery for childhood hepatoblastoma: A successful approach-results of the first prospective study of the international society of pediatric oncology. *J Clin Oncol* **18**, 3819–28.

Roebuck DJ, Aronson D, Clapuyt P, et al (2007) 2005 PRETEXT: a revised staging system for primary malignant liver tumours of childhood developed by the SIOPEL group. International Childrhood Liver Tumor Strategy Group. *Pediatr Radiol* **37**, 123–32.

Roebuck DJ, Sebire NJ, Pariente D (2007) Assessment of extrahepatic abdominal extension in primary malignant liver tumours of childhood. *Pediatr Radiol* **37**, 1096–100.

Trobaugh-Lotrario AD, Tomlinson GE, Finegold MJ, Gore L, Feusner JH. (2009) Small cell undifferentiated variant of hepatoblastoma: adverse clinical and molecular features similar to rhabdoid tumors. *Pediatr Blood Cancer*. Mar; **52**(3): 328–34.

Zimmermann A (2005) The emerging family of hepatoblastoma tumours: From ontogenesis to oncogenesis. *Eur J Cancer* **41**, 1503–14.

Zsíros J, Maibach R, Shafford E, et al. (2010) Successful treatment of childhood high risk hepatoblastoma with dose intensive multiagent chemotherapy and surgery—final results of the SIOPEL-3HR study of the childhood Liver tumor strategy group *J Clin Oncol* **28**, 2584–90.

Chapter 27

Retinoblastoma

Guillermo Chantada and Carlos Rodríguez-Galindo

Introduction

Retinoblastoma is a malignant tumour arising from the embryonic neural retina and occurs in about 1 in 14 000–18 000 live births. Thus, an estimated 8000 children develop retinoblastoma each year worldwide. Recent data from population-based studies showed a three to seven times increased incidence rate of retinoblastoma in some areas of Latin America. The reason for this is not known; environmental factors such as a decreased intake of fruits and vegetables during pregnancy as well as a putative role of the human papilloma virus in some areas may play a role. When retinoblastoma is diagnosed in the intraocular stage, as it usually occurs in the most affluent countries, disease-free survival has been over 80–90 per cent for the past decades. However, in less developed countries, retinoblastoma is diagnosed later, when the disease has disseminated to extraocular sites and survival is lower than 50 per cent for most affected children worldwide.

Presenting signs and symptoms

Retinoblastoma presents in two distinct clinical forms: (1) Bilateral or multifocal, hereditary (25 per cent of cases), characterized by the presence of germline mutations of the *RB1* gene. These may be the result of a new germline mutation in the 75 per cent or it may be inherited from an affected survivor, which accounts for the remaining 25 per cent of the cases. In less developed countries, familial cases are less common. (2) Unilateral (75 per cent of the cases) which are sporadic in about 90 per cent of the cases and the remaining 10 per cent have germline mutations. However, in the absence of a positive family history, it is not possible without genetic screening to determine which unilateral cases are inheritable (Fig. 27.1).

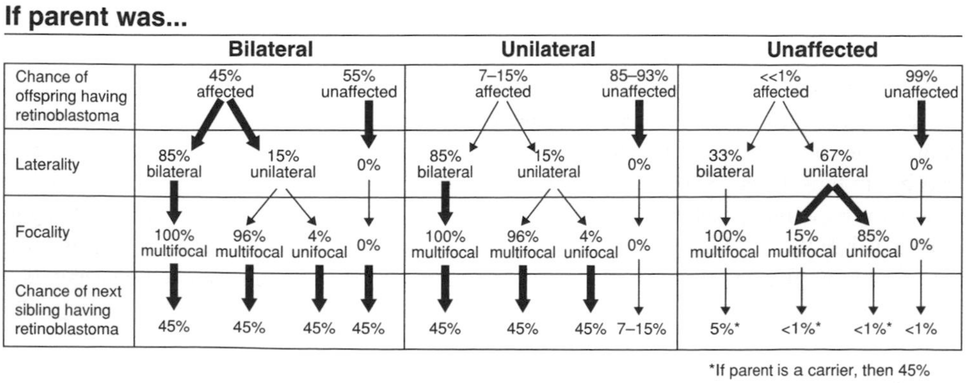

If parent was...

	Bilateral				Unilateral				Unaffected			
Chance of offspring having retinoblastoma	45% affected		55% unaffected		7–15% affected		85–93% unaffected		<<1% affected		99% unaffected	
Laterality	85% bilateral	15% unilateral	0%		85% bilateral	15% unilateral	0%		33% bilateral	67% unilateral	0%	
Focality	100% multifocal	96% multifocal	4% unifocal	0%	100% multifocal	96% multifocal	4% unifocal	0%	100% multifocal	15% multifocal	85% unifocal	0%
Chance of next sibling having retinoblastoma	45%	45%	45%	45%	45%	45%	45%	7–15%	5%*	<1%*	<1%*	<1%

*If parent is a carrier, then 45%

Fig. 27.1 Card for genetic counselling of retinoblastoma.
© David H. Abramson, MD, (1996), reproduced with permission.

Patients with bilateral retinoblastoma tend to present before 1 year of age and those with unilateral disease often present in the second or third year of life. However, there are wide variations in the age of diagnosis in different countries, according to the degree of socioeconomical development; children in less developed countries are diagnosed at a later age. It is uncommon for retinoblastoma to be diagnosed during the first month of life, except in familial cases where screening is performed; however, regardless of the family history, more than 90 per cent of neonatal cases have either bilateral disease at presentation or will develop asynchronous bilateral retinoblastoma.

The presenting features of retinoblastoma vary according to the level of socioeconomic development. In developing countries, late diagnosis is common and patients usually present with proptosis and an orbital mass, often with pre-auricular adenopathy (Fig. 27.2b). In developed countries, the most common presenting signs are the presence of a white reflex in the child's eye (leukocoria; Fig. 27.2a) which occurs in two-thirds of the cases or, less frequently, strabismus. Less common presenting signs include a painful red eye, glaucoma, poor vision, orbital cellulitis, hyphema or unilateral mydriasis. Even though leukocoria is frequently present, it may be overlooked since it may be only seen when the child looks sideways. It may also be noticeable in a flash photograph. Whilst leukocoria is a relatively specific sign with few differential diagnoses, strabismus is very common in children and often due to a benign cause. However, the occurrence of strabismus in a young child calls for a dilated examination of the retina with special attention given to the macula.

A syndrome associated with deletion of the long arm of chromosome 13 (the 13q deletion syndrome) has been reported with mental retardation and dysmorphic features. Identification of these anomalies may precede the recognition of concomitant retinoblastoma. Such children require karyotype analysis and retinal examination.

Trilateral retinoblastoma refers to the association of bilateral retinoblastoma with an asynchronous intracranial primitive neuroectodermal tumour. This association can occur in 3 to 9 per cent of patients with the genetic form, and appears to be more common in familial cases. The prognosis has until recently been almost uniformly fatal. The interval between the diagnosis of bilateral retinoblastoma and the diagnosis of the brain tumour is usually more than 20 months.

Biology

Retinoblastoma was the first cancer to be described as a genetic disease. In 1971, Knudson proposed the 'two-hit hypothesis', in which two mutational events in a developing retinal cell lead to the development of retinoblastoma. This hypothesis was subsequently extended to suggest that the two events could be mutations of both alleles of the *RB1* gene. *RB1* is located within chromosome 13q14; its product, pRb, is a key substrate for G1 cyclin-cdk complexes, which phosphorylate target gene products required for the transition of the cell through the G1 phase of the cell cycle. pRb is the major gatekeeper controlling growth regulation and the lack of pRb or its inactivation removes the constraint on cell cycle control. The *RB1* is a large gene, and mutations have been described in almost every exon. There are no mutational hot spots, although new germline mutations have an overwhelming preference for the paternal allele. This second hit occurs at a much higher frequency than the first hit, and it is more sensitive to environmental factors such as ionizing irradiation, thus explaining the increased risk of irradiation-induced malignancies in survivors of retinoblastoma.

Histology

Retinoblastoma is a tumour of neuro-epithelial origin consisting of small undifferentiated anaplastic cells with scanty cytoplasm and large nuclei that stain deeply with haematoxylin, arising

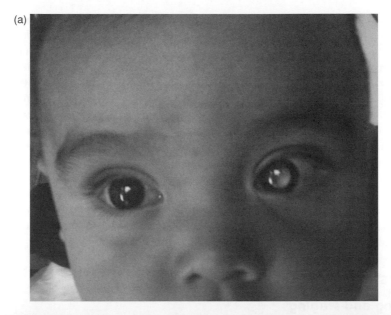

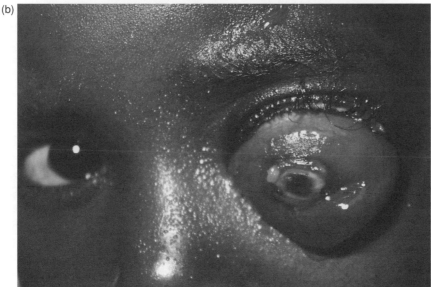

Fig. 27.2 Clinical presentation of retinoblastoma. (a) Leukocoria. (b) Massive orbital dissemination (Courtesy Dr Kahaki Kimani, Kenya).

from the nucleated layer of the retina. Calcification usually occurs in necrotic areas. Retinoblastoma cells often express photoreceptor-differentiation antigens, neuron-specific enolase and the ganglioside GD2, but not CD99, glial fibrillary acidic protein or S-100; it has been recently suggested that its cell of origin may be a cone precursor. Retinoblastoma cells may show features of photoreceptor differentiation and Flexner-Wintersteiner rosettes, which are characteristic of retinoblastoma but may be present in other ophthalmic tumours (medulloepithelioma). Alternatively, it may present with highly undifferentiated retinoblasts or a mixed pattern. The tumour may grow either in an endophytic pattern seeding the vitreous or in an exophytic form into the subretinal space. The active seeds of retinoblastoma can remain viable for long periods following chemotherapy or radiation. When the tumour grows from the retina outwards into the subretinal space (exophytic pattern), it produces a retinal detachment, sometimes with no clear view of the mass and can resemble Coats disease or other forms of exudative retinal detachment. Both vitreous and subretinal seeding are the major obstacles to cure intraocular tumours with chemoreduction because of the difficulty of chemotherapy to reach these areas with low vascular supply. Retinoblastoma can disseminate outside the eye, through the optic nerve and/or the subarachnoid space to the chiasm, the brain, and the meninges. It can also escape from the eyeball through the sclera and invade the orbit and beyond it to the surrounding structures. The tumour cells can also reach the choroid and, from there, may gain access to the systemic circulation giving rise to hematogenous metastasis involving the bone, bone marrow, or any other organ. Metastatic retinoblastoma usually involves the central nervous system (CNS), either as a solitary mass or multiple lesions, or with leptomeningeal dissemination. It can also invade facial structures such as the pre-auricular lymph nodes and the bones of the skull.

Diagnostic and extent of disease evaluation

Grouping and staging

The Reese-Ellsworth (R-E) grouping system was used for many years to group eyes according to the extension of disease and their likelihood of being preserved with radiotherapy treatment. It proved to be less useful for predicting tumour control after modern chemoreduction therapies and is being gradually substituted by a new system generated by international experts (Table 27.1). Until recently, there was no widely accepted staging system for patients with extraocular disease. However, in recent years, a group of international retinoblastoma experts developed a staging system by consensus that articulates with the intraocular grouping system proposed for the eye-conserving therapies with chemoreduction (Table 27.2).

Imaging studies

All children with retinoblastoma should undergo a gadolinium-enhanced magnetic resonance imaging (MRI) of the orbits and brain. MRI is preferred to computed tomography (CT) scan because it allows for a better estimation of the invasion to the optic nerve, it evaluates accurately the pineal area and it avoids the exposure to radiation in these susceptible patients. MRI is also helpful in the differential diagnosis with Coats disease and other inflammatory conditions, and with persistent hyperplastic primary vitreous (PHPV). Given the short interval between the diagnosis of retinoblastoma and the occurrence of trilateral retinoblastoma, routine screening with MRI every 6 months until 5 years of age might be recommended, yet it is not clear whether earlier diagnosis can impact survival.

Ancillary studies

Additional evaluation of metastatic disease needs to be considered only in patients with stage 1 and high-risk features and all patients with stage 2 onwards. These include bilateral bone marrow aspirates and biopsies, and lumbar puncture with examination of the cytospin. Since retinoblastoma cells may adhere to the tube, the examination of the cytocentrifuge should be done to improve the yield of this procedure. Bone scintigraphy is only recommended in children with confirmed metastatic disease or those with bone pain.

Table 27.1 The International Grouping System for intraocular disease

Group A

Small tumours away from foveola and disc

- Tumours <3 mm in greatest dimension confined to the retina, *and*
- Located at least 3 mm from the foveola and 1.5 mm from the optic disc

Group B

All remaining tumours confined to the retina

- All other tumours confined to the retina not in Group A
- Subretinal fluid (without subretinal seeding) <3 mm from the base of the tumour

Group C

Local subretinal fluid or seeding

- Local subretinal fluid alone >3 to <6 mm from the tumour
- Vitreous seeding or subretinal seeding <3 mm from the tumour

Group D

Diffuse subretinal fluid or seeding

- Subretinal fluid alone >6 mm from the tumour
- Vitreous seeding or subretinal seeding >3 mm from tumour

Group E

Presence of any or more of these poor prognosis features

- More than 2/3 globe filled with tumour
- Tumour in anterior segment
- Tumour in or on the ciliary body
- Iris neovascularization
- Neovascular glaucoma
- Opaque media from hemorrhage
- Tumour necrosis with aseptic orbital cellulitis
- Phthisis bulbi

Table 27.2 The International Staging for Retinoblastoma

Stage 0	Patients treated conservatively (subject to presurgical ophthalmologic classifications)
Stage I	Eye enucleated, completely resected histologically
Stage II	Eye enucleated, microscopic residual tumour
Stage III	Regional extension
	a) Overt orbital disease,
	b) Pre-auricular or cervical lymph node extension
Stage IV	Metastatic disease
	a) Hematogenous metastasis:1. Single lesion, 2. Multiple lesions;
	b) CNS extension, 1.Prechiasmatic lesion 2. CNS mass, 3. Leptomeningeal disease

Treatment

Retinoblastoma is special among pediatric tumours in that two different treatments goals are sought by treating physicians: patient survival, usually lead by a pediatric oncologist, and eye survival, usually led by a pediatric ophthalmologist;each need different parameters to be considered for treatment in the context of a multidisciplinary team. So, the treatment of retinoblastoma includes surgical procedures, local therapies, radiotherapy, and chemotherapy that can be given systemically or locally.

Surgery

Enucleation is the simplest and safest therapy for retinoblastoma. A prosthetic implant is fitted after the procedure to minimize cosmetic deficits. Enucleation should be performed by an experienced pediatric ophthalmologist in order to obtain a long optic nerve stump. Initial enucleation is indicated in all eyes with secondary glaucoma, invasion of anterior segment (anterior chamber, iris), rubeosis iridis, impossibility of close follow up or limitations for using local therapies and Reese-Ellsworth Group Vb (groups D and E) eyes in most unilateral non-hereditary patients. Secondary enucleation is indicated after failure of conservative approaches and after neo-adjuvant chemotherapy in extraocular disease. Even though enucleation is a curative treatment for retinoblastoma and it may be done in most settings regardless their complexity, it is not always accepted by the families, especially in less developed countries. Up to 50 per cent of the affected families opt out of enucleation as initial treatment in some countries; these children die of a potentially curable disease. Therefore, in settings with this problem, comprehensive strategies, including psychosocial support should be implemented to improve survival. Some surgical procedures such as pars plana vitrectomy, anterior chamber paracentesis, and orbital exenteration are not indicated in most children with retinoblastoma.

Focal therapies

Focal treatments are used for small tumours (<3–6 mm), usually in patients with bilateral disease, and in combination with chemotherapy. These include: photocoagulation with argon laser which is used for the treatment of tumours posterior to the equator; transpupillary thermotherapy, which applies focused heat at subphotocoagulation levels, usually with diode laser; and cryotherapy, which is used for the treatment of small anterior lesions.

Radiotherapy

Radiotherapy in combination with focal treatments can provide excellent tumour control. However, radiation therapy increases the risk of second malignancies in heritable retinoblastoma survivors, and so contemporary management of intraocular retinoblastoma is designed to avoid or delay its use; the role of radiation is mainly as salvage method for eyes that have failed chemotherapy and focal treatments, usually due to progression of vitreous and subretinal seeding. Radiation therapy continues to have a major role in the treatment of patients with extraocular disease.

Several techniques can be used, usually through lateral or anterior fields. Recommended total doses are 4000–4500 cGy, although doses of 3600 cGy are under investigation in conjunction with other techniques.

Radioactive plaque technique is useful when treating localized tumours, both because the procedure time is short, and because a high dose of irradiation is delivered to the areas of interest while minimizing radiation effects to the extraocular structures. The radioactive implant is placed on the sclera over the base of the tumour, and is kept for 2– 4 days, the time needed to deliver approximately

4000 cGy to the apex of the tumour. Different radioactive episcleral plaques can be used, although ^{125}I is the most widely used. Control rates of 85–90 per cent can be achieved.

Chemotherapy

The use of chemotherapy for the treatment of retinoblastoma include three different scenarios.

Chemoreduction for conservative treatment

Chemoreduction is used as primary treatment for intraocular disease not amenable for local therapy in order to decrease tumour size and make the tumours suitable for local therapy. Carboplatin in combination with vincristine and etoposide are the most frequently used agents. Most intraocular tumours usually show dramatic shrinkage; however, consolidation with local treatment is needed in most cases to prevent relapse. Tumour location, patient age, and size of tumour correlate with responsiveness to chemotherapy. Most patients with less advanced disease such as R-E groups I–III or IRSG groups A–C respond favourably to chemotherapy, so that enucleation and external beam radiotherapy are usually avoided. For patients with advanced intraocular tumours (R-E groups IV-V or group D), especially those with vitreous seeds, ocular salvage rates are not better than 50 per cent with chemoreduction and focal therapy, and consolidation with EBRT is usually required. Different treatment modalities such as periocular administration of carboplatin and the administration of intra-arterial melphalan via superselective administration in the ophthalmic artery have been employed, but to date no consensus exists on the best therapy.

Even though chemoreduction followed by local treatment became the standard therapy for intraocular retinoblastoma, there are several limitations for this approach. Its long-term safety is not known, especially as far as potential induction of secondary malignancies, especially treatment-induced leukemia. However, results with the use of carboplatin and vincristine without etoposide may be comparable in eyes with less advanced disease. Therefore, the optimal regimen and duration of treatment are still under investigation. Finally, this treatment is tedious and needs meticulous management; resources are only available in specialized centers. Chemoreduction regimens should be used with caution in less developed countries where patient compliance is poor or uncertain. Deaths after refusal of enucleation or toxicity have been published.

Adjuvant chemotherapy for high-risk stage 1 and stage 2 disease

After enucleation, the eye should be comprehensively evaluated by an experienced ocular pathologist: histopathological microstaging is essential to define groups with different risk of extraocular relapse. Invasion to the choroid, sclera, and optic nerve are considered as significant risk factors for extraocular relapse. The role of adjuvant chemotherapy for these patients to reduce the relapse rate is a matter of controversy. Their prognostic significance appears not to be influenced by the laterality of the tumour. Because these factors are infrequent in developed countries, there have been no randomized studies published in the literature as for other malignancies. There is almost universal agreement that there is no need of adjuvant chemotherapy for patients with intraretinal disease and in those with prelaminar optic nerve invasion. The role of chemotherapy in isolated choroidal invasion is controversial because the relapse rate, when there is no concomitant postlaminar optic nerve involvement is only about 3 per cent. Different degrees of choroidal invasion may have different prognostic implications and some subgroups, such as those with massive invasion, may benefit from adjuvant chemotherapy. However, a consensus definition for the different degrees of choroidal invasion has not been available until recently and results between different series are not comparable. Therefore, the effectiveness of adjuvant therapy in this subgroup will be difficult to prove.

Invasion to the optic nerve beyond the lamina cribrosa is a major risk factor for relapse and adjuvant therapy is recommended. When the cut end is free of tumour, most treatment groups recommend adjuvant chemotherapy alone. With the use of current high-resolution MR imaging, postlaminar optic nerve invasion may be presumed preoperatively by detecting contrast enhancement in the distal portion of the nerve. Some of these patients have received neo-adjuvant chemotherapy in an attempt to avoid the occurrence of a tumour residue at the resection margin. However, identifying post laminar optic nerve invasion through imaging studies is a challenge and the sensitivity of MRI when the optic nerve is not enlarged is about 60 per cent in centres with extensive experience. Patients with invasion of the cut end of the optic nerve are considered as stage 2 because a microscopic tumour residue is left behind after enucleation and they are uniformly considered for adjuvant therapy with chemotherapy and orbital radiotherapy. In recent series, about 70 per cent of these patients survive, albeit with important cosmetic and neuroendocrinological sequelae because of radiation. The importance of microscopic scleral invasion as a risk factor for relapse is less clear because it usually occurs with other concomitant factors. When there is evidence of microscopic trans-scleral invasion, these children should be considered as stage 2, but patients with only intra-scleral invasion (stage 1) need adjuvant chemotherapy as well. The chemotherapy regimens used for the adjuvant therapy of children with stage 1 disease and pathology risk factors and those with stage 2 disease include the combination of carboplatin and etoposide, or more intensive regimens including the same agents at higher doses together with alkylating agents such as cyclophosphamide or ifosfamide and an anthracycline as it is used in other centres. The use of more intensive regimens is reserved for children with stage 2 disease as per the COG strategy, but other groups showed that subgroups of Stage 1 patients such as those with postlaminar optic nerve or microscopical scleral invasion, also benefit from intensive regimens.

Treatment of overt extraocular retinoblastoma (stages 3 and 4)

In all these cases, neo-adjuvant chemotherapy is warranted. Extensive and mutilating surgeries such as orbital extenteration are of no use. About 70 per cent of the patients with stage 3 disease are curable with an aggressive approach using neo-adjuvant chemotherapy, enucleation of the residual mass and adjuvant chemo- and radiotherapy. The agents used are the same as those used for high-risk stage 1 and 2 disease. Orbital relapse after enucleation is also curable with the same approach.

However, even though a complete remission is usually achieved with conventional chemotherapy in patients with stage 4 disease, it is usually short lived and ultimate survival is infrequent. However, recent series report that metastatic retinoblastoma outside the CNS (Stage 4a) may be cured using high-dose chemotherapy and autologous stem cell rescue. Patients usually receive four to six cycles of conventional induction chemotherapy followed by high-dose chemotherapy and autologous stem cell rescue. Different preparative regimens have been used, but thiotepa-containing regimens appear to be effective because of its high penetration to the CNS. This modality has also been explored for children with CNS metastasis (stage 4b), but very few patients survive, even with this treatment. The Children's Oncology Group (COG) has launched an international study of multi-modality therapy for these children (COG ARET0321). Those with stage 4a and 4b metastatic disease (as well as those with trilateral retinoblastoma) receive aggressive conventional induction chemotherapy, have autologous stem cells harvested, receive high-dose carboplatin, thiotepa, and etoposide with autologous stem cell rescue, and then (depending on response) are considered for external beam radiation. Recent reports suggest that this strategy may also be effective for trilateral retinoblastoma.

Second malignancies in retinoblastoma survivors

The cumulative incidence of second cancers in patients with germline mutations of the *RB1* gene is greatly increased with the use and dose of radiation therapy, and this incidence is reported to increase steadily with age, to up to 40–60 per cent at 40–50 years of age, although more recent studies estimate a considerably lower risk. Patients with non-hereditary retinoblastoma are not inherently at an increased risk.

Almost any neoplasm has been described in survivors of retinoblastoma and 60–70 per cent of the tumours occur in the head and neck areas. The most common second tumours are osteogenic sarcoma, arising both inside and outside the irradiation field, soft tissue sarcomas and melanomas. Survivors of bilateral retinoblastoma are also at risk of developing epithelial cancers late in adulthood, particularly in the lung.

Further reading

Abramson DH, Dunkel IJ, Brodie SE, et al. (2008) A phase I/II study of direct intraarterial (ophthalmic artery) chemotherapy with melphalan for intraocular retinoblastoma initial results. *Ophthalmology* **115**, 1398–404.

Antoneli CB, Steinhorst F, de Cassia Braga Ribeiro K, et al. (2003) Extraocular retinoblastoma: a 13-year experience. *Cancer* **98**, 1292–8.

Brisse HJ, Guesmi M, Aerts I, et al. (2007) Relevance of CT and MRI in retinoblastoma for the diagnosis of postlaminar invasion with normal-size optic nerve: a retrospective study of 150 patients with histological comparison. *Pediatr Radiol* **37**, 649–56.

Canturk S, Qaddoumi I, Khetan V, et al. (2010) Survival of retinoblastoma in less-developed countries impact of socioeconomic and health-related indicators. *Br J Ophthalmol* **94**, 1432–6.

Chantada GL, Dunkel IJ, de Davila MT, et al. (2004) Retinoblastoma patients with high risk ocular pathological features: who needs adjuvant therapy? *Br J Ophthalmol* **88**, 1069–73.

Chantada GL, Fandino AC, Guitter MR, et al. (2010) Results of a prospective study for the treatment of unilateral retinoblastoma. *Pediatr Blood Cancer* **55**, 60–6.

Corson TW, Gallie BL (2007) One hit, two hits, three hits, more? Genomic changes in the development of retinoblastoma. *Genes Chromosomes Cancer* **46**, 617–34.

de Camargo B, de Oliveira Santos M, Rebelo MS, et al. (2010) Cancer incidence among children and adolescents in Brazil: first report of 14 population-based cancer registries. *Int J Cancer* **126**, 715–20.

Dunkel IJ, Alcdo A, Kernan NA, et al. (2000) Successful treatment of metastatic retinoblastoma. *Cancer* **89**, 2117–21.

Ganguly A, Shields CL (2010) Differential gene expression profile of retinoblastoma compared to normal retina. *Mol Vis* **16**, 1292–303.

Holladay DA, Holladay A, Montebello JF, Redmond KP (1991) Clinical presentation, treatment, and outcome of trilateral retinoblastoma. *Cancer* **67**, 710–5.

Khelfaoui F, Validire P, Auperin A, et al. (1996) Histopathologic risk factors in retinoblastoma: a retrospective study of 172 patients treated in a single institution. *Cancer* **77**, 1206–13.

Kleinerman RA, Tucker MA, Tarone RE, et al. (2005) Risk of new cancers after radiotherapy in long-term survivors of retinoblastoma: an extended follow-up. *J Clin Oncol* **23**, 2272–9.

Laurie NA, Donovan SL, Shih CS, et al. (2006) Inactivation of the p53 pathway in retinoblastoma. *Nature* **444**, 61–6.

Laurie NA, Gray JK, Zhang J, et al. (2005) Topotecan combination chemotherapy in two new rodent models of retinoblastoma. *Clin Cancer Res* **11**, 7569–78.

Leal-Leal CA, Rivera-Luna R, Flores-Rojo M, et al. (2006) Survival in extra-orbital metastatic retinoblastoma: treatment results. *Clin Transl Oncol* **8**, 39–44.

Lee EY, Chang CY, Hu N, et al. (1992) Mice deficient for Rb are nonviable and show defects in neurogenesis and haematopoiesis. *Nature* **359**, 288–94.

Lumbroso-Le Rouic L, Aerts I, Levy-Gabriel C, et al. (2008) Conservative treatments of intraocular retinoblastoma. *Ophthalmology* **115**, 1405–10.

MacCarthy A, Birch JM, Draper GJ, et al. (2009) Retinoblastoma: treatment and survival in Great Britain 1963 to 2002. *Br J Ophthalmol* **93**, 38–9.

Munier FL, Verwey J, Pica A, et al. (2008) New developments in external beam radiotherapy for retinoblastoma: from lens to normal tissue-sparing techniques. *Clin Experiment Ophthalmol* **36**, 78–89.

Sastre X, Chantada GL, Doz F, et al. (2009) Proceedings of the consensus meetings from the International Retinoblastoma Staging Working Group on the pathology guidelines for the examination of enucleated eyes and evaluation of prognostic risk factors in retinoblastoma. *Arch Pathol Lab Med* **133**, 1199–202.

Shields CL, Ramasubramanian A, Thangappan A, et al. (2009) Chemoreduction for group E retinoblastoma: comparison of chemoreduction alone versus chemoreduction plus low-dose external radiotherapy in 76 eyes. *Ophthalmology* **116**, 544–51.

van Dijk J, Oostrom KJ, Imhof SM, et al. (2009) Behavioural functioning of retinoblastoma survivors. *Psychooncology* **18**, 87–95.

Wilson MW, Haik BG, Liu T, et al. (2005) Effect on ocular survival of adding early intensive focal treatments to a two-drug chemotherapy regimen in patients with retinoblastoma. *Am J Ophthalmol* **140**, 397–406.

Xu XL, Fang Y, Lee TC, et al. (2009) Retinoblastoma has properties of a cone precursor tumor and depends upon cone-specific MDM2 signaling. *Cell* **137**, 1018–31.

Chapter 28

Other rare tumours

Beatriz de Camargo, Yves Reguerre and Daniel Orbach

Introduction

This chapter will describe rare tumours that occur in children and adolescents. This group comprises Group XI from the third edition of the International Classification of Childhood Cancer (ICCC-3) and reflects specific epidemiological interests in tumours with higher incidence in some parts of the world, such as adrenocortical carcinoma (XIa) in Southern Brazil, thyroid carcinomas (XIb) in Belarus and Ukraine, nasopharyngeal carcinoma (XIc) in Africa and China, and malignant melanoma in Australia and New Zealand. A combination of environmental and genetic factors may be responsible for these variations. This chapter will also describe tumours from the miscellaneous subgroup of unspecified malignant tumours in ICCC Group XI. The two most frequent histological types represented in this group are pleuro-pulmonary blastoma and pancreatoblastoma. These tumours can be challenging for clinicians and pathologists due to their rarity and often different epidemiology and patterns of behaviour and morphology.

Thyroid carcinomas

Epidemiology

Thyroid carcinomas are rare in children. These lesions represent 1.2 per cent of all childhood cancers in children younger than 15 years of age and 8.2 per cent in adolescents (15–19 years old). The age-standardized incidence rates for children (0–14 years old) vary from 0.5 to 1.2 per million in Europe. The incidence rates are much higher (4.4–11 per million) in adolescents compared to children. Data from the Surveillance, Epidemiology, and End Results (SEER) registry of the United States has identified an annual incidence of 5.4 per million children/adolescents (0–19 years old) between 1973 and 2004. A significant increase of 1.1 per cent per year has been observed. The highest incidence is seen in females, adolescents, and white patients, 95 per cent are older than 10 years and 2.4 per cent have been treated for a previous malignancy. Exposure to external medical radiation or external and internal radiation from atomic bomb explosions has been shown to lead to an increased risk of thyroid cancer. The exposure of children less than 4 years of age to fallout from the Chernobyl reactor accident led to a substantial increase in the incidence of childhood cancer in the affected countries (Belarus, Ukraine, and western parts of Russia). Extremely high incidence rates have been observed for thyroid cancer in the paediatric cancer registry of Belarus, 24 per million in all age groups. Thyroid cancer is the most common secondary malignancy in children treated with radiation of the neck region.

Diagnosis and staging

Clinical presentation is usually an anterior cervical adenopathy or palpable thyroid nodule. Hoarseness can occur and indicates compression or invasion of the recurrent laryngeal nerve.

Approximately 80 per cent of affected children have regional lymph node metastases, and 10–20 per cent distant metastases. The most common site for distant metastases is the lung, bones, and liver. The evaluation begins with thyroid function tests that usually confirm euthyroidism. Ultrasound provides information regarding whether the lesion is cystic or solid, thyroid size, and the presence of multiples nodules. Thyroid scintigrams performed with iodine-123 usually shows cold or hypofunctioning nodules. Hot functional nodules are usually benign. Conventional imaging with X-rays, computed tomography (CT), magnetic resonance imaging (MRI), and bone scans will demonstrate local spread and distant metastases. Octreotide scintigraphy is useful only for medullary thyroid carcinoma. Fine-needle aspiration biopsy is performed in children; though it is controversial if is as sensitive or specific as in adult. The differential diagnosis among benign and malignant follicular carcinoma may be difficult. Thyroid nodules containing follicular features have a 20–30 per cent malignancy rate. Stevens et al. (see Further Reading) performed a meta-analysis of 12 studies in a paediatric population and the accuracy, positive predictive value, and negative predictive value were 83.6 per cent, 55.3 per cent, and 98.2 per cent respectively, suggesting that fine needle biopsy is useful for excluding malignancy in the paediatric population. Staging should be evaluated by the American Joint Committee on Cancer (AJCC)/International Union Against Cancer (UICC) tumour-node-metastasis (TNM) staging system, which describes the size of the tumour (T0–T4), node metastasis to regional, ipsilateral, bilateral cervical nodes (N0, N1a,N1b), and distant metastases(M0–M1).

Several studies have shown that thyroid carcinoma in paediatric patients differs from adults with respect to its presentation and outcome. Although children tend to present with disease at a more advanced stage than adults, their prognosis is better. Mean tumour size, extra-thyroid spread, and node metastasis at presentation are more common in children. In a large series of 1753 paediatric patients with thyroid carcinoma, male gender, non-papillary subtype, distant metastases, and nonsurgical treatment were all independent factors for worse outcome. A clear biological explanation for differences in the behaviour of thyroid cancer in children is still not available.

Biology and pathology

The predominant histological patterns of thyroid malignancy are papillary, follicular, and medullary, which are seen with similar frequency in children/adolescents; 70 per cent are papillary, 20 per cent follicular, 5–10 per cent medullar, and anaplastic patterns are very rare. Rearrangements of the *RET* gene are common. *RET–PTC* rearrangements (PTC-1, PTC-2, PTC-3) are characteristic of papillary carcinoma. Medullary carcinoma in young patients is attributed to screening families with multiple endocrine neoplasia (MEN 2A, MEN 2B) familial cancer syndromes and familial medullary thyroid carcinoma. Type MEN 2A is associated with pheochromocytoma, hyperparathyroidism, cutaneous lichen amyloidosis, and Hirschsprung. Type MEN 2B is associated with pheochromocytoma, intestinal ganglioneuromatosis, and marfanoid features. Both syndromes are due to germline mutations in the *RET* proto-oncogene.

Treatment

The optimal surgical management of children with thyroid tumours is controversial. Some are in favour of an aggressive surgical approach utilizing total thyroidectomy because of the propensity of differentiated thyroid cancer to disseminate in this age group. On the other hand, others advocate a more conservative surgical procedure employing thyroid lobectomy, based on the fact that the mortality rate is low. Routine use of total or subtotal thyroidectomy does not improve the outcome in patients with localized tumours and is associated with an increased risk of complications.

Permanent hypocalcemia is the more common complication. Limited surgery is appropriate only for paediatric patients who do not exhibit lymphadenopathy. In localized tumours, male gender, advanced tumour, and clinical lymphadectomy are risk factors for disease-free survival and aggressive treatment should be performed in these patients, whereas a conservative or stepwise approach may be acceptable for other patients. A conservative approach with unilateral lobectomy alone and/or nodule excision can be appropriate for select patients without risk factors. Radioactive iodine after total thyroidectomy is recommended in metastatic disease, and total thyroidectomy facilitates [131] I imaging and treatment. The role of this treatment in localized disease is still unknown as there are no randomized trials evaluating the benefit of this procedure.

Children identified by *RET* screening to be at risk for the development of medullary thyroid cancer should be treated with prophylactic thyroidectomy before development of the disease. This genotype–phenotype relationship should be used to determine the optimal timing of prophylactic thyroidectomy in families with hereditary medullary thyroid cancer. The most common germline *RET* mutation, codon 634 in exon 11, is observed in two-thirds of patients with FMTC and MEN 2A. The exons found to harbor germline *RET* mutations (exons 10, 11, 13, 14, 15, and 16) encode either cysteine-rich or tyrosine kinase domains. *RET* mutations are classified into three levels according to the risk of developing cancer. Low risk refers to mutations in codons 768, 790, 791, 804, and 891, with a more variable penetrance and a later age of onset, which is usually not before 10 years. Intermediate risk is related to mutations in codons 609, 611, 618, 620, 630, and 634 and is associated with medullary thyroid cancer before age 5. High risk is related to mutations in codons 883, 918, and 922, which may cause medullary thyroid cancer as early as 6 months of age and are present in roughly 25 per cent of patients with sporadic medullary thyroid cancer as somatic mutations.

Adrenocortical carcinoma

Epidemiology

Adrenocortical carcinomas are very rare in children and adolescents. This lesion accounts for 0.2 per cent of all new cancers diagnosed each year in the United States and Europe. Incidence rates range from 0.5 to 2.0 cases per million children. A higher incidence of 1.5 per million has been observed in São Paulo, Brazil, more than three times the rate in most others regions. Unlike other paediatric carcinomas, most adrenocortical carcinomas are diagnosed before 6 years of age. Adrenocortical carcinoma has been reported in association with genetic diseases, such as congenital adrenal hyperplasia, Li-Fraumeni syndrome, and Beckwith–Wiedeman syndromes. In families with Li-Fraumeni syndrome, the frequency of adrenocortical tumours is 100 times that of the general population.

Diagnosis and staging

Typically, children present with signs and symptoms of increased production of androgens (virilization) and/or cortisol (hypercortisolism or Cushing syndrome). Virilization is the most common presentation and is often combined with features of Cushing syndrome. Signs of virilization include hirsutism, facial and pubic hair, increased muscle, rapid growth, and penile and clitoral enlargement. Children with Cushing syndrome present with moon face, obesity, hypertension, impaired glucose metabolism, and growth arrest. Hyperestrogenism (feminization) or aldosteronism (Conn syndrome) is seen more rarely. Non-functional tumours are rare. Other signs and symptoms include abdominal pain, large palpable mass, and weight loss. Distant metastases usually develop in the liver, lungs, and bone. At diagnosis, two-thirds of children have localized disease and completely resectable tumours. The recommended staging system is based on disease stage and tumour size as follows:

Stage I: Completely resected small tumours (<100 g and volume <200 cm^3) with normalized hormone levels after surgery

Stage II: Completely resected large tumours (≥100g or ≥200 cm^3) with normalized hormone levels after surgery

Stage III: Unresectable, gross or microscopic residual disease, tumour spillage, patients with stage I or II who fail to achieve normalized hormone levels after surgery or patients with retroperitoneal lymph node

Stage IV: Patients with distant metastases.

Biology and pathology

Histological differentiation of adenomas and carcinomas is not always easy. The histological score proposed by Weiss involves nine criteria: high mitotic rate, atypical mitoses, high nuclear grade, low percentage of clear cells, necrosis, capsular invasion, sinusoidal invasion, venous invasion, and diffuse tumour architecture. The presence of each criterion is given a score of 1, and a total score ≤2 is typically associated with adrenocortical adenoma, whereas a score ≥3 is indicative of adreno-cortical carcinoma. This score is useful but far from infallible. Other scores are also used, such as the Slooten and Hough systems. A germline mutation affecting R337H in the p53 domain was first reported in Brazilian children with adrenocortical carcinoma, and further studies have demonstrated that the mutation occurs in Brazilian families with Li-Fraumeni and Li-Fraumeni-like syndromes. A founder germline *TP53* mutation has been identified in Southeast Brazil at an unusually high prevalence. Analyses of several tumours diagnosed in families have shown that the presence of p53 R337H is associated with multiple cancers in the spectrum of Li-Fraumeni syndrome at a younger age, including soft tissue and bone sarcomas in adolescents, and breast carcinoma in young adults. The penetrance at age 30 years is approximately 50 per cent, with a greater than 90 per cent lifetime risk of developing cancer in carriers of the mutation.

Treatment

Surgery is the mainstay of treatment. Rupture of the capsule leading to tumour spillage occurs in approximately 20 per cent of cases. Infiltration of the vena cava by a tumour thrombus can occur, making radical surgery difficult. The role of lymphadectomy is unknown, but lymph node sampling should be performed. The use of systemic therapy is indicated in advanced disease. Mitotane, an insecticide derivative, causes adrenocortical necrosis and has been used in adrenocortical carcinoma. Several reports are available on the complete response, but prolonged use is limited by side effects that limit patient compliance, including severe gastrointestinal and neurologic toxicity. Chemotherapeutic agents, such as cisplatin, etoposide, 5-fluorouracil, and doxorubicin, have result in a response rate of 20–40 per cent.

Malignant melanoma

Epidemiology

Malignant melanomas are uncommon in children but increasing significantly in adolescents. In Europe, the incidence rate is 0.7 per million children and 12.9 per million adolescents. Factors contributing to melanoma in children include congenital melanoma, giant congenital melanocytic nevi, xeroderma pigmentosum, neurocutaneous melanosis, and family history. The most important risk factor for the development of adolescent melanoma is thought to be intermittent sun exposure during childhood.

Diagnosis and staging

Histological confirmation of melanoma in children is very difficult. Problems with over-diagnosis because of misinterpretation of benign Spitz nevus, as well as under-diagnosis because of a reluctance to diagnose a malignant melanoma in a child, are rare. The classifications of Breslow (depth of invasion described as less than 1 mm to greater than 4 mm) and Clark levels (invasion of the epidermis, papillary, papillary dermis, reticular dermis, and subcutaneous deep) should be used in children to evaluate prognosis and treatment.

Biology and pathology

Several criteria are assessed for differential diagnosis. Symmetry, maturation, few mitoses, absence of atypical mitosis, and no mitosis in the deeper portion of the lesion are in favour of Spitz nevus. None of the factors are specific and diagnosis is made based on a combination of features. Sometimes distinction between Spitz nevus and melanoma is impossible and may lead to a diagnosis of Spitz Tumor of Uncertain Malignant Potential (STUMP).

Treatment

All lesions should be managed by complete excision with clear surgical margins. Systemic treatment is recommended for disseminated disease.

Nasopharyngeal carcinoma

In Europe, undifferentiated carcinoma of the nasopharyngeal type UCNT represents only about 1 per cent of all childhood cancers, but it nevertheless represents one-third of all malignant tumours of the nasopharynx. Nasopharyngeal tumours are deeply situated, under the base of the skull, which explains the varied and often late clinical features related to invasion of adjacent structures. UCNT usually arises in the pharyngeal recess. The presenting sign is usually cervical lymphadenopathy, as the nasopharyngeal lesion may remain clinically silent for a long time. At diagnosis, the disease is often locally advanced. However, metastases are initially rare (one case in a series of 34 paediatric patients). When metastases are present, the most frequent metastatic sites are the lungs, mediastinum, bone, and liver. Staging is currently based on the fifth AJCC classification. Depending on the extent of the tumour, the child may present one or several symptoms at diagnosis, none of which are specific, such as headache, hearing loss, nasal obstruction, anosmia, epistaxis, trismus related to invasion of masticatory muscles, disorders of deglutition due, among other things, to invasion of the hypoglossal nerve (XII), dysphonia due to invasion of the vagus nerve (X) or diplopia due to invasion of the abducens nerve (VI). Cervical lymphadenopathy is also a frequent presenting sign (30 per cent). It typically involves the spinal or superior jugulo-carotid chains.

Epidemiology

This tumour mainly affects adolescents and young adults. In paediatric populations, the age of diagnosis is between 12 and 15 years. The geographical distribution of nasopharyngeal carcinoma represents one of the major characteristics of the disease, as this tumour is much more frequent in China and North Africa, suggesting a genetic association an associated viral cause (Epstein–Barr virus, EBV) or the role of certain dietary habits (excessive salt intake, vitamin C deficiency).

EBV is frequently detected in the genome of tumour cells by immunohistochemistry hybridization using the EBER 1 probe.

Histopathology

UCNT is one of the rare paediatric tumours of epithelial origin (carcinoma). The diagnosis, often very strongly suspected on analysis of the cell smear derived from lymph node aspiration cytology, is confirmed by histological examination after cervical lymphadenectomy or biopsy of the nasopharyngeal mass. The most frequent histological type of carcinoma of the nasopharynx in childhood is the undifferentiated form Type III of the WHO classification in >90 per cent of cases.

Treatment

Surgery has no place in the curative treatment of UCNT, apart from biopsy during the initial assessment to obtain adequate histological material for diagnosis. The radiosensitivity of the tumour has been clearly established and local external beam radiotherapy of the nasopharynx and lymph nodes remains the standard treatment of this disease (at doses between 50 and 65 Gy). Radiotherapy is mainly delivered to the nasopharynx (including the base of the skull when initially invaded). Bilateral cervical lymph node chains are also systematically treated with curative intent in the case of initial invasion or preventively when they are not initially invaded. The usual doses are delivered by fractions of 1.8 Gy per session, 5 days a week, but dose reduction allows improved tolerance and decreased sequelae. The use of modern techniques such as intensity modulation radiotherapy (IMRT) or tomotherapy protects the salivary glands, parotid, and cochleas and should decrease the late sequelae in these organs. Sometimes distinction between Spitz nevus and melanoma is impossible and may lead to a diagnosis of Spitz Tumor of Uncertain Malignant Potential (STUMP).

The overall survival and relapse-free survival (RFS) after only radiotherapy in children are less than 40 per cent and sometimes even lower. Patients in relapse have a very poor prognosis regardless of the treatment proposed. UCNT is an extremely chemosensitive tumour and neo-adjuvant chemotherapy also improves the conditions of radiotherapy by decreasing neck pain and stiffness, thereby facilitating positioning of the child for irradiation. It also improves radiation fields by delineating the irradiation margins between the tumour and adjacent structures. Although the value of chemotherapy on long-term survival has not been formally demonstrated in this tumour by comparative studies, the great majority of paediatric teams recommend a combination of chemotherapy and radiotherapy in the management of children with UCNT both in the neo-adjuvant setting, concomitantly and sometimes as adjuvant therapy after radiotherapy. Recent series reporting the results of chemotherapy and radiotherapy combinations show an improvement of overall survival by about 77 per cent. Most paediatric protocols therefore combine several drugs, including cisplatin, with a high response rate to chemotherapy exceeding 75 per cent. Due to the major sequelae and good overall prognosis of this disease, current treatment protocols are designed to decrease the total doses of irradiation delivered to the neck and nasopharynx, particularly following a good response to neo-adjuvant chemotherapy.

Pleuropulmonary blastoma

Pleuropulmonary blastoma (PPB) is a rare malignant neoplasm of the lung presenting in early childhood. PPB is a dysembryonic malignancy believed to arise from pleuropulmonary mesenchyme. It is recognized as the pulmonary analogue of more common childhood developmental neoplasms. PPB is divided into three pathologic subtypes representing a progression of the disease along an age-related biologic continuum from birth to around age72 months (93 per cent of cases).

Type I PPB is an air-filled purely cystic neoplasm (median diagnosis age: 10 months)

Type II PPB is a cystic and solid neoplasm (median age at diagnosis: 36 months)

Type III PPB (solid) is an aggressive sarcoma (median age at diagnosis: 43 months)

PPB is a strongly genetic disease. Familial association of pleuropulmonary blastoma with cystic nephroma and other renal tumours is frequent and occurs in almost 25 per cent of cases. Inherited *DICER1* mutations have been recently discovered in familial pleuropulmonary blastoma.

Metastasis in type I PPB has not been reported. Types II and III metastasize most frequently to brain parenchyma. In fewer than 5 per cent of cases, PPB metastasizes to bone, liver, and lung parenchyma. Metastasis documented at the time of diagnosis is rare but does occur. Most metastases occur within 24–36 months of diagnosis; metastasis more than 36 months after diagnosis is unusual.

Therapy

Due to its rarity, treatment of this disease has not been clearly defined. For all types of PPB, complete surgery (segmentectomy, lobectomy or rarely total pneumonectomy) is the cornerstone of therapy. In case of initial incomplete resection, resection should be completed by immediate redo surgery. The need for systematic total pleurectomy in addition to total or partial pneumonectomy in these very young patients should be discussed by a multidisciplinary team. In case of initial unresectable lesion, the diagnosis may be based on true-cut or surgical biopsy. PPB is a chemosensitive tumour. The need for adjuvant chemotherapy after complete resection of a type I tumour is a subject of debate. The decision should take into account the patient's age, the family history, the quality of surgery and the possibility of ensuring strict follow up. For instance, in view of the relatively low event-free survival (EFS) in type I (50 per cent) with surgery only, French guidelines include systematic adjuvant vincristine–actinomycin D after surgery. Types II and III should be considered as aggressive blastomas and treated with at least surgery and chemotherapy. For types II–III, neo-adjuvant chemotherapy should be used in initially unresectable tumours. Systematic adjuvant chemotherapy is commonly given for 6–9 months even after complete resection. The regimens most frequently used are IVA, IVAdO or VAIA (ifosfamide, vincristine, actinomycin D with or without doxorubicin). The role of radiotherapy is more difficult to define as patients are very young and the high total dose of radiotherapy required may lead to severe late effects (thoracic growth defect, cardiac dysfunction, pulmonary dysfunction). In our opinion, radiotherapy should be considered in the case of persistent incomplete resection, after multiple surgery or after locoregional relapses. The International Pleuropulmonary Blastoma Registry (www.ppbregistry.org) reports a 5-year overall survival of 85–90 per cent in type I and 45–60 per cent in types II and III.

Pancreatoblastoma

Pancreatoblastoma is a rare pancreatic malignancy in infancy. This tumour mostly occurs in patients less than 10 years old (78 per cent of all cases). Median age at diagnosis is 5 years. It predominantly affects males with a sex ratio of 1.6. Most cases occur sporadically but this tumour may also occur in a context of Beckwith–Wiedemann syndrome. This tumour was first described by Becker in 1957 and was finally named pancreatoblastoma by Horie in 1977. This tumour is considered to have an embryonic origin. Evidence of an endocrine component, with acinar cells containing zymogen granules and the presence of alpha fetoprotein (AFP), suggests that this tumour arises from pluripotent stem cells.

Diagnosis

The most frequent presenting sign is an abdominal mass associated with pain in half of cases. The mass is usually very large with a rough surface. One-third of patients present associated asthenia or diarrhea and vomiting. Jaundice is rare (less than 10 per cent of cases). Asymptomatic tumour is also possible. At diagnosis, metastases are rare (17 per cent) and mostly involve the liver (88 per cent of cases) or lymph nodes (portal or splenic hilum). Other distant metastases may be observed in the lungs or mediastinum. Sixty per cent of patients present elevated AFP levels at diagnosis. In laboratory studies, AFP levels are often elevated as both the liver and the pancreas arise from the same primitive cells. AFP assay is useful at diagnosis to confirm the suspected diagnosis and during follow up to detect early relapses.

Therapy

Pancreatoblastoma is less aggressive in infants and children than in adults. The treatment of choice is complete resection, which is often curative. More than 95 per cent of patients with disease confined to the pancreas are cured by complete surgical excision, but unresectable tumour is associated with a poor prognosis. According to the initial site, cephalic duodenopancreatectomy or corporeo-caudal pancreatectomy may be necessary. This fairly radical surgery is generally well tolerated in children.

Only retrospective data are available to assess the value of chemotherapy in this tumour and they confirm that pancreatoblastoma is a chemosensitive tumour. Many drugs had been used, such as ifosfamide, doxorubicin, cyclophosphamide, and etoposide. The most commonly used regimen is the cisplatin–doxorubicin combination. In the case of unresectable tumour or distant metastases, neo-adjuvant chemotherapy is used to reduce tumour bulk, avoid distant progression, and allow subsequent complete surgery.

Similarly, retrospective data have shown that pancreatoblastoma is also sensitive to radiotherapy. This treatment may be used in the case of persistent unresectable tumour after failure of chemotherapy or after macroscopic incomplete surgery and after local relapse despite chemotherapy. The total doses used range from 30 to 46 Gy.

The 5-year overall prognosis is about 45 per cent. Prognosis appears to be better in patients under the age of 16, after complete resection and with localized tumour.

Further reading

Achatz MI, Hainaut P, Ashton-Prolla P (2009) Highly prevalent TP53 mutation predisposing to many cancers in the Brazilian population: a case for newborn screening? *Lancet Oncol* **10**, 920–5.

Achatz MI, Olivier M, Le Calvez F, et al. (2007) The TP53 mutation, R337H, is associated with Li-Fraumeni and Li-Fraumeni-like syndromes in Brazilian families. *Cancer Lett* **245**, 96–102.

Boman F, Hill DA, Williams GM, et al. (2006) Familial association of pleuropulmonary blastoma with cystic nephroma and other renal tumors: a report from the International Pleuropulmonary Blastoma Registry. *J Pediatr* **149**, 850–4.

Boussen H, Bouaouina N, Mokni-Baizig N, et al. (2005) [Nasopharyngeal carcinoma. Recent data]. *Pathol Biol (Paris)* **53**, 45–51.

Calva D, O'Dorisio TM, Sue O'Dorisio M, et al. (2009) When is prophylactic thyroidectomy indicated for patients with the RET codon 609 mutation? *Ann Surg Oncol* **16**, 2237–44.

Defachelles AS, Martin De Lassalle E, Boutard P, et al. (2001) Pancreatoblastoma in childhood: clinical course and therapeutic management of seven patients. *Med Pediatr Oncol* **37**, 47–52.

Dhebri AR, Connor S, Campbell F, et al. (2004) Diagnosis, treatment and outcome of pancreatoblastoma. *Pancreatology* **4**, 441–51.

Drut R, Jones MC (1988) Congenital pancreatoblastoma in Beckwith–Wiedemann syndrome: an emerging association. *Pediatr Pathol* **8**, 331–9.

Garritano S, Gemignani F, Palmero EI, et al. (2010) Detailed haplotype analysis at the TP53 locus in p.R337H mutation carriers in the population of Southern Brazil: evidence for a founder effect. *Hum Mutat* **31**, 143–50.

Gingalewski CA, Newman KD (2006) Seminars: controversies in the management of pediatric thyroid malignancy. *J Surg Oncol* **94**, 748–52.

Hill DA, Ivanovich J, Priest JR, et al. (2009) DICER1 mutations in familial pleuropulmonary blastoma. *Science* **325**, 965.

Hogan AR, Zhuge Y, Perez EA, et al. (2009) Pediatric thyroid carcinoma: incidence and outcomes in 1753 patients. *J Surg Res* **156**, 167–72.

Jaksic T, Yaman M, Thorner P, et al. (1992) A 20-year review of pediatric pancreatic tumors. *J Pediatr Surg* **27**, 1315–7.

Kowalski LP, Goncalves Filho J, Pinto CA, et al. (2003) Long-term survival rates in young patients with thyroid carcinoma. *Arch Otolaryngol Head Neck Surg* **129**, 746–9.

Orbach D, Brisse H, Helfre S, et al. (2008) Radiation and chemotherapy combination for nasopharyngeal carcinoma in children: Radiotherapy dose adaptation after chemotherapy response to minimize late effects. *Pediatr Blood Cancer* **50**, 849–53.

Priest JR, Hill DA, Williams GM, et al. (2006) Type I pleuropulmonary blastoma: a report from the International Pleuropulmonary Blastoma Registry. *J Clin Oncol* **24**, 4492–8.

Ribeiro RC, Sandrini F, Figueiredo B, et al. (2001) An inherited p53 mutation that contributes in a tissue-specific manner to pediatric adrenal cortical carcinoma. *Proc Natl Acad Sci USA* **98**, 9330–5.

Steliarova-Foucher E, Stiller C, Lacour B, Kaatsch P. (2005) International Classification of Childhood Cancer, third edition. *Cancer* **103**, 1457–67.

Steliarova-Foucher E, Stiller CA, Pukkala E, et al. (2006) Thyroid cancer incidence and survival among European children and adolescents (1978–1997): report from the Automated Childhood Cancer Information System project. *Eur J Cancer* **42**, 2150–69.

Stevens C, Lee JK, Sadatsafavi M, Blair GK (2009) Pediatric thyroid fine-needle aspiration cytology: a meta-analysis. *J Pediatr Surg* **44**, 2184–91.

Stiller CA (1994) International variations in the incidence of childhood carcinomas. *Cancer Epidemiol Biomarkers Prev* **3**, 305–10.

Wada N, Sugino K, Mimura T, et al. (2009) Treatment strategy of papillary thyroid carcinoma in children and adolescents: clinical significance of the initial nodal manifestation. *Ann Surg Oncol* **16**, 3442–9.

Wada N, Sugino K, Mimura T, et al. (2009) Pediatric differentiated thyroid carcinoma in stage I: risk factor analysis for disease free survival. *BMC Cancer* **9**, 306.

Index